AF768362

Handbook of Embodied Cognition and Sport Psychology

Handbook of Embodied Cognition and Sport Psychology

edited by Massimiliano L. Cappuccio

The MIT Press
Cambridge, Massachusetts
London, England

© 2019 Massachusetts Institute of Technology

All rights reserved. No part of this book may be reproduced in any form by any electronic or mechanical means (including photocopying, recording, or information storage and retrieval) without permission in writing from the publisher.

This book was set in Stone Serif by Westchester Publishing Services. Printed and bound in the United States of America.

Library of Congress Cataloging-in-Publication Data
Names: Cappuccio, Massimiliano, editor.
Title: Handbook of embodied cognition and sport psychology / edited by Massimiliano L. Cappuccio.
Description: Cambridge, MA : The MIT Press, 2019. | Includes bibliographical references and index.
Identifiers: LCCN 2018004433 | ISBN 9780262038508 (hardcover : alk. paper)
Subjects: LCSH: Sports—Psychological aspects. | Athletes—Psychology. | Cognition.
Classification: LCC GV706.4 .H365 2018 | DDC 796.01/9—dc23
LC record available at https://lccn.loc.gov/2018004433

10 9 8 7 6 5 4 3 2 1

The editor dedicates this book to his wife, Raquel.

Contents

Foreword 1

Rich S. W. Masters

I play golf with my son sometimes. He is only twelve. On long summer evenings, when the course is quiet, we wander from tee to green enjoying our time together. As do all talented youngsters, my son expects to play every shot exquisitely, so at some point our enjoyment is usually spoiled because he does not make the perfect swing that he intended or misses a putt that he expected to make. Emotions take over … his shoulders slump, his head goes down, gestures ensue, and inevitably more bad shots follow. Naturally, my mirror neurons notice and, sure enough, I usually emulate him with my own bad shots!

Afterward, I explain to my son that everyone hits bad shots, even the great players; he cannot expect to have the game of an expert (yet). He informs me that he can't stop himself from feeling down. I explain that a body with slumped shoulders and downcast eyes tells its brain to feel down. I tell him that if he walks with his shoulders back and his head held high, his body will tell his brain that all is good with his game.

My son has his own interpretation of what I tell him; he is far too young to understand the complexities of embodiment in sport. How can he *grasp* that what he thinks, how he feels—note the metaphor—is a function of the on-flowing interactions between his body and his mind and the environment in which they are situated; that these mental processes are the upshot of his history as an embodied agent that is tightly coupled with, and continuously adapting to, its environment?

How can he understand that his ability to walk the course on warm summer evenings is made less computationally complex by the manner in which his body has evolved to exploit the environment, or that when he waggles his club before a shot his body is providing him information about the "dynamical" affordances for ball hitting, just as when hefting a stone to throw?

How can he comprehend the futility of trying to replicate a perfect swing, when variability and degeneracy underpin so much of what is remarkable about his motor abilities ... and I wonder if ever he will hold a pencil between his gritted teeth in order to force his body to tell his brain to smile!

I hope that when he is older my son reads this handbook and realizes that the psychologists, philosophers, neuroscientists, psychiatrists, sociologists, anthropologists, educators, movement scientists, sport doctors, and coaches who wrote the twenty-six sweepingly insightful chapters that make up its content—and his Dad—were "on the ball," so to speak!

Foreword 2

David Papineau

Sport and the study of the human mind might not seem natural bedfellows. Indeed most people would probably think of them as diametrically opposed. Kipling's references to "flannelled fools" and "muddied oafs" express a widespread attitude. Athletes might be admired for their bodily attributes and physical achievements, but as a class they are not generally considered mentally noteworthy.

Over the past couple of decades, however, a significant number of writers have come to realize that sporting prowess has much to teach us about the workings of our minds. In truth, accomplished athletes are mentally as well as physically exceptional, and the extreme sophistication of the skills they have mastered poses a challenge to many conventional assumptions about the mind.

Until recently, cognitive science and empirically oriented philosophy of mind were dominated by the computer model of the mind. Sensory "transducers" imported detailed information about the environment into the brain, where it was combined with standing "data bases," analyzed by "central processors," and generated "outputs" in the form of motor instructions. In this conception of the mind, all the intelligent action occurred internally, in the computational inferences performed by the central processor.

This model does not fit at all well with sporting skills, especially those involving extreme temporal constraints. There's simply no time for all that processing. In bat-ball games like tennis, cricket, baseball, squash, and table tennis, elite athletes typically have less than 500 milliseconds to tailor their reactions to the approaching ball. Even so, their responses are by no means inflexible. The same stimulus engenders different reactions in different tactical situations, and moreover, athletes are capable of producing novel responses in real time when faced with new challenges.

The contributions in this volume explore a range of mental mechanisms that make such sporting achievements possible, drawing in a variety of ways on an existing tradition of work on embodied cognition. One important strand is an understanding of perception deriving from J. J. Gibson, which replaces the idea of abstract object-oriented information that needs to be processed to yield motor instructions with an account of perception that is action-orientated from the start. A related insight is that unfolding sequences of actions are often directly guided by the environment, via processes that monitor and control action-environment relations. These two thoughts come together in connection with sporting skills that involve interactions with other athletes, either as teammates or as opponents; here the perception of others' actions can activate responses directly, with the help of dedicated motor neurons, thereby facilitating the ongoing production of coordinated activity.

These last remarks are only a superficial indication of the wide range of insights to be found in this volume. Time and again the contributors show how sports offer a unique window into the human mind. I have come to think of sports as playing the same role in psychology as particle accelerators in physics. Just as particle accelerators allow physicists to find out how matter behaves in exceptional high-energy conditions, so sports show us things about the human mind that aren't normally apparent in less testing circumstances. The articles that follow are a testament to the fertility of this approach. They mark a significant step in our understanding of the mind and point the way to further progress.

Introduction

Massimiliano L. Cappuccio

> Although sport is played with the body, it is won in the mind.
>
> —Aidan Moran, *Sport and Exercise Psychology*, 2004

1

With the sentence quoted above, Aidan Moran opens the introduction of his well-known textbook, *Sport and Exercise Psychology*, which in many ways represents an inspiration for the present volume. His words eloquently define the distinctive domain in which sport psychology operates: physical training and exercise are not sufficient to excel in a competition, if certain key elements of the athlete's preparation—traditionally labeled as "mental"—are not perfectly tuned for the challenge.

These elements involve the cognitive, attentional, motivational, and affective dimensions of the athlete's mind. They are often affected by psychological and situational dynamics involving self-perception, confidence, and distracting worries that operate deeply in the mind of the athlete. The expertise of sport psychologists is indispensable for recognizing and regulating these dynamics. This is how sport psychologists primarily help coaches and trainers to maximize athletes' performances. But their professional intervention can be applied also to other forms of preparation that, although only indirectly related to competition, are no less important for winning: talent identification and development; optimization, acceleration, and diversification of training methods; team-building and conflict resolution; life-coaching through the highs and lows of the athlete's career; and ethical pedagogy and appreciation of sport values for a positive way of living. That is how sport psychology makes itself indispensable for winning, as winning has to do with the athlete's *mind* no less than his or her *body*.

That said, how do we concretely delineate the domain of the mental in contrast to that of the merely physical? Practicing a preperformance relaxation technique, perfecting a gymnastic maneuver, implementing a complex tactical scheme in rugby or basketball: Are these accomplishments of the body or the mind? And where exactly do we draw the distinction? Insofar as the scope of sport psychology depends on a demarcation between mind and body, this philosophical question is not only speculatively but also professionally and deontologically significant. However, not only is the right answer difficult to provide, but the question itself might be the wrong one to ask—if formulated in dualistic terms. For centuries, in fact, philosophers have been trying to explain the mind-body relation utilizing metaphysical concepts (substances, properties, and events) and rationalistic narratives that most often build on explicitly dualistic oppositions (spirit/matter, thought/action, intention/movement, judgment/affect, and so on). Common sense and everyday language are still confounded by the many misunderstandings generated by the Cartesian manner of construing the mind-body relationship.

The advent of cognitive science as an integrated interdisciplinary framework for the naturalistic study of the mind has the potential to change—and has already started changing—our philosophical perspective on this foundational issue. Cognitive science is the field of theoretical, empirical, and technological inquiry that studies intelligent systems (brains, artificial neural networks, computers, swarms, societies, and so on) and mental functions (memory, perception, attention, sensorimotor control, language production and processing, problem solving, and the like). As an intrinsically interdisciplinary endeavor, cognitive science research involves shoulder-to-shoulder collaborations among cognitive psychologists, cognitive linguists, cognitive anthropologists, and so on. Together, they study how cognition works at the level of the underlying processes and mechanisms (for example, informational and predictive processes). This teamwork involves also cognitive philosophers, that is, the philosophers of mind and philosophical psychologists who operate within the cognitive-science paradigm. Cognitive philosophers have never stopped asking the kinds of normative and foundational questions that were important to their predecessors but, unlike them, try to answer such questions considering the functional, logico-causal, and informational architecture of complex systems and processes, using a combination of empirical, synthetic, and phenomenological methods that involve both quantitative and qualitative analyses. That is why many traditional metaphysical questions have been at least partly replaced by, or redefined through, a more concrete demand for rich experimental data sets, powerful computational simulations and reliable explanatory/predictive models, and accurate protocols for the collection and the comparison of first-person experiential reports.

Today, to clarify the mission and the scope of sport psychology requires understanding the deep intertwinement of "body" and "mind" within the framework of cognitive science and cognitive philosophy. That is one of the reasons a joint venture between sport psychologists and cognitive scientists—including, importantly, cognitive philosophers—is a must. The protocols of practical intervention adopted by practitioner psychologists must be validated scientifically and based on evidence, in accord with the theoretical models, the empirical data, and the integrative methods introduced by cognitive science research: this is quite a sophisticated and powerful conceptual toolbox, as illustrated by Rich Masters in his suggestive foreword, one that today's sport psychologist must be equipped with.

In turn, cognitive science relies deeply on the work of sport psychologists and needs their knowledge to gain a richer characterization of human expertise and a more concrete grasp of all forms of adaptive intelligence based primarily on sensorimotor capabilities and skillful engagement with the environment. Sport, indeed, offers to cognitive science a privileged perspective from which to study the limits and the potential of the mind "in action," through the examination of the feats of ability accomplished by sportsmen and sportswomen—when humans are required to make the most out of cognitive faculties like perception, motor control, action planning, and decision in complex, possibly fast-changing, real-life scenarios. As remarked in David Papineau's insightful foreword, sport performance allows us to observe these cognitive faculties under a magnifying lens: competition and other sport challenges expose them when they are both extraordinarily developed, nearing the edge of human perfection, and extraordinarily under stress, approaching the verge of exhaustion and collapse. Cognitive science can use the lens provided by sport psychology to recognize the kinds of mental resources that are needed by well-trained humans to accomplish their superior feats of ability, but aims to generalize these observations by modeling the skillful abilities of typical humans.

2

Sport psychology importantly helps cognitive scientists also in another way: it can help them identify and critically discuss their own intellectualist assumptions and transcend them. This primarily means rediscussing classical *cognitivism*, elaborating a viable alternative to it: cognitivism is the traditional approach to cognition that construes the scientific study of the mind on internalist, instructionist, symbolicist—and, to a large extent, intellectualist—assumptions, reducing even the most basic and practical forms of intelligence and knowledge to temporally abstract formal functions, amodal information processing, and acontextual models of the world stored in the brain and detached from real-life experiential contingencies. Cognitivism lacks the conceptual resources—and probably also the motivation—necessary to see that athletic skill (for example, wrestling) *is* a legitimate form of intelligence, involving cognitive faculties not less sophisticated and complex than—say—mathematical reasoning (Matthen 2014).

The shortcomings of the cognitivist approach are today pointed at by the proponents of the embodied cognition theory. The embodied cognition program—especially the radical trends that defend anti-computationalist, anti-representationalist, and dynamicist views (e.g., Hutto and Myin 2017; Chemero 2009)—opposes many of the assumptions of cognitivism and offers an alternative to them. The fundamental principle of embodied cognition is that the reach and the very nature of mental functions constitutively depend on the material and temporal details of their implementation, including the history of interactions between the embodied agent and its world (Gallagher 2005, 2011).

This means, first of all, that many "low-level" physiological, regulatory, and adaptive processes involving the nonneural body and the environment actively participate in the most basic forms of cognition (sensorimotor, affective, adaptive), structurally scaffolding them and shaping them. Not only are perception and action intrinsically intelligent, but also the hormonal and immune systems (Marin and Kipnis 2013), autonomic and peripheral responses (Aranyosi 2013), and highly selective saccadic reflexes (Mann, this volume) can play an intelligent role in certain tasks. Even the anatomical and postural specificity of the body, with its inherent material properties (hardness, elasticity, and so on) and the intrinsic biomechanical and morphological constraints of the actuators (degrees of freedom, weight distribution, and the like), can play a cognitive role: for example, the pendulum-like configuration of one's body parts can contribute to reducing the computational complexity of a task of bipedal motion (Pfeifer, Iida, and Lungarella 2014).

This secondarily means that competent embodied dispositions and habitual patterns of perception and action, emerging from dynamic forms of adaptive coupling between embodied agents and their environment, importantly contribute to scaffold and shape "higher" forms (inferential, linguistic, representational) of cognition. In this picture, cognitive functions such as strategic control and decision, perceptual discrimination, linguistic representation, memory, judgment, and creativity are not to be understood just as informational contents centrally stored in the brain or abstract programs detached from their material implementers: on the contrary, cognitive functions can correctly be modeled and understood only considering the fine-grained specificity of the physical and biological systems that instantiate them and the real-life circumstances in which they have been developed and trained.

As famously illustrated by how physical encumberment modifies geographical slant perception (Proffitt et al. 1995) and hunger influences judges' rulings (Danziger, Levav, and Avnaim-Pesso 2011), bodily affects can dramatically curb perception and objective judgment. Accordingly, in his phenomenological account, Gallagher (2005) emphasizes that bodily dispositions and affordances in the environment can determine the outcome of evaluative and decisional processes more than any representation of the world internally stored by or manipulated within the central nervous system. Intelligent know-how, athletic skill, and physical expertise emerge from the consolidation and diversification of a larger and larger repertoire of habitual interactions and affective patterns, which constitute the cognitive agent's structural coupling with real-world scenarios (Chiel and Beer 1997).

In the last three decades, the theorists of embodiment have proposed several more-specific, and at times conflicting, interpretations of the theory of embodiment (Gallagher 2011). Despite the diversity (and, sometimes, the contraposition) of these different declinations of the core notion of embodiment, the fundamental principles of embodied cognition theory can be effectively summarized referring to a handful of general theses. Kirchhoff (forthcoming) lists four of them:

1. The *constitutive thesis*: "Cognitive systems ... are realized in patterns of sensorimotor activity nonlinearly coupled with the embedding environment."
2. The *cognitive-affective inseparability thesis*: "Patterns of affectivity are part and parcel of perception, action and thinking," which implies that intelligent and adaptive behavior could hardly be understood in isolation from the living phenomenology of first-person experience.
3. The *meta-plasticity thesis*: Mentality emerges over and is situated in "a plastic network of processes spanning brain, body, and world." This thesis is also accompanied by the claims that the very physical structure of the body acts as a natural distributor, a constrainer, and a regulator of mental processes, as described by Wilson and Foglia 2011.
4. Last, but not least, the *nonrepresentational thesis*, which is not endorsed with equal force by all the trends of embodied cognition theory: "The sensorimotor profile of organisms is sufficient for at least some kinds of cognitive activities, thus replacing the need for organisms to construct complex internal mental representations of the outside environment."

The chapters in this collection discuss the numerous implications and applications of these theses, referring to different approaches and doctrines that claim affiliation to the embodied cognition program (see Shapiro and Spaulding, this volume). Most of the current debate is polarized by the contraposition between the two most influential declinations of the embodied mind theory: the *enactive* (or "sensorimotor") and the *extended* (or "distributed") approach.

The enactive approach, generally oriented toward biological and dynamical accounts of the mind, stresses that mental faculties are neither physically localized nor representational, but emerge holistically on the continuous adaptive interplay between the organism and its ecological surroundings. The genetic/constitutive role played by the sensorimotor coupling between the agent and his/her world environment is particularly emphasized over off-line forms of intelligence.

The extended approach, on the other hand, is typically more sympathetic than its counterpart to functionalist and computationalist accounts of the mind, as it stresses that intracranial (neuronal, usually organic) and extracranial (nonneuronal, possibly artificial) vehicles of cognition are in principle complementary or even interchangeable as they can—at times—complete, augment, or replace one another.

Many of the chapters in this volume are explicitly or implicitly aligned with either the enactive or the extended approach. Chapter 6's introduction (by Christensen and Sutton) and chapter 9 (by Francesconi and Gallagher) offer a richer characterization of these two approaches and discuss their implications for sport psychology.

3

Remarkably, most of the psychologists and cognitive scientists who work on sport and performance seem naturally inclined to embrace at least the core general tenets of embodied cognition and tend to endorse one variant or the other of the theory (see Beilock 2008, 2015; Gray 2014). Such proximity is not merely coincidental, as sport psychology and embodied cognitive science share a communal theoretical and historical root.

For example, the characterization of skill acquisition as progressive automatization of complex action patterns, offered by some of the precursors of the contemporary embodied program (Dreyfus and Dreyfus 1980), was in substantial accord with the view expressed by one of the classical works by Fitts and Posner (1967) that contributed to define sport psychology as a scientific discipline: namely, the view that a less cognitively demanding motor execution is one of the distinctive marks of expertise itself, which is why only experts can deliver their skillful performances in the form of unreflective habitual action (i.e., through automatic routines).

Also, some of the key ideas put forward by *The Embodied Mind* (Varela, Thompson, Rosch 1991), one of the seminal texts of embodied cognition theory, resonate deeply with influential doctrines in developmental psychology and ecological psychology that paved the way to the foundation of sport psychology. These key ideas are well known and appreciated by sport psychologists, who inherited them primarily from the

Piagetian and neo-Piagetian tradition (with the preeminence attributed to "enactive learning" during early cognitive development) and the Gibsonian and post-Gibsonian tradition (with the ecological concepts of "affordances" and "direct perception"). These traditions historically contributed to the theoretical foundation of both sport psychology, as an academic discipline and as an applied practice, and embodied cognition theory, as a new integrative approach to research and theoretical modeling, and represent their communal root.

First, Piaget's genetic epistemology program (1954) took the understanding of cognitive development in the direction of the theories that focus on the dominance, during the first three to six years of life, of knowledge derived from sensorimotor experience. Bruner (1966) purified Piaget's proposal, suggesting that the first few years of life were entirely experienced, learned, and remembered in sensorimotor ("enactive") coordinates. Finally, the "neo-Piagetian" movement, exemplified by Pascual-Leone (1970) and Case (1985), added the emergence and growth of working memory as a control structure to this sensorimotor foundation.

The influence of ecological psychology on sport psychology and embodied theory is even more remarkable and can be traced back to the approach called "direct perception" or "direct realism" proposed by James J. Gibson (1966, 1979). In many senses, this approach stemmed from a reaction against the "computational" or "functionalist/information processing" approach that had been growing in the 1960s, largely inspired by Putnam's theory of machine-state functionalism in philosophy of mind (Putnam 1960). Putnam's theory presupposed both the computational theory of mind (the thesis that cognitive processes are fundamentally algorithmic in nature), and the principle of multiple-realizability (which states that a cognitive function, like any other algorithmic function, can be implemented by any material support capable to physically instantiate the relevant formal operations of symbolic manipulation (see Putnam 1967). This computational and functionalist/information-processing approach is often associated with the internalist and neuro-reductionist view that human cognition is entirely realized and carried out by the central nervous system alone, and the extra-neural body and the extra-bodily environment don't play any properly cognitive or informational role. This view is illustrated by Putnam's famous "brain-in-a-vat" scenario, although attributing this view to the American philosopher would be incorrect (see Putnam 1981).

The ecological approach proposed by Gibson firmly rejected these functionalist, computationalist, and internalist assumptions and proposed an alternative set of principles. First, human sensory capabilities evolved in the service of the actions that humans needed to perform in their environments to live their lives. Hence, human cognition is to be characterized as an integrated set of interactions among the sensory and motoric systems, coordinated to generate intelligent actions that may only rarely require the intervening representational machinery of abstract thinking and detached problem solving. In its most radical version, the Gibsonian argument cut out the middleman altogether—rejecting all behavioral explanations based on internal representations and touting direct connections from perception to action. (The idea that recurrent perception/action feedback loops constitute the most fundamental building blocks of cognition, and scaffold higher forms of intelligence, is one of the precursors of the enactive/sensorimotor account of the mental; see O'Regan and Noë 2001; Noë 2005).

Following Gibson, many theorists of action control and movement science that have deeply influenced the field of sport and performance psychology have focused specifically on the anatomical and physiological properties of the body to explain skillful action and expertise—minimizing the role of information processing and even de-emphasizing the importance of brain processes altogether. These approaches, as exemplified by researchers like Michael Turvey (1973), Peter Kugler (Kugler and Turvey 1987), and Claudia Carello (Carello and Turvey 2016), suggest that much of human performance—its physical and dynamic properties, with the possibilities, impossibilities, trajectories, and timing of limb movements—are determined primarily by the physics and biology of human anatomy (the muscular and skeletal physiognomy, the geometry and degrees of freedom of the effectors), and only secondarily by the processes of perception, planning, and control. Hence, according to the action theorists inspired by the Gibsonian tradition, we need to understand more about the body itself and pay less attention to psychological processes and internal representations of the external world.

4

The strong theoretical link between the ecological approach and embodied mind theory is testified by the remarkable preeminence of Gibson's notion of affordance in most of the chapters included in this collection. However, the relationship between Gibsonian theory and embodiment is multifaceted (see Chemero 2009; and Wilson and Golonka 2013). The embodied cognition program has tried to expand or revise certain elements of the ecological approach: the naïve realist epistemology implied by direct perception theory was replaced by the constructivist principle that cognition is a tentative process of unfinished negotiation and precarious adaptation to a world-environment that can make sense only to a living organism structurally coupled with it. Embodied theory has also worked to update some of the key ecological notions, to keep pace with the emerging neurosciences and their empirical discoveries: for example, the notion of motor affordance was updated and expanded to accommodate the new data and models of action execution and motor control coming from neuropsychological research, such as the discovery of canonical and mirror neurons in the premotor cortex.

In this updated framework, embodied cognition theory emphasizes not only the action possibilities enabled by the physical structure of the body and the objects in the environment, but also the emotional, intentional, and motivational forces that fuel these actions. These forces are not just accessory to the origin of mental functions. They are seen as fundamental components of the living mind: built-in saliency detection and discrimination filters; powerful anticipatory mechanisms; adaptive systems for priority selection and allocation of interest, attention, and motivation; and flexible response habits—all play a legitimately cognitive role, constituting the foundation of mental development and the evolutionary expression of intelligence in the world.

Despite some controversial points still debated by opposing schools of ecological psychologists and embodied cognition theorists, the Gibsonian legacy within the tradition of embodied cognition is robust and represents a primary source of inspiration for many of the authors who wrote for the present *Handbook*. This legacy revives through the embodied cognition program, which offers sport psychologists updated theoretical tools, informed by the advances made during the last few decades by all the relevant branches of the cognitive sciences (clinical neuropsychology, neurolinguistics, robotics, cognitive archeology and anthropology, and so on).

An example particularly cited by sport psychologists (Beilock 2015) as evidence that neurocognitive functions and their bodily realizers must be studied together is that reading comprehension and memory improve if the subject, while reading the descriptions of certain physical activities (e.g., baseball actions), performs physical manipulations that are consistent with them (Glenberg 2011). The "action-based" theory of reading comprehension, confirmed by neuroimaging studies, asserts that the sensory and motor systems are involved during the process of understanding, imagining, and remembering an action described in a written story, as if the reader was actually perceiving or executing that action (Glenberg and Gallese 2012).

This investigation of the embodied scaffoldings of language confirms the results of Beilock et al. (2008), who demonstrated in neuroimaging examinations of brain activation that fans of a sporting activity with scarce experience "on the field" and athletes who actually play the sport show different patterns of brain activation when watching videos of game play. Compared with fans, players' brains show much more activation in motor-planning and motor-control regions—the areas that would be active if the subjects were actually playing rather than merely watching a match.

This result (and similar ones, for example those concerning motor resonance during observation of basketball tasks: Aglioti et al. 2008; Abreu et al. 2012) have been interpreted as evidence for a communal embodied root of motor execution, imagination, and action understanding (Gallese 2007; Beilock 2015). According to this interpretation, TV sports fans reflectively evaluate those actions in a way detached from its motoric dimension, while expert players rely on their own motor repertoire to mentally simulate the execution of the actions they are watching, reenacting the very performative experience they would have lived firsthand during the execution of those very actions.

Thus, motor expertise, and performative familiarity with the execution of skilled action, matter to judgment and comprehension, and this shows up in brain activation: according to Gallese (2007), what can be lived out in imagination and in remembering depends crucially on an internal "embodied" simulation of what has been previously experienced, which employs one's established reservoir of sensorimotor memories and the relevant actional know-how (for a similar conclusion suggested by a different body of evidence, see Witt, South, and Sugovic 2014; for a review of the literature on embodied simulation informed by mirror neurons theory, see Ferrari and Rizzolatti 2015; for a review more specifically related to sport and athletic skills, see Abreu, Esteves, and Aglioti this volume, and Ikegami, Nakamoto and Ganesh this volume).

Not only the embodied nature of skill expertise is reflected by the capability to remember and imagine already experienced actions. Embodiment also projects onto the capability to creatively improvise new actions, strategically interpreting the current circumstances and adapting to unprecedented sensorimotor contingencies. The notion of "enactive creativity" is useful for clarifying this capability (Rucińska and Aggerholm, this volume; see also Hutto and Myin 2017 for an enactivist account of imagination). This enactivist account highlights that creative performers can push and expand their skills to new and higher levels. The embodied/enactive approach to cognition sees creativity as a capacity for active exploration of the limits of one's know-how. This capacity can be strengthened by practice, if training is designed to push the performer to diversify his/her experiences and master the opportunities arising from unusual or particularly challenging situations.

5

This volume is composed of seven sections. With the help of multidisciplinary teams of researchers, each section explores a particular area of thematic interest situated at the intersection of embodied cognitive science and sport psychology. The authors of the chapters are prevalently psychologists with varying specializations (sport and performance, sport and exercise, developmental, social psychology) and philosophers (philosophers of mind, philosophers of science, cognitive philosophers and AI theorists, psychological philosophers, epistemologists, phenomenologists, ethicists, and, of course, sport philosophers). The book's authors include also neuroscientists, psychiatrists, sociologists, anthropologists, educationalists, kinesiologists, sport doctors, and professional coaches and trainers. Their scientific interest in sport is often accompanied by a strong personal passion, as many among them successfully participate in agonistic competitions as practitioners or just as fans. The titles of the sections reflect, at the same time, some of the theoretical issues most debated by cognitive scientists and some of the main domains of practical intervention in sport psychology.

Section 1 presents the key notions and concepts necessary to lay the theoretical foundation of our interdisciplinary discourse. The very meaning of embodied cognition, and the reasons that make it relevant to the theory and practice of sport psychology, are introduced and discussed. Chapter 1, by philosophers Lawrence Shapiro and Shannon Spaulding, carefully introduces the distinctive theses of embodiment and explains how they are relevant in correctly interpreting some of the essential notions and models utilized by sport psychologists.

The athlete's emotions can damage her/his performance or lead her/him to victory, hence the importance of dominating them rather than suppressing them. Chapter 2, coauthored by philosophical psychologists Dan Hutto and Michael Kirchhoff and exercise scientist Ian Renshaw, offers the radically enactive/embodied cognition view on emotions and suggests the need to appropriately train them. The embodied/enactive theory construes emotions as a key component (as opposed to a mere accident) of cognition and emphasizes the deep link between affects, performance, expertise, and training.

Chapter 3, written by sport psychologist Paula Silva, kinesiologist Adam Kiefer, experimental psychologist Michael A. Riley, and philosopher of science Tony Chemero, expands the radically enactivist background, introducing conceptual tools such as affordances and dynamical systems, which link the legacy of ecological psychology to both embodied/enactive cognition and movement science.

If the first three chapters offer a theoretical introduction to embodied cognition, chapter 4, by sport psychologist Geir Jordet and movement scientist Gert-Jan Pepping, represents its applied and pragmatic counterpart: it describes a human-centered and discipline-specific approach to sport performance, which sees athletes as unique embodied individuals developing specific proficiencies (and specific problems) in particular disciplinary settings.

Section 2 tackles one of the issues that most seriously concerns athletic performance: the nature of embodied skill, its cognitive preconditions, and the factors that disrupt it. A correct understanding of the roles played by attention, self-awareness, and consciousness is key to developing a consistent theoretical account of both sport performance in optimal conditions and its failure in pressure-filled environments (the so-called choking effect). Chapter 5 combines the different scientific views of four experts of choking effect (sport psychologists Rob Gray, Christopher Mesagno, Denise Hill and cognitive scientist Tom Carr) and a philosopher (Massimiliano Cappuccio) to offer a comprehensive review of the theories inspired by Roy Baumeister's idea that self-consciousness is a general factor of performance disruption. The chapter explores different dimensions (sensorimotor, affective, narrative) and degrees of self-awareness, documenting how they undermine the execution of well-trained actions. The three chapters that follow offer various opportunities to critically reexamine the explanation of choking centered on self-consciousness, considering the most valuable alternatives to it.

Chapter 6 introduces an anti-dualistic theory of cognitive control and skillful performance—called *Mesh* by the authors—subsuming both automatized behaviors and strategic awareness under an integrated system that relies on the same working memory resources. Among other things, *Mesh* aspires to unify the comprehension of several instances of performance disruption, whether caused by self-focus or distraction. The chapter reproduces a paper originally written for *Mind & Language* by cognitive philosophers Wayne Christensen and John Sutton and personality psychologist Doris McIlwain, preceded by a new introduction by Christensen and Sutton.

Chapter 7 criticizes the distinction between unreflective action and cognitive control, arguing that peak performance requires self-focus and careful attention to movement execution. The critical analyses conducted in this chapter by philosopher Barbara Montero and sport psychologists John Toner and Aidan Moran mainly target Gabriele Wulf's theory of attentional focus, which states that attention to one's own movements is always detrimental to performance. The authors question the breadth of its domain of applicability.

Chapter 8 explores a related issue from a different point of view, as it questions the cliché that sees professional athletes as "mindless agents" or "consciousnessless" automata capable only of routine and habitual movement. On the contrary, the embodied and phenomenological approach put forward by the authors (sport philosophers Jens Birch, Vegard Fusche Moe, and Gunnar Breivik) highlights the reflective and deliberative dimension of performing experience, and the active role of the athlete as an aware intentional agent.

If skill disruption theory is central to the work of sport psychologists, skill acquisition is not less important—as every model of performance under pressure inevitably builds on a theory of training and motor learning. Theories of learning and skill development are the focus of section 3, which explores how the improvement of complex sensorimotor capabilities links to the development of other mental skills in the athletes.

Section 3 opens with chapter 9, coauthored by education theorist Denis Francesconi and phenomenologist Shaun Gallagher, who provided a general account of sport pedagogy inspired by the embodied theory. Their account examines two major theories of embodiment (the enactive and the extended cognition approaches), and two complementary notions of embodiment (body schema and body image), discussing their practical implications for physical education and sensorimotor learning, with original insights on the use of contemplative practices and attentive presence to facilitate skill training.

Chapter 10 develops this discourse, documenting how cognitive enhancement, including the expansion of general intelligence and problem-solving capacities, is facilitated—especially in children—when accompanied by an appropriate regime of physical exercise and training. The chapter combines the expertise of cognitive neuroscientist David Moreau and kinesiologist Phillip D. Tomporowski to explain how brain plasticity mechanisms disclose opportunities of cognitive enhancement during the age of development, when the creation of new neural networks benefits most from sensorimotor activity.

Chapter 11 investigates an issue that is hotly debated by scientists and various categories of people working in the sport business: What is talent, and how can it be identified? Is it an inherited gift or the result of long and hard training? According to the authors, philosopher Mirko Farina and sport psychologist Alberto Cei, the answer suggested by embodied cognition is articulated and complex: appropriate practice and intense experience during optimal periods of development, characterized by higher rates of neuroplasticity, can express and maximize the innate potential if accompanied by environments conducive to learning and well-designed training methods.

Can technology improve training practices by artificially augmenting the natural cognitive endowment of the athletes and accelerating the rate of sensorimotor skills learning? Chapter 12 addresses this question. Various studies reviewed there, including the research personally conducted by the author, neuropsychologist Miriam Reiner, suggest that neurofeedback-based (EEG) training methods (in combination with specially designed learning environments using virtual/augmented reality) can be used to hasten and improve supervised training methods.

Even when performing solo tasks or training in isolation, the athlete is never entirely alone. Section 4 is dedicated to the intersubjective and social dimension of sport skills, with a particular emphasis on team sports and other competitive athletic disciplines: our approach to social cognition is affected by the consideration of these sport activities, in which instinctive capabilities of empathic attunement and coordination with the teammates, no less than quick understanding and anticipation of the opponents' moves, are crucial for winning.

Chapter 13, written by sport neuropsychologist Ana Maria Abreu, sport scientist Pedro Tiago Esteves, and social neuroscientist Salvatore Maria Aglioti, opens the section with a neuroscientific model of goal understanding and action anticipation that is relevant to sport: that is, the "embodied simulation" theory. In accord with the principles of embodied and grounded cognition, this theory maintains that one's motor system is recruited during the observation of actions executed by others, and that this internal reenactment helps expert performers understand the others' actions and predict their motor outcome. Various bodies of experimental evidence are reviewed, and the main aspects of the theory are discussed.

Whereas chapter 13 focuses on the benefits of embodied simulation in team sport (coordination among teammates and fast communal responses to the opponents), chapter 14 discusses some ramifications of embodied simulation that the athlete might not desire. In particular, certain forms of motor contagion seem to confirm the general theory: the mere observation of poor performances is capable of priming, in a deficient way, the motor systems of expert athletes, increasing their chances of failure. The chapter, coauthored by neuroscientist Tsuyoshi Ikegami, neuroscientist and engineer Gowrishankar Ganesh, and sport scientist Hiroki Nakamoto, carefully distinguishes among different forms of contagion and critically discusses the main hypotheses about their neurocognitive underpinnings.

Can sport scientists accept the philosophical notions of shared intentionality and decisional processes distributed among multiple agents? This question is addressed by chapter 15, where cognitive neuropsychologist Lincoln Colling offers a systematic review of the experimental literature on joint action. The chapter provides an articulated portray of the cognitive systems underlying shared knowledge and co-planning of actions, with particular reference to action coordination in team sports.

Sport people are not anonymous participants in well-coordinated joint actions: they are members of a society with an identity and a communal history made out of traditions, norms, beliefs, and values. For this reason, section 5 discusses the best research methods in the social sciences for developing the sociological, anthropological, and cultural side of sport practices. These methods allow researchers to refine their capability to assess how skills are construed in different cultural and societal contexts and why stereotypes arise.

The centrality of bodily experience becomes evident in chapter 16, written by sport philosophers Jesús Ilundáin-Agurruza and Kevin Krein and sport psychologist Karl Erickson. The chapter, dedicated to performance in extreme sports, focuses on the ethos of martial arts and the East Asian sapiential doctrines that historically accompanied their development. The chapter is a source of fascinating insights concerning the phenomenological and existential meaning of those risky sport activities in which not only victory, but survival, is at stake.

Chapter 17 addresses the issue of cultural representation of gender in sport. No less destructive than explicitly discriminatory practices, sexist stereotypes constitute a well-known threat to the performances of female professional athletes. The chapter, coauthored by a diverse and well-coordinated team of women excelling in both academia and sport (philosophers Michele Merritt and Audrey Yap, sociologist of sport Cassie Comely, and applied sport psychologist Caren Diehl), affirms the phenomenological significance of the gendered body in the athletic context.

Understanding beliefs, stereotypes, and sociocultural forms of organization and decision requires the development of accurate scientific tools. Chapter 18, therefore, coauthored by a sociologist of sport (Raúl Sánchez-García), a sociologist of social interaction (Giolo Fele), and an ethnomethodologist (Kenneth Liberman), is dedicated to the development and application of reliable ethnomethodological protocols. The social sciences can adopt these protocols to shed light on the sociocultural dimension of sport practices and how they affect the cognition of professional athletes.

I have already mentioned that "affordance" is a crucial notion in our discourse. Section 6 deepens the theoretical background: according to the ecological approach to perception, objects are not just neutral sources of visual information, but "invite" the actions allowed by their shapes and their intrinsic possibilities of manipulation. Embodied cognition expands this notion to account for the specific motor skills and interactive attitudes of the observers, emphasizing the reciprocal coupling between skillful embodied agents, with their sensorimotor predispositions, and the environmental contingencies that solicit them.

Chapters 19 and 20 provide the foundation for a correct application of the notion of affordance in sport psychology. In chapter 19, sport psychologist Duarte Araújo, movement scientist Keith Davids, and philosopher of science Patrick McGivern investigate how adaptive behaviors are modulated across various contexts of interaction:

the conduct of the agent is described as a precarious equilibrium dynamically emerging on the surface of biomechanical and environmental constraints, modulated by task boundaries and perceptual information available to the agent.

Chapter 20, coauthored by Duarte Araújo and Keith Davids with sport and exercise psychologist Matt Dicks, investigates the mechanisms that allow expert athletes to competently select among various affordances. Here, intentional decision is not determined by the intellectual representation of goals and reasons, but emerges dynamically from the tension between contextual constraints to action and opportunities of variation available to an embodied agent.

Chapter 21 focuses on throwing as a particular kind of affordance that is highly characteristic of the human evolutionary background. Not only is throwing objects (for long distances or accuracy) a key action in many athletic disciplines, but it also defines the distinctively human embodied cognitive endowment. Cognitive psychologists Andrew D. Wilson and Geoffry P. Bingham and kinesiologist Qin Zhu explore the ecological and embodied meaning of this fascinating, and only apparently simple, action on which many sport disciplines are based.

Chapter 22, by cognitive philosopher Wayne Christensen and cognitive scientist Kath Bicknell, expands the notion of affordance to include not only present but also anticipated action opportunities, which are disclosed by the prediction of the action's outcomes. Mountain biking is examined as the perfect case study to richly describe how action control and sense of agency extend to imminent future experiences.

To deepen this theme, section 7 inquires about the source of the mind's predictive capabilities. This inquiry, central for both the tradition of philosophical psychology and the future of embodied cognition, is particularly debated now that predictive processing theory promises to unify the understanding of various mental functions (perception, imagination, memory, inference) under the same general Bayesian mechanics: the brain's fundamental goal is to reduce the mismatch between sensory input and the corresponding predictions generated by feed-forward systems.

Chapter 23 applies this idea by addressing the functioning of visual and motor imagery. As described by the authors (sport psychologists Tadhg E. MacIntyre, Noel E. Brick, Jürgen Beckmann, and Aidan P. Moran, and cognitive neuroscientist Christopher R. Madan), imagination can prepare professional players to face intimidating competitions, as it regulates the perception of the task-related pressure and the mental rehearsal of the relevant action routines. At the neurocognitive level, visualization techniques rely on the reenactment of previous sensorimotor experience and allow the anticipation of possible environmental changes.

Authored by vision scientist David L. Mann, chapter 24 describes the astounding predictive powers of ocular saccades: that is, very fast eye movements unconsciously produced by the eye to track perceptual changes in present objects and anticipate their future trajectories. Even if semiautonomous from the central nervous system, saccadic movements are intelligently adaptive and recognize with great flexibility goal-related features in accord with the interactive context.

Chapter 25, written by philosophers Zuzanna Rucińska and sport scientist Kenneth Aggerholm, explores the dimension of anticipation that underlies the creation of original movements when a strategic approach to challenging situations is necessary. According to enaction theory, expertise is more than just adaptive responsiveness to familiar situations; it also comprises the strategic anticipation of uncertain situations based on the capability to creatively recombine previous experiences to envision unprecedented forms of resolution.

The conclusion of this volume is entrusted to chapter 26, which offers an intellectually stimulating characterization of improvisation as a fundamental instinct at the service of creative talent, no less than an evolutionary force needed for survival and adaptation: a semi-paradoxical power of intuition at the verge of past and future, combining interpretation of the familiar and anticipation of the unknown. Referring to both martial arts and musical performance, the authors (psychiatrist and phenomenologist Nelson Mauro Maldonato, cognitive neuroscientist Alberto Oliverio, and computer scientist Anna Esposito) offer a rich phenomenological analysis of the peculiar temporal structure of the improvisational experience, combined with a detailed cartography of the anatomical and neurocognitive substrates that make this miracle possible.

6

The purpose of this book is not to build a bridge between two islands, but to create awareness that these territories have never been really separated. Sport psychology research has always dwelled on the themes, the notions, and the models of embodied cognition theory. Embodied cognition, in turn, has often found the most striking confirmations of its theoretical claims in the psychological accounts of sport performance and athletic skill. Because of their close analogies and correspondences, these two disciplines have had many chances to cross each other's paths and become acquainted, but were rarely offered the opportunity to establish a horizon of programmatic cooperation. An explicit integration of their respective philosophies would allow them to share a mutually beneficial experience of scientific investigation and critical reflection while affirming their irreducible specificities and their distinctive backgrounds. I am grateful to the authors of this volume because they have contributed to creating the conditions for an encounter of this kind, indicating a promising path for interdisciplinary cooperation and intellectual exploration.

Acknowledgments

This volume was realized as part of the activities sponsored by the UAE National Research Foundation through the UPAR grant "Sport and Brain Science: Technological Applications for Peaking Performances" (grant code 31H087-UPAR (3) 2014). The idea of this book was inspired by the rewarding experience of interdisciplinary collaboration inaugurated by the First International Conference in Sport Psychology and Embodied Cognition, held in February 2014 at UAE University with the generous sponsorship of the Abu Dhabi Sports Council. I am deeply in debt to Tom Carr for the many suggestions about the precursors of embodied cognition theory: although the sole responsibility for the views expressed in this introduction is mine, some of the passages included here benefited significantly from the long discussions we had over e-mail. Also, I am grateful to the researchers who contributed to the process of blind review and revision of the chapters: in addition to the authors who acted as referees for the other chapters, I must also deeply thank Omar AlHelalat, Fausto Carauna, Gunjan Khera, Mark Scott, Mog Stapleton, Christian Swann, and Ricarda Wullenkord. A special thanks to Alya Faisal for her continuous support during the revision of the chapters.

References

Abreu, Ana Maria, E. Macaluso, R. T. Azevedo, Paola Cesari, Cosimo Urgesi, and Salvatore Maria Aglioti. 2012. "Action Anticipation beyond the Action Observation Network: A Functional Magnetic Resonance Imaging Study in Expert Basketball Players." *European Journal of Neuroscience* 35 (10): 1646–1654.

Aglioti, Salvatore M., Paola Cesari, Michela Romani, and Cosimo Urgesi. 2008. "Action Anticipation and Motor Resonance in Elite Basketball Players." *Nature Neuroscience* 11 (9): 1109–1116.

Aranyosi, István. 2013. *The Peripheral Mind: Philosophy of Mind and the Peripheral Nervous System.* Oxford: Oxford University Press.

Beilock, Sian L. 2008. "Beyond the Playing Field: Sport Psychology Meets Embodied Cognition." *International Review of Sport and Exercise Psychology* 1 (1): 19–30.

Beilock, Sian L. 2015. *How the Body Knows Its Mind.* London: Hachette.

Beilock, Sian L., Ian M. Lyons, Andrew Mattarella-Micke, Howard C. Nusbaum, and Steven L. Small. 2008. "Sports Experience Changes the Neural Processing of Action Language." *Proceedings of the National Academy of Sciences of the United States of America* 105 (36): 13269–13273.

Bruner, Jerome S. 1966. *Toward a Theory of Instruction*. Cambridge, MA: Harvard University Press.

Carello, Claudia, and Michael Turvey. 2016. "Dynamic (Effortful) Touch." In *Scholarpedia of Touch*, edited by Tony Prescott, Ehud Ahissar, and Eugene Izhikevich, 227–240. Amsterdam: Atlantis Press.

Case, Robbie. 1985. *Intellectual Development: Birth to Adulthood*. New York: Academic Press.

Chemero, Anthony. 2009. *Radical Embodied Cognitive Science*. Cambridge, MA: MIT Press.

Chiel, H. J., and R. D. Beer. 1997. "The Brain Has a Body: Adaptive Behavior Emerges from Interactions of Nervous System, Body and Environment." *Trends in Neurosciences* 20 (12): 553–557.

Danziger, Shai, Jonathan Levav, and Liora Avnaim-Pesso. 2011. "Reply to Weinshall-Margel and Shapard: Extraneous Factors in Judicial Decisions Persist." *Proceedings of the National Academy of Sciences of the United States of America* 108 (42): 6889–6892.

Dreyfus, Stuart E., and Hubert L. Dreyfus. 1980. "A Five-Stage Model of the Mental Activities Involved in Directed Skill Acquisition." Berkeley: University of California Operations Research Center. https://www.scribd.com/document/23103065/A-Five-Stage-Model-of-the-Mental-Activities-Involved-in-Directed-Skill-Acquisition.

Ferrari, Pier Francesco, and Giacomo Rizzolatti. 2015. *New Frontiers in Mirror Neurons Research*. Oxford: Oxford University Press.

Fitts, P. M., and M. I. Posner. 1967. *Human Performance*. Pacific Grove, CA: Brooks/Cole.

Gallagher, Shaun. 2005. *How the Body Shapes the Mind*. New York: Oxford University Press.

Gallagher, Shaun. 2011. "Interpretations of Embodied Cognition." In *The Implications of Embodiment: Cognition and Communication*, edited by W. Tschacher and C. Bergomi, 59–70. Exeter, UK: Imprint Academic.

Gallese, Vittorio. 2007. "The Shared Manifold Hypothesis: Embodied Simulation and Its Role in Empathy and Social Cognition." In *Empathy in Mental Illness and Health*, edited by Tom F. D. Farrow and Peter W. R. Woodruff, 448–472. Cambridge: Cambridge University Press.

Gibson, James J. 1979. *The Ecological Approach to Visual Perception*. Boston: Houghton Mifflin.

Gibson, James Jerome. 1966. *The Senses Considered as Perceptual Systems*. Boston: Houghton Mifflin.

Glenberg, Arthur M. 2011. "How Reading Comprehension Is Embodied and Why That Matters." *International Electronic Journal of Elementary Education* 4 (1): 5–18.

Glenberg, Arthur M., and Vittorio Gallese. 2012. "Action-Based Language: A Theory of Language Acquisition, Comprehension, and Production." *Cortex: A Journal Devoted to the Study of the Nervous System and Behavior* 48 (7): 905–922. doi:10.1016/j.cortex.2011.04.010.

Gray, Rob. 2014. "Embodied Perception in Sport." *International Review of Sport and Exercise Psychology* 7 (1): 72–86.

Hutto, Daniel D., and Erik Myin. 2017. *Evolving Enactivism: Basic Minds Meet Content.* Cambridge, MA: MIT Press.

Kirchhof, Michael D. Forthcoming. "The Body in Action: Predictive Processing and the Embodiment Thesis." In *Oxford Handbook of Embodied Cognition: Embodied, Extended and Enactive,* edited by Albert Newen, L. De Bruin, and Shaun Gallagher. Oxford: Oxford University Press.

Kugler, Peter Noble, and Michael T. Turvey. 1987. *Information, Natural Law, and the Self-Assembly of Rhythmic Movement.* London: Routledge.

Marin, Ioana, and Jonathan Kipnis. 2013. "Learning and Memory … and the Immune System." *Learning and Memory* 20 (10): 601–606.

Matthen, Mohan. 2014. "Debunking Enactivism." *Canadian Journal of Philosophy* 44 (1): 118–128.

Moran, Aidan P. 2004. *Sport and Exercise Psychology: A Critical Introduction.* London: Routledge.

Noë, Alva. 2005. *Action in Perception.* Cambridge, MA: MIT Press.

O'Regan, J. K., and A. Noë. 2001. "A Sensorimotor Account of Vision and Visual Consciousness." *Behavioral and Brain Sciences* 24 (5): 939–973; discussion 973–1031.

Pascual-Leone, Juan. 1970. "A Mathematical Model for the Transition Rule in Piaget's Developmental Stages." *Acta Psychologica* 32 (January): 301–345.

Pfeifer, Rolf, Fumiya Iida, and Max Lungarella. 2014. "Cognition from the Bottom up: On Biological Inspiration, Body Morphology, and Soft Materials." *Trends in Cognitive Sciences* 18 (8): 404–413.

Piaget, Jean. 1954. *The Construction of Reality in the Child.* New York: Basic Books.

Proffitt, D. R., M. Bhalla, R. Gossweiler, and J. Midgett. 1995. "Perceiving Geographical Slant." *Psychonomic Bulletin & Review* 2 (4): 409–428.

Putnam, Hilary. 1960. "Minds and Machines." In *Dimensions of Mind,* edited by S. Hook, 148–180. New York: University of New York Press. Reprinted in H. Putnam, 1975, 362–385.

Putnam, Hilary. 1967. "Psychophysical Predicates." In *Art, Mind, and Religion,* edited by W. Capitan and D. Merrill. Pittsburgh, PA: University of Pittsburgh Press. Reprinted as "The Nature of Mental States," in Putnam (1975), *Mind, Language, and Reality,* 429–440. Cambridge: Cambridge University Press.

Putnam, Hilary. 1981. "Brains in a Vat." In *Reason, Truth and History,* edited by Hilary Putnam, 1–21. Cambridge: Cambridge University Press.

Turvey, Michael T. 1973. "On Peripheral and Central Processes in Vision: Inferences from an Information-Processing Analysis of Masking with Patterned Stimuli." *Psychological Review* 80 (1): 1–52.

Varela, Francisco J., Evan Thompson, and Eleanor Rosch. 1991. *The Embodied Mind: Cognitive Science and Human Experience*. Cambridge, MA: MIT Press.

Wilson, Andrew D., and Sabrina Golonka. 2013. "Embodied Cognition Is Not What You Think It Is." *Frontiers in Psychology* 4 (February): 58.

Wilson, Robert A., and Lucia Foglia. 2011. "Embodied Cognition." *Stanford Encyclopedia of Philosophy*. https://stanford.library.sydney.edu.au/entries/embodied-cognition/.

Witt, Jessica K., Susan C. South, and Mila Sugovic. 2014. "A Perceiver's Own Abilities Influence Perception, Even When Observing Others." *Psychonomic Bulletin and Review* 21 (2): 384–389.

I Concepts and Applications of the Embodied Approach to Sport Science: Foundational and Methodological Notions

1 Embodied Cognition and Sport

Lawrence Shapiro and Shannon Spaulding

1 Introduction

Successful athletic performance requires precision in many respects. A batter stands behind home plate awaiting the arrival of a ball that is smaller than three inches in diameter and moving close to 100 miles per hour. His goal is to hit the ball with a bat that is also smaller than three inches in diameter. This impressive feat requires extraordinary temporal and spatial coordination. The sweet spot of the bat must be at the same place, at the same time, as the ball. A basketball player must keep a ball bouncing as she speeds from one end of the court to the other, evading defensive players. She may never break pace as she lifts from the ground, throwing the ball fifteen feet toward a hoop eighteen inches in diameter.

Familiarity with professional-level play might lead one to lose sight of the exactness of the skills involved. For a good and amusing remedy to this, watch a few minutes of the Robocup. This annual soccer tournament matches teams consisting of the most technologically advanced robots on Earth. The robots shuffle around the field, slowly. They occasionally bump into each other, causing one or both to fall down. Whereas a human soccer player moves smoothly toward a ball, never breaking stride as she controls it with her foot until lofting a pass to a player downfield, the robot's encounter with the ball is anything but fluid. It stops in front of the ball, inspecting it as though it's some unknown object that has just fallen from outer space. It bounces from foot to foot before carefully orienting itself *just so*. The kick, when it finally comes, sends the ball rolling a few feet, typically in a random direction. If it hasn't fallen on its butt, the robot freezes, its work done.

Although athletes differ from nonathletes in the finesse they bring to particular situations, we must all move our limbs and torso and head so that we walk smoothly, reach accurately, bend and twist appropriately, and keep our eyes fixed on objects as they move past us. Thus, one task facing a psychologist involves explaining how the body does such things within the sometimes very demanding spatial and temporal constraints that a given task imposes. Part of the goal of this chapter is to sketch the commitments of an *embodied* approach to such an explanation. We shall see that an embodied account of motor skills draws concepts that depart radically from more traditional cognitivist theories of motor activity. Similarly, because an embodied approach to cognition introduces new ways to understand the human capacity for social interaction, it also promises to shed new light on how athletes coordinate their actions with each other.

2 Themes of Embodiment

"Embodied cognition" is best understood as a label for a diverse research program that spans work across the cognitive spectrum, including memory (Glenberg 1997), perception (O'Regan and Noë 2001), language (Kaschak et al. 2005), and emotion (Barrett 2012) (see Shapiro 2014a for a representative collection). Additionally, it takes as its subject matter not just human beings, but also simple organisms such as crickets (Webb 1996), simulated agents (Beer 2003), and robots (Brooks 1991). Given its breadth, the job of offering a succinct characterization of embodied cognition faces obvious difficulties.

Yet another challenge besets efforts to articulate the distinctive character of embodied cognition. Traditional cognitive psychology, not to mention many of its scientific predecessors, recognized the body's significance in thought processes. Indeed, Descartes, famous for his distinction between mind and body, nevertheless denied that the relationship between mind and body is simply like that of sailor in a ship. Rather, he insisted, "I am most tightly joined and, so to speak, commingled with it, so much so that I and the body constitute one single thing" ([1641] 1993, 53). Granting that investigations of cognition have, for centuries, acknowledged close ties between mind and body, a natural question arises: What new or novel connections between mind and body has embodied cognition discovered?

One of us (Shapiro 2007, 2010, 2012) has sought to respond to both worries above—how to limn the boundaries of embodied cognition, given its wide scope, and how to isolate those features of embodied cognition that mark it as a new approach to psychology—by describing various "themes" that pop up repeatedly in the various areas that embodied cognition researchers investigate. The first such theme is *conceptualization*. Research that supports conceptualization reveals that the properties of a body constrain and thus influence how an organism conceives of its world. This idea builds on the Gibsonian notion of an affordance (Gibson 1979). Gibson argued that organisms perceive their environments in terms of how they may interact with the objects they encounter.

Thus, a branch that a bird perceives as something to perch on might be perceived by a monkey as something to swing from. A prominent area of embodied cognition—enactivism—takes this Gibsonian suggestion further, arguing that the perceived world is a consequence of the actions the body takes toward it (O'Regan and Noë 2001; Noë 2004). Thus, insofar as different kinds of organisms have different kinds of bodies, and different kinds of bodies interact with the world in different ways, differently embodied organisms perceive, and thus conceive, of the same world in different ways. We shall take up the conceptualization theme in the final section of this chapter, where we discuss work that reveals athletes to possess special perceptual abilities as a result of their training.

A second theme of embodiment Shapiro describes is *constitution*. Claims concerning constitution are especially common in an area of embodied cognition devoted to showing how cognition might extend beyond the brain. Much of this research focuses less on the body's actual contribution to cognition and more on the use of external "props," such as calculators or diaries, to enhance cognition. For instance, Clark and Chalmers (1998) imagine a scenario involving a man, Otto, who relies extensively on his diary to compensate for the loss of his "natural" memory. In their view, the entries in the diary constitute actual memories, no less authentic than those that once would have been stored in Otto's hippocampus. More generally, those who pursue the idea of constitution seek to show how parts of the world might be recruited to become parts (constituents) of a cognitive system. The challenge these researchers face is in defending the claim that parts of the world qualify as actual *constituents* of cognition rather than as mere causal influences on cognitive processes that remain completely "brain bound" (see Adams and Aizawa 2008 and Rupert 2009 for criticisms). Failure to make the case for constitution over causation opens these researchers to the second worry we expressed above: they have not identified anything novel about embodied cognition because psychologists have long known that the world causally contributes in numerous ways to cognitive processes.

The third theme, *replacement*, is the focus of the section below. The basic idea behind replacement is that features of embodiment work to facilitate cognition in previously unrecognized ways. Replacement departs from traditional cognitive psychology in eschewing its strong commitment to a computational theory of mind, according to which cognition is an entirely computational process that involves the operation of algorithms over representational states, and in seeking to replace computationalism with something else (e.g., dynamical systems theory). In its most radical form, replacement advances the idea that thought processes involve no representational states at all, and thus have no need for computational processes (Shapiro 2013). Surely this claim goes too far, offering no positive account of how to construe cognitive capacities such as memory or planning in a nonrepresentational format (see Shapiro 2014b for discussion). More mildly, and promisingly, advocates of replacement see the body as "stepping in" to do work that once would have been attributed to computational processes. It is to this milder strain of replacement we now turn.

3 From Programs to Bodies

As the behaviorism that dominated psychology in the middle part of the twentieth century gave way to computational theories of cognition, psychologists interested in bodily movement endorsed the idea that such movements were under the control of a *motor program* (Keele 1968; Schmidt 1976). Schmidt, a significant figure in the development of the motor program concept, summarizes the view: "The program is generally thought to contain a centrally stored, prestructured set of muscle commands that are capable of carrying out movement without feedback information about the achievement of the environmental goal. Viewed this way, the program must determine which muscles contract, in what order, with what force, and for how long" (1976, 242).

Although the motor program concept evolved over the course of continued investigation, the basic idea (still with us today, as in Neilson and Neilson 2005) maintains a strong commitment to a computational theory of cognition. The motor program is, in a fairly literal sense, a computer program. It contains instructions written in a language of thought that the nervous system must first read and then execute. "Before we reach out for an object," Ghez explains, "our nervous system must first select a motor program that specifies (1) the sequence of muscles needed to bring the hand to the desired point in space and (2) how much each muscle must contract" (1985, 494). Presumably, Ghez would claim, the nervous system of the batter we mentioned above would have selected a series of commands that caused the muscles in the batter's arms to flex and extend in just the right way to produce a base hit.

The motor program approach to explaining muscle control is in keeping with the more general computational theory of cognition that retains prominence in most psychology departments today. Memory, for instance, might be analyzed in terms of stored representations that are recalled for current inspection; processes of language production tap into representations of grammatical rules that dictate the form of linguistic structures; vision involves the application of algorithms to information derived from the retinal image. Although proponents of embodied cognition have sought to challenge computationalism as it plays out across the broad domain of psychology, of special interest in the present context is the embodied response to motor programs. If muscle control is not under the direction of a program that the nervous system executes, from where does the control come?

Crucial to answering this question, from an embodied perspective, is rejection of the idea that control must come from a controller. Various research programs within embodied cognition seek to show that muscle control emerges from tight interactions among the body, the nervous system, and the environment. Notions central to the computational theory of cognition—*program, representation, executor*—are discarded, to be replaced with notions better suited for describing the continuous interactions between brain, body, and world. Often, these new notions draw from the conceptual resources of dynamical systems theory.

Well studied in this context is the development of stepping behavior in infants. A behavior such as walking requires delicate coordination between two legs. It is easy to take for granted that the legs of walking bipeds must move 180 degrees out of phase relative to each other (Thelen and Ulrich 1991, 60). But, of course, there are many more ways for stepping to go wrong than to go right. The legs might move in parallel, as they would if hopping. One leg might move at a slower frequency than the other, or with larger amplitude. Moreover, each leg contains over a dozen muscles. There are joints at the hip, the knee, and the ankle. Designing a motor program that maintains control of all these factors, coordinating them with the precision necessary to produce a fluid gait, would be no easy task.

Progress in understanding how the nervous system accomplishes this difficult feat begins with the realization that a leg can be treated as a spring with a certain tension and weighted by a specific mass. Just as a spring will equilibrate to the same length given any initial stretching or compression, so too the musculature of the leg ensures that it will tend toward a particular orientation regardless of its displacement. Thelen and Ulrich (1991) tested this idea with seven-month-old infants, who, when held above a treadmill so that the soles of their feet could touch the moving belt, engaged in stepping behavior. They conjecture that "the mechanical pulling of the leg backward stretches the leg muscles and allows them to store energy, much like stretching a spring beyond its equilibrium point. When the leg is stretched to its anatomical limit, it uses this stored energy to spring forward" (1991, 43).

Of course, the development and production of stepping behavior in human beings cannot be attributed solely to the interaction of the spring-loaded legs with the environment, as it might be in the "passive walkers" that roboticists have created (Collins et al. 2005). The effect of the moving treadmill belt on the legs does not account for why the legs adopt a pattern of stepping with the necessary 180-degree out-of-phase motion. The nervous system must be involved in such calibration. But the contribution the nervous system makes to stepping behavior should not be taken to diminish the extent of the departure from a motor program explanation of motion that work like Thelen and colleagues present.

In the first place, conceiving of the legs as weighted springs that, in effect, oscillate like pendula opens the way for recruiting a new explanatory framework for understanding limb movements. In particular, the language of dynamical systems, with its reference to state spaces, attractors, and control variables—concepts useful for characterizing the behavior of systems like pendula that change over time—lends insight into behavior that would otherwise have been forced into a computational framework of dubious appropriateness. Thelen and Ulrich, for instance, identified the alternating pattern of stepping behavior on the treadmill into which seven-month-old infants settled as an attractor point. Because the behavior of a dynamical system heads toward an attractor point from various initial conditions, Thelen and Ulrich predicted that infants' stepping would "resolve" into the alternating step pattern despite perturbations to the system. After inducing several perturbations—one in which the treadmill speed was increased, another in which a split treadmill caused the infants' legs to move at different speeds—Thelen and Ulrich confirmed their prediction. The alternating step attractor "pulled" the initially disrupted stepping behavior back into stability (1991). This example displays how dynamical systems theory can be applied to a domain once thought to be most fruitfully investigated from a computational perspective.

The example also highlights a prominent theme within embodied cognition literature. We mentioned above that the nervous system remains an important contributor to stepping behavior. Maintenance of the anti-phase motions of the legs seems to require that information about the state of one leg regulate the state of the other (Thelen and Ulrich 1991, 61). But, even if a computational description of how such information is processed turns out, in the end, to offer the best understanding of this particular feature of stepping behavior, one must not lose sight of how recognition of the body's physical properties constrains and minimizes candidate motor program explanations. This idea illustrates the replacement theme we introduced in the previous section.

Replacement, in this case, involves the elimination of computational processes in favor of simple mechanics. We noted already that the leg contains over a dozen muscles and three joints. A motor program that succeeded in controlling the behavior of these components and synchronizing them with the same number of components in the other leg would, doubtless, require sophisticated and elaborate neural computations. How much simpler the task becomes when conceiving of the legs as simple springs.

Because springs behave as they do by virtue of their tension and mass, there is no need for a motor program to guide their behavior—no more need than there is for a motor program to guide the behavior of a slinky as it descends a staircase. And, to the extent that computation is necessary for tasks such as calibration of the two legs, the conception of the legs as single springlike units reduces the complexity of the algorithms needed to control their behavior. As Thelen, Kelso, and Fogel note, "The dynamic conceptualization allows, in short, for much less information to be abstractly represented, and much more information in the sense of a wide variety of trajectories to come 'for free'" (1987, 45).

We see, then, one way in which an embodied approach to cognition might contribute to an understanding of athletic performance. Examination of the mechanical properties of the body suggests ways in which certain tasks, once thought to require computational solutions, might be better explained with a noncomputational alternative. Such an explanation replaces computational talk with descriptions of the dynamical behavior of the body. The batter who connects with the ball speeding toward his chest does something fantastically complicated, no doubt; but, it turns out, the task is less computationally demanding than one might first have supposed. The batter's arms are, after all, physical objects whose motion is subject to the same sort of dynamical analysis that emphasizes the mechanical—in contrast to computational—forces at work in an infant's stepping behavior. In this conception, the role of the motor program shifts from omniscient planner, responsible for controlling the contraction and extension of individual muscles, to opportunistic cobbler, taking advantage of the dynamical properties that muscles, bones, and joints bring for free.

If an embodied perspective on bodily movement reveals how the brain's computational burden might be reduced by taking advantage of the body's natural dynamics, so too does a focus on embodiment show perceptual processes to be far less computationally expensive than traditional cognitive science would suppose. Wonderfully illustrative of this embodiment-inspired shift from computational explanations of perception is research that investigates how an outfielder manages to catch a fly ball. That outfielders—amateurs as well as professionals—seem to have little difficulty tracking a ball from the instant of its impact with a bat to the second before it hits the ground, which may involve a distance of more than 100 meters, appears to be quite a marvel. Somehow, the outfielder manages to position himself exactly where he needs to be to intercept the ball. Moreover, given the initial distance between the outfielder and the ball, cues that might be useful for depth perception, such as parallax and disparity, are ineffective.

One way to explain how the outfielder maneuvers his body to just where it needs to be treats the task as a difficult computational problem. The idea is that the outfielder makes a prediction about the trajectory the ball will take after impact with the bat. The inputs to the computation include such things as the force with which the ball was hit, its direction as it leaves the bat, and its speed. But also included in the computation must be factors like wind direction, air resistance, and the ball's spin. This so-called trajectory prediction explanation of the outfielder's performance assumes that all these inputs feed into various cognitive systems that then grind through the appropriate computations, returning as output the location where the ball will drop, which is then used to guide the movement of the outfielder.

Of course, this computation-heavy explanation of how an outfielder intercepts a fly ball is possible in principle. But research suggests that outfielders are in fact not very good at predicting the trajectory a ball will take (Shaffer and McBeath 2005). Psychologists who study the outfielder problem have largely abandoned computational solutions in favor of those that assign a prominent role to the outfielder's ability to track continuously a single variable. The outfielder moves his body in such a way as to keep this variable constant, or invariant.

One such explanation, linear optical trajectory (LOT), requires that the outfielder positions himself so that the fly ball, which in fact has a parabolic trajectory, will appear to ascend in a straight line from home plate (see figure 1.1). Once situated in a position from which the ball's trajectory appears as a straight line, the outfielder will be in the exact location he needs to be in to catch the ball. As Andy Clark describes the LOT method, "Instead of using sensing to get enough information inside, past the visual bottleneck, so as to allow the reasoning system to 'throw away the world' and solve the problem wholly internally, it uses the sensor as *an open conduit allowing environmental magnitudes to exert a constant influence on behavior*" (Clark 2007, 266, emphasis original).

Competing with LOT is an alternative explanation that, while sharing LOT's emphasis on the outfielder's need to track a single variable, chooses a different variable. According to optical acceleration cancellation (OAC), the outfielder must position himself so that the upward acceleration of the ball is fixed at a constant rate. Deviation from a constant rate provides the outfielder with cues that allow him to adjust his location relative to the ball. If the ball's acceleration appears to slow as it climbs upward, the outfielder must move forward to catch it. On the other hand, if the ball's acceleration appears to increase, the outfielder must move backward to catch it (see figure 1.2).

Recent evidence suggests that OAC is more likely the strategy that outfielders actually use (Fink, Foo, and Warren 2009), but in the present context, less important than which, between LOT and OAC, is the correct explanation of the outfielder's performance is the sense that these explanations offer an embodied alternative to computationally heavy ones. An explanation such as trajectory prediction, we saw, conceives

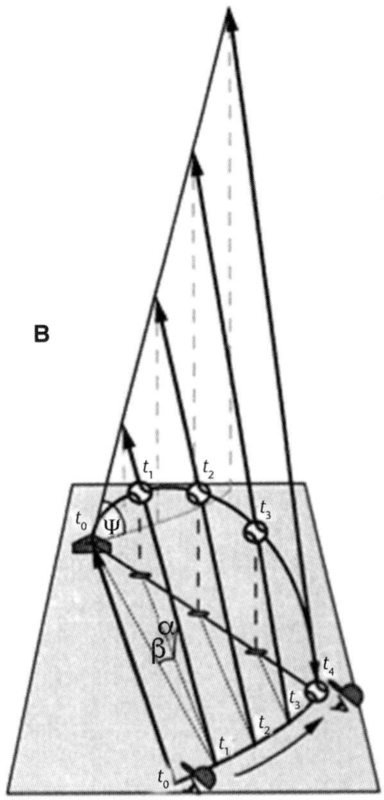

Figure 1.1
The ball's trajectory is parabolic, but the outfielder's motion can make it appear linear and ascending.
Source: McBeath, Shaffer, and Kaiser (1995).

of the outfielder's problem as demanding a solution consisting of computations over representations of a large number of variables. The output of the computations will be a prediction of the ball's trajectory, and the outfielder's job is then to move his body to the precise location at the end of the trajectory.

In contrast, both LOT and OAC seek to replace a computational explanation of the fielder's behavior with one that integrates the outfielder's motion into the solution. Through his motion, the outfielder establishes and then maintains continuous contact with a single variable (linear motion or constant acceleration). There is simply no need to represent such things as the ball's initial direction and speed. Factors like wind and air resistance are rendered irrelevant insofar as they become subsumed within linear

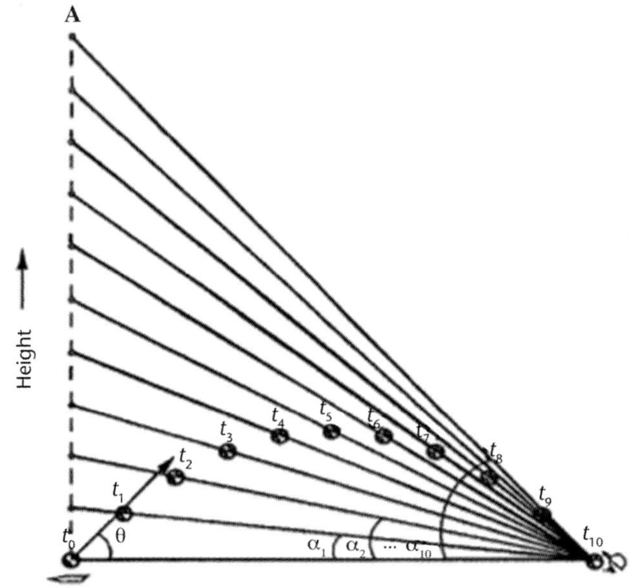

Figure 1.2
The outfielder will intercept the ball when making its upward acceleration appear constant, that is, to be rising equal distances in equal time intervals.
Source: Shaffer and McBeath (2002).

motion or constant acceleration. All that matters to the embodied strategies is that the outfielder keeps his body in a position where the ball appears to be moving straight up or with a constant acceleration.

We have seen two examples now in which an embodied perspective on sport performance—and performance more generally—marks a departure from more traditional computational accounts. In the case of calculating limb movements, the idea of a motor program that computes how muscles must flex and extend in order to move a limb is replaced by dynamical systems approaches that conceive of muscles and limbs as spring masses or oscillators. As such, limbs will exhibit, "for free," certain kinds of behavior, and the job of the nervous system shifts from one of designing and selecting precise motor programs to a vastly simpler one of governing the actions of simple machines with latent patterns of motion that need only to be released and coordinated. In the second example, we see how a body in motion can establish and maintain contact with a single variable, rendering unnecessary the sophisticated computations that a stationary observer would otherwise require to accomplish a task such as catching a fly ball. Embodied cognition, as we understand it, thus invites sport psychologists to hunt for explanations of athletic performance that minimize the computational demands on a nervous system that seems better conceived of as a source of control for a body already primed for movement and perception.

4 The Social Aspect of Sports

Above we distinguished three themes of embodied cognition: conceptualization, constitution, and replacement. The discussion of motor programs illustrates the fruitfulness of *replacing* traditional computational explanations with explanations that focus on bodily mechanics and motions. Here we focus on the social aspect of sports, which provides nice examples of conceptualization and builds further connections between embodied cognition and sport psychology.

Many sports involve interpreting and anticipating the behavior of other athletes. In basketball, for example, an athlete not only must execute actions in light of her immediate goals and overall game strategy, she also must coordinate her actions with her teammates' complementary actions and opponents' disruptive, incompatible actions. Coordinating her actions with teammates and opponents requires interpreting their behavior and anticipating what they will do next. For instance, she must recognize when an opponent is driving to the basket (as opposed to faking a drive to open enough space to shoot), she must anticipate the positions her teammates will be in when the opponent is driving to the basket, and decide whether to pursue the driving opponent or let a better-positioned teammate step in to defend against the drive. This dynamic interaction happens very quickly, and superior athletes are more highly skilled at coordinating their behavior with teammates and opponents' behavior.

Coordination between executing one's own actions and anticipating others' actions is not unique to team sports. Even in so-called individual sports, such as running, boxing, and karate, the athlete's actions are influenced by what she understands other athletes to be doing. Take running, for example. In a track race, a runner approaches the competition with a general race plan. In most cases, executing the race plan will depend on other athletes' performances. Suppose the race plan is to finish in the top two spots (in order to advance to the next round of competition, for example). The athlete must determine whether the runners around her are struggling more than she is and whether runners that pass her can sustain their pace. She must moderate her own effort so that she has enough energy left to finish strongly at the end of the race, all the while making sure she is well positioned in terms of place and effort in relation to the other athletes. As this example shows, individual sports involve coordination between one's own actions and competitors' actions as well.

Given that many sports involve this social element, the following question arises: How do we coordinate our actions with others' actions in sports? Neuroscientists have discovered that action execution and action observation recruit some of the same neurological systems. More specifically, research on mirror neurons has shown that parts of the sensorimotor system that are responsible for producing planned actions are also partly responsible for interpreting and anticipating others' actions, which suggests that performing a particular action and perceiving that action are closely related skills, realized by the same neural mechanism (Fogassi et al. 2005; Gallese 2009; Gallese, Keysers, and Rizzolatti 2004). We describe the action mirror neuron system in more detail below.[1]

The action mirror neuron system consists of the premotor cortex and parts of the posterior parietal cortex, specifically, the rostral part of the inferior parietal lobule and the lower part of the precentral gyrus plus the posterior part of the inferior frontal gyrus. These areas are involved in sensory guidance of movement and the production of planned movements. Scientists have discovered two kinds of mirror neurons in these areas: strictly congruent and broadly congruent mirror neurons (Rizzolatti and Craighero 2004). Strictly congruent mirror neurons fire for the execution or observation of particular narrowly construed behaviors. For example, a group of strictly congruent mirror neurons will fire only when a subject observes or executes a pincer grasp to pick up an object. These same neurons will not fire when the subject executes or observes a full-hand grasp. Other groups of strictly congruent mirror neurons fire only for full-hand grasps. Broadly congruent mirror neurons, in contrast, fire for the same action less narrowly construed. For example, a particular group of broadly congruent mirror neurons will fire when the subject observes or executes both pincer grasps or full-hand grasps. The same group of neurons will fire when the subject uses the hand to pick up a piece of food to eat or observes another subject use a tool to pick up the food to eat. Broadly congruent mirror neurons are both visuo-motor, as the previous examples show, and audio-motor. If a subject *hears*, for example, someone eating food, mirror neurons that correspond to mouth-related actions will fire.

A subset of broadly congruent mirror neurons, so-called logically related mirror neurons, is particularly important for action perception (Csibra 2007; Iacoboni 2005; Rizzolatti and Sinigaglia 2010). These neurons have all the features of broadly congruent mirror neurons and one interesting additional feature: they fire for the end-state of an action sequence even when the end-state is unobserved. For example, logically related mirror neurons fire for the act of grasping an object or, upon observing another's grasping motion, they fire for the motor act of eating. In the first-person case, the neurons fire while executing a certain action, *A*, but in the third-person case they fire in expectation of *B*, the probable next behavior in the sequence. Thus, these mirror neurons *predict* or *anticipate* the target's next behavior.

Although there is no consensus on the precise role of mirror neurons in action understanding, the evidence suggests that mirror neurons are at least *part* of the neural substrate of action interpretation and anticipation (Rizzolatti and Sinigaglia 2010). The activation of strictly congruent mirror neurons provides information about the precise details of the observed action (e.g., that it is a whole-handed grasp), and broadly congruent mirror neurons provide more general information about the observed action (e.g., that it is an eating-related grasp). Logically related mirror neurons function as predictive mechanisms for familiar behaviors (e.g., they fire in expectation of eating), thus providing information about the probable next behavior in a sequence. Each kind of mirror neuron provides different information about the observed action, and this information facilitates action interpretation and anticipation of others' actions.[2]

Of course, the patterns of neural activation for action execution and observation do not completely overlap. For example, the observer's brain exhibits various inhibitory responses that prevent the observer from actually performing the action, the actor's brain receives and processes proprioceptive information that the observer's brain does not, and the neural activity in the actor's mirror neuron system is stronger than that in the observer's mirror neuron system. Although motor mirror neuron activity may be strong enough to produce covert, unconscious movements, in normal cases the observer does not act exactly as the observed target acts. Nevertheless, the discovery that action observation and execution recruit the very same neurons is an intriguing finding, and it has significant implications for sport psychology.

Putting all of this together, the neuroscientific research on mirror neurons suggests that action observation and execution share a common neural basis, namely, the mirror neuron system. Thus, we have at least a partial answer to our question about how action coordination occurs: the same system underlies both production and observation of action. Mirror neurons are deployed one way (in conjunction with other neural systems) when executing an action, and they are deployed another way (in conjunction with other neural systems) when observing others execute that action.

To illustrate how mirror neurons work, we described relatively simple actions, but the same lessons apply to the more complex actions involved in sports. Driving toward the basket and observing an opponent drive toward the basket activate the same neural system. One interesting implication of this tight coupling between motor and perceptual processes is that the more skilled one becomes at performing a particular action, the better one will be at interpreting and anticipating the outcome of that action. For example, these findings imply that expert golfers should be better at putting, but they also should be better at perceptually discriminating and predicting the trajectory of others' putts. This implication is empirically substantiated in the literature on sport psychology.

As it turns out, the ability to perceive athletic behaviors differs according to one's experience in producing those behaviors (Shiffrar and Heinen 2010). Expert athletes are better than novice athletes and mere spectators at interpreting and predicting the outcome of athletic behaviors that are similar to the ones they perform. For example, a professional basketball player can judge more accurately than a novice or spectator whether a player is faking a drive to the basket and whether a shot will go in the basket. Female ballet dancers can perceptually discriminate the choreography of female ballet dancers better than male ballet dancers can, even though male ballet dancers frequently observe female ballet choreography. In both of these examples, the motor expertise seems to bring about perceptual expertise. And this is just what one would expect, given that the same neural system underlies action production and perception.

Focusing on how one's body influences one's perception illustrates a central theme of embodied cognition we introduced above, namely conceptualization. The idea begins with recognition that, through extended practice, athletes' bodies become more adept at executing particular skills. In turn, the brains of these athletes, and in particular their mirror neurons, become tuned to recognizing actions of a particular kind. This tuning enables athletes to perceive movements, or patterns of movement, that remain invisible to novices. Insofar as these perceptual feats reflect abilities to categorize certain motions such as, for example, driving to the basket or, in ballet, a *saute*, they illustrate the idea of conceptualization. The athletes see or conceive of the world (or of the motions of individuals in the world) differently than do nonathletes. Were we to focus just on explicating computational motor programs underwriting athletic performance, we would miss this insight.

Importantly, this coupling between athletic performance and perception has implications for sport psychology, as well. The effects of this tight coupling between motor and perceptual processes explain why novice athletes and spectators substantially overestimate their own athletic abilities, a phenomenon known as the Dunning-Kruger effect. The Dunning-Kruger effect is a cognitive bias in which the more knowledgeable and competent one is, the more accurately one assesses one's knowledge and competence. Individuals who are not knowledgeable or competent with respect to some issue egregiously overestimate their own knowledge and competence and fail to recognize others' equal or superior knowledge and competence (Kruger and Dunning 1999). For example, people who have poor social skills tend to overestimate their ability to figure out what other people are thinking or feeling, whereas those who are more socially skilled give a more accurate assessment of their ability to "read" other people (Ames and Kammrath 2004; Realo et al. 2003). In general, the deficiency of the less competent is invisible to them because recognizing their deficiency requires the very competency they lack.

In sports, this effect can be observed in the difference between an elite athlete's assessment of his athletic skills and the self-assessment of novices or spectators. The preceding discussion can help us explain how this bias arises. Performing athletic maneuvers in a particular sport increases one's ability to perceptually discriminate athletic maneuvers in that sport. Thus, putting practice makes one better able to assess the difficulty of a particular putt, visually analyze and predict the outcome of the putt, and more accurately assess one's ability to make this putt. Novice golfers and spectators are less adept at visually analyzing the difficulty of the putt and less able to accurately assess their ability to make the putt. Thus, for novice golfers and spectators, a particularly difficult putt literally looks easier.

The discussion so far explains the correlation between motor and perceptual abilities and a cognitive bias that results from this. The previous findings focus on elite athletes, novices, and spectators' passive observations of athletic behaviors. In most sporting events, however, athletes must interpret and anticipate others' behavior while at the same time executing their own athletic behaviors. The coupling between motor and perceptual processes also helps us to understand what happens when athletes interacting in an athletic competition have to balance the production of their own behavior while perceiving the behavior of others.

In this interactive context, because motor and perceptual processes are realized in part by the same neurological system, action perception and production compete for the same neurological resources. In other words, focus on producing athletic behavior may impair one's ability to perceive athletic behaviors, and focus on perceiving athletic behaviors may impair one's ability to produce athletic behaviors. The skills that are disrupted will depend on the skill level of the athlete.

As a novice basketball player, one must focus one's attention and effort on dribbling the basketball properly; that is, pushing the basketball to the ground at the right angle, force, and cadence. As one practices more, the simple skill of dribbling becomes easier and one does not need to focus on it to do it well. At the intermediate level, one masters dribbling in more challenging contexts, for example, running and dribbling, dribbling with a defender trying to get the ball, and so on. For expert basketball players, dribbling becomes automatized and requires no conscious attention. Indeed, attention to dribbling may in fact disrupt performance. The automation of basic skills like dribbling frees up the expert's attention for more complex athletic moves and strategic plays (Christensen, Sutton, and McIlwain 2016).

Given the nature of skill mastery, impairments in perceiving and executing athletic behaviors are relative to one's skill level. For novices, observing others dribble may disrupt attempts at dribbling, and focusing on dribbling may make it difficult to observe others dribbling. Indeed, for this reason it is amusing to watch a group of children learn how to dribble basketballs. For intermediate-level athletes, dribbling itself requires no conscious attention. Driving to the hoop, however, is more challenging, and doing this while perceiving a defender may disrupt one's ability to execute the drive. For expert basketball players, the previous skills are relatively easy and more or less automated. This frees up the expert's attention to focus on strategy: for example, running plays to orchestrate a height mismatch between an offensive and defensive player. Executing a more complex athletic move may interfere with the expert athlete's ability to interpret and anticipate opponents' moves, thereby disrupting her ability to run effective strategic plays.

A further consequence of how production and perception are coordinated is that interacting athletes sometimes are so focused on executing their own actions that they do not perceive opponents' overt disruptive actions. As sports fans can attest, it is baffling to see elite athletes miss glaring opportunities. In these instances, an athlete's perception of another athlete's behavior may be impaired even in comparison to what spectators see. Though perplexing to sports fans, this impairment is a straightforward consequence of how perception and motor production are coordinated in the sensorimotor system. Given that action execution and perception involve the same neurological resources, when one of these tasks is much more demanding, it diminishes the ability to achieve the other task.

5 Conclusion

The body contributes to cognition in surprising ways—ways that more standard computationally oriented approaches to cognition often fail to appreciate. In this chapter we have focused on how the mechanics of the body can *replace* the need for computational solutions to various motor and perceptual tasks. We have also examined the neural basis for social cognition, which can result in perceptual and conceptual refinements that reflect an individual's specific history of interaction with objects, including other individuals, in her environment. Sport psychologists have been quick to notice the significance of these ideas in their efforts to understand athletic performance. Indeed, some sport psychologists have been instrumental in expanding and developing research programs within embodied cognition (see especially Beilock 2008). We believe that continued erosion in the disciplinary boundaries between embodied cognition and sport psychology will bring tremendous benefits to both fields.

Notes

1. For more comprehensive overviews of the mirror neuron system, see Rizzolatti and Craighero (2004), Pineda (2009), and Rizzolatti and Sinigaglia (2010).

2. See Spaulding (2013) for an extended defense of these claims.

References

Adams, Frederick, and Kenneth Aizawa. 2008. *The Bounds of Cognition*. Malden, MA: Wiley-Blackwell.

Ames, Daniel R., and Lara K. Kammrath. 2004. "Mind-Reading and Metacognition: Narcissism, Not Actual Competence, Predicts Self-Estimated Ability." *Journal of Nonverbal Behavior* 28 (3): 187–209.

Barrett, Lisa Feldman. 2012. "Emotions Are Real." *Emotion* 12 (3): 413–429.

Beer, Randall D. 2003. "The Dynamics of Active Categorical Perception in an Evolved Model Agent." *Adaptive Behavior* 11 (4): 209–243.

Beilock, Sian L. 2008. "Beyond the Playing Field: Sport Psychology Meets Embodied Cognition." *International Review of Sport and Exercise Psychology* 1 (1): 19–30.

Brooks, Rodney A. 1991. "Intelligence without Representation." *Artificial Intelligence* 47 (1–3): 139–159.

Christensen, Wayne, John Sutton, and Doris J. F. McIlwain. 2016. "Cognition in Skilled Action: Meshed Control and the Varieties of Skill Experience." *Mind & Language* 31 (1): 37–66.

Clark, Andy. 2007. "Re-Inventing Ourselves: The Plasticity of Embodiment, Sensing, and Mind." *Journal of Medicine and Philosophy* 32 (3): 263–282.

Clark, Andy, and David Chalmers. 1998. "The Extended Mind." *Analysis* 58 (1): 7–19.

Collins, Steve, Andy Ruina, Russ Tedrake, and Martijn Wisse. 2005. "Efficient Bipedal Robots Based on Passive-Dynamic Walkers." *Science* 307 (5712): 1082–1085.

Csibra, Gergely. 2008. "Action Mirroring and Action Understanding: An Alternative Account." In *Sensorimotor Foundations of Higher Cognition*, edited by Patrick Haggard, Yves Rossetti, and Mitsuo Kawato, 435–459. Attention and Performance Series 22. Oxford: Oxford University Press.

Descartes, R. [1641] 1993. *Meditations on First Philosophy*. 3rd ed. Translated by D. Cress. Indianapolis, IN: Hackett.

Fink, Philip W., Patrick S. Foo, and William H. Warren. 2009. "Catching Fly Balls in Virtual Reality: A Critical Test of the Outfielder Problem." *Journal of Vision* 9 (13): 1–8.

Fogassi, Leonardo, Pier Francesco Ferrari, Benno Gesierich, Stefano Rozzi, Fabian Chersi, and Giacomo Rizzolatti. 2005. "Parietal Lobe: From Action Organization to Intention Understanding." *Science* 308 (5722): 662–667.

Gallese, Vittorio. 2009. "Motor Abstraction: A Neuroscientific Account of How Action Goals and Intentions Are Mapped and Understood." *Psychological Research* 73 (4): 486–498.

Gallese, Vittorio, Christian Keysers, and Giacomo Rizzolatti. 2004. "A Unifying View of the Basis of Social Cognition." *Trends in Cognitive Sciences* 8 (9): 396–403.

Ghez, C. 1985. "Voluntary Movement." In *Principles of Neural Science*, 2nd ed., edited by E. Kandel and J. Schwartz, 493–501. New York: Elsevier Science.

Gibson, James J. 1979. *The Ecological Approach to Visual Perception.* Boston: Houghton-Mifflin.

Glenberg, A. M. 1997. "What Memory Is For." *Behavioral and Brain Sciences* 20 (1): 1–19; discussion 19–55.

Iacoboni, Marco. 2005. "Understanding Others: Imitation, Language, Empathy." In *Perspectives on Imitation: From Cognitive Neuroscience to Social Science*, edited by S. Hurley and N. Chater, 77–99. Cambridge, MA: MIT Press.

Kaschak, Michael P., Carol J. Madden, David J. Therriault, Richard H. Yaxley, Mark Aveyard, Adrienne A. Blanchard, and Rolf A. Zwaan. 2005. "Perception of Motion Affects Language Processing." *Cognition* 94 (3): B79–89.

Keele, Steven W. 1968. "Movement Control in Skilled Motor Performance." *Psychological Bulletin* 70 (61): 387–403.

Kruger, J., and D. Dunning. 1999. "Unskilled and Unaware of It: How Difficulties in Recognizing One's Own Incompetence Lead to Inflated Self-Assessments." *Journal of Personality and Social Psychology* 77 (6): 1121–1134.

McBeath, M. K., D. M. Shaffer, and M. K. Kaiser. 1995. "How Baseball Outfielders Determine Where to Run to Catch Fly Balls." *Science* 268 (5210): 569–573.

Neilson, Peter D., and Megan D. Neilson. 2005. "An Overview of Adaptive Model Theory: Solving the Problems of Redundancy, Resources, and Nonlinear Interactions in Human Movement Control." *Journal of Neural Engineering* 2 (3): S279–312.

Noë, Alva. 2004. *Action in Perception.* Cambridge, MA: MIT Press.

O'Regan, Kevin, and Alva Noë. 2001. "A Sensorimotor Account of Vision and Visual Consciousness." *Behavioral and Brain Sciences* 24 (5): 939–973; discussion 973–1031.

Pineda, Jaime A. 2009. "Mirror Neuron Systems." *The Role of Mirroring Processes in Social Cognition.* New York: Humana/Springer.

Realo, Anu, Jüri Allik, Aire Nõlvak, Raivo Valk, Tuuli Ruus, Monika Schmidt, and Tiina Eilola. 2003. "Mind-Reading Ability: Beliefs and Performance." *Journal of Research in Personality* 37 (5): 420–445.

Rizzolatti, Giacomo, and Laila Craighero. 2004. "The Mirror-Neuron System." *Annual Review of Neuroscience* 27:169–192.

Rizzolatti, Giacomo, and Corrado Sinigaglia. 2010. "The Functional Role of the Parieto-Frontal Mirror Circuit: Interpretations and Misinterpretations." *Nature Reviews: Neuroscience* 11 (4): 264–274.

Rupert, Robert D. 2009. *Cognitive Systems and the Extended Mind.* Philosophy of the Mind. New York: Oxford University Press.

Schmidt, R. A. 1976. "Control Processes in Motor Skills." *Exercise and Sport Sciences Reviews* 4:229–261.

Shaffer, Dennis M., and Michael K. McBeath. 2005. "Naive Beliefs in Baseball: Systematic Distortion in Perceived Time of Apex for Fly Balls." *Journal of Experimental Psychology: Learning, Memory, and Cognition* 31 (6): 1492–1501.

Shapiro, Lawrence. 2007. "The Embodied Cognition Research Programme." *Philosophy Compass* 2 (2): 338–346.

Shapiro, Lawrence. 2010. *Embodied Cognition.* London: Routledge.

Shapiro, Lawrence. 2012. "Embodied Cognition." In *The Oxford Handbook of Philosophy of Cognitive Science,* edited by E. Margolis, R. Samuels, and S. Stich, 118–147. New York: Oxford University Press.

Shapiro, Lawrence. 2013. "Dynamics and Cognition." *Minds and Machines* 23 (3): 353–375.

Shapiro, Lawrence. 2014a. *The Routledge Handbook of Embodied Cognition.* London: Routledge.

Shapiro, Lawrence. 2014b. "Radicalizing Enactivism: Basic Minds without Content, by Daniel D. Hutto and Erik Myin." *Mind: A Quarterly Review of Psychology and Philosophy* 123 (489): 213–220.

Shiffrar, Maggie, and Thomas Heinen. 2010. "Die Fähigkeiten von Athleten Verändern Deren Wahrnehmung von Handlungen." *Zeitschrift Für Sportpsychologie* 17 (4): 130–142. http://econtent.hogrefe.com/doi/full/10.1026/1612-5010/a000018.

Spaulding, Shannon. 2013. "Mirror Neurons and Social Cognition." *Mind & Language* 28 (2): 233–257.

Thelen, Esther, J. A. Scott Kelso, and Alan Fogel. 1987. "Self-Organizing Systems and Infant Motor Development." *Developmental Review* 7 (1): 39–65.

Thelen, Esther, and B. D. Ulrich. 1991. "Hidden Skills: A Dynamic Systems Analysis of Treadmill Stepping during the First Year." *Monographs of the Society for Research in Child Development* 56 (1): 1–98; discussion 99–104.

Webb, Barbara. 1996. "A Cricket Robot." *Scientific American* 275 (6): 94–99.

2 Emotions on the Playing Field

Daniel D. Hutto, Michael D. Kirchhoff, and Ian Renshaw

> Learn to control your emotions or they will control you.
>
> —Edgar Martinez

1 Introduction

Skillful performance in sport involves more than technical proficiency. How an athlete feels—whether he or she is confident, elated, nervous, or fearful—also matters to how they perform in certain situations. Taking stock of this, some sport psychologists have begun to develop techniques for ensuring more robust, reliable performances by focusing on how athletes respond emotionally to situations while, at the same time, training their action-oriented skills. In this chapter we add theoretical insight to those efforts, offering reasons to endorse a radically enactivist framework when it comes to thinking about the basic characteristics of emotions; how emotions are involved in skilled performance; and how they integrate with the sort of intelligence that informs the skilled execution of action exhibited in embodied expertise.

The chapter divides into five main parts. Following this introduction, part 2 explicates how recognition that emotional attunement may play a central role in the acquisition of expertise has led to the development of the Affective Learning Design (ALD) approach to training in sport psychology—an approach that aims to promote what we dub *embodied virtues*. Part 3 considers how the emotions might be brought into the mix under the auspices of classical cognitivist visions of mind, but highlights problems for the intellectualist characterization of the emotions that such approaches sponsor. Part 4 proposes a radically enactive approach to the emotions that can overcome the problems that plague more purely intellectualist theories. Part 5 shows how our preferred account of the emotions can combine neatly with a radically enactive account of the sort of intelligence that imbues sporting performances. It is concluded that an integrated, radically enactive account of emotion and cognition serves as an appropriate theoretical framework for understanding the constraint-based approach to training in sports assumed by ALD.[1]

2 Sporting Expertise as the Acquisition of Embodied Virtues

Traditionally sport training tends to bench or sideline the emotions. This is because it is typically assumed, in line with the long-standing philosophical tradition of rationalism, that emotions—whether positive or negative—are not only separate from but interfere with and have the potential to pervert the kinds of purely cognitive thinking needed for executing the technical skills embodied in sporting expertise. Hence, so such thinking goes, "it is necessary to suppress or remove emotions in order to make more rational decisions (i.e. cold cognition)" (Headrick et al. 2015, 85).[2] For this reason, actively quelling or keeping emotions out of the mix while training sport skills is advisable. Training regimes that adopt this approach can be said to subscribe to a kind of cognition-emotion separatism.

Alternatively, training technical skills might be thought to be—like it or not—necessarily a matter of training emotions, since emotions are always, one way or another, part of the development of technical skills. This is the signature idea of cognition-emotion integrationism. For anyone who adopts cognition-emotion integrationism, emotions can never be left on the sidelines when training technical expertise in sports; it is just that emotional contributions can be more or less ignored or focused on during training. Consequently, the resultant practical choice is clear: ignore the emotions or explicitly train them.

Against this backdrop, some sport scientists argue that more attention should be given to the emotions and how they are bound up with cognition during training and performance. ALD approaches to training are interested in the "holistic development of expertise" (Headrick et al. 2015, 87). Thus they adopt an approach to the acquisition of expertise that seeks to understand "integrated emotional and behavioural tendencies of athletes during learning" (88).[3] The driving assumption behind ALD is that performance outcomes can be enhanced, at least in some cases, by manipulating affective aspects of learning experiences.

In deciding how to construct such learning experiences, ALD builds on the Representative Learning Design, or RLD, assumption that "the development of expertise is predicated on the accurate simulation of key performance constraints during practice/learning" (Headrick et al. 2015, 85). Yet ALD goes further than RLD in extending the latter's basic logic to the emotions, ensuring that these too are taken into account in training at a ground-floor level. Consequently, ALD has the practical goal of understanding "how affective constraints on behaviour may be included during the acquisition of expertise in sport" (Headrick et al. 2015, 83). In other words, it is concerned with understanding "how perceptions, actions, intentions, feelings and thoughts continuously emerge under … constraints" (84). In sum, ALD seeks to create learning environments that promote better functional outcomes by introducing affective constraints on behavior so as to bring about better emotional attunement during the training and subsequent execution of sport skills.

The ALD approach is motivated not solely by the intuition that emotions matter in sporting performances but by empirical findings that emotions can make a significant difference during both training and competition. For instance, in a comparative study of novice and elite ice climbers, Seifert and Davids (2012) found that novices deliberately adopted a so-called X-position with their arms and legs when having to climb an ice wall quickly. The X-position gives more stability, but comes at the cost of losing energy and reduces competitive performance. So why do it? Apparently, this coordination tendency was the result of novice's initial fear and apprehension in dealing with the icy surface. Indeed, as reported by Headrick et al. (2015), the authors of the original study concluded that this "emotion was a major constraint on their particular cognition, perceptions and actions" (86). Confirming what we might intuitively expect, other studies reveal correlations between displays of nervousness on the part of gymnasts and decreases in their performance when they attempted routines on balance beams of increasing heights (Cottyn et al. 2012).

The types of emotions experienced and their intensity vary according to circumstance and appear to be modulated by an athlete's level of experience. In line with this observation, a five-year longitudinal study of an elite female shooter, her coach, and two ALD consultants revealed a need to shift emphasis, over time, in the focus that is placed on the emotions, mastery of specific actions, and their combination (Hanin et al. 2016). The athlete in question used a mix of emotion-centered, action-centered, and mixed coping strategies during performance, answering to her developing needs in self-control as she became more experienced, moving from junior to more senior categories.

Taking such findings on board, ALD isn't a blunt instrument. Using its methods, coaches and trainers can create learning environments that are sensitive to different kinds of coping strategies at different stages of an athlete's career. Designing appropriate learning experiences using ALD principles requires investigating how best to enable individuals to acquire robust expertise by using strategies that foreground emotions, actions, or a mix of both at different stages of their skill acquisition. Notably, in enacting such strategies, an athlete might be concerned with gaining mastery, in more or less explicit ways, over performance-related emotions: those that are more transient and episodic; those tied to an athlete's relatively long-standing and stable tendencies and dispositions; and those of a more reflective, meta-cognitive sort, involving explicit awareness and second-order attitudes about more basic states of mind (Hanin 2007, 33).

It has been reported that this general type of approach to training has, to date, been "successfully used in practice during the last decade in 14 different sports (track-and-field, swimming, diving, rhythmic gymnastics, alpine skiing, etc.)" (Hanin et al. 2016, 21). All these cases highlight the ways that emotions appear to be centrally involved in the training of expertise in sport, whatever an athlete's level of ability. Indeed, this is hardly surprising given that emotions are "often involved with moving out of a 'comfort zone' when confronted with a new or more challenging task" (Headrick 2015, 86).

The underlying assumption is that "through practice and experience in sport, athletes ... increase their resistance to perturbations, including negative thoughts, and emotions" (Headrick 2015, 84). Yet ALD need not focus solely on negative emotions: indeed, it shouldn't, since it is widely acknowledged that emotions "such as happiness, excitement and enjoyment permeate successful endeavor in sport" (McCarthy, Allen, and Jones 2013, 505). Recognizing the importance of both negative and positive emotions to the mastery of expertise, Hanin et al. (2016) observe that performance-related emotions are "always either functional or dysfunctional and not limited to pleasant and unpleasant categories" (21).[4]

There is an obvious parallel between this approach and venerable traditions in philosophy that regard the development of emotional responsiveness as part and parcel of the acquisition of virtues. For example, according to Aristotle, acquiring virtue (*areté*) quite generally requires tuning the emotions so as to have them "at the right times, with reference to the right objects, towards the right people, with the right aim, and in the right way" (1984, 21–24). Becoming virtuous in the Aristotelian sense, in any practical endeavor, necessitates attuning one's emotions properly to situations until such responsiveness becomes second nature. In this light we might understand the processes of situated embodied practice that integrate emotional attunement with the training of technical skills in sport as the acquisition of embodied virtues.[5]

Importantly, as with Aristotle's approach to the virtues, when modifying constraints ALD does not seek to discover general rules that apply to everyone but to adjust the patterns and tendencies of response to the developing needs of individual athletes. The training programs are "carefully matched to each individual's intrinsic dynamics, or predispositional behavioural tendencies" (Headrick et al. 2015, 85).

The end product of such training is appropriately "intertwined emotions, cognitions, and actions" (Headrick et al. 2015, 86). Thus, taking ALD seriously requires getting a practical grip on how cognition and emotion "constrain each other interactively" (85). Theoretically speaking, this approach to embodied expertise invites investigating "how emotions might continuously interact with intentions, cognitions, perception and actions" (85).

3 Problems with Intellectualist Accounts of the Emotions

On the assumption that emotions matter to training and performance we might wonder, how do they make a difference? A possible answer could be to think of the emotional aspects and technical intelligence involved in sporting expertise in classical cognitivist terms: interacting as two causally related streams and grounded in a set of orderly transitions of mental states—a set of transitions triggered by characteristic inputs and leading to characteristic outputs.

Classical cognitivist approaches to cognition are intellectualist. They subscribe to rationalism insofar as they think of cognitive processes in representational-cum-computational terms—conceiving of such processes as transitions between nonmental and contentful mental states that take the form of serial or sequential steps: first sensing, then perceiving, then thinking or reasoning, and finally acting.

There are well-known limitations in modeling the intelligence of minds in performance in terms of classic reasoning processes involving the manipulation of structured conceptual representations that express propositions (Sutton et al. 2011; Sutton and McIlwain 2015). Even assuming that such reasoning may be tacit, that style of processing is deemed too slow and rigid to properly account for the dynamically updated, on-the-fly character of intelligent responses.

A related worry about old-school cognitivist approaches is that they fail to accommodate the interactive complexity of cognition because they think of it in overly linear terms. Although there have been attempts to address these issues by proposing theories that build feedback into cognitivist stories in various ways, arguably, such developments are epicyclical patches at best and lack the advantage of making a much more radical overhaul to cognitivist thinking (see Clark 2016). We will explore what adopting a more radical enactive line on the intelligence behind sporting expertise looks like in part 4.

For now, we focus here on the stumbling blocks of providing a classical cognitivist account of the emotions. In this vein, it is clear to see why such an account is sorely needed. For example, Baron-Cohen's confession below about how his account of mindreading fails to say anything about the emotions is indicative of how classical cognitivist accounts have tended to handle the emotions in general. Thus, by swapping "embodied expertise" for "mindreading," we get a sense of the recognized need for a developed classical cognitivist account when thinking about how the emotions might make a difference to the technical mastery of embodied expertise.

> My model of [embodied expertise] says very little about the role of emotion. In part this reflects my view that we are long way from having a good theory of emotion. Clearly, future models of [embodied expertise] will need to give a full account of the role of emotion in this domain, since it is self-evident that human beings are not "cold" computational devices. (Baron-Cohen 1995, 136)

What might such an account look like? Cognitivist theories of emotions understand emotions as contentful states of mind that are directed at specific targets and which essentially involve evaluative appraisal (see, e.g., Nussbaum 2001; Solomon 2003).[6] As evaluative states of mind with specific targets, emotions are inherently intelligent and normative. Cognitivists take them to exist within the rational space of reasons and, as such, regard emotional states of mind as standing in normatively constrained relations to other contentful attitudes.

It follows, according to such theories, that having certain feelings could not suffice for having an emotion, since, as evaluative content is the defining feature of an emotion, it isn't possible to individuate an emotion even by "a unique feeling associated with it" (Gaut 2003, 17).

Nevertheless, there is some latitude in how cognitivists might understand the sort of contentful attitudes that are assumed to constitute emotions. The attitudes might be thought to be explicitly formed propositional attitudes, such as beliefs or judgments. Or they might be thought to be some other kind of pre-reflective, implicit contentful attitudes (for a detailed discussion of this point, see Morag 2016, 31ff.). Either way, emotions are conceived as content-bearing mental states of some kind.

In particular, emotions are thought to be or embed structured propositional attitudes bearing conceptual content—content that makes them, by their very nature, "rationally assessable and reason-sensitive" (Morag 2016, 152). Crucially, emotions are open to revision through reasoning. Indeed, what makes cognitivism about emotions initially attractive is that it satisfies "a deep intuition that emotions are meaningful. They ... inform us about our relationship to the world, they embody our convictions, and they factor intelligibly into our decisions in life" (Prinz 2004, 16).

All the features of cognitivist theories of the emotions just mentioned make it possible to understand emotions along classical cognitivist lines, by supposing that the relevant emotional targeting and appraisals are conducted at the sub-personal level and result "from 'computational' inferences and equally 'computational' reasons" (Morag 2016, 152).

Despite the popularity of cognitivist theories of the emotions in some quarters, there are compelling reasons to doubt their adequacy. A fundamental objection to this entire class of theories is the "emotionality problem" (Morag 2016, 33; see also Clark 2016, 233). Pure cognitivist accounts of the emotions seem woefully incomplete in that they underrate the importance of feelings: it is easy to imagine that types of contentful attitudes that cognitivists assume to be constitutive of emotions might take the form of "cold," "detached," and, wholly, "unemotional" assessments. Thus a much-discussed downside of purely cognitivist accounts of the emotions is that they can't be the whole story about emotions. It follows that "an emotion thus cannot be merely a fittingness judgment.... Something has to be added"; "emotions are not just evaluative judgments" (Morag 2016, 33).

The standard verdict is that cognitivist accounts leave out something essential. They need to supply an extra ingredient; they need to try—as directors like to say—"once more, with feeling." But such accounts lack the resources to account for the phenomenology of emotional responsiveness—the embodied experiences of anger, frustration, or happiness—as anything other than mere accidental afterthoughts or add-ons to cognition. Certainly, as long as one stays within the confines of pure cognitivism there is no easy fix for this problem. For example, as Morag (2016) notes, adding in a care and concern factor won't help if "we regard the care-factor as an additional judgment, [for] then we encounter the same problem of unemotional judgment" (37).

Beyond this, cognitivist theories of emotion take emotions to be evaluative states of mind in a way that entails that emotions are answerable to semantic and rational and social norms—namely, that all emotions are constitutively normative in a strong sense; emotions are taken to have semantic contents that determine what they target, and emotional appraisals are answerable to norms of reason and fittingness. In making these assumptions cognitivism does not merely advance the view that having certain contentful attitudes can influence our emotions but also that having the right kinds of contentful states of mind *is what makes it the case* that we are undergoing a certain emotion on a certain occasion. For example, I may be ashamed of my action only insofar as I believe I have done something wrong; if I come to believe I did not do anything wrong then I will no longer be ashamed.

A major problem for cognitivist approaches that conceive of emotions as constitutively content involving is, as Morag (2016) observes, that they are obliged "to explain where this ... content comes from" (61). Yet, as things stand, we currently lack a credible story about the natural origins of emotional content and norms.

Inspired by cognitivist approaches, some philosophers have sought to answer this challenge and to account for normative structure of emotions in naturalistic terms that suit cognitive science. For example, Hufendiek (2016) has sought to account for the normative dimension of emotions—their inherent semantic, rational, and social norms—by appeal to standards set by biology that fix how things ought to be with regard to the organism's well-being. According to her analysis, the contentful evaluative attitudes that constitute emotions requires "representing things as true or false, appropriate or inappropriate, good or bad, pretty or ugly [and that] presupposes norms with regard to which something is true or false, and so on" (2016, 7). In particular Hufendiek calls on biosemantics to account for the normative dimension of emotions. Thus, for her, various norms emotions are subject to "can be explained by taking emotions to be embodied action-oriented representations" (10). By appeal to biosemantics she aims to show "how a naturalist theory of representation can account for emotions' being subject to rational norms" (94).

Any attempt to account for such norms by appeal to biosemantics is not likely to succeed, since classic biosemantic theories face the crippling problem that there is "a root mismatch between representational error and failure of biological function" (Burge 2010, 301; see also Hutto and Myin 2013, ch. 4; Hutto and Myin 2017, ch. 5).

It might be thought that, if this is so, we need only look elsewhere for the requisite account of emotional contents and norms. But in fact there is no need to provide a strongly normative account of basic characteristics of emotions, since, on close inspection, it turns out they are not subject to semantic, rational, and social norms—at least not in their raw or natural state.

Consider again the claim that having the right kinds of contentful states of mind is what makes it the case that we are undergo a certain emotion on a certain occasion. As the example of shame reveals, our beliefs and emotion are often at least causally linked together. However, sometimes our contentful evaluations of a situation and our emotional responses to it come apart. Consider a case in which you feel insulted by a perceived slight. According to cognitivism, that feeling of emotional upset should only persist as long as you believe that you have been insulted. Yet such feelings can persist, albeit without reason, even after you come to believe that you were not insulted. And that's the rub—for if contentful attitudes and emotions *can ever* come apart then they cannot be constitutively related.

This problem for cognitivist theory has been dubbed the "problem of recalcitrant emotions" (Morag 2016, 38). It shows its face most obviously in cases in which people are subject to particular phobias, prejudices, and implicit biases. But there are plenty of mundane cases too. Our emotions can and do often outlast changes to our relevant contentful evaluative attitudes. Thus Jane's seething anger and feelings of outrage at what she takes to be some transgression of Jill's might not immediately subside, even upon her discovery that Jill is innocent of that of which she is accused. And even if, as a consequence of this discovery, Jane no longer directs her anger at Jill, it need not follow that Jane's anger will entirely or immediately dissipate. Cases like this reveal that Jane's particular contentful attitudes do not constitute her emotional state.

Considerations of this sort reveal that, in essence, emotions "are not reasons in the standard normative sense" (Morag 2016, 57). Emotions are not—at root—rational; they are not inherently tied to deliberation in any constitutive sense. The fact is that certain things set us off in ways we cannot often directly rationally control; this is captured in the idea that we often experience an "upwelling of emotion." In short, "whatever affective processes are, they are not rational processes, that is they are not inferential processes done in reference to norms of fit" (57).

Yet even though emotional episodes are not in essence products of deliberation or under rational control or direction, it does not follow that they should be understood in terms of a "law-like causal mechanism" (Morag 2016, 58). Indeed, we must recognize that different individuals will respond differently to situations, and even that the same individual can respond differently to similar situations such that "people vary in their reactions and may react in different ways on different occasions" (58).

Still, in retreating from intellectualist renderings of the emotions that cast them as essentially involving rational inference, we should beware of going too far in the other direction—of holding that emotion "does not include an activity of evaluation at all" (Morag 2016, 153). In moving away from the intellectualism of cognitivist theories, some have developed an account of the emotions that does not "presuppose intentionality or targeting" (9), but which instead understands emotions as operating "blindly" by means of associative processes that, though not very intelligent, are "not entirely 'dumb'"(154). In contrast we think that emotions can be targeted and thus world-involving, and that emotional appraisals take the form of embodied evaluations that aren't dumb at all, and that it is possible to make sense of these ideas even if emotional intentionality and appraisal are not constituted by any kind of contentful attitude.

4 Radically Enactive Emotions

There is another way to make sense of the basic characteristics of the emotions that is more embodied and enactive. Indeed, the effort to overcome the "emotionality problem" discussed in the previous section has made various somatic feeling theories of the emotions appear attractive down the ages. According to the classic somatic theory, emotions are just feelings of bodily changes as they occur (James 1884; Lange 1885). The basic James-Lange idea has been revamped and updated in the somatic perception theory advocated by Damasio (1994) and others. Accordingly, the original James-Lange idea has been revised to allow for emotions to occur, even without the relevant bodily changes, just in case the relevant brain activity that monitors the bodily changes is present. Hence, on this updated view, "as if" feelings triggered by central processes in the brain suffice for having certain emotions.[7]

Classic somatic and updated somatic-perception theories of emotions overcome the emotionality problem by putting feelings center stage. Yet a problem for both kinds of somatic theories is that they "have little to say about the processes by which external stimuli are evaluated for ecological and social significance" (Hill 2009, 199). Basically, if emotions are reduced to targeting bodily feelings or perceptual states of such emotions, then they would lack the right kind of reach and focus. Prinz (2004) puts his finger on the problem, noting that "emotions promote behavioural responses. We run when we are afraid. If emotions represented bodily changes this would be unintelligible. We should flee when our hearts race" (59).

What this shows is that if emotions are to play an appropriate role in our world-directed activity, we need a good account of the world-directed intentionality of the emotions: how there can be attitudes of "feeling towards" in which the objects of emotions target "a particular thing or person (that pudding, this man), an event or an action (the earthquake, your hitting me) or a state of affairs (my being in an aeroplane)" (Goldie 2000, 17). Consequently, we need to provide an adequate account of the emotions that avoids making a false choice between pure cognitive theories and pure somatic, bodily feeling theories and that supplies an account of "how emotions can be sophisticated cognitive states and, at the same time, have bodily feelings as a major component" (Ratcliffe 2008, 17).

To get this account we must overhaul some deeply entrenched and constraining assumptions; indeed, ultimately, "central to this overhaul is the abandonment of the distinction between cognition and affect" (Ratcliffe 2008, 17). Prinz (2004) takes a major step in the right direction by asking us to conceive of emotions as gut reactions that "use our bodies to tell us how we are faring in the world" (69).

However, a serious drawback of Prinz's (2004) embodied appraisal theory of the emotions—like all cognitivist theories—is its assumption that "to show that emotions are appraisals, one must first establish that they are mental representations" (52). Equally problematic is the fact that Prinz's theory relies on a classical biosemantic theory of content to do its heavy lifting when it comes to explaining how such mental representations get their content. Thus, just like Hufendiek's (2015) embodied theory of the emotions, Prinz's account suffers if it turns out, as appears to be the case, that classical biosemantic theories fail to deliver those promised goods (once again, for developed arguments that biosemantic theories do, in fact, fail in this regard, see Hutto 2012; Hutto and Myin 2013, ch. 4).

The good news is that it is possible to salvage what is promising about embodied appraisal theories by avoiding the crippling problems faced by biosemantic theories of representational content. Going this way requires abandoning the ambition of using such theories to explain semantic contents that introduce conditions of satisfaction into the mix. Instead the basic resources of theories that lay stress on the importance of biological functions provide a way of understanding how minds target specific worldly items without involving or entailing the existence of representational contents per se. Using the basic resources of biosemantic theories for a different purpose, it is possible to explicate the world-directed character of embodied attitudes—namely, their basic intentionality—in a way that does not presuppose the existence of contentful attitudes (Hutto 2008; Hutto and Myin 2017; Hutto and Satne 2015).

A nonrepresentational account of emotional intentionality built along these lines gives us the resources to make sense of the phenomenon of "feeling towards." Goldie (2000) introduced the notion to highlight the way that emotions are both intentional and involve feelings, but he also stressed the need to recognize "an intentional element which is neither belief nor desire, and which is, in many respects more fundamental to emotional experience than either of these" (19).

The capacity for "feeling towards" something is thus a central feature of basic episodes of emotional experience. We can understand this rudimentary kind of intentionality—this feeling towards—by thinking of basic emotional responses as target-directed instead of as inherently content-involving.

In adopting such a view of emotional intentionality, it is natural to move away from the representationalism that defines classical cognitivism in another key respect. Thinking of emotional intentionality as a kind of "feeling towards" along radically enactive lines is to conceive of emotional attitudes as embodied attitudes of whole creatures and not just as contentful properties of inner mental states or vehicles. The intentionality of emotional attitudes is not, by these lights, understood to be a property of some functionally specified and semantically individuated mental state that is internal to emotional beings.

The proposed view of intentionality fits with enactivist views of the emotions and emotional appraisals that make much of the "mounting evidence that the body isn't as dumb as all that" (Howell 2016, 147). As Colombetti (2014) discusses, neuroscientists have discovered that regions of the brain that were once thought to be dedicated solely to emotion, such as the amygdala, are in fact involved in "memory, action tendencies, arousal, and attentional orientation" (99). Contrariwise, brain areas such as the lateral prefrontal cortex that have been traditionally deemed purely cognitive have been "shown to be sensitive to the emotional character of stimuli" (99). Going beyond the brain, affective science "has been confirming that several changes take place in expression, autonomic nervous system activity and muscular tension when people undergo an emotion or are in a specific mood" (Colombetti 2014, xv). This is to adopt a full-bodied approach to the emotions, where the notion of body is a comprehensive notion—that includes the "wetter and bloodier self-regulatory dimensions of embodiment" (15). Enactivist theories of the emotions go further still, focusing on embodied activity that reaches further than the skin and into the world and back again. By enactivist lights, emotions are extensive spatiotemporally dynamic and loopy processes that span brains, bodies, and the world.

As highlighted above, there are reasons to think that the intentionality of basic emotions is neither based in nor entails the existence of contentful attitudes. Consistent with this, radical enactivists hold that the evaluative aspects of basic emotions should not be understood as rooted in contentful mental states that are anything like conceptually grounded judgments. Enactive theories of the emotions accept that "organisms do not merely 'get aroused' in emotional episodes but also evaluate the world and their relationship to it" (Colombetti 2014, 111). Even so, they deny that the evaluations are based in mental representations, holding that embodied emotional evaluations are best understood as embodied organismic activity that is "constitutive of the activity of appraising" (101).

When fearful, a person responds to and treats some target object or situation as if it were dangerous in ways that are manifest in the pattern of their embodied activity—they approach it with caution, avoid it where possible, and so on. Hence, Jessica may respond with fear when tasked with climbing quickly up an ice wall even if she does not form any contentful attitudes at all (e.g., when fearful appraisal takes the form of embodied states such as shaking, sweating, and so forth). Her fearful response to the situation of having to climb an ice wall that she is unprepared to climb can be evaluative in embodied ways even if she does not form any contentful attitudes at all, on any level. Importantly, if embodied evaluations are not contentful attitudes of any kind, then basic emotional modes of responsiveness are not to be understood as already existing in the space of reasons. Still, even so, full-bodied appraisals made on the basis of gut feelings are still appraisals.

Of course, it is also possible for Jessica to respond with fear to the very same situation in ways that are bound up with a range of contentful attitudes—her specific thoughts, beliefs, hopes, and so on.[8] The common denominator in both of these cases is the emotional attitude of fear that is non-contentfully directed at the particular objects and situations, usually with attention focused on specific aspects of the object or situation. It is just that in some cases of emotional responding, one also forms contentful thoughts about the situation in addition to having non-contentful world-involving embodied, emotional responses.

Putting all of this together, the end product of going radically enactive about emotion is that we have all we need to understand the cognitive-emotion package deal we have been looking for. It is possible that emotions pervade the sort of intelligent activity and appraisal that underpins sporting performances. We are now in a better position to understand how seizing opportunities on the playing field, or failing to, can be inherently emotional, especially when the actions in question do not rest on rational inference or decision making but are spontaneously drawn from us in response to particular situations.

5 Integrated Minds in Performance

How might the radically enactive account of the emotions sketched above combine with an account of the intelligence displayed in sporting performances? There is a natural fit with an ecologically dynamic approach to skill development favored by ALD.

Ecological dynamics seeks to combine basic principles of ecological psychology and dynamical systems theory. On the one hand, it draws heavily on ideas central to Gibson's (1979) ecological psychology, assuming that there is a tight fit between animals and their environment and that perception is fundamentally bound up with and is for action. For Gibsonians, perceiving is an active, dynamic process in the service of getting an effective, practical grip on the world. Accordingly, perception takes the form of targeted interactions with aspects of the world, and thus it is extended in both time and space. Notoriously, Gibsonians are adamant that perceiving, so conceived, can be fully explained without the need to posit any intervening inferences or mental representations.

The constraints-led approach augments these core ideas from ecological psychology by calling on unique explanatory resources from dynamical systems theory (Davids, Button, and Bennett 2008; Chow et al. 2011, 2015). Dynamical systems theory is the perfect partner for the Gibsonian conception of perceiving as an embodied activity. This is because it employs differential equations to explain and predict how the states of nonlinear systems evolve over time. It begins by taking stock of a number of variables that describe the state of a system at a particular point in time. It then makes use of its special mathematical tools to chart the trajectory of changes in the states of such systems as they move through a space of possibilities, which is known as a phase space. In the language of dynamical systems theory, nonlinear systems move toward regions that attract them and away from regions that repel them, traversing a landscape known as a topology.

The equations of dynamic systems theory describe the tendencies of such complex systems, including their tendencies for interacting with other such systems. What makes complex, nonlinear systems special is that they are self-organizing—they exhibit an order that is produced and constrained by mutual and reciprocal influence of their components. Yet, crucially, the factors that shape the trajectory of the system do not do so "in the sense of 'instructing' how it should behave or of 'monitoring' its evolution" (Colombetti 2014, 36). Moreover, the effects of such influence are not reliably proportional: "a small (large) change in some variable or family of variables will not necessarily result in a small (large) change in the system" (Rickles, Hawe, and Shiell 2007, 934).

In these key respects, dynamical systems are importantly unlike linear systems. Linear systems can be functionally decomposed and analyzed in terms of their structural parts and respective operations. Functional decomposition of a linear system into the sum of its parts makes it possible to analyze each part separately and thereby to explain and predict how the whole system, taken as the sum of those parts, will behave over time. Since nonlinear, dynamical systems are not amenable to such decomposition, their evolution over time requires the special mathematical techniques described above.

Combining central ideas from ecological psychology with the special mathematical tools of dynamical systems theory (as in Chemero 2009) has opened the way for fruitfully investigating the complex self-organizing responsiveness of learners acquiring skills in embodied activities. From a constraints-led perspective, the processes involved in the mastery of embodied skills can be characterized by a number of interacting variables, and the continuous, temporal, and interdependent changes in their unfolding patterns can be captured by a set of differential equations. Importantly, although it is possible to focus on the dynamics of the parts of complex systems for various purposes, the basic unit of analysis for ecological dynamics is the nonlinearly coupled organism-environment system.

Crucially, from the vantage point of a constraints-led approach, individuals are understood as situated dynamical systems that are open simultaneously to influence and intervention on multiple scales. Training is focused on the self-organizing antics of such dynamical systems, which are always open to reconfigurations enabling them to self-organize quickly and flexibly to the contextual demands (Kelso 1995). Therefore trainers working within this paradigm selectively modify specific bodily, environmental, emotional, and other task constraints—for example, changing the size of playing fields, adjusting distances between players, fatiguing players—to shape and control the emergence of skills and expertise over time.

Skilled performance is explained in terms of embodied activity that involves dynamic processes that span brain, body, and environment. Accordingly, cognitive processes are not, for example, conceived of as mechanisms that exist only inside individuals. Instead they are identified with nothing short of bouts of extensive, embodied activity that take the form of more or less successful organism-environment couplings. Likewise, embodied skills are acquired and emerge as a consequence of a history of interactions between learners and their embedding environments in ontogeny and phylogeny. Through sustained, context-sensitive, active engagements with worldly offerings, organisms are changed so as to be able, in Clark's (2015) apt formulation, to get "a grip on the patterns that matter for the interactions that matter" (5).

Getting a grip on the patterns that matter in skillful performance is not mindless, blind, or automatic; rather it is context-sensitive in ways that reveal it to be "highly disciplined mental activity" (Sutton et al. 2011, 78). Consider that

> an elite cricketer, for example, with less than half a second to execute an ambitious cover drive to a hard ball honing directly in at 140 km/h, draws not only on smoothly-practised stroke-play, but somehow also on experience of playing this fast bowler in these conditions, and on dynamically-updated awareness of the current state of the match and of the opposition's deployments, to thread an elegant shot with extraordinary precision through a slim gap in the field. It's fast enough to be a reflex, yet it is perfectly context-sensitive. (Sutton et al. 2011, 80)

That is all well and good, but there are serious problems with classical cognitivism's vision of the character of this intelligence, construed in terms of symbolic reasoning, as mentioned in passing in part 1. Those problems have driven those seeking to understand what lies at the roots of embodied expertise to ask, "Is there a kind of knowledge that is less like a clunky set of internalised propositions, and that could explain the dynamics of interactive movement in high-speed expert sport?" (Sutton and McIlwain 2015, 100).

Clark (2016) has made significant headway in answering this challenge, showing how the increasingly influential predictive processing accounts of the brain dovetail "perfectly … with work on the embodied mind and environmentally situated mind" (295). In this vein, Clark discusses the role of anticipatory attention in ball sports and how it integrates with and informs the complex, looping interplay of perception and action in embodied performance (65–67).

In tune with constraints-led approaches, the explanation that Clark recommends revives "many ideas explicit in the continuing tradition of J. J. Gibson and ecological psychology" (2016, 246). Consider the now-classic example of how baseball outfielders position themselves in order to catch fly balls. Ecological theorists hold that, rather than making propositionally based predictions involving complex calculations over conceptually structured representations in their heads, it appears that outfielders get where balls are by running so as to keep the trajectories looking reliably straight, and "making moment-by-moment self-corrections that crucially involve the agent's own movements" (Clark 2016, 247). The strategy employed in situated acts of embodied expertise—as in the outfielder case—is to use various sensory channels as "an open conduit allowing environmental magnitudes to exert a constant influence on behaviour" (248). Thus outfielders apparently solve the problem of getting to the right place at the right time—of anticipating where they need to be—by being sensitive to environmental information in ways that enable them to adjust their embodied activity without having to form rich, contentful, inner models of the world.

Returning to the case of the anticipatory expertise exhibited in cricket, it too fits a similar profile. It is well known that despite persistent coaching folklore, experts in fast ball sports—baseball, cricket, table tennis, and squash—do not "keep their eye on the ball." Instead they make predictive saccades that, literally, put them ahead of the game (Mann, Spratford, and Abernethy 2013). Or rather, after comparing the visual-motor performances of elite cricket batters with less-skilled club-level batters, Mann and colleagues discovered that "elite batters directed their gaze ahead of the flight-path of the ball immediately prior to bat-ball contact, whereas the gaze of the club-level batters tended to be behind the ball" (6).

Whereas the saccadic behavior of the non-elite players was less regimented, elite cricket batters, by contrast, were discovered to closely align their head with the location of the ball and use two specialized eye-movement strategies that focused on (1) the location of ball-bounce and (2) the location of bat-ball contact. These combined head- and eye-movement strategies allow the elite players to direct their gaze toward the ball as they hit it so as to "'park' their gaze ahead of the ball so that gaze could 'lie-in-wait' for the ball to arrive" (Mann, Spratford, and Abernethy 2013, 6).

Although the eye movements of the best batter were reported to be initiated only a fifth of a second earlier than the worst batter's, these differences in the embodied profiles displayed by club-level and elite cricketers explain why elite players have more time to respond to information about the ball's movement at the bounce point.

A central feature of the above cases of embodied expertise is that the cognitive tasks are solved in a shared way that exploits a "golden opportunity to spread the problem-solving load between brain, body and world" (Clark 2016, 246). Crucially, adopting this sort of ecological stance on embodied expertise is to understand perception-action couplings in an entirely different way than that of classical cognitivist accounts.

Taking a step away from that tradition, Clark (2016) holds that the big lesson we should take away from Gibson is that sensing is not all about "getting enough information inside ... so as to allow the reasoning system to 'throw away the world' [and] to solve the problem *wholly* internally" (247; emphasis added). Hence, seen by Clark's lights, the coordinated sensorimotor engagement with the environment exhibited in embodied expertise—the self-generated motor activity—acts as a "*complement* to neural information processing" (Clark 2016, 248; emphasis added; see also Lungarella and Sporns 2005, 25).

The sort of story Clark tells about how predictive processing theories of neural activity can be united with enactive and embodied approaches is attractive. It has the right tools for answering the Sutton and McIlwain challenge—namely, the challenge of finding something other than "clunky propositions" to explain the embodied intelligence we deploy in sporting performances.

Yet Clark does not go far enough. His tendency is to intellectualize enactivism. This is most evident from the fact that Clark posits mental representations to play a central role on multiple levels in his predictive processing story (see, e.g., Clark 2016, 39, 47, 291–294). When it comes to explicating the kind of content such mental representations are meant to have, Clark (2016) turns to and relies on Millikan's notion of pushmi-pullyu representations (see 187, and also 133). We won't rehearse, for a third time, why we think this move is unsatisfactory and unnecessary. Suffice it to say, we think that it is possible to provide a nonrepresentational account of predictive processing that makes that story's vision of the anticipatory brain safe for radical enactivists (see Hutto 2015; Hutto and Myin 2017, ch. 3 and ch. 7).

Another unfortunate feature of Clark's (2016) account is his suggestion that information is picked up, acquired, and used by cognitive systems. Thus Clark speaks about "sampling the environment so as to yield reliable information" (64). In discussing the outfielder case he tells us that "information is typically retrieved *just-in-time* for action, in ways that leave the information in the environment *until* just the right moment" (65, emphases added). And, elsewhere again, that action serves to "deliver *fragments of information 'just in time'* for use, and that information guides action, in an ongoing circular embrace. Perception thus construed need not yield a rich, detailed and action-neutral inner model awaiting the services of 'central cognition' to deduce appropriate action" (Clark 2016, 250; emphasis added).

Retaining the idea that any information is literally collected from the world—that information somehow gets inside the perceiver's head and is neurally processed—is a very un-Gibsonian position. Ecological psychology was inspired by an attempt to provide explanatory tools for a nonrepresentationalist cognitive science that breaks faith with these sorts of commitments. It makes central use of the notions of direct perception of environmental affordances in ways that do not assume or require positing inferences involving mental representations or the literal pickup of information.

Van Dijk, Withagen, and Bongers (2015) provide an analysis that reveals that on a Gibsonian account "there need not be any content involved at all, as information for affordances cannot be evaluated as being more or less true or accurately corresponding to an affordance—there are no conditions to satisfy it being about the affordances.... Information can be more or less useful for adapting to the environment, that is all" (213). But if we abandon the problematic idea of informational content (as we should), then we should also steer clear of using the metaphor of brains storing information that is collected from the environment (see Hutto and Myin 2017, ch. 2).

Finally, again showing his cognitivist colors, Clark (2016) everywhere talks of the installation of "learned models" through extended experience, holding that through learning and training we acquire "bodies of knowledge" (68; see also 6, 17, 22, 25, 27, 79). Here too, insisting on taking this extra step of positing inner models and stored knowledge is precisely to wander into territory where metaphysical monsters lie (Hutto 2015; Hutto and Myin 2017)—and taking it is explanatorily unnecessary (see also Kirchhoff 2015). It is better to say that thanks to sustained adaptation and attunement through training we become knowledgeable bodies—we do not acquire bodies of knowledge.

Where Clark (2016) agrees with more full enactive, dynamic views of cognition and emotion is in understanding emotion and cognition as an intertwined package deal. As we have seen, enactive and embodied theories of mind understand cognition to be a spatiotemporally extended phenomenon that "unfolds as the continuous coevolution of acting, perceiving, imagining, feeling and thinking" (Thompson 2007, 43). Likewise, Clark too regards recent work on the James-Lange theory to have added to that story "an important predictive twist" (Clark 2016, 233). And, as Clark sees it, it is the predictive twist that "allows us to combine a core insight of the James-Lange theory (the idea that introspective self-monitoring is a key component in the construction of emotional experience) with a fully integrated account of the role of other factors, such as context and expectation" (235).

In the end, what is on offer is not a disintegrated account of cognition and emotion—not some kind of two-factor theory—but an entangled vision of cognition and emotions that sees them as parts of "a single, highly flexible process [that] fluidly combines top-down predictions with all manner of bottom-up sensory information" (Clark 2016, 235). Contextualized thus, the predictive processing account of emotion belongs "in the same broad camp as the so-called 'enactivist' camps ... that reject any fundamental cognition/emotion divide and that stress continuous reciprocal interactions between brain, body and world" (235).

Viewing the brain as a dynamic anticipatory organ aligns neatly with the claim that intelligent responding and emotionality are integrated. Consider Barrett and Bar's (2009) affective prediction hypothesis. It implies that emotional appraisal of an object's salience or relevance does not take place after object identification or recognition. Instead, affectivity is inherent to visual processing such that to perceive is also to perceive in an affectively charged fashion. For Barrett and Bar, external "sensations do not occur in a vacuum, but in a context of internal sensations from the body," including "sensations from organs, muscles, [and] joints (or 'interoceptive' sensations)" (1325). What this suggests is that perceivers are always affectively attuned when perceiving and acting: emotions are part of the microscale constraints from which macroscale activities emerge, and as such cannot be separated from embodied activity in the world. On this view, then, synergetic self-organization provides a robust link between intelligent responding and emotionality that is in line with a radically enactive understanding of how emotions and technical intelligence come together in embodied expertise in a way that lends theoretical support to ALD.

We can see this coming together in the design of the Battle Zone concept, an example of constraints-led training, developed by Renshaw and colleagues (Renshaw, Chappell, et al. 2010; Renshaw, Jia Yi Chow, et al. 2010). The AIS Cricket Australia Centre of Excellence adopted the Battle Zone as an antidote to the tendency of formal cricket practice to focus on what is called "net practice" as its main way of developing technique (Renshaw, Jia Yi Chow, et al. 181). A criticism of net practice is that it facilitates training situations in which players are not being confronted with situations that are representative of real-time match conditions and scenarios. While players are encouraged to imagine scenarios and make guesses about possible game situations, doing so in relatively artificial circumstances fails to prepare them for the demands of actual game conditions. As Renshaw, Jia Yi Chow, et al. (2010) report, "Nets are failing cricketers in helping them develop decision-making skills and it is no wonder that coaches are critical of the 'game sense' of young players" (181).

The Battle Zone design was proposed to address this problem and to set up training conditions that align closely with match conditions, ensuring not only to increase technical skill levels, but also to constantly challenge players emotionally as well. The Battle Zone enables "realistic practice" and allows for a better transition from skill acquisition to the real game, "creating players who can solve problems via exploration of their own constraints" (Renshaw, Jia Yi Chow, et al. 2010, 182). All the variables of the Battle Zone can be manipulated or intervened upon. For example, bowlers can be moved closer to the batter, increasing tension. Or, more runs can be awarded for hitting balls into selected areas. When appropriately used, the Battle Zone shifts the responsibility back to the learner, improving autonomy and enhancing feelings of competence as they gain "vital experiences that are representative of real match conditions" (Renshaw, Jia Yi Chow, et al. 183).

6 Conclusion

In this chapter we have taken the first steps toward providing an understanding of how emotions and technical intelligence integrate in acts of embodied expertise that underwrite skilled performances in sport. The chapter's theoretical exploration was inspired by important work by sport psychologists who are keen to ensure that emotions are not left out of the equation when training such expertise. Our collaboration shows how practice and theory can be mutually informing in this domain and sets the stage for future research. Our proposed integrated framework paints a picture of embodied expertise that supports new thinking about how to train for emotional attunement in practice—through the cultivation of embodied virtues—and offers a new twist on how to think about the dynamical architecture of our brains, bodies, and the world and the role they each play in making emotionally charged, cognition-in-action possible.

Notes

1. The authors acknowledge that Hutto's and Kirchhoff's contributions to this chapter were supported by the Australian Research Council Discovery Project "Minds in Skilled Performance" (DP170102987). Kirchhoff's work on this chapter was also made possible in part through the support of a grant from the John Templeton Foundation. The opinions expressed in this publication are those of the authors and do not necessarily reflect the views of the ARC or the John Templeton Foundation. We thank an anonymous reviewer for helpful comments on an earlier version of this chapter. Thanks also to Farid Zahnoun for proofreading the final version.

2. Another reason given for keeping emotions under wraps during training is that it is assumed by some that the mastery of expertise in sport is best done by decomposing practice tasks with the aim of reducing overall cognitive load (Headrick et al. 2015, 83).

3. Practically speaking, ALD assumes that "an important question for sport psychologists and coaches concerns how practice programmes can be designed to provide athletes with learning experiences that help them to exploit functional coordination tendencies ... under the affective constraints of sport performance" (Headrick et al. 2015, 84).

4. Hanin et al. (2016) speak of cases in which athletes reported feeling a wide range of emotions, describing their condition as nervous; upset; angry; fearful; tense; frightened; uncertain; confident; excited; wanting to fight; content; calm; and well-focused (see pp. 3 and 4).

5. Asian philosophical traditions have a venerable history of viewing performance and emotional attunement as deeply intertwined. For example, the performative practices of Japanese *dō*, the arts of self-cultivation, build finely attuned emotional responsiveness into training and performance (Ilundáin-Agurruza 2016).

6. So conceived, emotions are "intentional states with conceptual content—evaluative states of mind" (Morag 2016, 152). Gaut (2003) explains how, according to cognitive-evaluative theory, intentionality and evaluation are assumed to be connected: "An emotion … has an intentional object: I am afraid of something. I pity someone. According to the dominant (and I would argue correct) cognitive-evaluative theory of the emotions, an emotion not only has an intentional object, but also *essentially* incorporates an evaluation of that object. So to be afraid of something *essentially* involves evaluating that thing as dangerous; to pity someone *essentially* involves construing her as suffering, [and so on]" (Gaut 2003, 16; emphases added).

7. Clark (2016, 233) reports, "The basic James-Lange story has … been extended and refined in important work such has Critchley (2005), Craig (2002, 2009), Damasio (1999) … and Prinz (2004)."

8. The enactive, embodied responsiveness that constitutes emotional appraisal is rooted in our biological history but it can be educated through training and culture, through participation in various practices. Thus while basic emotional attitudes exhibit intentionality without content, according to a radically enactive view of the emotions, some emotional attitudes can also be content-involving, at least for beings that have mastered certain discursive, narrative practices; namely, for those whose minds have been socioculturally scaffolded in the right kind of ways (Hutto and Satne 2015; Hutto and Myin 2017).

References

Aristotle. 1984. "Nicomachean Ethics." In *The Complete Works of Aristotle*, edited by Jonathan Barnes. Princeton, NJ: Princeton University Press.

Baron-Cohen, Simon. 1995. *Mindblindness*. Cambridge, MA: MIT Press.

Barrett, Louise F., and Moshe Bar. 2009. "See It with Feeling: Affective Predictions during Object Perception." *Philosophical Transactions of the Royal Society of London B: Biological Sciences* 364 (1521): 1325–1334.

Burge, Tyler. 2010. *The Origins of Objectivity*. Oxford: Oxford University Press.

Chemero, Anthony. 2009. *Radical Embodied Cognitive Science*. Cambridge, MA: MIT Press.

Chow, Jia Yi, Keith Davids, Chris Button, and Ian Renshaw. 2015. *Nonlinear Pedagogy in Skill Acquisition: An Introduction*. London: Routledge.

Chow, Jia Yi, Keith Davids, Robert Hristovski, Duarte Araújo, and Pedro Passos. 2011. "Nonlinear Pedagogy: Learning Design for Self-Organizing Neurobiological Systems." *New Ideas in Psychology* 29 (2): 189–200.

Clark, Andy. 2015. "Predicting Peace: The End of the Representation Wars—A Reply to Michael Madary." In *Open MIND* 7(R), edited by T. Metzinger and J. M. Windt, 1–7. Frankfurt am Main: MIND Group. doi:10.15502/9783958570979.

Clark, Andy. 2016. *Surfing Uncertainty: Prediction, Action, and the Embodied Mind.* Oxford: Oxford University Press.

Colombetti, Giovanna. 2014. *The Feeling Body: Affective Science Meets the Enactive Mind.* Cambridge, MA: MIT Press.

Cottyn, Jorge, Dirk De Clercq, Geert Crombez, and Matthieu Lenoir. 2012. "The Interaction of Functional and Dysfunctional Emotions during Balance Beam Performance." *Research Quarterly for Exercise and Sport* 83 (2): 300–307.

Craig, A. D. Bud. 2009. "How Do You Feel—Now? The Anterior Insula and Human Awareness." *Nature Reviews: Neuroscience* 10 (1): 59–70.

Craig, Arthur D. 2002. "How Do You Feel? Interoception: The Sense of the Physiological Condition of the Body." *Nature Reviews: Neuroscience* 3 (8): 655–666.

Damasio, Antonio. 1994. *Descartes' Error.* New York: Harper Collins.

Damasio, Antonio. 1999. *The Feeling of What Happens.* New York: Harcourt Brace.

Davids, Keith, Chris Button, and Simon Bennett. 2008. *Dynamics of Skill Acquisition.* Champaign, IL: Human Kinetics.

Gaut, Berys. 2003. "Reasons, Emotions and Fictions." In *Imagination, Philosophy and the Arts,* edited by Matthew Kieran and Lopes D. McIver, 15–34. London: Routledge.

Gibson, James J. 1979. *The Ecological Approach to Visual Perception.* Boston: Houghton Mifflin.

Goldie, Peter. 2000. *The Emotions: A Philosophical Exploration.* Oxford: Oxford University Press.

Hanin, Yuri L. 2007. "Emotions in Sport: Current Issues and Perspectives." In *Handbook of Sport Psychology*, 3rd ed., edited by G. Tenenbaum and R. C. Eklund, 31–58. Hoboken, NJ: John Wiley and Sons.

Hanin, Yuri, Muza Hanina, Hrvoje Šašek, and Ana Kobilšek. 2016. "Emotion-Centered and Action-Centered Coping in Elite Sport: Task Execution Design Approach." *International Journal of Sports Science and Coaching* 11 (4): 566–588.

Headrick, Jonathon, Ian Renshaw, Keith Davids, Ross A. Pinder, and Duarte Araújo. 2015. "The Dynamics of Expertise Acquisition in Sport: The Role of Affective Learning Design." *Psychology of Sport and Exercise* 16 (January): 83–90.

Hill, Christopher. 2009. *Consciousness.* Cambridge: Cambridge University Press.

Howell, Robert J. 2016. "Extended Virtues and the Boundaries of Persons." *Journal of the American Philosophical Association* 2 (1): 146–163.

Hufendiek, Rebekka. 2016. *Embodied Emotions: A Naturalist Approach to a Normative Phenomenon*. London: Routledge.

Hutto, Daniel D. 2008. *Folk Psychological Narratives: The Sociocultural Basis of Understanding Reasons*. Cambridge, MA: MIT Press.

Hutto, Daniel D. 2012. "Truly Enactive Emotion." *Emotion Review* 4 (2): 176–181.

Hutto, Daniel D. 2015. "REC: Revolution Effected by Clarification." *Topoi: An International Review of Philosophy* (December): 1–15.

Hutto, Daniel D., and Erik Myin. 2013. *Radicalizing Enactivism: Basic Minds without Content*. Cambridge, MA: MIT Press.

Hutto, Daniel D., and Erik Myin. 2017. *Evolving Enactivism: Basic Minds Meet Content*. Cambridge, MA: MIT Press.

Hutto, Daniel D., and Raúl Sánchez-García. 2015. "Choking RECtified: Embodied Expertise beyond Dreyfus." *Phenomenology and the Cognitive Sciences* 14 (2): 309–331.

Hutto, Daniel D., and Glenda Satne. 2015. "The Natural Origins of Content." *Philosophia* 43 (3): 521–536.

Ilundáin-Agurruza, Jesus. 2016. *Holism and the Cultivation of Excellence in Sports and Performance: Skillful Striving*. London: Routledge.

James, William. 1884. "What Is an Emotion?" *Mind: A Quarterly Review of Psychology and Philosophy* 9:188–205.

Kelso, J. A. Scott. 1995. *Dynamic Patterns: The Self-Organization of Brain and Behavior*. Cambridge, MA: MIT Press.

Kirchhoff, Michael D. 2015. "Experiential Fantasies, Prediction, and Enactive Minds." *Journal of Consciousness Studies* 22 (3/4): 68–92.

Lange, Carl Georg. 1885. *Om Sindsbevaegelser; et Psyko-Fysiologisk Studie*. Sweden: Lund.

Lungarella, M., and O. Sporns. 2005. "Information Self-Structuring: Key Principle for Learning and Development." In *Proceedings: The 4th International Conference on Development and Learning*, 25–30.

Mann, David L., Wayne Spratford, and Bruce Abernethy. 2013. "The Head Tracks and Gaze Predicts: How the World's Best Batters Hit a Ball." *PLoS ONE* 8 (3): e58289.

McCarthy, Paul J., Mark S. Allen, and Marc V. Jones. 2013. "Emotions, Cognitive Interference, and Concentration Disruption in Youth Sport." *Journal of Sports Sciences* 31 (5): 505–515.

Morag, Talia. 2016. *Emotion, Imagination, and the Limits of Reason*. London: Routledge.

Newell, Karl M. 1986. "Constraints on the Development of Coordination." In *Motor Development in Children: Aspects of Coordination and Controls*, edited by M. G. Wade and H. T. A. Whiting, 341–361. Amsterdam: Martinus Nijhoff.

Nussbaum, Martha C. 2001. *Upheavals of Thought: The Intelligence of Emotions*. Cambridge: Cambridge University Press.

Prinz, Jesse J. 2004. *Gut Reactions: A Perceptual Theory of Emotion*. New York: Oxford University Press.

Ratcliffe, Matthew. 2008. *Feelings of Being: Phenomenology, Psychiatry and the Sense of Reality*. Oxford: Oxford University Press.

Renshaw, Ian, Greg Chappell, David Fitzgerald, John Davison, and Brian McFadyen. 2010a. "The Battle Zone: Constraint-Led Coaching in Action." In *1 of 1-Conference of Science, Medicine and Coaching in Cricket*, 181. Queensland: Australia.

Renshaw, Ian, Jia Yi Chow, Keith Davids, and John Hammond. 2010. "A Constraints-Led Perspective to Understanding Skill Acquisition and Game Play: A Basis for Integration of Motor Learning Theory and Physical Education Praxis?" *Physical Education and Sport Pedagogy* 15 (2): 117–137.

Rickles, Dean, Penelope Hawe, and Alan Shiell. 2007. "A Simple Guide to Chaos and Complexity." *Journal of Epidemiology and Community Health* 61 (11): 933–937.

Seifert, Ludovic, and Keith Davids. 2012. "Intentions, Perceptions and Actions Constrain Functional Intra- and Inter-Individual Variability in the Acquisition of Expertise in Individual Sports." *Open Sports Sciences Journal* 5 (1): 68–75.

Solomon, Robert C. 2003. "On Emotions as Judgments (1988)." In *Not Passion's Slave: Emotions and Choice*, 92–113. New York: Oxford University Press.

Sutton, John. 2007. "Batting, Habit and Memory: The Embodied Mind and the Nature of Skill." *Sport in Society* 10 (5): 763–786.

Sutton, John, and Doris McIlwain. 2015. "Breadth and Depth of Knowledge in Expert versus Novice Athletes." In *The Routledge Handbook of Sport Expertise*, edited by Damion Farrow and Joe Baker, 95–105. London: Routledge.

Sutton, John, Doris McIlwain, Wayne Christensen, and Andrew Geeves. 2011. "Applying Intelligence to the Reflexes: Embodied Skills and Habits between Dreyfus and Descartes." *Journal of the British Society for Phenomenology* 42 (1): 78–103.

Thompson, Evan. 2007. *Mind in Life: Biology, Phenomenology, and the Sciences of Mind*. Cambridge, MA: Harvard University Press.

Van Dijk, Ludger, Rob Withagen, and Raoul M. Bongers. 2015. "Information without Content: A Gibsonian Reply to Enactivists' Worries." *Cognition* 134 (January): 210–214.

3 Trading Perception and Action for Complex Cognition: Application of Theoretical Principles from Ecological Psychology to the Design of Interventions for Skill Learning

Paula Silva, Adam Kiefer, Michael A. Riley, and Anthony Chemero

> For many actions, we are aware of nothing between the conception and the execution. All sorts of neuromuscular processes come between ... but we know absolutely nothing of them. We think the act, and it is done.
>
> —James, *The Principles of Psychology*, 1890

1 Introduction

A brief observation of an athlete in action readily reveals the seamless flow between intention formation and intention enactment highlighted in the quote above by William James. Consider, as an example, the set of tasks performed by a soccer player in the pursuit of scoring a goal: she moves toward the ball, intercepts it while avoiding the opponent, navigates through the field, passes the ball to an unguarded teammate, navigates closer to the left side of the goal through a gap between defenders, watches the ball as it flies back toward her, jumps up and forward at just the right time, and heads the ball toward the right upper corner of the goal, avoiding the goalkeeper who is jumping leftward. If asked about the play, the athlete would likely be able to identify, in retrospect, the sequence of enacted intentions leading to goal satisfaction. The processes underlying the selection, from indefinitely many choices, of the particular movement solutions that realize these intentions are, in contrast, typically immune to conscious inspection. These processes are among the primary targets of theories of motor behavior. Hypotheses about them, whether explicit and clearly articulated or implicit and unarticulated, drive decision making of managers, trainers, coaches, and clinical sport professionals whose jobs include the challenge of facilitating the development of motor skills to optimize performance and prevent injuries. An articulated theoretical framework is preferred because the explanatory and predictive features of theory should promote the judicious selection of optimal principles for practice and interventions, including the design of training technologies.

In this chapter, we present and discuss the ecological approach to motor behavior, which provides a radically embodied and embedded perspective on the processes that support the flow between intention formation and action execution (Chemero 2009). This approach is contrasted with the more traditional information-processing approach to motor behavior, with two particular aims. The first is to provide evidence that the hypothesized, complex cognitive processes implicated by the latter approach can be greatly simplified, if not fully dismissed, when we consider the constitutive role of perception and action in intention formation and action execution. The second is to demonstrate how this principle (which is the power of an embodied, embedded perspective) can inspire innovative and transformative approaches to skill learning in sport settings and beyond. We do so by elucidating how the different views on the processes supporting motor behavior lead to very different proposals for how to use visual feedback to promote learning of optimal movement execution.[1]

2 Explaining Motor Behavior: What Is the Challenge for Theory?

Skilled motor performance is supported by movement patterns characterized by two related features of movement: effectiveness and efficiency (Guthrie 1952). Movement effectiveness is determined by the extent to which it promotes accurate and consistent achievement of the intended functional outcomes. Movement efficiency is determined by the level of physical and mental effort involved in the achievement of those outcomes. Physical effort has been indexed, for instance, by the energy expenditure or biomechanical stress associated with a movement pattern supporting task performance (Lay et al. 2002; Sparrow et al. 1999; Sparrow and Newell 1998). Mental effort relates to cognitive demands (attention, memory, etc.) involved in movement organization, and has been indexed by the level of performance on a secondary task (Smith and Chamberlin 1992). Any theoretical account of the processes supporting motor behavior must explain how individuals successfully achieve movement solutions for task performance that are both effective and efficient.

The seemingly automatic link between action conception and execution that is a hallmark of our daily experiences does not help us see the complexity of the problem biological movement systems evolved to solve. Bernstein (1967), better perhaps than anyone else before him, envisioned such complexity and, consequently, set specific challenges for theories of motor behavior (Turvey 1990). First and foremost, he drew attention to the fact that any activity, from mundane to highly skilled, involves a very large number of components (neural, muscular, skeletal, etc.) that vary in structure and function and that operate at various temporal and spatial scales. The movement pattern required to effectively and efficiently achieve a desirable functional outcome has to be produced through the organization of these many components that together constitute our action system. Importantly, the number of dimensions that defines the action system implicated in a given task (e.g., the arm for reaching) is much higher than the number of dimensions that defines the task. For example, reaching with the arm for a particular object while placing the hand at a particular orientation yields a task space that is six-dimensional, defined by three spatial dimensions of position and orientation about three spatial axes. The arm, described at the coarse scale of the joints, consists of seven spatial degrees of freedom (rotation about three axes in the shoulder, one in the elbow, two in the wrist, and pronation-supination of the forearm). The implication of this kinematic redundancy is that there are indefinitely many combinations of joint movements and related neuromuscular patterns (hereafter simply "movement solutions") that could be used to realize a particular intention. Put differently, there is a many-to-one mapping between potential movement solutions and functional outcomes. In light of the abundance of choices the movement system can make (Gelfand and Latash 1998), what constrains selection of a particular pattern?

Task performance, particularly in athletic and sport contexts, is embedded in dynamic environments. Reliably achieving intended outcomes (i.e., movement effectiveness) thus implies that contextual conditions must necessarily constrain the processes supporting flexible and adaptive selection of movement solutions. For example, a soccer player intercepting the ball with the head will do so using very different body movements every time depending, for instance, on their position with respect to the ball and to players from the opposing team. Controlled experimental studies have consistently demonstrated this phenomenon in the laboratory: movement solutions displayed by expert performers exhibit context-sensitive variability (Kelso et al. 1984; Steen and Bongers 2011; Wilson et al. 2016). Variability is structured so as to stabilize relevant performance outcomes (Latash 2012; Latash, Scholz, and Schöner 2002), and action organization seems to imply selection of a family of movement solutions, not just a particular one (Latash 2010).

Movement solutions will be efficient in addition to effective if they exploit (and not simply compensate for) forces provided "for free" by the body and task environment. Examples of these forces include the gravitational field and the elastic field of the body created by muscles and connective tissues. Effective gait patterns, for instance, exploit pendular dynamics in a way that optimally conserves potential energy from cycle to cycle (Holt, Fonseca, and LaFiandra 2000; Holt, Hamill, and Andres 1991). Similarly, the mass-spring dynamic characteristic of running patterns optimally exploits the elastic properties of muscles and connective tissues to reduce the need for metabolic energy generation (Farley, Glasheen, and McMahon 1993). The charge of processes supporting movement effectiveness and efficiency is, therefore, to "bend" the force field provided "for free" by the context to generate the overall force structure that is required for successful behavior (Bernstein 1967; Turvey, Fitch, and Tuller 1982). A key question to be answered by theories of motor behavior can, therefore, be formulated as follows: What is the nature of the processes supporting movement effectiveness and efficiency across variable and dynamic contexts?

3 The Information-Processing Approach to Motor Behavior

The information-processing approach to motor behavior maintains logical coherence with the classical view of cognition (Chomsky 1975; Fodor 1975; Pylyshyn 1980) in that it assumes that the processes supporting movement effectiveness and efficiency implement computations over representations. Consider, as an example, theories of motor behavior inspired by engineering control theory principles, such as optimality (Flash and Hogan 1985; Harris and Wolpert 1998; Kawato 1999; Wolpert and Kawato 1998). According to these theories, skilled performance of a particular task is the product of (a) the computation of a family of movement solutions to achieve a *represented* goal state (e.g., the coordinates in space where a soccer ball must be intercepted); (b) selection of the one solution that minimizes a predetermined optimality criterion (e.g., jerk, effort, noise); and (c) execution of the motor plan by the peripheral neuromuscular system. This style of control predicates a purely cognitive planning stage that precedes and is logically independent from the action execution stage (e.g., Glover 2004). As a result, the dynamics of action execution cannot directly inform or shape the planning process.

Representational structures hypothesized to be involved in motor planning have been variously referred to as motor engrams, programs or schemas (Keele 1968; Schmidt 1975), and internal inverse (Kawato, Furukawa, and Suzuki 1987; Shadmehr and Mussa-Ivaldi 1994) and forward models (Kawato 1999). The idea common to these various approaches is that the nervous system drives the movements of body segments during task performance by deploying a largely preconceptualized plan. It does so supported (in the more recent variations on the original motor program theory) by sensory input about contextual conditions. Because processing sensory input takes time, information available for selecting the course of behavior at a given moment is always about something that happened a few milliseconds earlier. To circumvent this problem, more recent theories of motor performance that fall under the information-processing approach conceptualize the brain as a predictive device. Those approaches postulate that the nervous system builds representations of the world and models of the body that are used to continuously generate predictions of what will happen next and parameterize movements accordingly (see, e.g., Jordan and Wolpert 1999). These predictions take the form of sensory states that would be expected to occur in the future (the anticipated future state of the movement system) based on a copy of the motor commands issued to muscles and internalized knowledge about the body and task environment. The course of behavior is proposed to be selected by a neural implementation of an estimator, such as a Kalman filter (Denève, Duhamel, and Pouget 2007; Todorov 2004). The key property of this filter is its ability to combine the estimated future state with (delayed) sensory feedback to provide a basis for computing motor commands that will be appropriately adjusted to upcoming conditions (Denève, Duhamel, and Pouget 2007). The effectiveness of the estimator in predicting changes in context and their consequences for movement outcomes in real time depends on two factors: the fidelity of the representations of the world and the body supporting the predictions, and the accuracy of the (often complex and nonlinear) calculations of the muscular torques required to achieve a desired spatial trajectory. Therefore, the quality of performance depends on the quality of the representations and of the computations over these representations.

In sum, according to the information-processing approach to motor behavior, movement effectiveness and efficiency is achieved by a neural implementation of an inference engine that distills a *future-looking* rule. This rule is a particular sensory-motor transformation (or sensory input–motor output relation) that sustains the desired functional outcome under variations in context. The computational processes generating these inferences can be expected to be quite complex considering (a) the high dimensionality of the action system, (b) the nonlinear and context-dependent relation between a motor command or muscle activation and the resulting movement, and (c) the presupposed ambiguous mapping of sensory input to the contextual conditions that generated them (see Ostry and Feldman 2003, for an extensive critique of internal model approaches). Importantly, the computational processes supporting control of motor behavior proposed by modern information-processing accounts are considerably more flexible in comparison with the processes proposed by the original motor program approach (Keele 1968). Modern accounts do not assume, for example, that all motor behavior is open-loop. The gain in flexibility, however, comes at the cost of greater computational and representational demands. In other words, the gain in flexibility can be attributed to increasing the complexity and sophistication of the cognitive processes proposed to explain successful movement planning (Jordan and Wolpert 1999; Kawato 1999). In the pages that follow, we present an alternative theoretical approach that emphasizes the constitutive role of perception and action in intention formation and action execution. The approach does not require invoking complex cognitive processes and related representational content, and thus stands to offer a more parsimonious account of movement effectiveness and efficiency than the cognitive approaches described thus far.

4 The Ecological Approach to Motor Behavior

The ecological approach to skilled motor performance, proposed by James Gibson (1979) and subsequently developed by others (Lee 1976; Michaels and Carello 1981; Shaw, Kugler, and Kinsella-Shaw 1990; M. T. Turvey and Carello 1986; Michael T. Turvey et al. 1981; Warren Jr. 1998; Warren 2006), stands in sharp contrast to the information-processing approach just described. In particular, the ecological approach attempts to explain the organization of action without resorting to representations or internal models. Two key concepts carry most of the load in meeting this challenge: affordances and information (Fajen et al. 2009).

Affordances are opportunities for action offered by the environment to an individual when certain relevant individual-environment relations are obtained (Michaels and Carello 1981). Therefore, affordances can be considered a source of knowledge, off-loaded onto the environment, about the means to accomplish a task. For the sake of illustration, consider again the set of actions taken by the soccer player described at the beginning of the chapter. The particular choices she made reflect the affordances that emerged and were discovered as she engaged with the dynamic task environment: an opponent struggling to control the ball after a bad pass afforded ball stealing; an unmarked teammate afforded passing the ball as she approached opponents; a gap between opponents afforded moving through to approach the goal; the ball reaching the peak of its trajectory in front of her afforded heading the ball to score a goal. Notice that we listed the affordances in shorthand, that is, without mentioning the characteristics required of the individual for their actualization. For example, a soccer ball arcing through the air affords heading to the goal only to individuals with the ability to jump to a particular height at a particular time. Therefore, an individual's capabilities relative to the environment determine what behaviors are afforded in a particular situation (Kadar and Shaw 2000; Shaw 2001). If affordances can be perceived—which a large body of research suggests is the case (see Fajen et al. 2009)—then it is possible that they support a continuous flow from intention formation to action execution, leading to goal satisfaction.

Perception of affordances requires information about them. Information, in the ecological approach, refers to ambient energy fields (optical, mechanical, acoustic) that are structured by objects and surfaces in the environment and by perceivers' dynamical relations to them created during activity (Gibson 1979). The structure in ambient energy arrays is lawfully determined. For example, the patterning of optical energy available at a point of observation (i.e., the optic array) is not ambiguous; it is specific to a particular relation of the observer to the environmental layout and, therefore, can be reliable information about affordances. The implication is that perception of affordances does not need to be construed—as is needed from a traditional information-processing perspective (Fodor 1975; Knill and Richards 1996; Marr 1982)—as the process of inferring the most likely distal stimulus based on an ambiguous proximal stimulus (e.g., in the case of vision, a distorted, upside-down, two-dimensional retinal image). Instead, perception can be *direct*, meaning that it is based on the detection of information that unambiguously specifies the animal-environment system (Gibson 1966, 1979). If the information available to perceivers is not ambiguous, as has been traditionally assumed, then there is no theoretical motivation for computational and representational processes that are supposed to assign meaning to ambiguous sensory data, and perceivers can be said to be in epistemic contact with the world rather than with a mental representation that stands in place of the world. In this view, neural processes are involved in the active detection of information, but they do not create meaning.

The research program of the ecological approach involves determining what informational variables could regulate behaviors, such as catching, hitting, and locomotion. Again, information is viewed as regulating action directly, in a task-specific manner. Many studies provide empirical support to this idea (Fajen 2005a, 2005b; Fajen et al. 2003; Michaels, Jacobs, and Bongers 2006; Peper et al. 1994; Warren et al. 2001; Zaal and Bootsma 1995). Results of these studies show that movement solutions can be mapped to optical patterns (informational variables) that emerge when an individual engages with a particular task environment. For example, control of forward and backward displacement when catching a ball can be mapped to the acceleration or trajectory of the ball in the visual field—catchers move so as to cancel optical acceleration or to linearize the optical trajectory of the ball; by doing so, they arrive at the right place, at the right time, to catch the ball (Chapman 1968; Oudejans et al. 1996). Action selection can be understood, from this view, as the selection of a set of movement solutions that creates and sustains a desired low-dimensional pattern of stimulation—the pattern of stimulation specifying the animal-environment relation that leads to goal satisfaction.

The power of the ecological approach comes from an understanding of information that both regulates and is generated by the activity of animals. For instance, when an individual navigates toward an object, she controls her locomotion by keeping the optical contour of the object at the center of optical expansion. At the same time, optical expansion is generated by the individual's motion toward the object, and the center of optical expansion changes in a one-to-one manner with changes in locomotor direction. This information, therefore, is about both the individual and her actions and about the environment in which the actions are occurring. Importantly, because the informational patterns available to the actor's perceptual systems are lawfully structured by and specific to the animal-environment interaction, no computation or inference is required to perceive direction of heading or to use information originating in optical outflow to control the direction of locomotion. The information (about direction of heading) must be detected, but heading direction does not need to be computed on the basis of incomplete sensory data. The information is in the optic flow pattern, and is not created in the organism's nervous system (Zhao and Warren 2015).

This example illustrates how when individuals are learning a new skill they actively engage their environments and discover stable relations with it that get the task done. These actor-environment relations, in turn, select and reinforce the movement patterns that created them (Kelso and Fuchs 2016). Importantly, the lawful structuring of stimulus energy by the actor-environment relation implies that individuals can discover how to move to create particular patterns of stimulation, even without any explicit, conscious knowledge of how their movements relate to them.

To summarize, the relations between an individual and the environment supported by information about affordances allow for noncomputational explanations to action organization (see Warren 2006, for a review on noncomputational accounts). Importantly, the individual that is part of such relations can rely on stable aspects of the world (in particular its affordances) to arrive at the right movement solutions that support task performance. It is, therefore, the embedding of an individual in her environment that allows the ecological approach to sidestep the need for complex cognitive processes and related representational content implicated by the information-processing approach.

5 Affordances at Work: An Empirical Illustration

The argument that individuals perceive affordances and use them to organize context-sensitive movement solutions finds support in empirical work (Fajen 2005a, 2005b; Michaels, Jacobs, and Bongers 2006; Wilson et al. 2016). Wilson et al. (2016), for instance, demonstrated that expert throwers perceive the affordance for hitting a target by measuring how their actions changed as the affordance changed. These authors used a task-dynamic approach (Saltzman and Kelso 1987) to define the affordance space. This strategy entails a definition of the task in a way that allows the identification, through simulations, of the set of motor outputs that relate to successful performance. This set constitutes the "functional space" (or affordance) that an individual intending to perform the task must perceive.

Wilson and colleagues (2016) characterized the task of throwing for distance and accuracy as the task of generating a projectile motion that intercepts a particular target. The task-relevant motor outputs in question were a combination of release parameters: release angle, release speed, and release height. The possible combinations of release parameters that result in hitting the target are what the target offers a to-be-thrower (or the affordance of *hitability*). Accordingly, these combinations defined the affordance space for throwing. These combinations were identified in the study in question through simulations of projectile motions. A functional, or affordance, space for throwing was created for each parameter set: a target, placed at a particular distance, orientation, and height, to be hit by a tennis ball undergoing projectile motion. Results showed that movement solutions (here a particular combination of release parameters) of expert throwers consistently fell within the defined affordance space. This finding was not a function of throwers consistently using one particular solution. Manipulations of contextual conditions that shaped the affordance space (target distance and orientation) were associated with changes in movement solutions. The results of this study are consistent with the idea that individuals perceive affordances and control their actions based on them.

The work just described illustrates how affordances can refer to the action system of an individual performing the task and provide resources for action selection. The affordance of throwing resides in a space (a manifold) defined by three functionally relevant parameters of the dynamics of throwing and is defined in intrinsic, action-relevant units that fall directly out of the task-dynamical analysis. Therefore, affordances are properties that can in principle guide both learning and real-time action selection and execution after learning, without resorting to complex computations and representations.

6 Can Affordance-Based Control *Really* Substitute for Complex Cognition?

One might argue that the case of throwing is not strong enough evidence that perception of affordances can substitute for the complex computational processes implicated by the information-processing approach to motor behavior. A better test case would require a "representation hungry" problem (Clark 1997; Clark and Toribio 1994), one that supposedly cannot be solved with only ongoing, available information to perceptual systems. A paradigmatic example of a representation-hungry problem is anticipation of future states. Computational approaches have postulated internal models to explain anticipation (e.g., Miall and Wolpert 1996). However, research shows that there is an alternative to appealing to such computational-representational structures and processes. With the right kind of information, an individual can be coupled to her task environment in a way that supports behavior about forthcoming events without explicit prediction (McBeath, Shaffer, and Kaiser 1995; McLeod and Dienes 1996; Oudejans et al. 1996; Peper et al. 1994; Zhao and Warren 2015). This idea can be illustrated with a paradigmatic example from sports, the outfielder problem: How does the outfielder get to the right place at the right time?

For this particular problem, the ball-in-flight is the relevant aspect of the outfielder's environment. One way for the outfielder to catch the ball is to explicitly compute where and when the ball will land and select the speed and direction of locomotion to arrive at the correct location and time. This requires neural implementation of the equations of parabolic motion and a set of internalized statements of facts about the environment (the size, mass, and shape of the ball, air resistance, initial position and velocity, etc.). The solutions, therefore, resort to very complex cognitive processes of computation over representations, whether the calculations are explicit or implicit. The ecological alternative assumes the use of on-line information that specifies stable relations between the outfielder and the ball in the present that, if sustained, will direct the outfielder to the right place at the right time—in other words, information about ball *catchability* in the immediate future. This information must point to action strategies that result in successful performance. Two candidate information-based strategies have been delineated: run so as to cancel optical acceleration (McLeod and Dienes 1996; Oudejans et al. 1996) and run so as to create a linear optical trajectory (McBeath, Shaffer, and Kaiser 1995). A fly ball affords catching to actors with the set of skills to execute these strategies. Both strategies can be traced back to Chapman's nonanalytic strategy for catching a baseball (Chapman 1968).

The two identified strategies are competing hypotheses. However, they share a feature that is crucial to the argument that information-based control can *really* substitute for complex cognition: the actions of the outfielder trying to catch a ball creates optical information about her relation to the ball. If a particular relation is achieved and sustained, the outfielder will end up at the right place and time to catch the ball. The strategies presented suggest that acting in the present so as to stabilize a particular relation specified by ongoing information (either optical acceleration or optical trajectory) will result in successful ball catching at a future time. No explicit modeling or computation is required. Therefore, complex solutions to problems that seem to require representations might be greatly simplified by capitalizing on regularities that emerge as an individual actively engages with the environment in which she is embedded.

At this juncture, we hope to have provided evidence that explanations in terms of complex computational processes implicated by the information-processing approach can be greatly simplified if we consider the constitutive role of perception and action in intention formation and action execution. We now turn our attention to the implications of this understanding to the design of interventions to promote skill learning.

7 Skill Learning: Traditional Model of Practice

One of the primary tasks of coaches and rehabilitation professionals is to facilitate skill learning. The traditional model of practice to achieve this challenge was developed based on the information-processing approach to motor behavior, and in particular the motor programing theories proposed in the 1960s and 1970s (Keele 1968; Schmidt 1975). The most influential of these theories attributed skilled performance to (a) a generalized motor program whose charge was to specify a general, abstract movement solution to a particular class of tasks, and (b) motor schemas whose charge was to parameterize the solution according to extant conditions (Schmidt 1975). Accordingly, skill learning was defined as the process of acquiring (a) and (b) (Schmidt 1975). Traditional models of practice were, therefore, designed to facilitate this process. In particular, to facilitate acquisition of (a), instructors prescribe and demonstrate an idealized movement solution for the to-be-learned skill. To facilitate acquisition of (b), instructors create opportunities for learners to practice the prescribed movement solution under various task conditions with knowledge of results. This model of practice has been guided by results of research in the area of motor behavior and cognition designed to determine, for instance, the best way to structure practice (e.g., random or blocked) and/or the optimal scheduling for providing knowledge of results (Schmidt 1991; Schmidt and Young 1991). The findings of this research program continue to be applied in sport and rehabilitation settings to promote skill learning (Durham et al. 2009; Porter, Wu, and Partridge 2010). But is this a justifiable approach?

To answer this question, we consider a key feature of such a practice model. It requires an internal focus of attention by the learner. That is, an explicit focus on the prescribed movement form (or body movements). Can this be considered best practice in promoting skill learning?

8 The Evidence: Is There a Case for Promoting Internal Focus of Attention?

The evidence is overwhelming that models of training that promote an internal focus of attention during learning cannot be considered best practice, at least not in the general case. First, motor skills that are acquired explicitly tend to be less resilient if the individual is under either psychological (Beilock and Carr 2001; Gray 2004) or physiological fatigue (Poolton, Masters, and Maxwell 2007). Skills also tend to be less robust when a fast response is required (Turner and Fischler 1993). On the other hand, studies have shown that promoting an external focus of attention results in greater movement effectiveness in a wide range of tasks and contextual conditions (see Wulf 2013; Wulf and Prinz 2001, for reviews). For example, when soccer players were given the instruction to set a goal for the task of dribbling a ball around cones, those who chose a goal requiring an internal focus of attention, such as optimal dribbling technique, performed more slowly than those who set a goal requiring an external focus of attention, such as maintaining the position of the ball in relation to the cones (Jackson, Ashford, and Norsworthy 2006). Promoting an external focus of attention improves not only movement effectiveness but also movement efficiency. Examples include production of greater force magnitudes for a particular level of muscle activation (Wulf and Dufek 2009), greater muscular resistance against fatigue (Porter, Wu, and Partridge 2010), greater speed (Fasoli et al. 2002), and more efficient muscular coordination patterns (Lohse and Sherwood 2011).

The traditional model of practice to promote skill learning cannot be sustained based on the available evidence just reviewed. Training instructions should promote an external attentional focus on relevant components of the task environment and not on body movements. This evidence should inform the development of new, more effective models of practice. The particulars of these new models are not, however, fully determined by the evidence. What is the most effective means to promote an external focus? To answer this question, we must evaluate the available evidence, which requires reference to theory. Particularly relevant in this case are theories of motor behavior such as the ones just described. Different theories might support different interpretations of the evidence, which in turn lead to qualitatively different answers to the question just posed. The consequence is that qualitatively different training strategies may emerge. The effectiveness of new strategies should, of course, be verified by appropriate scientific methods before judicious application can be warranted.

9 Analyzing Evidence through the Prism of Theory: Explaining the Advantage of an External Focus of Attention

Wulf and Prinz (2001) articulated the "constrained action hypothesis" to explain higher gains in movement effectiveness and efficiency with an external focus of attention. Their explanation states that when an individual practices a skill with an internal focus of attention, she explicitly constrains the motor system in ways that disrupt "automatic processing." Directing attention to the effects of the movement in the task environment, in contrast, allows the more automatic and unconscious processes to operate, and performance improves. The conscious and automatic processes described in that hypothesis were not clearly defined, however. If different theories provide different definitions of those processes, then they might lead to very different kinds of learning protocols and different instructions to promote an external focus of attention. This is precisely the case we will illustrate here. Ecological and information-processing approaches to motor behavior have very different views on what this "automatic processing" is. We briefly recap such views and then close the chapter by showing that these different views result in very different ways of using visual feedback as a means to promote skill learning.

The information-processing approach makes a distinction between controlled and automatic processes (Shiffrin and Schneider 1977). Novel or difficult tasks require explicit attention and cognitive control, which taxes working memory, which has long been thought to be limited to approximately seven pieces of information at a time (Miller 1956). Practice can lead multiple pieces of information or motor instructions to be neutrally implemented as a single chunk. For example, learning to drive a car with a manual transmission requires careful attention to a sequence of actions, something like "release gas pedal, while almost simultaneously pressing clutch, then move gear stick, then release clutch, while almost simultaneously pressing gas pedal." After significant practice, this now-automatic sequence of events can become a single chunk "shift," which takes up much less working memory. This provides a possible explanation for the performance deficits caused by an internal focus of attention: focusing on the components of an automatic process can break the chunk into parts, which increases cognitive load and hurts performance (Rosenbaum, Kenny, and Derr 1983; Sakai, Kitaguchi, and Hikosaka 2003).

The ecological approach would equate automatic processing with the (self-ordering) dynamics promoted by the informational coupling of an individual's movements with the relevant aspects of the environment supporting task performance. When learning a new skill, individuals actively engage with their environments and discover stable relations with it that support task performance. These actor-environment relations, specified by simple informational variables, select the movement patterns that created them (Kelso and Fuchs 2016). Therefore, it makes sense that focusing on body movements would disrupt this process, because the information that directs the selection of movement patterns is in the task environment. Consider the case of the outfielder running to catch a fly ball. If she focuses on her body movements, she might not be able to couple her running to the ball's trajectory in a way that will lead her to the right place and time to intercept the ball. An ecological approach to learning would, therefore, naturally lean toward promoting an external focus of attention.[2] In the following section we discuss how the two different views are related to different motor learning strategies by considering different ways of using visual feedback to promote "implicit" learning of biomechanically efficient movement form.

10 Theory-Inspired Strategies to Promote Skill Learning: Providing Implicit "Instructions" through Visual Displays

Teaching proper form during sport maneuvers is the goal of sport coaches and rehabilitation professionals because of the increased risk of injury associated with less efficient movement solutions. For example, increased risk of anterior cruciate ligament (ACL) injury has been associated with employment of kinetic and kinematic patterns that increase stresses to the ACL, such as large amplitudes of knee valgus characterized by inward movement of the knees (Boden et al. 2000; Krosshaug et al. 2007; Olsen et al. 2004). Injury to this ligament has devastating consequences, including limited function, reduced levels of physical activity, and the development of disabling secondary knee conditions such as osteoarthritis (Barenius et al. 2014; Engström et al. 1990; Gottlob and Baker Jr. 2000; Gottlob et al. 1999; Kessler et al. 2008; Lohmander et al. 2004; Myer et al. 2014; Von Porat, Roos, and Roos 2004). Recovering from ACL injury is challenging, despite advances in surgical and rehabilitation techniques. Therefore, prevention is essential. Prevention typically involves efforts to improve movement form to reduce biomechanical risk factors (Hewett, Ford, and Myer 2006; Yoo et al. 2010).

Most interventions designed to facilitate optimal form still promote an internal focus of attention, despite the evidence and perhaps because of lack of other available options. For instance, there are a number of ACL injury prevention programs using explicit instructions regarding desired landing positions by emphasizing proper alignment of the hip, knee, and ankle (Di Stasi, Myer, and Hewett 2013; Myer, Brent, et al. 2008; Myer, Chu, et al. 2008; Myer et al. 2011; Myer et al. 2005; Paterno et al. 2004). More recently, there has been a push for the development of alternative strategies because of the demonstrated negative consequences of an internal focus of attention. Particularly relevant is the reduced resilience of motor skills learned explicitly in the context of higher physiological and psychological stress during competition (Beilock and Carr 2001; Poolton, Masters, and Maxwell 2007). The expectation is that movement form will suffer more in stressful game situations when it has been taught explicitly during practice, which might explain the limited success of prevention programs in reducing the incidence of ACL injury over time (Benjaminse and Otten 2011).

As implicit learning has proven to be effective in improving movement effectiveness (Wulf 2013), researchers in the area of sport medicine have hypothesized that it might also be effective in modifying the biomechanical features of movement that have been related to increased risk of injury (Benjaminse and Otten 2011; Kiefer et al. 2015). The challenging question is how to promote movement solutions that are biomechanically efficient without explicit instruction. Two different strategies, related to the two different theoretical views on the processes supporting action selection, have been proposed to prevent ACL injury and are presented here.

10.1 Information-Processing-Inspired Strategy: Action Imitation through Video Overlay

The information-processing approach to motor behavior espouses the idea that computational processes select and drive the execution of movement solutions for task performance. If this is the case, then learning might be facilitated by training methods that implicitly prime the neural mechanisms that instantiate these processes. There is evidence that the same visuomotor neurons (called mirror neurons) fire when an action is performed and when a similar or identical action is passively observed (Fadiga et al. 1995; Lotze et al. 1999). That is, observation of a particular action activates neural mechanisms involved in producing it. Therefore, action observation might be a good strategy to prime neural circuitries supporting effective and efficient movement solutions for task performance without the need for explicit instructions about the movement solutions themselves.

The empirical findings about neural activation during action observation inspired the proposition of a new general method for prevention of ACL injury that is consistent with the information-processing approach: action imitation through video overlay (Benjaminse et al. 2015; Benjaminse and Otten 2011; Gokeler et al. 2013). Essentially, the learner attempts to imitate a model producing biomechanically ideal movement solutions during training of risky sport maneuvers. To facilitate that, athletes receive visual feedback about the position of their body and that of a model. In particular, the learner sees in a visual display the contour of the model's body ("goal pattern") overlaid with the contour of her own body. The learner quite literally "steps into" a template of a gender- and size-matched model on the screen. The contour of the model works as a target and the only instruction is to replicate the model's movement as closely as possible. Of notice is the fact that learners still have to focus on producing a very complex contour—the visual feedback is as complex as the to-be-acquired pattern. This means that they have to potentially attend to many parameters at the same time. There is evidence that individuals have a hard time correcting more than three movement parameters at a time when employing an internal focus of attention (see review of biofeedback technology by Shull et al. 2014). Therefore, this might limit the success of the approach. The hope, however, is that shifting the learner's attention to the visual display and away from her own body movements will activate neural mechanisms that support the selection and execution of sought-after movement solution. This practice model is built on the assumption that biomechanically efficient movement solutions are embodied in neural mechanisms that can be "awakened" and reinforced through action imitation. The efficacy of this approach in optimizing movement patterns and preventing ACL injury still needs to be tested. In any case, it demonstrates the benefit of analyzing evidence in light of theory for the development and application of new and existing technologies to support skill learning.

10.2 A Strategy Inspired by the Radically Embodied-Embedded Ecological Approach: Augmented Neuromuscular Feedback

According to the ecological approach, expertise follows from our ability to discover movement solutions, in terms of low-dimensional patterns of stimulation that emerge in the context of task performance. Any strategy for learning inspired by the ecological approach, therefore, starts with the assumption that giving explicit, body-focused movement solutions to the learner for a particular task does not help them become experts in it. Instead, practice instructions should provide task-appropriate problems that encourage the learner to discover the solutions. Strategies to improve movement efficiency inspired by the ecological approach will, therefore, necessarily look very different from those inspired by the information-processing approach.

A model of training inspired by the ecological approach should foster skill learning by promoting sensitivity to information about the affordance space that supports task performance. Of relevance for present purposes is the fact that the affordance space for a particular task (e.g., landing from a jump) contains the entire set of movement solutions that leads to successful performance, including the ones that increase the risk of injury. For example, success in landing is determined by the ability to generate force to counteract downward acceleration of the center of mass. This can be done successfully using large magnitudes of trunk lean and knee valgus, despite the fact that these solutions increase stress on the ACL. There is no question that athletes usually are able to successfully perform sport maneuvers. Thus, to prevent ACL injury, attunement to information about their affordance spaces is not sufficient. The challenge is to design a training method to push experts to regions of the space that reduce their risk of exceeding biomechanical tolerance for sustaining an injury.

Augmented neuromuscular feedback (Kiefer et al. 2015) is a strategy, consistent with this logic, that has been conceptualized to promote biomechanically efficient movement patterns. The idea is to create implicit visual feedback during task performance about key biomechanical parameters characterizing safe movement solutions. What these parameters are will depend on the type of task and the type of injury to be prevented. This can be done by coupling the learner's movements to shapes in a visual display and relating the sought-after biomechanically efficient solution to an easily identifiable goal shape. The idea is to artificially create easily detectable information in the environment (e.g., in a visual display) about the portion of the affordance space that should drive action selection and execution. The instructions to the learner are not to simply imitate a pattern. Instead, the instruction identifies a perceptual goal that is simpler than the movement solution, per se: perform the task (squat, jump, etc.) so as to create a simple shape in the stimulus, for instance a rectangle. Biomechanically efficient solutions naturally emerge if learners achieve the goal shape; if they do so repeatedly, over the course of practice through mechanisms of implicit learning, then the learners may develop robust movement patterns that protect them from injury when transfer to the performance environment occurs.

Normally, a given action reliably produces a nonarbitrary perceptual outcome. However, the implementation of the proposed training strategy requires manipulation of the natural action-perception relation in artificial feedback displays. This can be done using motion-capture data, processed in near real time, to generate the display of visual images on a screen or portable augmented-reality display. Using that technological approach, a desired movement pattern—however complex in terms of segmental motion, kinetics, or joint rotations—can be mathematically transformed into a simple visual feedback pattern. Individuals can learn difficult movements in terms of the simplified visual pattern. In other words, they can implicitly discover the sought-after biomechanically efficient movement solutions through their attempts to create the desired, low-dimensional visual feedback. The required knowledge is "off-loaded" to the visual display. That is a prime example of how perception and action can substitute for complex cognition.

The power of the proposed approach to prevent ACL injury is gained through the abstract relation between movement patterns and visual feedback. Pointedly, the visual display does not showcase the to-be-acquired movement patterns themselves. By capturing the high-dimensional patterns in a perceptually available low-dimensional shape, the proposed augmented neuromuscular feedback has the potential to truly simplify movement control. This approach finds support in research showing that extremely difficult patterns can be learned if they are tied to simple perceptual outcomes. For example, it is nearly impossible to perform 4:3 bimanual coordination (the right hand completes four cycles of a circular movement while the left hand completes three cycles at the same time) while subjects view their hand movements directly. Yet this pattern is easily achieved when subjects cannot see their hands and instead are tasked with controlling the motion of two virtual feedback dots. Crucially, each dot is tied to the motion of one hand, but the dots' movements are mathematically transformed so that a successful 4:3 hand pattern makes the dots appear to move synchronously in a 1:1, phase- and frequency-locked pattern (Mechsner et al. 2001). When subjects in that protocol are instructed to move their hands to externally focus on the coordination of the dots in a 1:1 pattern in the display instead of internally focus on their actual hand movements, a previously nearly impossible 4:3 movement pattern becomes relatively easy to master. In this case, the movement was learned implicitly using "knowledge" off-loaded to the task environment (Brenner and Smeets 2011; Shea et al. 2001). This type of motor learning is fast, robust, may improve retention, and leads to excellent transfer as demonstrated in prior studies employing this feedback principle (Fernandez and Bootsma 2008; Fowler and Turvey 1978; Kovacs, Buchanan, and Shea 2008; Kovacs, Buchanan, and Shea 2009; Mechsner 2004; Pawlak and Vicente 1996; Wang et al. 2013).

That the motor learning benefits of mapping movement variables onto simple feedback extend to learning complex, whole-body, closed-chain movement tasks is well supported (cf. Faugloire et al. 2005; Varoqui et al. 2011). In the experiment of Faulgoire and colleagues, subjects were tasked with in-phase or 180° anti-phase coordination of rhythmic rotations of the lower leg and trunk about the ankle and hip joints, respectively. Rather than being instructed explicitly to perform those coordination patterns, subjects were simply instructed to view a real-time feedback display and move the body so as to create either a circle or downward-sloping line. The feedback was, unbeknownst to subjects, an angle-angle diagram (ankle vs. hip joint rotations). In the joint angle space, a circle corresponded to in-phase and a diagonal line to anti-phase coordination. Subjects quickly learned to produce ankle-hip coordination patterns by an external attentional focus on "controlling" the desired shapes in the feedback display. Those who had this feedback available produced more stable postural coordination faster than those who did not. Moreover, when stroke patients performed this task as a balance intervention they showed long-lasting improvements in balance performance (Varoqui et al. 2011).

The proposed augmented neuromuscular feedback utilizes well-established visual feedback strategies to promote efficient, rapid, and robust learning of complex movements. However, the effectiveness of this form of training in promoting biomechanically efficient movement solutions and injury prevention also requires empirical support. Studies are under way to test it. The description of the training strategy is sufficient to indicate that analyzing evidence through the prism of a radically embodied, embedded account to motor behavior can lead to innovative and potentially transformative models of practice to promote skill learning. Augmented neuromuscular feedback is but one example. The key to transformative practice, in our view, is in the logic behind it: capitalizing on information revealed as an individual engages with her task environment to promote emergence of effective and efficient movement solutions.

11 Conclusion

There is no question that the design of new strategies to promote skill learning should be based on available empirical evidence. Less obvious is the idea presented above that advancing new models of practice and the development, or leveraging, of technology to support it could greatly benefit from analyses of empirical evidence in the light of theory. There are at least two benefits of explicitly tying the new training strategies proposed to theory. First, it promotes a rational, logical process for deriving new hypotheses from available evidence that has a greater chance to promote truly innovative and transformative interventions than does commonsense thinking or coaching lore. Second, scientific studies designed to test the effects of new forms of interventions on skill learning can provide an empirical basis that concurrently informs practice and furthers the theoretical understanding of motor behavior and learning. As this understanding develops, new propositions arise, and this cyclical process allows for more effective cross-fertilization between theory and practice.

In this chapter, two qualitatively different strategies were proposed to promote learning of biomechanically efficient movement solutions with the overarching goal of preventing ACL rupture, a serious sport injury. These strategies were derived from the analysis of the same empirical evidence (the benefit of an external focus of attention) through the prism of two different theoretical views on the processes supporting action selection. The prism provided by the information-processing approach led to a method of training aimed at priming the complex brain mechanisms involved in the production of the desired movement solutions: action imitation using video overlay. The idea of imitating a model is not new. The innovation refers to how the new technology allows the learner to shift her focus of attention to a visual display in the task environment and away from her own body movements, which is expected to facilitate learning. The prism provided by the ecological approach led to a method that encapsulates the sought-after movement solutions onto simple perceptual forms projected onto the task environment, trading perception and action for complex cognition. By focusing on creating and sustaining simple forms on a visual display, learners can implicitly discover and produce biomechanically efficient movement solutions without any explicit knowledge about the mapping between visual feedback and body movements. The training method promoted by the ecological approach is innovative in all of its aspects, from the logic behind it to the technology involved. If the effectiveness of this training in preventing ACL injury is verified by appropriate scientific studies, it can truly transform models of practice in the field of sport medicine.

Notes

1. In this chapter, we contrast an ecological approach to motor behavior with an information-processing approach. Another contrast, one we do not make here, could be drawn between ecological and enactive approaches. The relationship between these two approaches is one of great current interest. One of us has written about this in the past (Chemero 2009, 2012). We know of two conferences that were devoted to this relationship in 2016 alone ("Moving Cognition beyond Its Basic Ecology," University of Antwerp, May 2016; "Pluralism in the Cognitive Sciences," University College Dublin, June 2016). We cannot settle the issue in this chapter. That said, we think that although the philosophical commitments of the ecological and enactive approaches are quite different, their relationships to scientific practice and data are very similar. That is, although there are disagreements, they are "merely philosophical." We believe that enactive movement scientists will endorse the models and interventions we discuss in what follows.

2. Note that this is an example of the philosophical differences between the enactive and ecological approaches. Enactive theorists tend toward an idealist metaphysics, which could make them uncomfortable with the distinction between internal focus of attention and external focus of attention (e.g., Thompson 2007). Ecological theorists embrace a realist metaphysics and do not feel this discomfort. This is a genuine philosophical disagreement. That said, enactivists should be just as unhappy with what we (following the jargon of the literature) call "internal focus of attention" as we are, and should prefer what we (again, following the motor control literature) call "external focus of attention," even if they do not like these terms.

References

Barenius, Björn, Sari Ponzer, Adel Shalabi, Robert Bujak, Louise Norlén, and Karl Eriksson. 2014. "Increased Risk of Osteoarthritis after Anterior Cruciate Ligament Reconstruction: A 14-Year Follow-up Study of a Randomized Controlled Trial." *American Journal of Sports Medicine* 42 (5): 1049–1057.

Beilock, Sian L., and Thomas H. Carr. 2001. "On the Fragility of Skilled Performance: What Governs Choking under Pressure?" *Journal of Experimental Psychology: General* 130 (4): 701–725.

Benjaminse, Anne, Alli Gokeler, Ariel V. Dowling, Avery Faigenbaum, Kevin R. Ford, Timothy E. Hewett, James A. Onate, Bert Otten, and Gregory D. Myer. 2015. "Optimization of the Anterior Cruciate Ligament Injury Prevention Paradigm: Novel Feedback Techniques to Enhance Motor Learning and Reduce Injury Risk." *Journal of Orthopaedic and Sports Physical Therapy* 45 (3): 170–182.

Benjaminse, Anne, and Egbert Otten. 2011. "ACL Injury Prevention, More Effective with a Different Way of Motor Learning?" *Knee Surgery, Sports Traumatology, Arthroscopy* 19 (4): 622–627.

Bernstein, Nicholai A. 1967. *The Co-Ordination and Regulation of Movements*. London: Pergamon.

Boden, Barry P., G. Scott Dean, John A. Feagin Jr., and William E. Garrett Jr. 2000. "Mechanisms of Anterior Cruciate Ligament Injury." *Orthopedics* 23 (6): 573–578.

Brenner, Eli, and Jeroen B. J. Smeets. 2011. "Quickly 'Learning' to Move Optimally." *Experimental Brain Research* 213 (1): 153–161.

Chapman, Seville. 1968. "Catching a Baseball." *American Journal of Physics* 36 (10): 868–870.

Chemero, Anthony. 2009. *Radical Embodied Cognitive Science*. Cambridge, MA: MIT Press.

Chemero, Anthony. 2012. "Modeling Self-Organization with Nonwellfounded Set Theory." *Ecological Psychology* 24 (1): 46–59.

Chomsky, Noam. 1975. *Reflections on Language*. New York: Pantheon Books.

Clark, Andy. 1997. "The Dynamical Challenge." *Cognitive Science* 21 (4): 461–481.

Clark, Andy, and Josefa Toribio. 1994. "Doing without Representing?" *Synthese* 101 (3): 401–431.

Denève, Sophie, Jean-René Duhamel, and Alexandre Pouget. 2007. "Optimal Sensorimotor Integration in Recurrent Cortical Networks: A Neural Implementation of Kalman Filters." *Journal of Neuroscience* 27 (21): 5744–5756.

Di Stasi, Stephanie, Gregory D. Myer, and Timothy E. Hewett. 2013. "Neuromuscular Training to Target Deficits Associated with Second Anterior Cruciate Ligament Injury." *Journal of Orthopaedic and Sports Physical Therapy* 43 (11): 777–792, A1–11.

Durham, Katherine, Paulette M. Van Vliet, Frances Badger, and Catherine Sackley. 2009. "Use of Information Feedback and Attentional Focus of Feedback in Treating the Person with a Hemiplegic Arm." *Physiotherapy Research International* 14 (2): 77–90.

Engström, B., M. Forssblad, C. Johansson, and H. Törnkvist. 1990. "Does a Major Knee Injury Definitely Sideline an Elite Soccer Player?" *American Journal of Sports Medicine* 18 (1): 101–105.

Fadiga, Luciano, Leonardo Fogassi, Giovanni Pavesi, and Giacomo Rizzolatti. 1995. "Motor Facilitation during Action Observation: A Magnetic Stimulation Study." *Journal of Neurophysiology* 73 (6): 2608–2611.

Fajen, Brett R. 2005a. "Calibration, Information, and Control Strategies for Braking to Avoid a Collision." *Journal of Experimental Psychology: Human Perception and Performance* 31 (3): 480–501.

Fajen, Brett R. 2005b. "The Scaling of Information to Action in Visually Guided Braking." *Journal of Experimental Psychology: Human Perception and Performance* 31 (5): 1107–1123.

Fajen, Brett R., Michael A. Riley, and Michael T. Turvey. 2009. "Information, Affordances, and the Control of Action in Sport." *International Journal of Sport Psychology* 40 (1): 79–107.

Fajen, Brett R., William H. Warren, Selim Temizer, and Leslie Pack Kaelbling. 2003. "A Dynamical Model of Visually-Guided Steering, Obstacle Avoidance, and Route Selection." *International Journal of Computer Vision* 54 (1–3): 13–34.

Farley, C. T., J. Glasheen, and T. A. McMahon. 1993. "Running Springs: Speed and Animal Size." *Journal of Experimental Biology* 185 (December): 71–86.

Fasoli, Susan E., Catherine A. Trombly, Linda Tickle-Degnen, and Mieke H. Verfaellie. 2002. "Effect of Instructions on Functional Reach in Persons with and without Cerebrovascular Accident." *The American Journal of Occupational Therapy* 56 (4): 380–390.

Faugloire, Elise, Benoît G. Bardy, Omar Merhi, and Thomas A. Stoffregen. 2005. "Exploring Coordination Dynamics of the Postural System with Real-Time Visual Feedback." *Neuroscience Letters* 374 (2): 136–141.

Fernandez, Laure, and Reinoud J. Bootsma. 2008. "Non-Linear Gaining in Precision Aiming: Making Fitts' Task a Bit Easier." *Acta Psychologica* 129 (2): 217–227.

Flash, T., and N. Hogan. 1985. "The Coordination of Arm Movements: An Experimentally Confirmed Mathematical Model." *Journal of Neuroscience* 5 (7): 1688–1703.

Fodor, Jerry A. 1975. *The Language of Thought*. Cambridge, MA: Harvard University Press.

Fowler, Carol A., and Michael T. Turvey. 1978. "Skill Acquisition: An Event Approach with Special Reference to Searching for the Optimum of a Function of Several Variables." In *Information Processing in Motor Control and Learning*, edited by George E. Stelmach, 1–40. New York: Academic Press.

Gelfand, Israel M., and Mark L. Latash. 1998. "On the Problem of Adequate Language in Motor Control." *Motor Control* 2 (4): 306–313.

Gibson, James Jerome. 1966. *The Senses Considered as Perceptual Systems*. Boston: Houghton Mifflin.

Gibson, James Jerome. 1979. *The Ecological Approach to Visual Perception*. Boston: Houghton Mifflin

Glover, Scott. 2004. "Separate Visual Representations in the Planning and Control of Action." *Behavioral and Brain Sciences* 27 (1): 3–24; discussion 24–78.

Gokeler, Alli, Anne Benjaminse, Timothy E. Hewett, Mark V. Paterno, Kevin R. Ford, Egbert Otten, and Gregory D. Myer. 2013. "Feedback Techniques to Target Functional Deficits Following Anterior Cruciate Ligament Reconstruction: Implications for Motor Control and Reduction of Second Injury Risk." *Sports Medicine* 43 (11): 1065–1074.

Gottlob, C. A., and C. L. Baker Jr. 2000. "Anterior Cruciate Ligament Reconstruction: Socioeconomic Issues and Cost Effectiveness." *American Journal of Orthopedics* 29 (6): 472–476.

Gottlob, Charles A., Champ L. Baker Jr., James M. Pellissier, and Lisa Colvin. 1999. "Cost Effectiveness of Anterior Cruciate Ligament Reconstruction in Young Adults." *Clinical Orthopaedics and Related Research* 367 (October): 272–282.

Gray, Rob. 2004. "Attending to the Execution of a Complex Sensorimotor Skill: Expertise Differences, Choking, and Slumps." *Journal of Experimental Psychology: Applied* 10 (1): 42–54.

Guthrie, E. R. 1952. *The Psychology of Learning*. Rev. ed. New York: Harper and Row.

Harris, C. M., and D. M. Wolpert. 1998. "Signal-Dependent Noise Determines Motor Planning." *Nature* 394 (6695): 780–784.

Hewett, Timothy E., Kevin R. Ford, and Gregory D. Myer. 2006. "Anterior Cruciate Ligament Injuries in Female Athletes: Part 2, a Meta-Analysis of Neuromuscular Interventions Aimed at Injury Prevention." *American Journal of Sports Medicine* 34 (3): 490–498.

Holt, Kenneth G., Sergio T. Fonseca, and Michael E. LaFiandra. 2000. "The Dynamics of Gait in Children with Spastic Hemiplegic Cerebral Palsy: Theoretical and Clinical Implications." *Human Movement Science* 19 (3): 375–405.

Holt, Kenneth G., Joseph Hamill, and Robert O. Andres. 1991. "Predicting the Minimal Energy Costs of Human Walking." *Medicine and Science in Sports and Exercise* 23 (4): 491–498.

Jackson, Robin C., Kelly J. Ashford, and Glen Norsworthy. 2006. "Attentional Focus, Dispositional Reinvestment, and Skilled Motor Performance under Pressure." *Journal of Sport and Exercise Psychology* 28 (1): 49–68.

James, William. 1890. *The Principles of Psychology*, Vol. 2. New York: Holt.

Jordan, Michael I., and Daniel M. Wolpert. 1999. "Computational Motor Control." In *The Cognitive Neurosciences*, edited by Michael S. Gazzaniga, 601–620. Cambridge, MA: MIT Press.

Kadar, Endre E., and Robert E. Shaw. 2000. "Toward an Ecological Field Theory of Perceptual Control of Locomotion." *Ecological Psychology* 12 (2): 141–180.

Kawato, M. 1999. "Internal Models for Motor Control and Trajectory Planning." *Current Opinion in Neurobiology* 9 (6): 718–727.

Kawato, M., K. Furukawa, and R. Suzuki. 1987. "A Hierarchical Neural-Network Model for Control and Learning of Voluntary Movement." *Biological Cybernetics* 57 (3): 169–185.

Keele, Steven W. 1968. "Movement Control in Skilled Motor Performance." *Psychological Bulletin* 70 (6 Pt 1): 387–403.

Kelso, J. A. Scott, and Armin Fuchs. 2016. "The Coordination Dynamics of Mobile Conjugate Reinforcement." *Biological Cybernetics* 110 (1): 41–53.

Kelso, J. Scott, Betty Tuller, E. Vatikiotis-Bateson, and Carol A. Fowler. 1984. "Functionally Specific Articulatory Cooperation Following Jaw Perturbations during Speech: Evidence for Coordinative Structures." *Journal of Experimental Psychology: Human Perception and Performance* 10 (6): 812–832.

Kessler, M. A., H. Behrend, S. Henz, G. Stutz, A. Rukavina, and M. S. Kuster. 2008. "Function, Osteoarthritis and Activity after ACL-Rupture: 11 Years Follow-up Results of Conservative versus Reconstructive Treatment." *Knee Surgery, Sports Traumatology, Arthroscopy* 16 (5): 442–448.

Kiefer, Adam W., Adam M. Kushner, John Groene, Christopher Williams, Michael A. Riley, and Gregory D. Myer. 2015. "A Commentary on Real-Time Biofeedback to Augment Neuromuscular

Training for ACL Injury Prevention in Adolescent Athletes." *Journal of Sports Science and Medicine* 14 (1): 1–8.

Knill, David C., and Whitman Richards. 1996. *Perception as Bayesian Inference*. Cambridge: Cambridge University Press.

Kovacs, A. J., J. J. Buchanan, and C. H. Shea. 2008. "Perceptual Influences on Fitts' Law." *Experimental Brain Research* 190 (1): 99–103.

Kovacs, Attila J., John J. Buchanan, and Charles H. Shea. 2009. "Bimanual 1:1 with 90° Continuous Relative Phase: Difficult or Easy!" *Experimental Brain Research* 193 (1): 129–136.

Krosshaug, Tron, Atsuo Nakamae, Barry P. Boden, Lars Engebretsen, Gerald Smith, James R. Slauterbeck, Timothy E. Hewett, and Roald Bahr. 2007. "Mechanisms of Anterior Cruciate Ligament Injury in Basketball: Video Analysis of 39 Cases." *American Journal of Sports Medicine* 35 (3): 359–367.

Latash, Mark. 2010. "Motor Control: In Search of Physics of the Living Systems." *Journal of Human Kinetics* 24:7–18.

Latash, Mark L. 2012. "The Bliss (Not the Problem) of Motor Abundance (Not Redundancy)." *Experimental Brain Research* 217 (1): 1–5.

Latash, Mark L., John P. Scholz, and Gregor Schöner. 2002. "Motor Control Strategies Revealed in the Structure of Motor Variability." *Exercise and Sport Sciences Reviews* 30 (1): 26–31.

Lay, Brendan. S., William A. Sparrow, K. M. Hughes, and Nicholas J. O'Dwyer. 2002. "Practice Effects on Coordination and Control, Metabolic Energy Expenditure, and Muscle Activation." *Human Movement Science* 21 (5/6): 807–830.

Lee, David N. 1976. "A Theory of Visual Control of Braking Based on Information about Time-to-Collision." *Perception* 5 (4): 437–459.

Lohmander, L. S., A. Ostenberg, M. Englund, and H. Roos. 2004. "High Prevalence of Knee Osteoarthritis, Pain, and Functional Limitations in Female Soccer Players Twelve Years after Anterior Cruciate Ligament Injury." *Arthritis and Rheumatism* 50 (10): 3145–3152.

Lohse, Keith R., and David E. Sherwood. 2011. "Defining the Focus of Attention: Effects of Attention on Perceived Exertion and Fatigue." *Frontiers in Psychology* 2 (November): 332.

Lotze, Martin, Pedro Montoya, Michael Erb, Ernst Hülsmann, Herta Flor, Uwe Klose, Niels Birbaumer, and Wolfgang Grodd. 1999. "Activation of Cortical and Cerebellar Motor Areas during Executed and Imagined Hand Movements: An fMRI Study." *Journal of Cognitive Neuroscience* 11 (5): 491–501.

Marr, D. 1982. "Vision." In *Vision: A Computational Investigation into the Human Representation and Processing of Visual Information*, 41–98. New York: W. H. Freeman.

McBeath, Michael K., Dennis M. Shaffer, and Mary K. Kaiser. 1995. "How Baseball Outfielders Determine Where to Run to Catch Fly Balls." *Science* 268 (5210): 569–573.

McLeod, Peter, and Zoltan Dienes. 1996. "Do Fielders Know Where to Go to Catch the Ball or Only How to Get There?" *Journal of Experimental Psychology: Human Perception and Performance* 22 (3): 531–543.

Mechsner, Franz. 2004. "A Psychological Approach to Human Voluntary Movements." *Journal of Motor Behavior* 36 (4): 355–370.

Mechsner, Franz, Dirk Kerzel, Günther Knoblich, and Wolfgang Prinz. 2001. "Perceptual Basis of Bimanual Coordination." *Nature* 414 (6859): 69–73.

Miall, R. Christopher, and Daniel M. Wolpert. 1996. "Forward Models for Physiological Motor Control." *Neural Networks* 9 (8): 1265–1279.

Michaels, Claire F., and Claudia Carello. 1981. *Direct Perception*. Englewood Cliffs, NJ: Prentice-Hall.

Michaels, Claire F., David M. Jacobs, and Raoul M. Bongers. 2006. "Lateral Interception II: Predicting Hand Movements." *Journal of Experimental Psychology: Human Perception and Performance* 32 (2): 459–472.

Miller, G. A. 1956. "The Magical Number Seven Plus or Minus Two: Some Limits on Our Capacity for Processing Information." *Psychological Review* 63 (2): 81–97.

Myer, Gregory D., Jensen L. Brent, Kevin R. Ford, and Timothy E. Hewett. 2008. "A Pilot Study to Determine the Effect of Trunk and Hip Focused Neuromuscular Training on Hip and Knee Isokinetic Strength." *British Journal of Sports Medicine* 42 (7): 614–619.

Myer, Gregory D., Jensen L. Brent, Kevin R. Ford, and Timothy E. Hewett. 2011. "Real-Time Assessment and Neuromuscular Training Feedback Techniques to Prevent ACL Injury in Female Athletes." *Strength and Conditioning Journal* 33 (3): 21–35.

Myer, Gregory D., Donald A. Chu, Jensen L. Brent, and Timothy E. Hewett. 2008. "Trunk and Hip Control Neuromuscular Training for the Prevention of Knee Joint Injury." *Clinics in Sports Medicine* 27 (3): 425–448.

Myer, Gregory D., Avery D. Faigenbaum, Kim Barber Foss, Yingying Xu, Jane Khoury, Lawrence M. Dolan, Teri M. McCambridge, and Timothy E. Hewett. 2014. "Injury Initiates Unfavourable Weight Gain and Obesity Markers in Youth." *British Journal of Sports Medicine* 48 (20): 1477–1481.

Myer, Gregory D., Kevin R. Ford, Joseph P. Palumbo, and Timothy E. Hewett. 2005. "Neuromuscular Training Improves Performance and Lower-Extremity Biomechanics in Female Athletes." *Journal of Strength and Conditioning Research* 19 (1): 51–60.

Olsen, Odd-Egil, Grethe Myklebust, Lars Engebretsen, and Roald Bahr. 2004. "Injury Mechanisms for Anterior Cruciate Ligament Injuries in Team Handball: A Systematic Video Analysis." *American Journal of Sports Medicine* 32 (4): 1002–1012.

Ostry, David J., and Anatol G. Feldman. 2003. "A Critical Evaluation of the Force Control Hypothesis in Motor Control." *Experimental Brain Research* 153 (3): 275–288.

Oudejans, R. R., C. F. Michaels, F. C. Bakker, and M. A. Dolné. 1996. "The Relevance of Action in Perceiving Affordances: Perception of Catchableness of Fly Balls." *Journal of Experimental Psychology: Human Perception and Performance* 22 (4): 879–891.

Paterno, Mark V., Gregory D. Myer, Kevin R. Ford, and Timothy E. Hewett. 2004. "Neuromuscular Training Improves Single-Limb Stability in Young Female Athletes." *Journal of Orthopaedic and Sports Physical Therapy* 34 (6): 305–316.

Pawlak, William S., and Kim J. Vicente. 1996. "Inducing Effective Operator Control through Ecological Interface Design." *International Journal of Human-Computer Studies* 44 (5): 653–688.

Peper, L., R. J. Bootsma, D. R. Mestre, and F. C. Bakker. 1994. "Catching Balls: How to Get the Hand to the Right Place at the Right Time." *Journal of Experimental Psychology: Human Perception and Performance* 20 (3): 591–612.

Poolton, Jamie M., Richard S. W. Masters, and Jonathan P. Maxwell. 2007. "Passing Thoughts on the Evolutionary Stability of Implicit Motor Behaviour: Performance Retention under Physiological Fatigue." *Consciousness and Cognition* 16 (2): 456–468.

Porter, Jared, Will Wu, and Julie Partridge. 2010. "Focus of Attention and Verbal Instructions: Strategies of Elite Track and Field Coaches and Athletes." *Sport Science Review* 19 (3/4): 77–89.

Pylyshyn, Zenon W. 1980. "Computation and Cognition: Issues in the Foundations of Cognitive Science." *Behavioral and Brain Sciences* 3 (1): 111–132.

Rosenbaum, David A., Sandra B. Kenny, and Marcia A. Derr. 1983. "Hierarchical Control of Rapid Movement Sequences." *Journal of Experimental Psychology: Human Perception and Performance* 9 (1): 86–102.

Sakai, Katsuyuki, Katsuya Kitaguchi, and Okihide Hikosaka. 2003. "Chunking during Human Visuomotor Sequence Learning." *Experimental Brain Research* 152 (2): 229–242.

Saltzman, E., and J. A. Kelso. 1987. "Skilled Actions: A Task-Dynamic Approach." *Psychological Review* 94 (1): 84–106.

Schmidt, Richard A. 1975. "A Schema Theory of Discrete Motor Skill Learning." *Psychological Review* 82 (4): 225–260.

Schmidt, Richard A. 1991. "Frequent Augmented Feedback Can Degrade Learning: Evidence and Interpretations." In *Tutorials in Motor Neuroscience*, edited by Jean Requin and George E. Stelmach, 59–75. NATO ASI Series 62. Amsterdam: Springer Netherlands.

Schmidt, Richard A., and Douglas E. Young. 1991. "Methodology for Motor Learning: A Paradigm for Kinematic Feedback." *Journal of Motor Behavior* 23 (1): 13–24.

Shadmehr, Reza, and Ferdinando A. Mussa-Ivaldi. 1994. "Adaptive Representation of Dynamics during Learning of a Motor Task." *Journal of Neuroscience* 14 (5 Pt 2): 3208–3224.

Shaw, Robert. 2001. "Processes, Acts, and Experiences: Three Stances on the Problem of Intentionality." *Ecological Psychology* 13 (4): 275–314.

Shaw, Robert E., Peter N. Kugler, and Jeffrey Kinsella-Shaw. 1990. "Reciprocities of Intentional Systems." In *Perception and Control of Self-Motion*, edited by Rick Warren and Alexander H. Wertheim, 579–619. Hillsdale, NJ: Erlbaum.

Shea, Charles H., Gabriele Wulf, Chad A. Whitacre, and Jin-Hoon Park. 2001. "Surfing the Implicit Wave." *Quarterly Journal of Experimental Psychology A: Human Experimental Psychology* 54 (3): 841–862.

Shiffrin, Richard M., and Walter Schneider. 1977. "Controlled and Automatic Human Information Processing II: Perceptual Learning, Automatic Attending and a General Theory." *Psychological Review* 84 (2): 127–190.

Shull, Pete B., Wisit Jirattigalachote, Michael A. Hunt, Mark R. Cutkosky, and Scott L. Delp. 2014. "Quantified Self and Human Movement: A Review on the Clinical Impact of Wearable Sensing and Feedback for Gait Analysis and Intervention." *Gait and Posture* 40 (1): 11–19.

Smith, Matthew D., and Craig J. Chamberlin. 1992. "Effect of Adding Cognitively Demanding Tasks on Soccer Skill Performance." *Perceptual and Motor Skills* 75 (3 Pt 1): 955–961.

Sparrow, W. A., Kirstie M. Hughes, Aron P. Russell, and Peter F. Le Rossignol. 1999. "Effects of Practice and Preferred Rate on Perceived Exertion, Metabolic Variables and Movement Control." *Human Movement Science* 18 (2/3): 137–153.

Sparrow, W. A., and K. M. Newell. 1998. "Metabolic Energy Expenditure and the Regulation of Movement Economy." *Psychonomic Bulletin and Review* 5 (2): 173–196.

Steen, M. Marieke C. van der, and Raoul M. Bongers. 2011. "Joint Angle Variability and Co-Variation in a Reaching with a Rod Task." *Experimental Brain Research* 208 (3): 411–422.

Thompson, Evan. 2007. *Mind in Life: Biology, Phenomenology, and the Sciences of Mind*. Cambridge, MA: Harvard University Press.

Todorov, Emanuel. 2004. "Optimality Principles in Sensorimotor Control." *Nature Neuroscience* 7 (9): 907–915.

Turner, Carl W., and Ira S. Fischler. 1993. "Speeded Tests of Implicit Knowledge." *Journal of Experimental Psychology: Learning, Memory, and Cognition* 19 (5): 1165–1177.

Turvey, M. T. 1990. "Coordination." *American Psychologist* 45 (8): 938–953.

Turvey, M. T., and Claudia Carello. 1986. "The Ecological Approach to Perceiving-Acting: A Pictorial Essay." *Acta Psychologica* 63 (2): 133–155.

Turvey, M. T., Hollis L. Fitch, and Betty Tuller. 1976 "The Bernstein Perspective I: The Problems of Degrees of Freedom and Context-Conditioned Variability." In *Human Motor Behavior: An Introduction*, 239–252. Hillsdale, NJ: Erlbaum.

Turvey, Michael T., Robert E. Shaw, Edward S. Reed, and William M. Mace. 1981. "Ecological Laws of Perceiving and Acting: In Reply to Fodor and Pylyshyn (1981)." *Cognition* 9 (3): 237–304.

Varoqui, Deborah, Jérôme Froger, Jacques-Yvon Pélissier, and Benoît G. Bardy. 2011. "Effect of Coordination Biofeedback on (Re)Learning Preferred Postural Patterns in Post-Stroke Patients." *Motor Control* 15 (2): 187–205.

Von Porat, A. R. E. M., E. M. Roos, and Harald Roos. 2004. "High Prevalence of Osteoarthritis 14 Years after an Anterior Cruciate Ligament Tear in Male Soccer Players: A Study of Radiographic and Patient Relevant Outcomes." *Annals of the Rheumatic Diseases* 63 (3): 269–273.

Wang, Chaoyi, Deanna M. Kennedy, Jason B. Boyle, and Charles H. Shea. 2013. "A Guide to Performing Difficult Bimanual Coordination Tasks: Just Follow the Yellow Brick Road." *Experimental Brain Research* 230 (1): 31–40.

Warren, William H. 2006. "The Dynamics of Perception and Action." *Psychological Review* 113 (2): 358–389.

Warren, William H., Bruce A. Kay, Wendy D. Zosh, Andrew P. Duchon, and Stephanie Sahuc. 2001. "Optic Flow Is Used to Control Human Walking." *Nature Neuroscience* 4 (2): 213–216.

Warren, William H., Jr. 1998. "Visually Controlled Locomotion: 40 Years Later." *Ecological Psychology* 10 (3/4): 177–219.

Wilson, Andrew D., Andrew Weightman, Geoffrey P. Bingham, and Qin Zhu. 2016. "Using Task Dynamics to Quantify the Affordances of Throwing for Long Distance and Accuracy." *Journal of Experimental Psychology: Human Perception and Performance* 42 (7): 965–981.

Wolpert, Daniel M., and Mitsuo Kawato. 1998. "Multiple Paired Forward and Inverse Models for Motor Control." *Neural Networks* 11 (7/8): 1317–1329.

Wulf, Gabriele. 2013. "Attentional Focus and Motor Learning: A Review of 15 Years." *International Review of Sport and Exercise Psychology* 6 (1): 77–104.

Wulf, Gabriele, and Janet S. Dufek. 2009. "Increased Jump Height with an External Focus due to Enhanced Lower Extremity Joint Kinetics." *Journal of Motor Behavior* 41 (5): 401–409.

Wulf, Gabriele, and Wolfgang Prinz. 2001. "Directing Attention to Movement Effects Enhances Learning: A Review." *Psychonomic Bulletin and Review* 8 (4): 648–660.

Yoo, Jae Ho, Bee Oh Lim, Mina Ha, Soo Won Lee, Soo Jin Oh, Yong Seuk Lee, and Jin Goo Kim. 2010. "A Meta-Analysis of the Effect of Neuromuscular Training on the Prevention of the Anterior Cruciate Ligament Injury in Female Athletes." *Knee Surgery, Sports Traumatology, Arthroscopy* 18 (6): 824–830.

Zaal, Frank T. J. M., and Reinoud J. Bootsma. 1995. "The Topology of Limb Deceleration in Prehension Tasks." *Journal of Motor Behavior* 27 (2): 193–207.

Zhao, Huaiyong, and William H. Warren. 2015. "On-Line and Model-Based Approaches to the Visual Control of Action." *Vision Research* 110 (Pt B): 190–202.

4 Flipping Sport Psychology Theory into Practice: A Context- and Behavior-Centered Approach

Geir Jordet and Gert-Jan Pepping

1 Introduction

Sport psychology, as an academic field, has come a long way since its infancy, with the launch of the first designated peer review journals almost forty years ago. Today, much of the research published in leading sport psychology journals is based on well-validated theories, is conducted in highly sophisticated laboratories, and employs advanced multilevel statistics. However, as theory and methodology become increasingly sophisticated, there is a risk that researchers will focus more on narrow questions raised in the exclusive context in which the theories and methods were developed, and consequently remove their focus from the questions asked by people operating in actual real-world sport contexts. In doing so, contemporary and dominant paradigms within sport psychology may fail to fully or effectively address questions of concerns for elite athletes, coaches, and others involved in elite-level sport.

This is a concern that in large part has been addressed by the accounts from experienced sport psychology practitioners (e.g., Collins and Cruickshank 2015; Gilbourne and Richardson 2006; McDougall, Nesti, and Richardson 2015; Nesti 2010), who report that sport psychology education does not adequately prepare students for the questions that they end up working with in elite-sport environments. Consequently, the field of sport psychology may have a lot to gain from focusing more on the application of theories and empirical research to practice. In this chapter, we take a more radical point of view by arguing that sport psychology itself needs to change. This implies a new approach to theory production and the kinds of questions we ask in our research, as well as a new focus on how we apply the existing knowledge base in our field.

The field of sport psychology traditionally seems to be structured, to a large extent, with a primary focus on isolated and disembodied psychological processes or mechanisms, with only rarely any focus on actual behaviors associated with those mechanisms, and

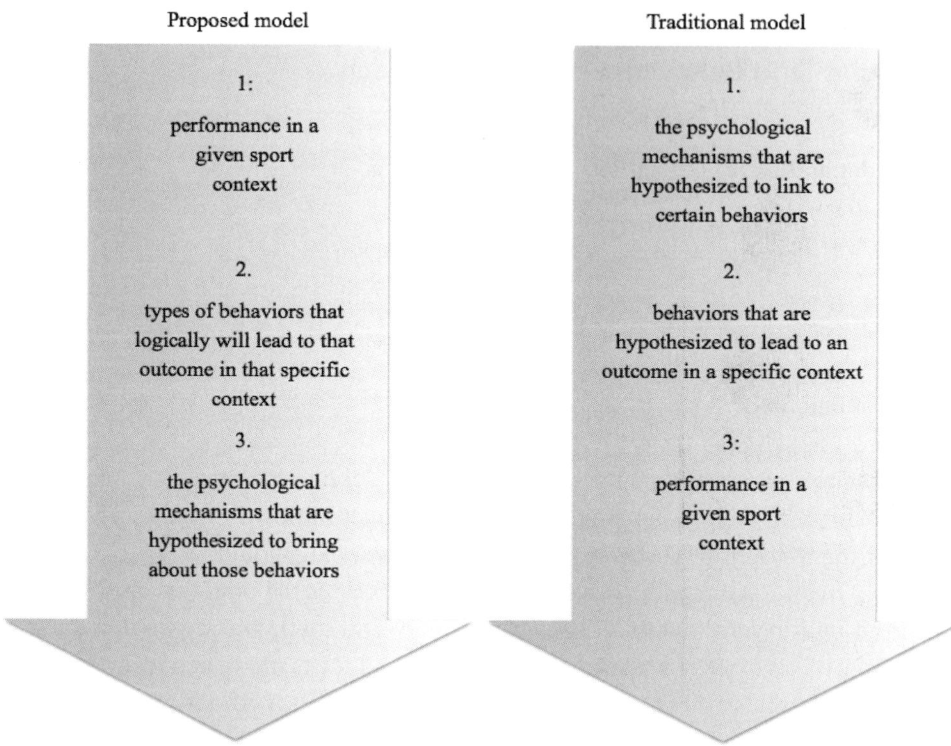

Figure 4.1
In this chapter we propose to approach research and practice initiatives by (1) reflecting on and addressing context and the desired outcome (performance) in this context, then (2) identifying the exact types of behaviors that logically will lead to that outcome in that specific context, and finally (3) addressing the psychological mechanisms that are hypothesized to bring about those behaviors (proposed model, on left side). In the traditional model for research and practice in sport psychology, we argue that the opposite order is followed (traditional model, on right side).

hardly ever the embodied expression of knowledge and performance as the starting point (see figure 4.1).

One simple way to express this concept can be found in the table of contents of more or less any major sport psychology textbook, where the majority of the chapters typically are labeled with words based on cognitive or emotional mechanisms such as motivation, anxiety, concentration, self-confidence, group cohesion, aggression, and imagery (e.g., Cox 2012; Karageorghis and Terry 2011; Weinberg and Gould 2015). In the field of sport psychology, we rarely ask questions and focus on performance (the embedded and embodied expression of knowledge) before having considered the psychological mechanisms. Rather, a primary focus on "performance" belongs to entirely different subdisciplines of the sport science, such as "performance analysis" (e.g., McGarry et al. 2013) and "motor control" (e.g., Schmidt and Lee 2011). Ironically, motor control and learning used to be a part of the larger discipline of sport psychology, but the two were separated, arguably from the 1960s, something that may not have served the practical side of sport psychology (Collins and Cruickshank 2015).

Relatively recent research reviews, in both social psychology (Baumeister, Vohs, and Funder 2007) and sport psychology (Andersen, McCullagh, and Wilson 2007), show that leading journals in the respective fields hardly ever feature articles where actual behavior is a variable. Rather, the focus is on self-report variables, typically measured via questionnaires, and only rarely involving any type of overt behavior. In fact, the only type of behavior touched on by the majority of the publications in the fields of both social and sport psychology seem to be keystrokes on a keyboard or pen-writing in a questionnaire. From an embodied cognitive science viewpoint, this is problematic if we want to conceive of psychology as a field purporting to explain agency as *meaningful human behavior*. After all, most, if not all, human behavior is expressed through agency, meaningful *action* in the environment. Agency needs to be understood as an expression of knowledge that is embedded and embodied, with an emphasis on the interaction between the agent and the world (Dawson 2014).

Athletes and coaches, especially at the elite level, are intensely absorbed in concrete practical tasks and dilemmas related to how they can improve the athlete's performance in their given sport. In this chapter, it is argued that if sport psychology, as a field, is to provide a sound foundation for effective (performance development) practice, sport psychology researchers (and practitioners) need to reconsider the questions that are pursued. In short, we need to flip our approach and start the other way around from what is usually done when we conduct research and communicate our scholarship to students and athletes and coaches. Namely, this means starting with performance, context, and specific behaviors *before* addressing the psychological mechanisms that may be relevant to examine or affect those behaviors. In particular, we argue that we should (1) start our research and practice initiatives by reflecting on and addressing the specific context in question and the desired outcome in that context (e.g., performance in a given sport and with reference to the context it is embedded in), (2) identify the exact types of behaviors that logically will lead to the desired outcome in that specific context (e.g., behaviors related to coping with a specific problem, adaption to different types of contexts, and learning and improving one's sport skills), and (3) address the embodied psychological mechanisms that are hypothesized to bring about those behaviors (e.g., motivations, emotions, and perceptions) (see figure 1, left side).

A necessary but perhaps uncomfortable implication of such a position is the assertion that this means focusing on specific sports, with their unique contexts and specific behaviors, and using each specific sport as the point of departure. Further, we need to recognize the importance of the (social and emotional) environmental context in which meaningful agency takes place. In fact, it is this recognition that will provide us with the badly needed conceptual and theoretical framework that can assist us in effectively flipping sport psychology theory into practice.

In this chapter, we briefly present a historical background to the current state of sport psychology research and practice, arguing for the need of our flipped approach. We then present the theoretical underpinnings of such an approach. Conceptually, the flipped approach rests on foundations of ecological psychology (e.g., Gibson 1979; Bronfenbrenner 1979), which describes how cognition should be described in terms of agent-environment interactions and dynamics, rather than in terms of disembodied computation and representation (Chemero 2009). From this viewpoint, the environment is held as intrinsically meaningful, with sufficient information and meaning just waiting to be discovered in the athlete-environment interaction. As for practical implications, we use soccer as a case, to show a concrete way to structure and communicate psychology with an emphasis on performance development behaviors in this specific sport. Finally, we discuss the implications of such an approach for both research and practice in the field of sport psychology.

2 History

In this section, we show how some of the historical developments in psychology as an independent field of study can explain, at least partially, the higher status assigned by psychologists (and hence also sport psychologists) to disembodied internal mental processes—at the cost of drawing attention away from specific sport contexts, functions, and agency (performance and behavior). Further, we describe the manner in which ecological psychology provides an alternative way to structure both research and practice in sport psychology, with its focus on environmental opportunities for action (affordances) and constraints, and the actions and behaviors necessary to find and utilize value in the real world.

The inferior status of context and actions in contemporary sport psychology can be traced back to certain events in the historical development of the mother disciplines of philosophy and psychology. Since the mechanization of the worldview in the seventeenth century, when the contributions by the French philosopher Descartes were made popular, mind-body and man-environment dualisms have dominated different scientific disciplines (e.g., Reed 1996b; Lombardo 1987). As a result, the environment in which agency takes place was conceived as meaningless, consisting merely of matter in motion. A separation between the objective qualities of the environment and how humans can subjectively be in touch with them ensued. Properties of the environment that exist independently of the agent, "out there," such as form, mass, and speed (so-called primary qualities) were differentiated from qualities that could seemingly be inferred to exist only in the human mind, such as color, taste, smell, and meaning (secondary qualities, see e.g., Neisser 1967). Only the primary qualities, that is, the meaningless environment, could be directly measured. The secondary qualities, on the other hand, could not be measured, and hence required a separate methodology to be accessed. This paved the way for the pencil and paper methods that we now know to be so prevalent in social and sport psychology. In psychology, this further contributed to a prevalent mistrust, or at the very least disinterest, in everyday events, real behaviors, and experiences in the actual world.

The emergence of modern psychology in the 1860s commanded that the new scientific psychologists had to come up with both new theories and new methodologies to justify their own profession (Reed 1997). One way forward was to attempt to provide alternative views to commonsense and everyday experience, to advance an entirely new route that could lead to what would be perceived as new knowledge. Many psychologists then became interested in disembodied and hypothetical constructs like mental sensations, memory, and information processing (the basics of modern cognitive psychology). These processes may have become more valuable to researchers than the experience of the more concrete events and behaviors that actually take place.

3 An Ecological Alternative

There seems to be a need for an alternative basis for our psychological understanding. Here we argue that an embedded and more context-specific or sensitive perspective can rest on ecological foundations (e.g., Gibson 1979; Bronfenbrenner 1979). Reed (1996a) characterized ecological psychology as a theoretical perspective "in which the psychological experiences and activities of persons and animals is placed firmly at the center of our field" (6). This approach to agency and the coordination of animate motor behavior has two reciprocities at its core: (1) the reciprocity of agent and environment, and (2) the reciprocity of perception and action. An agent can only be properly understood as living in and interacting with an environment in which it eats, sleeps, breathes, moves, and so on. An environment, on the other hand, exists by virtue of the agent that it is inhabited by. Hence, agent (athlete) and environment (context) form an *inseparable* pair.

Affordances take a very special place within the ecological psychology. The affordance of anything is defined as "a specific combination of the properties, of its substances and its surfaces taken with reference to an animal" (Gibson 1979, 67). In the context of sport, the environment of an athlete consists of the affordances of objects, other agents, places, and events for that athlete. With affordances, Gibson introduced the "what" of behavior. Affordances exist, regardless of whether they are being perceived; affordances are ecological *facts* of reality. In any athlete's environment there are features (objects, places, other athletes) that have potential consequences for behavior. Through the concept of affordances, *agent behavior* is placed firmly back to the center of psychology; perception is of behavior, rather than of properties. Athletes do not primarily perceive the track, the coach, or balls in their environment. They perceive places to run on, someone to talk or listen to, and things to catch, throw, or score goals with. Performance behaviors, or *agency,* follow from the athlete's use of the affordances in their environment (Reed 1993, 1996a; for a recent comprehensive account of affordances and agency, see Withagen et al. 2012).

An ecological approach to psychology suggests that the context in which athletes operate says more about behavior than do individual mental processes. In other words, the unique relationship between environmental information and the individual's perception of this information is the most important variable that psychologists should study (Gibson 1979). It is this notion that drives the need to flip our approach in sport psychology.

In his book from 1979, *The Ecological Approach to Visual Perception,* James J. Gibson repeatedly stressed that he had tried to provide a basis for understanding behavior (perception *and* action) in the real world. Inherent in this was a genuinely pragmatic view on the field of psychology, a view that probably originated from the time when Gibson worked with problems related to flying during World War II. This research forced him to think in terms of applied psychology (Reed 1988). Furthermore, he emphasized the information that is relevant to peoples' lives, and disregarded other types of information, such as the information that often is presented in many laboratories.

In an attempt to develop this further, we will specify how a general use of the philosophical aspects of affordances (from Gibson 1979) can support and inform applied sport psychology research and practice. From ecologically informed expertise research, we know that expert athletes are able to functionally adapt their behaviors to dynamic and complex performance environments; they do this by continuously perceiving information and regulating goal-directed actions (Davids et al. 2015).

Hence, the ecological approach produces a compelling rationale for an environmental and context-specific approach to sport psychology. The following section goes into more depth on the exact manner such a context-specific approach can be conceived, which we demonstrate in the context of soccer.

4 Embedded Agency in Soccer: Performance Behaviors in a Specific Context

Based on these theoretical considerations, one way to proceed is to explicitly take a starting point in the meaningful context in which practitioners, coaches, and athletes operate. An embedded, context-specific perspective would explicitly address the *unique* challenges of a sport and the way performers in that sport *experience* these challenges, followed by theoretically, empirically, and experientially founded recommendations to cope with these features.

Knowledge of a sport's unique features can help coaches and sport psychology consultants target the most critical variables to performance, thus increasing intervention effectiveness. In the past couple of decades, some of the psychological specifics of soccer and the ways to work with athletes in soccer have been described in the works of sport psychology practitioners (e.g., Beswick 2010; Bull and Shambrook 2004; Cale and Forzoni 2004; Morrow 2001). However, oddly, given the soccer-specific titles of these books, none are based on empirical research with soccer players, and some do not even refer to any studies conducted with soccer players. Rather, the contents seem to be based much more on generic (disembodied, cognitive, cognitive-behavioral, or emotional) psychological skills that seem to be the same regardless of what sport they are applied in, such as concentration/focus, motivation, self-confidence, stress control, relaxation, goal-setting, and communication. Following the traditional model outline, this generic set of processes is then articulated using sport-specific examples.

Thus, a crucial next step toward professional psychology service delivery in soccer is to merge practical experience with an established knowledge base founded in ecologically valid and representative research with soccer players, to provide a more genuine, as well as relevant and functional, psychology of this particular context. A practitioner-friendly review of some of this research was conducted by Jordet (2016). Here, we review the following eight broad categories of agency (and related behaviors) relevant to performance in soccer:

prospectively controlling game dynamics
purposeful effort mobilization and exertion
self-regulation of learning
regulating (balancing) total load

coping with adversity, success, and pressure
managing and adapting to new contexts
managing relationships
expressing individuality

These categories and behaviors are to be understood in the context of an ecological account of agency; that is, they are embedded (environment/context driven), and they follow from the player's use of the affordances in their environment. Each of the categories of agency can be facilitated by a series of psychological (i.e., cognitive, motivational, emotional, or perceptual) mechanisms; in each, we first address context, then agency, and finally psychological process.

4.1 Prospectively Controlling Game Dynamics

Context: A player in a soccer game constantly has to perceive and act based on information from other players and the ball. The concept of affordances says something about the opportunities to act, for a given performer in a given context. Affordances provide a meaningful and functional specification of the objects and events available to perceive and act on. Specifically, in this context, the players from the other team represent obstacles that have to be avoided, by use of passes, dribbles, and shots, all delivered in the openings between the opponents and/or to areas that are not occupied by opponents.

Agency: Game awareness, sport intelligence, vision, and decision making are all popular characteristics coaches tend to use when referring to players who effectively perceive, process, and act on such game information (e.g., Mills et al. 2012). In the research literature, there is much evidence that expert soccer players, compared with players at a lower level, have more effective visual search patterns (e.g., Cañal-Bruland et al. 2011; Roca et al. 2011; Williams et al. 1994), better peripheral vision (Williams and Davids 1998), and better anticipation (Bishop et al. 2013). Observing soccer players during actual games reveals that they engage in a wealth of behavior generated to obtain information—so-called exploratory behavior. In an ecological approach, perception is seen as a mode of activity rather than a mode of receptivity. Gibson (1966) distinguished performatory activity from exploratory activity. Performatory actions are activities that bring one closer to a goal, whereas explorations are activities that aim to reveal information that can help guide one toward a goal. The way actions thus influence cognition is highly consistent with an embodied cognition perspective. In the context of soccer, one can argue that players gather most information by use of their eyes, and visual exploratory behavior (VEB) can be described as the manner in which players physically move their bodies and heads to more efficiently perceive their surroundings. Videotaping players using a close-up focus, to capture the players in full figure, provides real-game footage that then can be analyzed and correlated with both context and performance. Results from investigations with this method suggest a positive relationship between VEB and performance, with expert soccer players exploring more frequently than nonexpert players; when players within a game engage in high-frequency VEB, they are more likely to reach their teammates with a successful pass (Jordet 2005a, 2005b; Jordet, Bloomfield, and Heijmerikx 2013).

Psychological mechanisms: Studying decision making in sport cannot ignore the study of real-game behavioral manifestations of decisions, but that is exactly the manner in which the academic study of decision making largely has proceeded until now, with studies on anticipation (Williams and Davids 1998), memory recall (Williams and Davids 1995), and, recently, an upsurge of studies on effective information processing or executive functioning (Bishop et al. 2013; Faubert 2013; Verburg et al. 2014; Vestberg et al. 2012). This is not to say that these studies in any way are irrelevant or unimportant. On the contrary, they have produced significant knowledge that illuminates processes that most likely are central to performance. However, for this knowledge to be really useful for practitioners, coaches, and players, it would be better if it was embedded more firmly into specific contexts and translated into actual game behaviors.

4.2 Purposeful Effort Mobilization and Exertion

Context: In a game, players are required to execute actions such as jumps, sprints, repeated runs, tackles, duels, dribbles, and shots with sufficient power to successfully solve the task in that game situation, and then repeat these actions multiple times, often with limited time for recovery. This requires high levels of effort exertion. Similarly, to develop optimally over time, young players may have to get up from bed early to do extra training, stay behind after team practice to work on weaknesses, or stay up to watch games on TV to learn from players in the same position. It is logical that players who are able to mobilize high amounts of effort and direct it in ways that optimize development, learning, and performance will have great benefits.

Agency: This category of behaviors encompasses the magnitude of effort that players are able to mobilize and exert from the short- as well as long-term perspectives. For short term, from research with elite Brazilian soccer players, we know that narrowly focusing one's mental and physical effort onto a very specific task, while conserving or reducing effort to other, less-relevant tasks, is associated with high performance (Naito and Hirose 2014; Tedesqui and Orlick 2015). Further, for more long term, the best players seem to persist in exerting effort, prioritizing the right things, and sacrificing giving in to short term impulses and rather continue to engage in the activities that will produce long-term benefits (Mills et al. 2012; van Yperen 2009; Toering and Jordet 2015).

Psychological mechanisms: Effort mobilization and exertion often is related to motivation. In a longitudinal study of young Dutch academy players, to see who would make it ten years after they were measured (van Yperen 2009), and in a study of 644 professional players, examining the difference between national team and nonnational team players (Toering and Jordet 2015), goal commitment, delayed gratification, and self-control (or self-discipline or will-power) have been identified to discriminate high performance in several studies. The same was found in interviews with expert development coaches (Mills et al. 2012). In short, it seems that the players who are able to focus on the goals and behaviors necessary to reach the goal and resist the temptation to give in to distractions or short-term emotional gratification are more likely to be successful. It is likely that these players exert high levels of effort, invest energy, and mobilize all possible resources to get where they want to go.

4.3 Self-Regulation of Learning

Context: Soccer is the largest sport in the world, with 265 million active players (FIFA 2001); because only 0.04 of these play in a professional league, making it in this sport is extremely demanding (Haugaasen and Jordet 2012). Young players are typically selected early for academies where they get access to the best coaches and play with and against the best players in their age group. If they are not constantly developing and performing at a progressively higher level to stay among the best players, they are cut from the teams.

Agency: Evidence suggests that, to remain competitive and constantly develop and advance in this system, one must deliver large quantities of practice hours (Ford et al. 2009; Ford and Williams 2012; Ward et al. 2007; Haugaasen, Toering and Jordet 2014). However, other evidence suggests that the quality of practice—effective learning and actively engaging in cognitive processes responsible for learning—may be equally if not more important (van Yperen and Duda 1999; Toering et al. 2009; Toering et al. 2011). Hence, self-regulation of learning, referring to the extent to which people are proactive participants in their own learning processes (Toering et al. 2009), is a gross type of behavior that seems to be of importance for elite, or prospective elite, players.

Psychological mechanisms: We have conducted several studies to reveal that young Dutch elite players engage more than their non-elite counterparts in self-regulatory learning activities and metacognitions, such as reflecting on practice (e.g., Toering et al. 2009). This has been found also among world-class professional soccer players from

Manchester United (Horrocks 2012) and elite female youth soccer players (Gledhill and Harwood 2014).

4.4 Regulating (Balancing) Total Load

Context: The game of soccer puts many physical constraints on players, including the need to accelerate, decelerate, change direction, jump, stand up to opponents, and strike the ball (Dupont and McCall 2016). With respect to simple running, up to about 10 percent of the distance elite players cover during a game is performed using high-intensity actions (Carling et al. 2008), and sometimes there is very little time for recovery before a new high-intensity action needs to be employed (Carling, Le Gall, and Dupont 2012). Further, when physical and mental fatigue is allowed to accumulate, it will affect performance (e.g., Carling and Dupont 2011), once more illustrating the concept of embodied cognition.

Agency: Hence, it is critical for players to regulate their physical output during games. Equally importantly, given the requirement to engage in incredibly high doses of daily deliberate practice to keep up with these game demands, and exerting the accompanying levels of mental and physical effort to become or continue to perform as an elite soccer player (see review, in Haugaasen and Jordet 2012), it is important to balance training with high-quality recovery and rest to avoid burnout or overtraining (Ericsson, Krampe, and Tesch-Romer 1993). Several studies show that lack of sufficient recovery during a season is associated with the accumulation of stress during and at the end of the season than can lead to overreaching and overtraining (Faude et al. 2011; Brink et al. 2012).

Psychological mechanisms: Several psychological mechanisms have been shown to underlie adaptive and maladaptive behaviors related to response to total load in soccer—thus, clearly showing how cognition is embodied. For example, players with perfectionistic tendencies are more vulnerable to burnout (Hill et al. 2008), whereas players with high levels of harmonious passion are more protected against burnout (Curran et al. 2011; Curran et al. 2013). There is similar evidence with respect to stress and injuries, with higher levels of stress, daily hassle, and anxiety predicting more injuries in soccer players (Ivarsson, Johnson, and Podlog 2013; Ivarsson and Johnsson 2010).

4.5 Coping with Adversity, Success, and Pressure

Context: Over the span of a long career in soccer, with up to seventy-five to eighty games each year, and tens of thousands of practice hours, a player's performance will undoubtedly vary, and a player will have both good and bad days. Sometimes even the best players are left out of the team, they are injured and cannot practice, and, of course, just like nonathletes, they will occasionally experience problems in life. Despite this, the expectation from fans and coaches to a professional soccer player will always be to perform. Given the massive focus devoted to the players on the scene in the biggest sport in the world, even at a very young age, it is logical that another important factor that potentially can hinder performance is the failure to cope with success, with the extra attention and recognition that comes with it from mass media, social media, agents, scouts, and people in general. Finally, pressure can be defined as the degree of perceived importance of a situation (Baumeister 1984; Beilock and Gray 2007). One can argue that the pressure involved in soccer, particularly at the elite level, is perpetually high as a function of the enormous interest this sport receives from people all over the world. To illustrate, the World Cup Final has been shown to reach live television numbers of more than a billion people (FIFA Marketing and TV 2002). The pressure to perform when almost one-fifth of the world population is watching is hard to imagine.

Agency: Coping with adversity is most likely a key factor for elite soccer players, in which the goal logically is to work through adversity, setbacks, and failure to maintain the same or more focus and energy in practice and games as one would have had without the adversity. A longitudinal study showed that both successful and unsuccessful players experienced stress as young players, but only the ones who were ultimately successful as adults reported employing problem-oriented coping strategies (in which they employ behavioral strategies to manage the situation that causes the stress, not just the resulting emotions) (van Yperen 2009). As for coping with success, it is logical that players who can respond to success by exerting more, and not less, energy in a productive direction for their development—as well as players who, after success, are able to focus better on their tasks at hand in a given game, will develop more effectively and perform better.

An illustrative soccer-specific case of coping with pressure, in which players occasionally engage in some highly maladaptive behaviors and consequently fail to cope, is the penalty shoot-out. In a study of all penalty shoot-outs ever held in the World Cup, European Championship, and the UEFA Champions League, when players are faced with shots where a miss will instantly cause their team to lose, players score on about 60 per cent of their attempts, whereas with shots where a goal will secure a win, they score on about 90 per cent of their shots (Jordet and Hartman 2008). This says something about how vulnerable even highly elite soccer players are to pressure and the potential negative implications of a failed performance. In addition, with players in the same tournaments, when expectations to perform for a specific individual are high, performance is low (Jordet 2009a); when team expectations are high, individual performance is low (Jordet 2009b); when the relative importance of a tournament and/or a kick is high, performance is low (Jordet et al. 2007); and when a team has a history of losing these events, individual current performance is also low (Jordet, Hartman, and Jelle Vuijk 2012). With respect to performance behaviors, several of our studies indicate that avoidance behaviors (e.g., rushing a shot, with the possible intention of simply getting the situation over with) play a role in several of these players' performance failures (Jordet and Hartman 2008; Jordet 2009a, 2009b).

Psychological mechanisms: High-level development coaches identify resilience as a critical factor needed for a young player to make it to the professional level (Mills et al. 2012). Another study found that successful players, as opposed to unsuccessful ones, had a wide repertoire of stress-coping strategies that could be used to address any situation (Holt and Dunn 2004; Holt et al. 2006).

Expert soccer development coaches acknowledge that the attitude of "having made it" can easily stop effective development (Mills et al. 2012), which is equivalent to elite professional players of the highest status underperforming more than others in highly pressure-filled penalty shoot-out situations (Jordet 2009a). Hence, effective development and performance can generally be characterized by the ability to not be distracted or swayed by the external influences associated with success, to relentlessly engage in continuous learning with a pure focus on the core behaviors necessary to deliver high-level performances.

Anxiety is perhaps the most important psychological mechanism involved in coping with pressure. With the example of the penalty shoot-out again, one of our studies indicates that when a player's perception of control over the situation is low, anxiety is high (Jordet et al. 2006). Anxiety can probably also vary throughout the shoot-out (Jordet and Elferink-Gemser 2012). With this said, further directly illustrating embodied cognition, there seems to be a potential to influence one's teammates in those moments immediately following one's own shot, where big enthusiastic displays of celebration are associated with higher probabilities of ultimate team success, possibly as a result of individual emotions affecting other people's emotions (Moll, Jordet, and Pepping 2010).

4.6 Managing and Adapting to New Contexts

Context: The rules of a game should logically secure constant and nearly identical conditions and contexts for players to perform under, from game to game. However, the relative contextual differences that indeed are in place may put important constraints on performance in this sport. One simple illustration of this is the home advantage research, showing that the home team consistently wins more games than the away team—a phenomenon that historically has been more pronounced in soccer than in other major professional sports (Courneya and Carron 1992; Pollard and Pollard 2005). In addition, players, including senior professionals, hardly ever spend their entire careers at only one club (Littlewood, Mullen, and Richardson 2011). Rather, a career usually consists of multiple moves to new clubs, new cities, and new countries, which forces the player to effectively transition and adapt to new and very different types of culture, lifestyle, language, coaching, and team norms.

Agency: Much recent evidence has accumulated to show the exact reasons and ways the home team gains such a clear advantage in soccer, including crowd size (e.g., Goumas 2014), venue familiarity (e.g., Hvattum 2015), distance/traveling fatigue (e.g., Pollard and Gomez 2014), playing strategy (e.g., Staufenbiel, Lobinger, and Strauss 2015) and referee bias (e.g., Constantinou, Fenton, and Hunter Pollock 2014). A logical goal for players and teams faced with new contexts is to behave and perform consistently, regardless of the conditions they operate under. Not much research has been conducted specifically on the behaviors associated with successful transition into new soccer teams.

Psychological mechanisms: As for the home advantage, there have been no consistent and equivocal findings about the role of psychological variables (e.g., Duffy and Hinwood 1997). However, with transition into a new team, such relocation has been shown to trigger a series of psychological responses, such as culture shock, isolation, homesickness, fear, and irritability (Littlewood and Nesti 2011; Richardson et al. 2012). Understanding these issues begins with understanding the context and the conditions that underlie undesired/maladaptive behaviors, and then addressing the various subsequent psychological processes that ensue. In contrast, addressing, for example, transition-related fear as an isolated emotional construct, which technically could be buffered via the use of well-known psychological techniques such as meditation and positive self-talk, would be severely misguided and provide neither a full understanding of the issue nor a good platform to help alleviate it.

4.7 Managing Relationships

Context: A soccer player relates to and is reliant on a series of other people, on and off the field, and all these people have the potential to distract focus away from performance or to support and facilitate performance. Several studies show that relationships and team cohesion are important for teams to achieve success in a soccer context (Filho, Tenenbaum, and Yang 2015; Pain and Harwood 2008).

Agency: Elite development coaches hold interpersonal skills as critical for a player's ability to maneuver through the different social situations that are present in a soccer club context (Mills et al. 2012). Moreover, research shows that youth players who become successful, more than their non-elite counterparts, seek out social (van Yperen 2009) and tangible (Holt and Dunn 2004; Holt et al. 2006) support from their parents.

Psychological mechanisms: With that said, open communication does not necessarily come naturally to elite soccer players, a situation that may be rooted in the relatively traditionalist and macho culture that still may permeate soccer. Hence, communication, sharing, and bonding interventions seem to have a positive impact on soccer players and teams (Evans et al. 2013; Pain and Harwood 2009; Prapavessis, Carron, and Spink 1996; Voight and Callaghan 2001), although it is not certain whether these interventions are more helpful in soccer than in other sports.

4.8 Expressing Individuality

Context: In soccer, where such a small proportion of the player population actually reaches the professional level (Haugaasen and Jordet 2012), one could argue that every ambitious player needs to stand out with a unique signature and his or her own way to play, to simply get noticed, scouted, and selected for the highest level.

Agency: Players can stand out by engaging in behaviors that are inventive, new, or creative. The ultimate level of expert performance has been described as that in which an individual expresses him- or herself to contribute something personal, new, and unique to their domain (Ericsson and Charness 1994).

Psychological mechanisms: There are considerable individual differences in the ways that soccer players adopt and develop creative and divergent tactical thinking (Memmert 2010). Ironically, to help players develop these qualities, a key may be to help players open up their attention and not listen too attentively to what others say or do—good advice for coaches, therefore, may be to not offer too many specific prescriptions about the specific decisions that players should make (Memmert 2011).

5 Implications for Researchers

We argue that events, challenges, and experiences that athletes regularly encounter in their particular sport should be used as the frame of reference for researchers of sport psychology in that sport. Even though a sport such as soccer is similar to other sports, particularly to team ball sports, it has a number of unique physical, social, and cultural features. Knowledge of how psychological processes specifically relate to these features can help researchers and students acquire a more complete understanding of the most important psychological variables in this particular sport.

Hence, sport psychology researchers should first establish the type of behaviors that can be observed under different types of contexts, and then document the different cognitions and emotions that may be involved to facilitate, support, or moderate these behaviors—not the other way around. Unfortunately, we know more from the context-isolated (relatively speaking) study of psychological mechanisms such as anxiety and motivation in sport than we know about the environmental and contextual conditions under which, for instance, anxiety and motivation affect athletes, and how this in turn is related to specific performance behaviors.

The possible benefits of the proposed flipped approach include a higher degree of relevance and functionality with respect to applied implications of one's research. Further, it is likely that researchers would be better able to communicate their research to people in the practice field, given that the research would be more clearly rooted in questions that people in the practice field care about. As a limitation, it can be argued that the flipped approach necessitates, or at least is facilitated by, certain degrees of contextual (sport) knowledge on part of the researcher, and this may be a limitation. There is also the question of generalizability, in which a highly behavior- or context-specific approach may be difficult to generalize across different sports and contexts.

6 Implications for Practitioners

The embedded, context-specific, and phenomenological manner in which the material is presented makes sport psychology content more meaningful to professionals with an interest in functional solutions to practical problems. Practitioners facing a particular performance obstacle will obtain immediate insights and advice expressively based on the current state of knowledge of how to deal with *this given situation*. The traditional alternative would be to take a detour via generic psychological processes and generalize this information to deduce an indirect answer to the practical problem. The functionalistic alternative proposed is simply more "user friendly"

With respect to practitioners working in applied sport psychology, a context-specific approach is not new. Several highly respected applied (senior) sport psychologists, people who have been paramount in developing the field of applied sport psychology, have devoted much of their time to one specific sport (e.g., Robert Rotella in golf, Kenneth Ravizza in baseball, and Jim Loehr in tennis). A closer examination of books by these particular practitioners (i.e., Rotella 1996; Ravizza and Hanson 1995; Loehr 1990), show that they all have articulated highly sport-specific advice and/or fundamentally changed or adapted conventional advice to their specific sport (e.g., Rotella's aiming for the smallest possible target, Ravizza's pre-pitch routine, and Loehr's guidelines for the pauses between tennis points). These practical recommendations, which go beyond traditional textbook sport-psychology knowledge to functionally target the most critical obstacles to performance in each sport, would not have been possible to effectively articulate without considerable levels of sport-specific knowledge. Although there are many examples of excellent senior consultants from the same generation who have successfully adopted a more generalist approach (e.g., Dan Gould and Terry Orlick), the efficacy of the functional orientation involved in a sport-specific approach should not be underestimated.

7 Conclusion

In this chapter we have attempted to describe a new, embodied-cognition-based approach to theory, empirical research, and applied practice in sport psychology. The knowledge embedded in a specific context, expressed by the starting point in specific behaviors engaged in within that context, is the point of departure for this approach. The context-specific and phenomenological manner in which the material is presented makes it more meaningful to professionals whose interest lies in functional solutions to practical problems. Practitioners facing a particular performance obstacle will obtain immediate insights and advice expressly based on the current state of knowledge of how to deal with *this given situation*. This should be reflected not only in how we view practice and train practitioners in the field but also in the way we conduct our research, build and test our theories, and communicate the knowledge base in our literature.

References

Andersen, Mark B., Penny McCullagh, and Gabriel J. Wilson. 2007. "But What Do the Numbers Really Tell Us? Arbitrary Metrics and Effect Size Reporting in Sport Psychology Research." *Journal of Sport and Exercise Psychology* 29 (5): 664–672.

Baumeister, Roy F. 1984. "Choking Under Pressure: Self-Consciousness and Paradoxical Effects of Incentives on Skillful Performance." *Journal of Personality and Social Psychology* 46 (3): 610–620. doi:10.1037/0022-3514.46.3.610.

Baumeister, Roy F., Kathleen D. Vohs, and David C. Funder. 2007. "Psychology as the Science of Self-Reports and Finger Movements: Whatever Happened to Actual Behavior?" *Perspectives on Psychological Science* 2 (4): 396–403. doi:10.1111/j.1745-6916.2007.00051.x.

Beilock, Sian L., and Rob Gray. 2007. "Why Do Athletes Choke under Pressure?" In *Handbook of Sport Psychology*, 3rd ed., edited by Gershon Tenenbaum and R. C. Eklund, 425–444. Hoboken, NJ: John Wiley and Sons.

Beswick, Bill. 2010. *Focused for Soccer*. 2nd ed. Champaign, IL: Human Kinetics.

Bishop, Daniel T., Michael J. Wright, Robin C. Jackson, and Bruce Abernethy. 2013. "Neural Bases for Anticipation Skill in Soccer: An fMRI Study." *Journal of Sport and Exercise Psychology* 35 (1): 98–109.

Brink, M. S., C. Visscher, A. J. Coutts, and K. A. P. M. Lemmink. 2012. "Changes in Perceived Stress and Recovery in Overreached Young Elite Soccer Players." *Scandinavian Journal of Medicine and Science in Sports* 22 (2): 285–292. doi:10.1111/j.1600-0838.2010.01237.x.

Bronfenbrenner, U. 1979. *The Ecology of Human Development: Experiments by Design and Nature.* Cambridge, MA: Harvard University Press.

Bull, Stephen John, and Christopher J. Shambrook. 2004. *Soccer: The Mind Game.* London: Reedswain.

Cale, Andrew, and Roberto Forzoni. 2004. *The Official FA Guide to Psychology for Football.* London: Hodder Education.

Cañal-Bruland, Rouwen, Simone Lotz, Norbert Hagemann, Jörg Schorer, and Bernd Strauss. 2011. "Visual Span and Change Detection in Soccer: An Expertise Study." *Journal of Cognitive Psychology* 23 (3): 302–310. doi:10.1080/20445911.2011.496723.

Carling, Christopher, Jonathan Bloomfield, Lee Nelsen, and Thomas Reilly. 2008. "The Role of Motion Analysis in Elite Soccer Contemporary Performance Measurement Techniques and Work Rate Data." *Sports Medicine* 38 (10): 839–862. doi:10.2165/00007256-200838100-00004.

Carling, Christopher, and Gregory Dupont. 2011. "Are Declines in Physical Performance Associated with a Reduction in Skill-Related Performance during Professional Soccer Match-Play?" *Journal of Sports Sciences* 29 (1): 63–71. doi:10.1080/02640414.2010.521945.

Carling, Christopher, Franck Le Gall, and Gregory Dupont. 2012. "Analysis of Repeated High-Intensity Running Performance in Professional Soccer." *Journal of Sports Sciences* 30 (4): 325–336. doi:10.1080/02640414.2011.652655.

Chemero, Anthony. 2009. *Radical Embodied Cognitive Science.* Cambridge, MA: MIT Press.

Collins, Dave, and Andrew Cruickshank. 2015. "Take a Walk on the Wild Side: Exploring, Identifying, and Developing Consultancy Expertise with Elite Performance Team Leaders." *Psychology of Sport and Exercise* 16 (P1): 74–82. doi:10.1016/j.psychsport.2014.08.002.

Constantinou, Anthony Costa, Norman Elliott Fenton, and Liam Jackson Hunter Pollock. 2014. "Bayesian Networks for Unbiased Assessment of Referee Bias in Association Football." *Psychology of Sport and Exercise* 15 (5): 538–547. doi:10.1016/j.psychsport.2014.05.009.

Courneya, K. S., and A. V. Carron. 1992. "The Home Advantage in Sport Competitions: A Literature Review." *Journal of Sport and Exercise Psychology* 14 (1): 13–27.

Cox, Richard H. 2012. *Sport Psychology: Concepts and Applications.* 7th ed. Boston: McGraw-Hill.

Curran, Thomas, Paul R. Appleton, Andrew P. Hill, and Howard K. Hall. 2011. "Passion and Burnout in Elite Junior Soccer Players: The Mediating Role of Self-Determined Motivation." *Psychology of Sport and Exercise* 12 (6): 655–661. doi:10.1016/j.psychsport.2011.06.004.

Curran, Thomas, Paul R. Appleton, Andrew P. Hill, and Howard K. Hall. 2013. "The Mediating Role of Psychological Need Satisfaction in Relationships between Types of Passion for Sport and Athlete Burnout." *Journal of Sports Sciences* 31 (6): 597–606. doi:10.1080/02640414.2012.742956.

Davids, Keith, Duarte Araújo, Ludovic Seifert, and Dominic Orth. 2015. "An Ecological Dynamics Perspective." In *The Routledge Handbook of Sport Expertise*, edited by Joe Baker and Damian Farrow, 130. London: Routledge.

Dawson, Michael. 2014. "Embedded and Situated Cognition." In *The Routledge Handbook of Embodied Cognition*, edited by Lawrence Shapiro, 59–67. London: Routledge.

Duffy, L. J., and D. P. Hinwood. 1997. "Home Field Advantage: Does Anxiety Contribute?" *Perceptual and Motor Skills* 84 (1): 283–286. doi:10.2466/pms.1997.84.1.283.

Dupont, G., and A. McCall. 2016. "Targeted Systems of the Body for Training." In *Soccer Science: Using Science to Develop Players and Teams*, edited by T. Strudwick, 221–246. Champaign, IL: Human Kinetics.

Ericsson, K. Anders, and N. Charness. 1994. "Expert Performance: Its Structure and Acquisition." *American Psychologist* 49 (8): 725–747.

Ericsson, K. Anders, Ralf T. Krampe, and Clemens Tesch-Romer. 1993. "The Role of Deliberate Practice in the Acquisition of Expert Performance." *Psychological Review* 100 (3): 363–406. doi:10.1037/0033-295X.100.3.363.

Evans, Andrew L., Matthew J. Slater, Martin J. Turner, and Jamie B. Barker. 2013. "Using Personal-Disclosure Mutual-Sharing to Enhance Group Functioning in a Professional Soccer Academy." *Sport Psychologist* 27 (3): 233–243.

Faubert, Jocelyn. 2013. "Professional Athletes Have Extraordinary Skills for Rapidly Learning Complex and Neutral Dynamic Visual Scenes." *Scientific Reports* 3 (January): 1154. doi:10.1038/srep01154.

Faude, O., M. Kellmann, T. Ammann, R. Schnittker, and T. Meyer. 2011. "Seasonal Changes in Stress Indicators in High Level Football." *International Journal of Sports Medicine* 32 (4): 259–265. doi:10.1055/s-0030-1269894.

FIFA. 2001. "FIFA Big Count 2000." *FIFA Communication Divisions*. http://www.fifa.com/mm/document/fifafacts/bcoffsurv/bigcount.statspackage_7024.pdf.

FIFA Marketing and TV. 2002. "2002 FIFA World CupTM TV Coverage." Accessed March 31, 2005. http://www.fifa.com/en/marketing/newmedia/index/0,3509,10,00.html (page discontinued).

Filho, Edson, Gershon Tenenbaum, and Yanyun Yang. 2015. "Cohesion, Team Mental Models, and Collective Efficacy: Towards an Integrated Framework of Team Dynamics in Sport." *Journal of Sports Sciences* 33 (6): 641–653. doi:10.1080/02640414.2014.957714.

Ford, Paul R., Paul Ward, Nicola J. Hodges, and A. Mark Williams. 2009. "The Role of Deliberate Practice and Play in Career Progression in Sport: The Early Engagement Hypothesis." *High Ability Studies* 20 (1): 65–75. doi:10.1080/13598130902860721.

Ford, Paul R., and A. Mark Williams. 2012. "The Developmental Activities Engaged in by Elite Youth Soccer Players Who Progressed to Professional Status Compared to Those Who Did Not." *Psychology of Sport and Exercise* 13 (3): 349–352. doi:10.1016/j.psychsport.2011.09.004.

Gibson, James J. 1966. *The Senses Considered as Perceptual Systems*. Boston: Houghton Mifflin.

Gibson, James J. 1979. *The Ecological Approach to Visual Perception*. London: Psychology Press.

Gilbourne, David, and David Richardson. 2006. "Tales from the Field: Personal Reflections on the Provision of Psychological Support in Professional Soccer." *Psychology of Sport and Exercise* 7 (3): 325–337. doi:10.1016/j.psychsport.2005.04.004.

Gledhill, Adam, and Chris Harwood. 2014. "Developmental Experiences of Elite Female Youth Soccer Players." *International Journal of Sport and Exercise Psychology* 12 (2): 150–165. doi:10.1080/1612197X.2014.880259.

Goumas, Chris. 2014. "Home Advantage in Australian Soccer." *Journal of Science and Medicine in Sport / Sports Medicine Australia* 17 (1): 119–123. doi:10.1016/j.jsams.2013.02.014.

Haugaasen, Mathias, and Geir Jordet. 2012. "Developing Football Expertise: A Football-Specific Research Review." *International Review of Sport and Exercise Psychology* 5 (2): 177–201. doi:10.1080/1750984X.2012.677951.

Haugaasen, Mathias, Tynke Toering, and Geir Jordet. 2014. "From Childhood to Senior Professional Football: A Multi-Level Approach to Elite Youth Football Players' Engagement in Football-Specific Activities." *Psychology of Sport and Exercise* 15 (4): 336–344. doi:10.1016/j.psychsport.2014.02.007.

Hill, Andrew P., Howard K. Hall, Paul R. Appleton, and Stephen A. Kozub. 2008. "Perfectionism and Burnout in Junior Elite Soccer Players: The Mediating Influence of Unconditional Self-Acceptance." *Psychology of Sport and Exercise* 9 (5): 630–644. doi:10.1016/j.psychsport.2007.09.004.

Holt, Nicholas L., and John G. H. Dunn. 2004. "Toward a Grounded Theory of the Psychosocial Competencies and Environmental Conditions Associated with Soccer Success." *Journal of Applied Sport Psychology* 16 (3): 199–219. doi:10.1080/10413200490437949.

Holt, Nicholas L., Tom Mitchell, and Others. 2006. "Talent Development in English Professional Soccer." *International Journal of Sport Psychology* 37 (2/3): 77–98.

Horrocks, David. 2012. "Brains in Their Feet?" *The Psychologist* 25 (1): 88–89.

Hvattum, Lars Magnus. 2015. "Playing on Artificial Turf May Be an Advantage for Norwegian Soccer Teams." *Journal of Quantitative Analysis in Sports* 11 (3): 183–192. doi:10.1515/jqas-2014-0046.

Ivarsson, Andreas, and Urban Johnson. 2010. "Psychological Factors as Predictors of Injuries among Senior Soccer Players: A Prospective Study." *Journal of Sports Science and Medicine* 9 (2): 347–352.

Ivarsson, Andreas, Urban Johnson, and Leslie Podlog. 2013. "Psychological Predictors of Injury Occurrence: A Prospective Investigation of Professional Swedish Soccer Players." *Journal of Sport Rehabilitation* 22 (1): 19–26.

Jordet, Geir. 2005a. "Applied Cognitive Sport Psychology in Team Ball Sports: An Ecological Approach." In *New Approaches to Sport and Exercise Psychology* 30, edited by R. Stelter and K. K. Roessler, 147–174. Aachen, Germany: Meyer and Meyer Sport.

Jordet, Geir. 2005b. "Perceptual Training in Soccer: An Imagery Intervention Study with Elite Players." *Journal of Applied Sport Psychology* 17 (2): 140–156. doi:10.1080/10413200590932452.

Jordet, Geir. 2009a. "When Superstars Flop: Public Status and Choking Under Pressure in International Soccer Penalty Shootouts." *Journal of Applied Sport Psychology* 21 (2): 125–130. doi:10.1080/10413200902777263.

Jordet, Geir. 2009b. "Why Do English Players Fail in Soccer Penalty Shootouts? A Study of Team Status, Self-Regulation, and Choking Under Pressure." *Journal of Sports Sciences* 27 (2): 97–106. doi:10.1080/02640410802509144.

Jordet, Geir. 2016. "Psychology and Elite Soccer Performance." In *Soccer Science: Using Science to Develop Players and Teams*, edited by T. Strudwick, 367–388. Champaign, IL: Human Kinetics.

Jordet, Geir, Jonathan Bloomfield, and Johan Heijmerikx. 2013. "The Hidden Foundation of Field Vision in English Premier League (EPL) Soccer Players." Presentation at MIT Sloan Sport Analytics Conference. http://www.sloansportsconference.com/wp-content/uploads/2013/02/The-hidden-foundation-of-field-vision-in-English-Premier-LeagueEPL-soccer-players.pdf.

Jordet, Geir, and Marije T. Elferink-Gemser. 2012. "Stress, Coping, and Emotions on the World Stage: The Experience of Participating in a Major Soccer Tournament Penalty Shootout." *Journal of Applied Sport Psychology* 24 (1): 73–91. doi:10.1080/10413200.2011.619000.

Jordet, Geir, Marije T. Elferink-Gemser, Koen A. P. M. Lemmink, and Chris Visscher. 2006. "The 'Russian Roulette' of Soccer? An Exploratory Examination of Perceived Control and Anxiety in a Major Tournament Penalty Shootout." *International Journal of Sport Psychology* 37 (2/3): 281–298.

Jordet, Geir, and Esther Hartman. 2008. "Avoidance Motivation and Choking Under Pressure in Soccer Penalty Shootouts." *Journal of Sport and Exercise Psychology* 30 (4): 450–457.

Jordet, Geir, Esther Hartman, and Pieter Jelle Vuijk. 2012. "Team History and Choking Under Pressure in Major Soccer Penalty Shootouts." *British Journal of Psychology* 103 (2): 268–283. doi:10.1111/j.2044-8295.2011.02071.x.

Jordet, Geir, Esther Hartman, Chris Visscher, and Koen A. P. M. Lemmink. 2007. "Kicks from the Penalty Mark in Soccer: The Roles of Stress, Skill, and Fatigue for Kick Outcomes." *Journal of Sports Sciences* 25 (2): 121–129. doi:10.1080/02640410600624020.

Karageorghis, Costas I., and Peter C. Terry. 2010. *Inside Sport Psychology*. Champaign, IL: Human Kinetics.

Littlewood, M. A., and Mark Nesti. 2011. "Making Your Way in the Game: Boundary Situations in England's Professional Football World." In *Critical Essays in Applied Sport Psychology*, edited by D. Gilbourne and M. B. Andersen, 233–249. Champaign, IL: Human Kinetics.

Littlewood, Martin, Chris Mullen, and David Richardson. 2011. "Football Labour Migration: An Examination of the Player Recruitment Strategies of the 'Big Five' European Football Leagues 2004–5 to 2008–9." *Soccer and Society* 12 (6): 788–805. doi:10.1080/14660970.2011.609680.

Loehr, James E. 1990. "Providing Sport Psychology Consulting Services to Professional Tennis Players." *Sport Psychologist* 4 (4): 400–408.

Lombardo, Thomas J. 1987. *The Reciprocity of Perceiver and Environment: The Evolution of James J. Gibson's Ecological Psychology*. Hillsdale, NJ: Lawrence Erlbaum.

McDougall, Michael, Mark Nesti, and David Richardson. 2015. "The Challenges of Sport Psychology Delivery in Elite and Professional Sport: Reflections from Experienced Sport Psychologists." *Sport Psychologist* 29 (3): 265–277. doi:10.1123/tsp.2014-0081.

McGarry, Tim, Peter O'Donoghue, António Jaime de Eira Sampaio, and Jaime Sampaio. 2013. *Routledge Handbook of Sports Performance Analysis*. London: Routledge.

Memmert, Daniel. 2010. "Testing of Tactical Performance in Youth Elite Soccer." *Journal of Sports Science and Medicine* 9 (2): 199–205.

Memmert, Daniel. 2011. "Creativity, Expertise, and Attention: Exploring Their Development and Their Relationships." *Journal of Sports Sciences* 29 (1): 93–102. doi:10.1080/02640414.2010.528014.

Mills, Andrew, Joanne Butt, Ian Maynard, and Chris Harwood. 2012. "Identifying Factors Perceived to Influence the Development of Elite Youth Football Academy Players." *Journal of Sports Sciences* 30 (15): 1593–1604. doi:10.1080/02640414.2012.710753.

Moll, Tjerk, Geir Jordet, and Gert-Jan Pepping. 2010. "Emotional Contagion in Soccer Penalty Shootouts: Celebration of Individual Success Is Associated with Ultimate Team Success." *Journal of Sports Sciences* 28 (9): 983–992. doi:10.1080/02640414.2010.484068.

Morrow, K. 2001. *"It's What's Up Here That Counts": Winning the Mental Game of Soccer*. Champaign, IL: Human Kinetics.

Naito, Eiichi, and Satoshi Hirose. 2014. "Efficient Foot Motor Control by Neymar's Brain." *Frontiers in Human Neuroscience* 8 (August): 594. doi.org/10.3389/fnhum.2014.00594.

Neisser, Ulric. 1967. *Cognitive Psychology*. New York: Appleton-Century-Crofts.

Nesti, Mark. 2010. *Psychology in Football: Working with Elite and Professional Players*. New York: Routledge.

Pain, Matthew, and Chris Harwood. 2009. "Team Building through Mutual Sharing and Open Discussion of Team Functioning." *Sport Psychologist* 23 (4): 523–542.

Pain, Matthew A., and Chris G. Harwood. 2008. "The Performance Environment of the England Youth Soccer Teams: A Quantitative Investigation." *Journal of Sports Sciences* 26 (11): 1157–1169. doi:10.1080/02640410802101835.

Pollard, Richard, and Miguel A. Gomez. 2014. "Components of Home Advantage in 157 National Soccer Leagues Worldwide." *International Journal of Sport and Exercise Psychology* 12 (3): 218–233.

Pollard, Richard, and Gregory Pollard. 2005. "Home Advantage in Soccer: A Review of Its Existence and Causes." *International Journal of Soccer and Science Journal* 3 (1): 28–38.

Prapavessis, Harry, Albert A. Carron, and Kevin S. Spink. 1996. "Team Building in Sport." *International Journal of Sport Psychology* 27 (3): 269–285.

Ravizza, K., and T. Hanson. 1995. *Heads-Up Baseball: Playing the Game One Pitch at a Time*. New York: McGraw-Hill Education.

Reed, Edward S. 1988. *James J. Gibson and the Psychology of Perception*. New Haven, CT: Yale University Press.

Reed, Edward S. 1993. "The Intention to Use a Specific Affordance: A Conceptual Framework for Psychology." In *Development in Context: Acting and Thinking in Specific Environments*, edited by R. Wozniak and K. Fisscher, 45–76. Hillsdale, NJ: Lawrence Erlbaum.

Reed, Edward S. 1996a. *Encountering the World: Toward an Ecological Psychology*. New York: Oxford University Press.

Reed, Edward S. 1996b. *The Necessity of Experience*. New Haven, CT: Yale University Press.

Reed, Edward S. 1997. *From Soul to Mind: The Emergence of Psychology, from Erasmus Darwin to William James*. New Haven, CT: Yale University Press.

Richardson, David, Martin Littlewood, Mark Nesti, and Luke Benstead. 2012. "An Examination of the Migratory Transition of Elite Young European Soccer Players to the English Premier League." *Journal of Sports Sciences* 30 (15): 1605–1618. doi:10.1080/02640414.2012.733017.

Roca, Andre, Paul R. Ford, Allistair P. McRobert, and A. Mark Williams. 2011. "Identifying the Processes Underpinning Anticipation and Decision-Making in a Dynamic Time-Constrained Task." *Cognitive Processing* 12 (3): 301–310. doi:10.1007/s10339-011-0392-1.

Rotella, Bob. 1996. *Golf Is Not a Game of Perfect*. New York: Simon and Schuster.

Schmidt, Richard A, and Timothy Lee. 2011. *Motor Control and Learning: A Behavioral Emphasis*. 5th ed. Champaign, IL: Human Kinetics.

Staufenbiel, Kathrin, Babett Lobinger, and Bernd Strauss. 2015. "Home Advantage in Soccer: A Matter of Expectations, Goal Setting and Tactical Decisions of Coaches?" *Journal of Sports Sciences* 33 (18): 1932–1941. doi:10.1080/02640414.2015.1018929.

Tedesqui, Rafael A. B., and Terry Orlick. 2015. "Brazilian Elite Soccer Players: Exploring Attentional Focus in Performance Tasks and Soccer Positions." *Sport Psychologist* 29 (1): 41–50. doi.org/10.1123/tsp.2014-0007.

Toering, T. T., M. T. Elferink-Gemser, G. Jordet, and C. Visscher. 2009. "Self-Regulation and Performance Level of Elite and Non-Elite Youth Soccer Players." *Journal of Sports Sciences* 27 (14): 1509–1517. doi:10.1080/02640410903369919.

Toering, Tynke, Marije Elferink-Gemser, Geir Jordet, Casper Jorna, Gert-Jan Pepping, and Chris Visscher. 2011. "Self-Regulation of Practice Behavior among Elite Youth Soccer Players: An Exploratory Observation Study." *Journal of Applied Sport Psychology* 23 (1): 110–128. doi:10.1080/10413200.2010.534544.

Toering, Tynke, and Geir Jordet. 2015. "Self-Control in Professional Soccer Players." *Journal of Applied Sport Psychology* 27 (3): 335–350. doi:10.1080/10413200.2015.1010047.

Van Yperen, Nico W. 2009. "Why Some Make It and Others Do Not: Identifying Psychological Factors That Predict Career Success in Professional Adult Soccer." *Sport Psychologist* 23 (3): 317–329.

Van Yperen, Nico W., and Joan L. Duda. 1999. "Goal Orientations, Beliefs about Success, and Performance Improvement among Young Elite Dutch Soccer Players." *Scandinavian Journal of Medicine and Science in Sports* 9 (6): 358–364. doi:10.1111/j.1600-0838.1999.tb00257.x.

Verburgh, Lot, Erik J. A. Scherder, Paul A. M. van Lange, and Jaap Oosterlaan. 2014. "Executive Functioning in Highly Talented Soccer Players." Edited by José César Perales. *PLoS ONE* 9 (3). doi:10.1371/journal.pone.0091254.

Vestberg, Torbjorn, Roland Gustafson, Liselotte Maurex, Martin Ingvar, and Predrag Petrovic. 2012. "Executive Functions Predict the Success of Top-Soccer Players." Edited by Antonio Verdejo García. *PLoS ONE* 7 (4): e34731. doi:10.1371/journal.pone.0034731.

Voight, Mike, and John Callaghan. 2001. "A Team Building Intervention Program: Application and Evaluation with Two University Soccer Teams." *Journal of Sport Behavior* 24 (4): 420.

Ward, Paul, Nicola J. Hodges, Janet L. Starkes, and Mark A. Williams. 2007. "The Road to Excellence: Deliberate Practice and the Development of Expertise." *High Ability Studies* 18 (2): 119–153. doi:10.1080/13598130701709715.

Weinberg, Robert S., and Daniel Gould. 2015. *Foundations of Sport and Exercise Psychology*. 6th ed. Champaign, IL: Human Kinetics.

Williams, A. Mark, and Keith Davids. 1995. "Declarative Knowledge in Sport: A by-Product of Experience or a Characteristic of Expertise?" *Journal of Sport and Exercise* 17 (3): 259–275.

Williams, A. Mark, and Keith Davids. 1998. "Visual Search Strategy, Selective Attention, and Expertise in Soccer." *Research Quarterly for Exercise and Sport* 69 (2): 111–128. doi:10.1080/02701367.1998.10607677.

Williams, A. Mark, Keith Davids, Les Burwitz, and John G. Williams. 1994. "Visual Search Strategies in Experienced and Inexperienced Soccer Players." *Research Quarterly for Exercise and Sport* 65 (2): 127–135. doi:10.1080/02701367.1994.10607607.

Withagen, Rob, Harjo J. de Poel, Duarte Araújo, and Gert-Jan Pepping. 2012. "Affordances Can Invite Behavior: Reconsidering the Relationship between Affordances and Agency." *New Ideas in Psychology* 30 (2): 250–258. doi:10.1016/j.newideapsych.2011.12.003.

II Theories of Skill and Skill Disruption: Awareness, Automaticity, and Control

5 The Many Threats of Self-Consciousness: Embodied Approaches to Choking under Pressure in Sensorimotor Skills

Massimiliano L. Cappuccio, Rob Gray, Denise M. Hill,
Christopher Mesagno, and Thomas H. Carr

1 Introduction

The phenomenon of choking under pressure (hereafter called "choking") has continued to fascinate sport practitioners, researchers (Beilock 2011), and people from many other backgrounds and pursuits. Each year seems to bring a new well-publicized example labeled a "choke," with perhaps the most recent being Jordan Spieth surrendering a five-stroke lead on the final nine holes of the 2016 US Masters golf tournament (O'Connor 2016). In this chapter we offer a critical review of the scientific research and the philosophic evaluations that bear on this very phenomenon.

According to Baumeister (1984), choking epitomizes a paradox many practitioners are familiar with: the situations that overemphasize the expectation to produce excellent results are those that most likely create below-standard performances. Choking seems to occur exactly when one desires the most to succeed, and that is why it is often feared by expert athletes, like a curse or a malicious spell. This phenomenon is usually construed by psychologists as the expert athletes' incapability to successfully perform actions that would otherwise be routine because of psychological factors such as increased desire to do well, increased anxiety and tension, and the changes in performance processes resulting from such increases (Carr 2015). However, the exact definition of choking varies significantly across different schools (reviewed by Christensen, Sutton, and McIlwain 2015), and there is no universal agreement about its nature and causes (e.g., Mesagno and Hill 2013), which relate to a multifaceted complexity of cognitive, motivational, and emotional dynamics that have been studied largely, but ultimately without consensus, by sport psychologists (Hill et al. 2010a; Mesagno, Guekes, and Larkin 2015).

This does not mean that no progress was ever achieved by psychological research or that our knowledge of choking has not improved. In fact, over the past thirty years, researchers have made several advances, including designing clever manipulations for creating pressure in the lab, developing theories about the cognitive processes that underlie choking, and using multi-method approaches that assess gaze behavior, movement kinematics, or brain activity along with performance outcomes (reviewed in Beilock and Gray 2007; Hill et al. 2010b; Gray 2011).

On the surface, these research efforts have led to a broadly accepted explanation for choking in sports (and sensorimotor skills more generally), an explanation that permeates both research journals and popular culture: namely, that choking occurs when an experienced athlete or skilled performer becomes "self-conscious" (Baumeister 1984). Critically re-elaborating Baumeister's idea and attempting to update his seminal approach to choking, this chapter aims to describe various levels and forms of self-consciousness (perceptual, emotional, motivational, narrative), exploring how they causally link to performance disruption and its underlying psychological dynamics.

Our account does not hide or minimize the difficulties associated with a reductive interpretation of the causal relationship between self-consciousness and performance: although broadly accepted, the explanation of choking based on Baumeister's notion of self-consciousness has also attracted a number of important and well-argued criticisms. If this chapter combines different views and discourses about choking, it is exactly to demonstrate that most of these objections apply only to the "one size fits all" approach that for too long has dominated choking research, propagating a reductive interpretation of the notion of self-consciousness.

We contend that such interpretation is misleading and does not capture the real potential contained in Baumeister's key intuition. Self-consciousness is not a monolithic, universal causal factor of performance disruption (because self-consciousness comes in different forms and degrees), and certainly is not the kind of factor that could *directly* cause performance disruption (because strategic thought and various regulatory processes are interposed between self-consciousness and the performance outcome). In other words, the way in which self-consciousness affects expert skills does not depend on a single linear causal chain, but is articulated at multiple parallel levels and can take several causal pathways depending on various possible interactions between intermediate variables.

A pluralistic and ecumenic approach is therefore indispensable to recognizing how multifaceted and layered the causal relationship between self-consciousness and performance disruption is. Ignoring this complexity, the bulk of previous research has failed to account for individual traits, perceptions, capabilities, and limitations of performers when understanding how they respond to pressure. Our complaint is best exemplified by how researchers identify whether "a choke" has occurred: namely, identification is based mainly, often purely, on extrinsic, objective criteria (there is some form of pressure present and the performance level is below the "typical" non-pressure level) without taking into account the individual characteristics of the performer, the phenomenology of his or her performative experience, or the situated circumstances of her or his actions (Mesagno and Hill 2013; Mesagno and Beckmann 2017).

The reductive, linear interpretation of self-consciousness as a universal trigger mechanism for choking stands in stark contrast to the rapidly growing "embodied" approach to perception and cognition in sport (reviewed in Gray 2014). The embodied approach to cognition (Varela, Thompson, and Rosch 1991) utilizes notions and methods that sport psychology research inherited from the traditions of ecological psychology (with the Gibsonian concepts of "affordances" and "direct perception"; see Gibson 1966, 1979) and developmental psychology (with the preeminence attributed to "enactive learning" by the Piagetian theories of early cognitive development, e.g., Bruner 1966). Embodied cognition applies these notions to explain how the reach and the very nature of mental functions largely depend on the details of their physical implementation and by the conditions of engagement and interaction offered to a situated agent by her or his environment. This means emphasizing the constitutive role played by fundamental forms of cognition (i.e., perceptual and motoric habits based on the consolidation of sensorimotor feedback loops) in scaffolding and shaping higher, more intellectual forms of cognition (i.e., propositional and conceptual competences based on explicit judgment and inference, logico-symbolic and linguistic representation, etc.)

In sport psychology, the embodied approach to cognition highlights that even "low-level" perceptual processes, like perceiving the size of a ball, seem to influence—and, reciprocally, to be influenced by—the individual capabilities and current state of the athlete: the perceptual, physical, emotional, and motivational condition of the athlete, as well as his epistemic, experiential, and cognitive situation.

We believe an embodied approach to choking can help see how the mechanisms that disrupt performance through self-consciousness are not just linear and top-down (as if choking was always originated by erroneous meta-representations and unnecessary beliefs accumulated in the mind of the athlete), but tend to emerge contextually, from the reciprocal interaction of complex and heterogeneous contingencies that depend largely on the athlete's perception of her own body and the environment in which the athlete with her body is situated (DeCaro et al. 2011 offers a similar suggestion). These considerations extend, for example, to how the current condition of the performer—on a roll or in a slump (Gray and Allsop 2013), tired or full of energy (Schnall, Zadra, and Proffitt 2010), physically burdened or feeling free and light (Bhalla and Proffitt 1999)—might matter to performance.

"This is embodied cognition in the raw," say Christensen, Sutton, and McIlwain (2015, 254), referring to a dramatic and unexpected episode of performance impairment in cricket, "with emotion and personality, kinesthesis and physiology, discipline and drives all affected together and on show" (254). In this spirit, we propose it is time to "embody" choking research by considering not just the perceptual and attentional dimension of self-consciousness that a performer brings to sensorimotor activity, but also the emotional, motivational, and narrative dimensions of self-consciousness and the particular ways in which each of these dimensions separately, and all of them as a whole, influence how the performer perceives and handles pressure.

For a long time, the research on choking has been dominated by the scientific approaches that impute performance disruption to the misallocation of the attentional resources available to the system (for a review, see Jackson and Beilock 2008). In the last few years, however, various explanatory narratives have focused on individual experiential circumstances, team dynamics, motivational backgrounds, and personal psychological profiles (e.g., Jordet 2009, 2010; Mesagno, Harvey, and Janelle 2012; Mesagno and Hill 2013; Carr 2015; Geukes et al. 2017). We recognize the complementarity of these approaches, and the deep interconnection between the causal factors that they study.

That is why, after some preliminary clarifications (part 2), the first half of the chapter (parts 3 to 7) reviews the experiments suggesting that performance disruption is engendered by perceptual and motoric self-consciousness (i.e., the condition in which the athlete overscrutinizes certain aspects of his own movements and actions, and their control, in the attempt to improve them), and the theories that try to make sense of these empirical results. The second half of the chapter (parts 8 to 14) explores a different aspect of self-consciousness, linked to how the psychological, motivational, and emotional backdrop of the athlete's experience under pressure influences self-presentation and self-esteem—an influence that can negatively affect performance through the mediation of disruptive personal narratives and social constructions of identity.

2 Some Preliminary Clarifications about Consciousness and Expertise

Baumeister (1982, 1984) identified a correlation between the performers' tendency to choke and their "dispositional self-consciousness." This full-fledged notion of self-consciousness aims primarily to describe the general inclination to see oneself as a socially evaluable object, or as psychological susceptibility to public judgment (see Mesagno, Harvey, and Janelle 2011). But Baumeister's theory can be applied to and account for multiple, partial dimensions of self-consciousness, including not only the sphere of personal identity and the intersubjective dynamics underlying narrative self-construction, but also more fundamental mechanisms of emotional awareness and reflective control of action. We recognize the mark of self-consciousness in every situation in which a cognitive system engaged in a challenging task seeks to gain explicit personal-level knowledge about its own psychophysical processes, states, and components: this happens when the system closely monitors its operations to access on-line information considered necessary to improve the precision and volume of its behavioral output.

This notion is a valid guide for a comprehensive study of performance disruption. Any notion of self-consciousness less multifaceted and articulated would be unable to capture all the nuanced meanings of skill and would inevitably fail to account for a complex phenomenon like choking. That is why rationalistic and aprioristic notions of "self-consciousness," mesmerized by the apparent contrast between abstract categories such as "thought" and "action," have recently attracted objections and criticisms. In particular, Dreyfus's model of skill acquisition (Dreyfus and Dreyfus 1980, often likened to Fitts and Posner's own model, 1967) recently became the polemical target of an interdisciplinary controversy concerning whether or not reflective awareness is a necessary and/or sufficient condition for choking, and whether expert, skillful execution of action allows explicit control or not (see Cappuccio 2015 for a collection of critical views; see also Breivik 2007, 2013; Montero 2010; Sutton et al. 2011; Toner, Montero, and Moran 2014, 2015).

For a long time, Dreyfus's model has represented the most influential phenomenological account of expert action as an unreflective, semiconscious, embodied routine. According to Dreyfus's model, a practitioner becomes an expert if and only if the explicit cognitive efforts necessary to control her actions decrease, when the execution of complex movements is automatized. Dreyfus has mainly been criticized for his nonrepresentational theory of unreflective action, or "absorbed coping," which is a corollary of his view on skill development as progressive automatization of motor habits (Dreyfus 2002). Absorbed coping explicitly states that proceduralized skillful activities not only *can* (characteristically), but *must* (necessarily) be "mindless" and "non-conscious," and that a state of decreased self-awareness is indispensable to deliver expert performance. That is why absorbed coping theory is associated with the categorical claim that conscious control ("reflective thought") and expert performance ("skillful action") are mutually exclusive. Despite the sophisticated anti-representationalist argumentation provided by Dreyfus, and his original phenomenology of embodiment (Dreyfus 2012), this claim is considered unpersuasive by many practitioners, psychologists, and philosophers, as it seems to deny the reflective dimension of expertise, which typically includes skillful capabilities of strategic planning and creative improvisation.

The debate concerning absorbed coping[1] is relevant to our discussion of choking insofar as some of the criticisms raised against Dreyfus's theory have been extended to Baumeister's, which represents the common denominator of the analyses conducted in this chapter. In fact, both Dreyfus's and Baumeister's theories can be categorized as "self-focus" approaches to performance disruption, as they agree that some forms of awareness of one's own condition and processes can damage performance. However, the two theories agree neither on the particular forms of self-consciousness responsible for choking, nor on the underlying cognitive mechanisms that cause skill disruption. Appreciating these nuanced differences is fundamental to correctly construing the complex relationship between peak performance and self-consciousness. What Christensen, Sutton, and McIlwain (2015) wrote about this relationship is insightful, and should be agreed on by all the supporters of Baumeister's theory:

> Skill experience is rich and various, and ... there are many forms of self-focus and self-awareness. Some of these can be damaging while other forms may be essential to good performance for some people in some contexts.... There are forms of "self-focus" which are distinct from body-focused attention, from technique-focused attention, and from skill or task focus. Likewise, ... not all forms of embodied self-awareness need involve full-scale self-consciousness. (255)

Accordingly, the primary goal of the researchers investigating the causes of choking should be to concretely distinguish between various types and degrees of self-awareness in skillful activity and empirically identify which attentional foci are detrimental to optimal action, when, and why. Such concrete analyses, more than abstract inferences based on an aprioristic definition of consciousness, can shed light on the complex, articulated involvement of explicit reflective knowledge in the impairment of skillful performance.

These analyses start with sensorimotor control: that is, the most fundamental embodied dimension of self-consciousness. That is why in the next sections we introduce an approach to skill disruption inspired by Baumeister's theory that—we believe—can effectively account for how motoric and perceptual self-consciousness typically causes underperformance. This approach seems immune from many of the criticisms that absorbed coping theory had to face because, unlike Dreyfus's theory, it presupposes neither that expert performance is necessarily "mindless" (or the performer unaware of her actions), nor that proceduralized execution necessarily excludes all forms of reflection and conscious control. On the contrary, we will see that the automatic execution of proceduralized action routines can be implemented during peak performance with the concurrent involvement of reflective strategic control, consistently with a dual cognitive architecture governed by virtually independent causal and informational systems (as theorized, for example, by Evans and Stanovich 2013).

3 Self-Consciousness as the Root of Sensorimotor Skill Disruption: Attentional Focus Theory and Execution Focus Theory

Let us investigate more closely the perceptual and motoric dimension of self-consciousness (i.e., the immediate awareness of one's own actions as they are executed). This dimension is captured by two questions that are considered crucial by both practitioners and researchers: What sensorimotor aspects of one's performance are relevant to choking? And, why does monitoring them too closely disrupt one's skills? A branch of the research on choking builds on Baumeister's key intuition to answer these questions. This branch has produced at least three well-elaborated theories, which have gained wide credence among sport psychologists during the last decades.

1. According to *reinvestment theory*, proposed by Masters and colleagues (Masters 1992; Masters, Polman, and Hammond 1993), "Automated motor processes can be disrupted if they are run using consciously accessed, task-relevant declarative knowledge to control the mechanics of the movements on-line" (Masters and Maxwell 2008, 160).
2. Resonating with Masters's seminal investigation, *execution focus theory* (EFT), proposed by Sian Beilock and colleagues, asserts that choking is caused by a "skill focus" or "execution focus" (e.g., Beilock and Carr 2001; Beilock et al. 2002; Beilock, Bertenthal, et al. 2008), which occurs when the athletes implement the cognitive goal structure of the task to be accomplished through a step-by-step level of explicit control.
3. According to *attentional focus theory* (AFT), proposed by Gabriele Wulf and colleagues, performance disruption is caused by an "internal focus" of attention (e.g., Wulf et al. 2000; Wulf and Prinz 2001), which occurs when the athletes exert explicit control over their body parts movements.

Here we focus only on AFT and EFT; reinvestment theory will be examined in part 13 (dedicated to the personality and psychology of frequent "chokers"). We must remark that, while both AFT and EFT impute performance disruption to explicit attention to one's own performance, some subtle differences characterize these two theories of performance disruption, not without implications for the etiology, the diagnosis, and the prognosis of choking.

To begin with, AFT and EFT do not fully agree on what counts as "self-components" of one's performance, and what those components are to be contrasted with. For AFT, internal foci comprise one's own body's movements, one's own body parts, and in general anything "near" the performing subject and close to the production of the movement; in turn, external foci comprise any unintentional effect of the movement, the movement's target or intended transformation in the environment, the tools or effectors moved by one's body to achieve one's goal and, in general, anything that is "far" from the performing subject and beyond the direct production of the movement, including elements in the environment that are not affected by one's actions. Note that, in some cases, the subject's whole body counts as an external focus, while singled-out body parts count as internal focus.

EFT, in contrast, claims that what damages performance is attention to execution of the component movements: that is, any form of explicit control that, analyzing a complex action into its constitutive sensorimotor elements, hinders the fluidity and automaticity of well-practiced routines. These two definitions often match, but not always: for example, according to AFT, whereas attention to wrist and shoulder movements during a golf-putting task is definitely an internal focus of attention (and as such is likely to decrease performance), attention to the tool (putter) used during the same task counts as an external focus, because the swing movement of the club is just an effect of one's body movements (Wulf et al. 2000; Wulf 2013). On the contrary, according to EFT, both attention to the body parts and attention to the club swing represent an execution focus, as they both imply an analysis of the constitutive elements of the familiar putting routine.[2]

Another difference between EFT and AFT is that they apply to partially different sets of activities and performers. For AFT, internal focus is universally detrimental to performance (Wulf 2015), as it systematically disrupts one's actions: (1) during both practice/learning and peak-performance conditions; (2) in both novices and experts (regardless of whether the activity has been fully automatized or not); and (3) independent of the degree of involvement of working memory.

EFT is more nuanced, as it claims that an execution focus is more detrimental than a distracting cue or secondary task only to experts in peak-performance conditions (not to novices rehearsing during practice or trying to perform as well as they can in a test), and only for automatized sensorimotor activities that do not heavily rely on working memory. EFT distinguishes between cognitive systems that do and do not utilize working memory to produce their output: after the proceduralization of the related sensorimotor skill (e.g., golf putting), the production of highly automatized sensorimotor routines involves no working memory; on the contrary, concurrent secondary tasks (e.g., memorizing/recognizing certain tones in a series) might involve a high usage of working memory. Regardless of their respective difficulty, the two tasks recruit two virtually independent systems that do not interfere with one another, as they utilize heterogeneous types of cognitive resources.

Accordingly, per EFT, the notion of choking as self-consciousness does not apply in the same way to skilled activities that necessarily require working memory to function properly, such as mathematical computation (Beilock, Bertenthal, et al. 2004; Beilock 2008b): in the specific case of dual tasks involving *only* activities of this kind, performance can be damaged more by distraction or cognitive overload than execution focus, because both tasks (whether involving automatized routines or not) draw cognitive resources from the same basin and will subsequently suffer from its depletion.

4 The Self-Monitoring/Execution-Focus Approach

In spite of these differences, the explanatory stories provided by AFT and EFT overlap significantly. Both theories (as well as reinvestment theory) can be considered varieties of an overarching approach to choking that we call "self-monitoring/execution-focus." This approach, broadly construed, maintains that control of performance execution by a well-practiced and highly integrated procedure (i.e., an automated motor program that can do the job on its own, without explicit intentional intervention on its operations) should be preferred to both internal focus and execution focus—when such a procedure is available: a well-practiced procedure is generally more fluent and reliable, presents fewer choice points at which the flow of performance can be interrupted or misdirected, and hence is less likely to lead to choking.

The mechanisms deemed important by the self-monitoring/execution-focus approach to choking are illustrated by Castaneda and Gray (2007) in a study of baseball batting. This study documented how, in a batting simulation, the performances of college baseball players were disrupted by four different attentional strategies, corresponding to four dual-task conditions: two strategies involve attention to skill execution (attention to one's own hand movements and attention to one's bat's movements, respectively), while the other two strategies involve attention to the external environment (attention to a series of tones, unrelated to the batting task, and attention to when the ball leaves the bat, respectively). The performance of expert players was damaged significantly more by the first two kinds of instructions, while the novices suffered more in the other two conditions. According to the authors, the study proves "that the optimal focus of attention for highly skilled batters is one that does not disrupt proceduralized knowledge and permits attention to the perceptual effect of the action, whereas the optimal focus of attention for less-skilled batters is one that allows attention to the step-by-step execution of the swing [including both attention to body movements and attention to the tool being moved]" (60).

Thus, for an experienced athlete attempting to perform his or her absolute best when executing a highly practiced act of sensorimotor skill under pressure, attention to self/execution (control and movement of the specific body parts involved in carrying out the action, or specific motions of a tool being used to implement the action) is less detrimental to performance than attention directed beyond the body parts moving and the tool being used (like the movement of the water generated by one's swimming). That is, if attention is directed toward the perceptual consequences of executing the action (what changed in the external environment that is relevant to my ultimate goal, and did it change for the better or for the worse?), then the damage to performance is smaller or less likely to occur. And (perhaps more surprising), even attention directed toward something completely irrelevant simply to occupy the conscious, intentional mind (e.g., singing a song to oneself, monitoring through headphones for a target in a stream of tones or words), thereby keeping conscious interventions and attempts at control occupied and out of the way of the proceduralized motor program, is less detrimental than attention to one's own bodily movements or movements of the tool one is using (as examples, see the experimental evidence collected by Mesagno, Marchant, and Morris 2009, testing for musical competences, and Gray 2004, testing for tones recognition).

5 An Opposite Explanation of Choking: The Distraction/Overload Approach versus the Self-Monitoring/Execution-Focus Approach

The self-monitoring/execution-focus approach is not the only cognitive theory of choking based on misallocation of attention: the main alternative to it within the same domain of explanation is represented by the distraction/overload approach to choking. These two approaches represent almost completely antithetical paradigms, as they respectively characterize choking as a form of *self-monitoring* (and a resulting focus on step-by-step *execution*: see Baumeister 1984; Beilock and Carr 2001; Wulf and Prinz 2001; Beilock, Kulp, et al. 2004) or a form of *distraction* (typically associated with *overload* of cognitive capacities, see Wine 1971). As previously mentioned, the self-monitoring/execution-focus approach imputes choking to the disruption of habitual motor routines that would be fluid and spontaneous if they were not hindered by the explicit, reflective control of the details of the execution. The distraction/overload approach, in contrast, imputes the negative effects of choking to the intrusion of external competing attentional stimuli or the overflow of demands on cognitive resources (caused, for example, by recurrent negative thoughts or worries). These two models differ remarkably because they identify opposite causes for choking: that is, either the excess or the lack of attention to action execution, respectively. But they also differ because they recommend contrary remedies to choking, presuppose discordant phenomenologies of skillful experience, and generate conflicting predictions on performance disruption.

One of the reasons both approaches are still popular is that each of them seems capable of telling sport scientists at least a part of the whole story about choking. The predictions generated by each approach within its own frame of reference have been tested empirically and confirmed in controlled laboratory settings using quantitative methodologies. We focus mainly on the studies supporting the self-monitoring/execution-focus model of choking, as they are particularly numerous and compelling and have been representing a significant stimulus for the whole scientific debate of the last fifteen years. Most of this debate revolved around the repeated attempts to either confirm or disprove the laboratory research that Beilock and her colleagues have conducted to investigate the formation and the application of the habitual skills that—per their theory—choking disrupts (for a review, see Jackson, Beilock, and Kinrade 2013).

In particular, three major empirical results collected by the researchers corroborate the self-monitoring/execution-focus model while simultaneously exposing the limits of the distraction/overload theory. These results suggest that performance disruption of highly practiced sensorimotor skills correlates more with the extent of attempts to explicitly control and/or monitor one's own component movements than with the degree of cognitive effort or working memory usage requested by the task.

1. Skill-focus instructions (i.e., attention instructions that emphasize the component processes of the performance, such as "keep the knees bent"), as well as skill-focused dual tasks (i.e., dual-task conditions in which the secondary task demands attentive analysis of the primary motor task, as under instructions like "keep the club head straight as you swing and say 'straight' when the club hits the ball" or "say when the swing movement is finished") damage the performance of experts much more than other kinds of instructions or dual-task conditions that do not solicit execution-monitoring (e.g., golf putting while trying to identify each occurrence of a target tone or word in a series played over headphones, see, e.g., Beilock and Carr 2001). This effect is not accounted for by distraction/overload theories of choking: such theories justify the opposite prediction, as they suggest that athletes are more likely to underperform when external stimuli compete with the task at hand, preventing the subject from concentrating on it (as in split-attention dual-task conditions with an extraneous target). That is why only the execution-focus theory, not the distraction/overload theory, explains why performance is damaged by conditions of focused

attention (when the athletes try hard to maintain total concentration on their task, as during a competition or tournament—i.e., the kind of situation in which choking most often occurs).

2. Expert performers are better at making skill-focused judgments when under pressure (e.g., Gray 2004). Namely, expert baseball players who bat under skill-focused dual-task conditions experience a more accentuated decrease in their primary task (motor performance) and a concurrent improvement in their secondary task (judgment about their primary task), when they perform in conditions of stress. This suggests that in situations of psychological distress and worry for one's own performance (prompted by social pressure and monetary incentives), attention tends to target the procedural components of one's movements (step-by-step analysis): consequently, the fluid execution of one's habitual action is disrupted while the judgment on those very actions becomes more accurate. The existence of this causal correlation is consistent with the self-monitoring/execution-focus theory and contributes to complete its explanatory paradigm, as it links the functional effects of choking to its psychological and contextual background. On the other hand, the same correlation does not find any justification within the distraction/overload theory, which supports the inverse type of prediction (i.e., higher attention to one's own component movements is supposed to increase the overall motor performances while reducing one's judgment capabilities for extraneous stimuli, not for task activities).
3. Distraction/overload theories struggle to explain why distractors and concurrent secondary tasks are consistently and successfully used as therapeutic interventions on athletes that are particularly prone to choke. Despite the heavier cognitive burden, the experts' performance is improved by those expedients that prevent them from attending to the details of their own movements (Jackson and Beilock 2008). This is achieved by redirecting their attention to external foci (Jackson, Ashford, and Norsworthy 2006, consistent with the attentional focus theories; see Wulf and Su 2007) or reducing the time they have available to perform (Beilock, Bertenthal, et al. 2004; Beilock, Bertenthal, et al. 2008). The fact that experts do not display a speed-accuracy trade-off in spite of the manipulations of the time constraints—indeed, they display the reverse—is particularly significant because it once again frustrates the predictions of the distraction/overload theories: the performance of experts is damaged much more by self-paced action instructions ("putt only when you think you are ready") than by fast action instructions ("putt as quickly as possible"). Distraction/overload theories cannot account for this result, as they support the opposite prediction: they assume that the performance level decreases when the

cognitive load increases, and that the cognitive resources are exhausted faster when the same task has to be processed in a shorter time. Self-monitoring/execution-focus theories, in turn, are well positioned to explain this result because they assume that the performance level depends on automatic routines, and automatic routines are damaged by attention instructions (which explicitly solicit execution-focus), not by speed instructions (which, in turn, facilitate automatic action routines; see Beilock, Bertenthal, et al. 2004).

Taken together, these results suggest that the disruption of the fluid course of familiar automatized routines is due to self-monitoring and/or execution focus, not to the exhaustion of working memory (as confirmed by the fact that even secondary tasks that heavily rely on working memory do not significantly affect the sensorimotor performances of the experts). Self/execution focus impairs the normal course of skillful actions not because it increases the computational burden, but because it decomposes the habitual action routines into disconnected segments and clumsy step-by-step procedures, preventing fluid and adaptive on-line control. That is why choking is occasionally characterized as "paralysis by analysis" (Jackson and Beilock 2008).

It is useful to remark that the execution focus component of self-monitoring/execution-focus theory has another advantage over both distraction/overload theories and also attentional focus theory taken by itself: execution focus theory seems in a better position to explain why choking is skill-level specific, or—in other words—why it threatens expert sport people while sparing novices (e.g., Beilock, Bertenthal, et al. 2004).[3] Split attention (dual tasks that do not involve execution focus) and fast action conditions (speed instructions) do not significantly damage the performances of expert athletes performing well-practiced sensorimotor skills, whereas novices experience a drop in their performance exactly under such conditions. On the contrary, skill-focus conditions (attention to movement execution or accuracy instructions) do not significantly decrease the performance of novices, while they can severely damage the performance of experts. In other words, distraction and heavy cognitive loads negatively affect the novices more than the experts, while self-monitoring and execution focus negatively affect the experts more than the novices. Self-monitoring/execution-focus theory can account for this inverted pattern of skill disruption in novices and experts because it assumes that only experts have automatized their motor routines, which is why only experts can experience a significant decrease in their performance when their motor routines are disrupted by execution focus. Distraction/overload theories cannot rely on an explanation of this kind, as they presuppose that choking depends on the exhaustion of the general cognitive resources available to the system (working memory), although there are no reasons to believe that experts have less cognitive resources than novices.

6 Objections and Challenges for the Self-Monitoring/Execution-Focus Approach

Despite its many merits, dissatisfaction with the self-monitoring/execution-focus approach to choking has been expressed on multiple levels. First, although the bulk of quantitative evidence from laboratory research supports the self-monitoring/execution-focus theory (Beilock and Gray 2007; Beilock 2011; Gray 2011), this explanation seems to be highly inconsistent with studies of athletes' experiences using qualitative methods (e.g., Hill et al. 2009; Oudejans et al. 2011).

Second, doubts have been raised (e.g., Toner and Moran 2015; Toner, Montero, and Moran 2016; Montero, Toner, and Moran, this volume) as to whether attention can be clearly dichotomized into internal states (i.e., exclusively focusing on the movements of one's own body or on the steps of how one is using a tool) versus external states (i.e., exclusively focusing on the goal-directed outcome of the movement or whether a goal is being achieved). The partial mismatch discussed earlier between internal focus and execution focus in describing the conditions that trigger choking reflects this difficulty.

Third, the ecological validity of laboratory studies that try to extrapolate results from the pressure induced by a small monetary reward to that from winning a major sporting event has been questioned (e.g., Christensen et al. 2015; Mesagno, Harvey, and Janelle 2011). Skeptics claim that laboratory experimentation inevitably fails to reproduce the pressure-filled environment of real competition in which choking typically occurs (Christensen, Sutton, and McIlwain 2015; Hill et al. 2010a). If this attribution to laboratory experimentation is correct, then the decreases in performance artificially produced under laboratory conditions might have little or nothing to do with the emotionally catastrophic effects engendered by choking in real-life competitions (or at best imitate them in only a very pale fashion).

That is why (fourth) it has been proposed that much of the supporting research has investigated "underperformance" rather than "choking," and that additional definitory efforts will be necessary to specifically characterize the intrinsic psychological features of choking to distinguish this phenomenon from other forms of performance disruption (Mesagno and Hill 2013; see also Carr 2015, for a discussion).

Finally, and perhaps most importantly, despite some efforts to relate individual personality traits to choking (e.g., Masters 1992; Otten 2009; Geukes et al. 2012; Geukes et al. 2017), in many ways we are apparently no closer to answering a central question:

Are there really "chokers" and "pressure players," and if so, why do some athletes fail in high pressure situations while others thrive?

These objections reach into the theoretical core of the self-monitoring/execution-focus approach to choking. The main inference underlying this theory is that performance anxiety typically solicits internal focus and/or execution focus in athletes during competition. Internal focus and/or execution focus, in turn, are likely to disrupt the continuous flow of automatic action by breaking its holistic and highly organic structure into an unnaturally detached, mechanical array of inflexibly juxtaposed, discrete kinematic components. This segmentation slows performance, makes it disjointed, and introduces many transition points from one component to the next at which planning and implementation errors can originate.

But this inference is not universally accepted; some researchers explicitly deny that anxiety is causally linked to self-monitoring, internal focus, or execution focus and argue that none of these is related to a consistent decrease in performance (e.g., Montero 2014, 2016; Montero, Toner, and Moran, this volume). This objection is accompanied by phenomenological accounts and qualitative reports suggesting that explicit control is not only possible but necessary to successfully complete many sport tasks, insofar as body awareness (including attention to one's own posture and movements) is needed to optimize action efficacy, effectively strategize, and make appropriate decisions during complex interactive sport activities (Sutton 2007; Toner and Moran 2015; Montero 2016; Birch, Fusche Moe, and Breivik, this volume), including not just game performance but training and repair after mistakes or slumps (Carr 2015).

Overall, these objections blame the self-monitoring/execution-focus theories of choking for assuming a simplistic notion of expertise, one that emphasizes the velocity and fluidity of routine skillful actions executed in familiar situations but does not recognize that expert skills are also characterized by superior capabilities of decision making, problem solving, and creative improvisation in problematic or unfamiliar situations (Sutton et al. 2011; Cappuccio 2015; Carr 2015; Rucińska 2014b; discontent with the dominant reductive picture of skill had already been raised by Csíkszentmihályi 1996).

Whether this characterization of the self-monitoring/execution-focus theories is correct or not, it reveals a theoretical polarization in the current scientific debate on the cognitive precursors of choking. While distraction/overload theories emphasize awareness, reflection, and explicit decision as the distinctive components of skillful expertise, the self-monitoring/execution-focus theories emphasize the habitual and adaptive components molded around familiar situations and repeated features of commonly encountered sporting environments. Neither provides a complete account of the many facets of expertise and its development. Can these two accounts be reconciled and a more complete and successful theory produced from their synthesis, or do they build on ultimately contradictory theoretical assumptions that are irreconcilable?

If possible, a unification of the two misallocation-of-attention approaches would certainly be desirable, as it would provide a fuller and more articulated understanding of choking. Important attempts to overcome this traditional dichotomy have already been made (e.g., *Mesh* theory, Christensen, Sutton, and McIlwain, this volume). The success of a truly unified approach to choking should be measured by its capability to account not only for the experimental results that support the attentional theories in laboratory research, but also for the large number of studies, both quantitative and qualitative, that focus on the experiential circumstances of individual athletes, their motivational backgrounds, and their personal psychological profiles (e.g., Jordet 2010; Mesagno, Harvey, and Janelle 2012; Mesagno and Hill 2013; Geukes et al. 2017).

The key to understand choking seems to be the complex interrelation between self-perception, motivation, emotion, sensorimotor control, and attention; that is why these components cannot be studied in isolation. A theoretical picture capable of systematically integrating all these components is still missing. This chapter does not aim to offer such theory, but provides at least some of the theoretical tools necessary to develop it, showing that multiple threats affect performance at different levels, and that all of them relate to some extent to some form of self-consciousness. Embodied cognition, broadly construed, provides the right kind of foundational narrative to appropriately recognize self-consciousness as a multifaceted and complex causal principle of performance disruption. Three notions offered by embodied cognition theory are particularly important:

1. Performance is affected by motor, perceptual, and judgment processes that are systemically integrated (they reciprocally influence one another and/or share the same neurocognitive resources). This is demonstrated by how even higher forms of decision and categorization are scaffolded by basic sensorimotor processes modulated by skill level.
2. Performance disruption cannot be understood without considering the role of emotions and feelings (primarily anxiety and its biophysical expressions) in governing choice and pursuit of goals, directing attention, and, more generally, shaping the cognitive landscape that determines better or worse performances.
3. Performance is not only affected by impersonal mechanisms, but also largely depends on the unique psychophysiological features of each performer as a situated agent with his or her anatomical configuration, motivations, beliefs, identity and self-presentation, and personality traits (e.g., narcissism and perfectionism).

These three notions are explored in the parts that follow, which cover particular aspects of self-consciousness and their undesired effects: part 7 focuses on the intertwinement of perceptual, motoric, and judgment processes; parts 8, 9, and 10 focus on the disruptive role played in performance by the appraisal of emotions like anxiety; and parts 11 to 14 deepen the motivational and psychological dimension of skill, examining how self-presentation and personality traits correlate to performance.

7 How Does Pressure Influence Performers' Perceptions of Their Environment?

In sport, it is common for athletes to describe how their perception of the environment can change from moment to moment and game to game. On the one hand, when an athlete is performing well, baseballs can look like "grapefruits" (Will 1990) and basketball hoops can look like "oceans" (Nobles 1995); "things slow down and you feel like you have more time" (McEnroe and Kaplan 2002, 57), and vision is "tunneled in" on the target (Swann et al. 2016). On the other hand, when an athlete is struggling, playing baseball can involve "swinging at aspirins" (Bradley 2003) and athletes notice "spectators and the presence of television" (Oudejans et al. 2011, 67). Are these comments just hyperbole or can perception really change so dramatically?

Embodied perception theory (EPT; see Proffitt 2006) proposes that perception is determined by the relationship between the physical characteristics of objects in a perceiver's environment and the perceiver's ability to act on them. EPT is a direct descendant of Gibson's (1966, 1979) ecological theories. EPT pursues the idea that our senses evolved into an integrated perceptual system to serve action (what is out there in the world, how can I with my own capabilities act in and on that world, and how do these affordances for action enable my goals or stand in their way). As Proffitt puts it in his 2006 paper, "Perception informs people about the opportunities for action and their associated costs" (110). To this end, explicit awareness of spatial layout varies not only with relevant optical and ocular-motor variables, but also as a function of the costs associated with performing intended actions. Although explicit awareness is mutable in this respect, visually guided actions directed at the immediate environment are not. When the metabolic costs associated with walking an extent increase—perhaps because one is wearing a heavy backpack—hills appear steeper and distances to targets appear greater. When one is standing on a high balcony, the apparent distance to the ground is correlated with one's fear of falling. Perceiving spatial layout combines the geometry of the world with behavioral goals and the costs associated with achieving these goals.

EPT is highly consistent with the subjective impressions of athletes, described earlier. Furthermore, recent laboratory experiments have essentially re-created the athletes' experiences illustrated in the quotes above. For example, researchers have shown that the perceived size of objects in a sporting environment is larger and the perceived speed is slower for more skilled compared with lesser skilled performers (for a review, see Gray 2014).

While the link between performance level (e.g., number of hits in a baseball game) and perception (e.g., size of the ball) is clear in these studies, an issue investigated less extensively is how pressure might alter athletes' perceptions. As we have seen, pressure can influence an athlete's ability to perform his or her sport (e.g., Baumeister 1984; Masters 1992; Beilock and Gray 2007; Mesagno, Harvey, and Janelle 2011; Carr 2015). But less evidence exists for the following questions: Does the presence of pressure or anxiety also change the perception of the size and speed of objects in the environment as would be predicted by EPT? Does this happen for all performers to the same extent, or might we be able to predict individual differences in performance or its control from individual differences in perceptual judgments? More generally, do any perceptual changes relate to and predict attentional control and/or performance outcomes? Below, we consider recent studies that have addressed these issues.

Cañal-Bruland, Pijpers, and Oudejans (2010) initially investigated how anxiety influences perception in a sporting context. In this experiment, participants threw darts at a target and produced a judgment of target size. Two conditions were compared: a low-anxiety condition in which participants threw darts while standing on the ground and a high-anxiety condition in which they threw while suspended 3.6 meters above the ground on a climbing wall. The size judgment task involved selecting one of nine circles that matched the size of the target on the dartboard. Results indicated that in the low-anxiety (on-the-ground, normal throwing posture) condition, a significant negative relationship between the mean radial error in dart throwing and the matched target size occurred. That is, participants that performed more accurately in the dart-throwing task estimated the target size to be larger. In the high-anxiety condition, there was no significant relationship between dart-throwing performance and judged target size. Cañal-Bruland et al. (2011) argued that the lack of effect in the high-anxiety condition was because the performer's attention was drawn away from the target.

One might well imagine that this conclusion is correct. People trying to cling to a climbing wall might be anxious, and either component of that situation—clinging to a climbing wall or feeling anxiety as a result—might influence performance. But whether this finding has anything to do with performance under pressure and choking or doing well is debatable. First, one might wonder whether the anxiety produced at heights while clinging to a wall is comparable to the anxiety produced by pressure to succeed in competition. Second, the anxiety manipulation did not actually significantly affect dart-throwing performance, though it did influence judged target size.

The distinction we just drew among various sources of anxiety and whether they work the same way is crucially important to understanding performance under pressure. Such a possibility can be seen in an incidental finding reported by Beilock, Bertenthal, et al. (2004), who found that while a self-report measure of "I felt pressure to perform" correlated with performance in their pressure condition, a widely used measure of situational anxiety did not. But this study was not intended to determine whether "pressure" and "anxiety" are the same or different, and it had very low power to discriminate. Several years later, Mesagno, Harvey, and Janelle (2011) found that different ways of imposing "pressure" on high-level field hockey players affected performance outcomes quite differently, and this finding, we believe, should figure heavily in how to think about pressure. Whereas the presence of an audience of peers and the prospect of being evaluated by a coach led to reduced performance relative to unpressurized practice, the prospect of earning money improved performance. Corroborative data from a widely used measure of anxiety showed that while reports of physiological symptoms (such as sweaty palms, racing hearts, shaky hands) *did not* predict performance, reports of worried thoughts about success or failure and their personal and social consequences—so called cognitive anxiety—*did* predict performance, and cognitive anxiety was higher when there was an audience or the prospect of evaluation. Finally, in the results of Mesagno, Harvey, and Janelle (2011) the negative impacts of social/evaluative pressure and the positive impact of monetary reward were approximately additive—as if they might have influenced different sets of processes to create effects that were somewhat independent (Carr 2015).

More recently, in light of these issues, Gray and Cañal-Bruland (2015) investigated the relationship among perceived target size, performance, and pressure in a golf-putting task. In this experiment, twenty-five experienced golfers completed three tasks on every trial: (1) putt a golf ball to a circular target on an indoor putting green from a distance of 2.5 m; (2) estimate the size of the target using drawing software on a computer screen; and (3) perform one of two secondary tasks (a "hole" task in which participants indicated whether a sound originated to the left or right of the hole during their putting stroke, and a "club" task in which participants indicated whether the sound occurred closer to the beginning or end of their backswing). The primary dependent variables were the final distance of the ball from the target, the percent correct for the two secondary tasks, and the perceived hole size. Performance was compared for three phases: (1) a low-pressure pretest; (2) a high-pressure phase, which involved both competitive (monetary reward) and social (results posted in public area) pressure applied together; and (3) a low-pressure posttest. Gray and Cañal-Bruland (2015) initially noticed large individual differences for several of the dependent measures including heart rate, putting kinematics, perceived hole size, percent correct in the two secondary tasks, and final distance from the target. Therefore, although there seemed to be links between the different dependent variables, these individual differences needed to be taken into account before traditional analyses could be done.

As we have been discussing, a challenge for researchers who investigate choking is how to take into account between-participant differences in responses to performance pressure. Should we lump all data together and analyze whether or not there was a "group choke" effect (e.g., Beilock and Carr 2001), or should we dichotomize the data and label all participants that showed significant performance decline as "chokers" and those who did not as "clutch" (e.g., Gray, Allsop, and Williams 2013), or should we treat the effect of pressure on performance as a continuum? Or perhaps there is yet another alternative: that laboratory impositions of pressure do not rise to the level that creates "choking" and hence these studies are examining a tendency to perform worse when the stakes are higher, but true "choking" is a different beast with different or additional mechanisms (see Mesagno and Hill 2013). Gray and Cañal-Bruland (2015), in their putting study, chose an option that falls between an attempt to find a bimodal distribution and a continuum in laboratory studies, which we describe next.

To make sense of their data, Gray and Cañal-Bruland (2015) performed a *k*-means cluster analysis using the pressure-manipulation check (heart rate) and two club-head kinematic variables (time to peak speed, TTPS, and velocity at impact, VI) as classification variables. The main goal of the study was to investigate the relationship among putting performance, perceived hole size, and attentional focus (as assessed by the secondary tasks); thus, these variables were not used in the classification. Similar to previous results (Beilock and Gray 2012), there were two distinct clusters: a group of eleven golfers, labelled the "choke" group, for which there were significant changes in HR, TTPS, and VI from the pretest to pressure phase, and a group of fourteen golfers, labelled the "clutch" group, for which there were no significant changes. Treating the "choke" and "clutch" groups as separate groups in the subsequent analyses, Gray and Cañal-Bruland found significant group differences for all three tasks the participants performed. Specifically, compared with the "clutch" group, the "choke" group putted worse (by 3 cm on average), estimated the target size to be smaller (by 3.8 cm on average), had lower accuracy for the "hole" secondary task (by 21 percent on average), and had higher accuracy for the "club" secondary task (by 23 percent on average).[4]

Why did the perceived size of the target decrease for the "choke" group under pressure, and what does this tell us about pressure-induced failures in performance? Based on the data from the secondary tasks, Gray and Cañal-Bruland (2015) proposed that this change in perception was essentially an artifact of changes in the performer's attention control. Consistent with self-monitoring/execution-focus theory, strong evidence exists of an inward shift of attention (i.e., inward toward skill execution per se, and away from the external environment and the targets of the execution) in the "choke" group because they performed worse at making the "hole" judgment and better at making the "club" judgment. When a person directs his attention to an object he intends to act on (e.g., a target he is aiming at or a ball he is about to strike), the task-relevant object becomes accentuated so that it stands out from other task-irrelevant objects, often making it appear larger (Bruner 1957). Conversely, shifting attention away from a target toward one's own body should make the target appear smaller (e.g., Cañal-Bruland et al. 2011). From this interpretation, it is unclear whether the change in perceived target size itself has any direct effect on performance under pressure or whether the changes in putting accuracy can all be explained by the effects of attentional control (e.g., disruption of automaticity with an internal self/execution focus of attention).

An attempt to simulate the effect of pressure through a contrast between speed instruction versus accuracy instruction in a putting task manipulated target size, but while speed-accuracy instructions affected performance considerably, the variation in target size had no significant effect (Beilock, Bertenthal, et al. 2008). However, a possible direct effect of perceptual changes on choking can be seen in a study of baseball batting (Gray 2013). In this study, experienced baseball batters performed two directional hitting tasks (hitting the ball to either the left or right side of the field—called "pull" or "opposite-field" hitting, respectively) in a batting simulator and made judgments about ball size between swings. The primary finding (as shown in figure 5.1, solid symbols) was an interaction between perceived ball size and the batting task. That is, when the pitch location was ideal for the batter's task (e.g., inside pitches for pull hitting and outside pitches for opposite-field hitting), perceived size was larger.

As first proposed by Cañal-Bruland and van der Kamp (2009), this effect can be explained by the attentional accentuation hypothesis, which claims that when a person intends to act on an object and directs her attention to it, the task-relevant object becomes accentuated so that it stands out from other task-irrelevant objects. The open symbols in figure 5.1 show unpublished data from a condition in which batters performed the same tasks under a combination of evaluative (being videotaped and evaluated by a coach) and competitive pressure (being entered into competition with a cash prize for performance). Consistent with Gray and Cañal-Bruland (2015), pressure seemed to eliminate the difference in perceived size for task-optimal and nonoptimal pitch locations. The data shown in figure 5.2 provide insight into how these perceptual effects might influence performance. Batters appeared to be using an effective hitting strategy of initiating more swing for task-optimal pitch locations in the low-pressure situation, while these advantageous behaviors essentially disappeared under pressure.

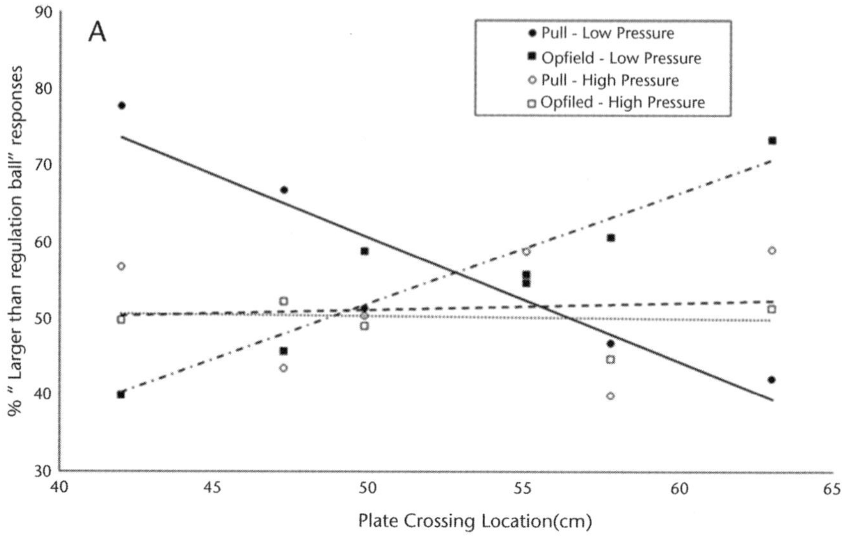

Figure 5.1
Mean percentage of "ball larger than a regulation baseball" response as a function of pitch crossing location. Data are shown for different combinations of batting task (pull hitting vs. opposite-field hitting) and pressure (low vs. high).
Source: Gray (2013).

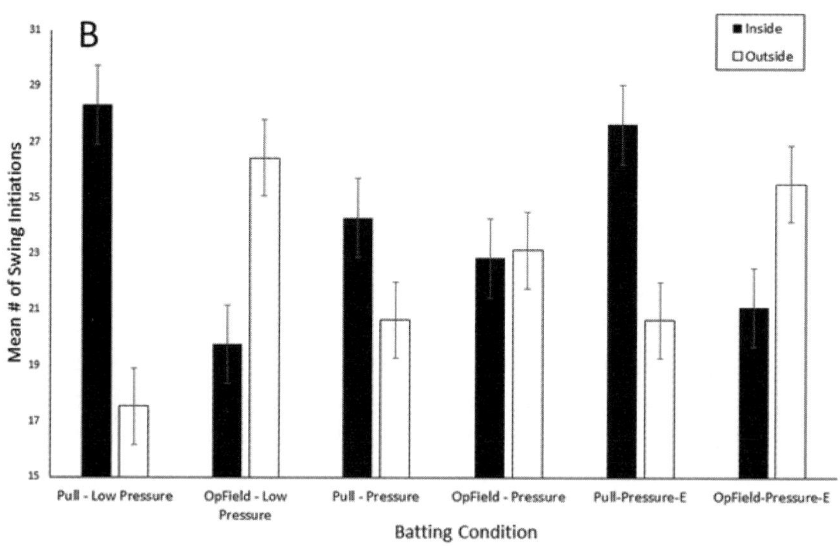

Figure 5.2
Mean number of swing initiations for different combinations of hitting task (pull hitting vs. opposite-field hitting) and pressure (low vs. high). Solid bars show data for pitches on the inside (i.e., close to the hitter's body), while open bars show outside pitches.
Source: Gray (2013).

Again, one might argue that these effects could be explained entirely at the level of attention control and are unrelated to the perceived ball size. That is, under low pressure the batter is attending to the optimal locations and is more likely to swing, while under pressure an inward shift in attention (focusing on the movement of the putter) eliminated this effect. However, the other two conditions presented in figure 5.2 (designated by an E at the end) show results from a condition in which the simulated diameter of the ball in the simulation varied as a function of pitch location. Specifically, when the batter's task was pull hitting, pitches with trajectories that crossed the inside of the plate had a simulated ball diameter of 8.4 cm, while for outside pitches it was the regulation size of 7.4 cm. The opposite was true when the batter's task was opposite-field hitting. These values were chosen based on the changes in perceived size observed for different pitch locations in low-pressure conditions (see Gray 2013 for details). Another way to think of this manipulation of varying the simulated ball size as a function of pitch location is that it is an attempt to cancel out the changes in perceived size resulting from pressure (shown in figure 5.1) by artificially manipulating the ball size. As can be seen in figure 5.2, this manipulation of simulated ball size effectively restored the batters' tendency to swing at pitches in locations that are task optimal. This in turn suggests that at least part of the change in behavior observed under pressure was due to the change in the perceived size of the ball. These results appear to be consistent with the proposed action selection role for embodied perception (Proffitt 2006). That is, perceiving objects as larger when action capability is higher makes one more likely to act.

In sum, recent research has shown that pressure can lead to reductions in the perceived size of target objects in a sporting environment. Whether these perceptual changes are directly related to how well a performer handles the pressure situation (e.g., by changing the likelihood they will act or act accurately) or are simply an artifact of changes in attentional control is an issue that needs additional future research. It will also be interesting to determine if pressure influences the perception of other aspects of the sporting environment, such as the perceived speed of objects and the perceived passage of time. Finally, because there again seems to be substantial individual variation in the perceptual effects of pressure, it is possible that changes in perception could be used as another objective, behavioral index of pressure effects. And, given extant arguments that the mechanisms of choking differ across task domains and levels of expertise (e.g., Beilock, Kulp, et al. 2004; Beilock and DeCaro 2007; DeCaro et al. 2011; Carr 2015; in general, the groundbreaking work done by Proffitt and colleagues deserves a particular mention in this context), research on perceptual changes as accompaniments and predictors (or even possibly causes) of performance changes under pressure needs to be pursued beyond the bounds of sporting environments.

8 How Do Emotions and Feelings Contribute to Performance Disruption?

As we have seen, there is a growing commitment to the idea that the mind must be understood in the context of its relationship to a physical body that interacts with the world (Beilock 2008a). According to this principle, in order to understand fully the phenomenon of choking in sport, it is essential to examine the athlete's psychological, emotional, and physiological response to the pressurized environment as a holistic and interacting unit. Consequently, a more detailed understanding of the causes, moderators, and consequences of choking may be gained that can inform evidence-based intervention designed to alleviate choking. Through the lens of embodied cognition, we next focus on the role of emotions in the experience of choking in sport. More specifically, we review the interplay among the athletes' emotions, cognitions, psychophysiological response, and the environment during acute sporting failure.

Emotions are subjective feelings that are a conscious response to the athlete's cognitive appraisal of an event (Fredrickson 2001, 2003). That is, by appraising the significance of a particular situation in terms of personal harm and benefits (Lazarus 2000), the athlete will experience an emotional response that triggers a physiological change (i.e., arousal, muscular tension, heart rate, and blood pressure) and action (i.e., approach and/or avoidance behaviors). Thereafter, such emotional and physical responses will be subjected to further appraisals (see Neil et al. 2011). Thus a continuous cycle of interaction and integration takes place among cognitions and emotions.

Emotions are classified according to their hedonic tone and functionality—with hedonic tone referring to whether the emotions are pleasant (e.g., happy) or unpleasant (e.g., anxiety), and functionality denoting whether the emotion has a positive (i.e., functional) or negative (i.e., dysfunctional) impact on the performance (Hanin 2000, 2007). Both pleasant and unpleasant emotions can have a functional or dysfunctional effect on performance, depending on the athlete's cognitive appraisal of those emotions (e.g., Totterdell 2000; Lane et al. 2011). For example, while the pleasant emotion of happiness often leads to optimal performance, it can also encourage performance failure if the athlete perceives the emotion is associated with satiated action tendency (Erez and Isen 2002). In this instance, athletes may lower effort when they are happy because they no longer feel the need to work hard. Conversely, the unpleasant emotion of anger can have a functional effect on performance, if the athlete believes the emotion is energizing, whereas anger can cause performance failure if it increases the athlete's perceptions of feeling out of control (Woodman et al. 2009). Thus, the appraisal of a pressurized situation will encourage an emotional response that affects attention (e.g., Eysenck et al. 2007), motor control (Coombes et al. 2009), perception (e.g., Vallerand and Blanchard 2000), decision making (Tenenbaum and Bar-Eli 1993), motivation (e.g., Kerr 2014), and, ultimately, performance (Gucciardi et al. 2010; Hill et al. 2010a; Neil et al. 2011).

With specific regard to choking in sport, anxiety has been identified as a central emotion (Hill and Shaw 2013; Mesagno and Hill 2013; Carr 2015), which is likely the principal emotion experienced by athletes in response to perceived pressure. Indeed, extensive evidence from experimental studies supports the role of high anxiety levels within the choking process (see Beilock and Gray 2007; Hill et al. 2010a for a review). Of the limited qualitative research available, anxiety has also been reported by athletes as being the dominant emotion they associate with their choking experience (Gucciardi et al. 2010; Hill et al. 2010b; Hill and Shaw 2013; Hill and Hemmings 2015). Critically, this work provides a further indication that athletes' appraisal of anxiety may be what determines performance outcomes, rather than the mere presence of the emotion. Hence, athletes who experience choking normally perceive their anxiety as debilitative, while those who appraise it as facilitative tend to excel under pressure (Gucciardi et al. 2010; Hill et al. 2010b; Hill and Shaw 2013). Furthermore, appraising their physiological responses to anxiety (i.e., muscular tension, increased heart rate, a tight chest, and palpitations) as debilitative also appears to encourage the likelihood of choking (Gucciardi et al. 2010).

While anxiety is an important determinant of choking in sport, it is concerning that researchers have failed to consider fully the potential influence of other emotions. This is despite evidence indicating that a broad range of emotions are likely to determine the outcomes of athletic performance (e.g., Totterdell 2000; McCarthy 2011; Uphill, Groom, and Jones 2014). Through qualitative research, many unpleasant emotions have been noted by athletes before and/or during their choking experience, which include (but are not limited to) embarrassment, shame, humiliation, fear, hate, inferiority, negativity, despondency, annoyance, anger, distress, or feeling overwhelmed, uncontrolled, or hopeless (see Gucciardi et al. 2010; Hill et al. 2010a; Hill et al. 2011; Mesagno, Harvey, and Janelle 2012). Since such emotions were not directly explored, it remains unclear which situational factors triggered each of the emotional reactions, how each emotion specifically affected the performer/performance, and whether any individual differences existed in terms of the emotional response and its effect. The only exception to date is Mesagno, Harvey, and Janelle (2012), who found that fear (of negative evaluation) led to choking in their study of basketball players (consistent with the findings reviewed earlier from Mesagno, Harvey, and Janelle 2011). Accordingly, while it cannot be doubted that anxiety can encourage choking in sport, researchers should also examine whether other emotions elicited as a result of perceived pressure can moderate choking.

9 Emotion, Motivation, and Choking in Sport

When placed in a meaningful situation, an athlete will experience an emotional response that enables him to prioritize his goals, generate a psychophysiological state of readiness, and become energized to act according to that situation (see Baumeister et al. 2007). While evolutionary psychology might presume emotions should have a benign and/or adaptive effect on human beings, evidence indicates that many self-defeating behaviors are fostered by emotion (Baumeister et al. 2007; Baumeister and Lobbestael 2011), including choking under pressure (Baumeister and Scher 1988). Emotions provide feedback regarding how well the athlete is moving toward a pertinent goal, with positive emotions tending to be experienced when appropriate progress is being made and negative emotions signaling progress is slower than expected (Carver and Scheier 1981; Carver, 2003). Thereafter, individuals are more likely to adjust their goals in order to avoid negative emotions and increase positive emotions. Consequently, if the athlete is moving effectively toward his or her goal and experiencing positive emotions, he or she is likely to become increasingly motivated to pursue that goal until it is reached. With choking in sport, however, athletes perceive they are unlikely to reach a pertinent goal, and so experience an intense negative emotional response (Hill et al. 2009). Initially, if the goal is important (e.g., winning a tournament), such negative emotions may initiate increased effort/motivation. Paradoxically, such efforts can lead to the misregulation of attention, whereby the athlete attempts to consciously control/monitor the explicit components of the skill (i.e., execution focus) and experiences choking as a result (see Baumeister and Heatherton 1996). Whereas, if the athlete continues to perceive she is not capable of reaching her goal, then the associated negative emotions will eventually cause her to cognitively disengage from the goal (Wrosch et al. 2003) and adopt avoidance motivation, as she removes herself from the situation causing the distress. Therefore, such avoidance-goal intentions and behaviors are also acknowledged determinants of choking in sport (Jordet and Hartman 2008; Jordet 2009; Carr 2015; Hill and Hemmings 2015).

Emotions can also direct the individual's attention to relevant aspects of the situation, allowing the opportunity to identify the appropriate action and/or reflect on lessons that can be learned for the next time they find themselves in the same situation (Baumeister et al. 2007). However, athletes with high trait anxiety, who are therefore prone to choking in sport (Baumeister and Showers 1986; Wang et al. 2004), are known to experience a narrowing of their attention and a sensitivity to threat stimuli in their environment when exposed to perceived pressure (Eysenck et al. 2007). As a result, when under pressure and experiencing high anxiety (and other unpleasant emotions), they are unable to look beyond the threat stimuli causing their unpleasant emotions. Consequently, during pressurized performance, those athletes with high trait anxiety will focus on removing themselves from the situation causing the negative emotions rather than assimilate relevant information and explore all appropriate options. Such avoidance motivation/behavior can not only lead to poor sporting performance (i.e., choking), but can also prevent the athlete from learning lessons from that situation to inform his or her self-management during future pressurized situations. This may go some way to explaining why some athletes continue to choke each time they are exposed to pressure (Hill et al. 2009, 2010b, 2011).

As a final comment, when individuals know they will experience negative emotions in the future when facing certain events (i.e., performing under pressure), they often begin to engage in proactive coping (i.e., efforts undertaken in advance of a stressful event to prevent or modify it) to minimize those emotions (Aspinwall and Taylor 1997). Such proactive coping efforts can include preventing the aversive event from occurring and/or minimizing its eventual impact. This hopefully can encourage the athlete to learn and develop a repertoire of coping strategies that can be employed to alter his or her appraisal of future pressurized situation and help him or her manage more effectively their emotional response (Hill et al. 2011; Hill and Hemmings 2015). However, in certain cases of choking, proactive coping has consisted of self-handicapping behavior, whereby the athlete attempts to lower his or her expectations of success by subconsciously undermining preparation for the pressurized event (see Hill et al. 2011). Indeed, such a coping approach may even cause the athlete to avoid high-value situations altogether (Hill et al. 2009).

Collectively, the above demonstrates that, for certain athletes, emotions can be counterproductive and lead to choking under pressure. Accordingly, the experience of choking is one in which the pressurized situation causes the athlete to suffer emotional distress, which in turn elicits goal intentions and motivational actions that prevent effective management of the self and situation. More work is needed to identify just which athletes might be more or less susceptible to the negative effects of emotions and consequent changes in motivation, strategy, and goal direction, and on how to intervene in the patterns to help athletes avoid or overcome those effects. Next we address one approach to such identification and intervention.

10 Choking under Pressure and Challenge/Threat Appraisals

A useful framework for understanding the interactions among an athlete's motivation, emotions, and performance outcomes that can lead to choking is the theory of challenge and threat states in athletes (TCTSA; see Jones et al. 2009). The TCTSA draws on the biopsychosocial model (Blascovich and Tomaka 1996), the model of adaptive approaches to competition (Skinner and Brewer 2004), and the control model of anxiety (Jones 1995), by proposing that when engaged in goal-driven performance events, athletes will appraise the situation as either a challenge or a threat (Blascovich 2008). Cognitive appraising of the event as a challenge occurs if they perceive they have sufficient resources to meet the situational demands, whereas they will appraise the event as a threat if they perceive insufficient resources to meet the situational demands (Blascovich and Mendes 2000).

Critically, each appraisal will lead to a challenge or threat motivational state (Jones et al. 2009), which have different associated physiological and emotional responses. Physiologically, a challenge state is characterized by an increased activation of the sympathetic-adreno-medullary (SAM) system and the release of epinephrine, which causes higher cardiac output and vasodilatation and decreased systemic vascular resistance. Combined, this leads to increased blood flow and the efficient mobilization of energy, which can facilitate action and coping responses (Blascovich et al. 2000). A threat state is also associated with SAM activity, yet there is an increased activation of the pituitary-adrenocortical system, which initiates the release of adrenocorticotropic hormone. Therefore, while cardiac activity increases, it is not accompanied by vasodilatation or decreased systemic vascular resistance. Accordingly, blood flow remains static and the athlete does not benefit from the efficient mobilization of energy as seen in a challenge state (Blascovich and Tomaka 1996).

Positive emotions are normally experienced by athletes in a challenge state, and negative emotions during a threat state. Nevertheless, it is accepted that the athlete's interpretation of his or her emotions will moderate this position. As an example, negative emotions (e.g., anxiety) can be interpreted as facilitative and therefore will exist in a challenge state (Mendes et al. 2008), while positive emotions (e.g., contentment), interpreted as debilitative for performance, can be experienced within a threat state.

The TCTSA also proposes that an athlete will appraise an event as a challenge or threat depending on his or her self-efficacy, perception of control, and goal orientation (Jones et al. 2009). Thus, athletes with high self-efficacy will perceive they have the capability to manage successfully the demands of the situation and will appraise the situation as a challenge. Conversely, those low in self-efficacy will appraise the event as a threat, for they are unsure whether they have the capability to meet those demands (Williams, Cumming, and Balanos 2010). Perceived control has a similar impact on athletes' appraisals, whereby if they believe they have sufficient control over themselves and the environment to achieve their performance goals, they will experience and benefit from a challenge appraisal. In contrast, those athletes lacking perceived control will appraise the situation as a threat. Finally, in terms of goal orientation, those who adopt approach goals (in particular, mastery approach) will view the upcoming event as a challenge, and those who hold avoidance goals will tend to have a threat appraisal. This is likely to be the result of self-referenced achievement goals increasing the athletes' self-efficacy and perceived control (Jones et al. 2009; Meijen et al. 2013; Turner et al. 2012).

There is an extensive evidence base to support the relationship between challenge and threat states, their associated cardiovascular indices (i.e., physiological response), and performance outcomes, which has been corroborated across tasks including perceptual-motor (Vine, Freeman, et al. 2013), cognitive (Turner et al. 2012), and sensorimotor skills (e.g., Moore et al. 2012). Hence, a challenge appraisal and motivational state has been linked to improved sport performance under pressure, with athletes in a threat state found to be more vulnerable to performance decrement and choking than those in a challenge state (Moore et al. 2012; Moore, Wilson, et al. 2013; Turner et al. 2012). By manipulating an athlete's appraisal and motivation state toward challenge (e.g., through manipulating gaze/reappraisal training), athletes are likely to experience enhanced performance under pressure and may, in turn, become increasingly resistant to choking (Moore, Vine, et al. 2013; Moore et al. 2015).

The precise mechanism through which challenge and threat appraisals affect performance remains somewhat unclear, although the most likely explanation is emotional and attentional control. Athletes in a challenge state experience facilitative emotions (Williams et al. 2010; Moore et al. 2012; Moore, Wilson, et al. 2013), which have an established relationship with optimal sport performance (Neil et al. 2011; Thomas, Maynard, and Hanton 2007). However, while challenge and threat states lead to differential emotional responses, those differences do not fully and consistently explain why athletes in a challenge state perform better than those in a threat state (see Moore et al. 2012). With regard to attentional control, individuals within a threat state are less able to remain focused on task-relevant information because they become distracted by threat stimuli in their environment (Vine, Freeman, et al. 2013). Furthermore, a longer quiet-eye duration (i.e., the final fixation located on an object for a minimum of 100 milliseconds, Vickers 2007, 280) has been noted with athletes in a challenge state (Vine, Moore, et al. 2013; Moore et al. 2012; Moore, Vine, et al. 2013), which is considered by some to benefit pressurized performance as it extends the critical period during which the motor response is selected and programmed. Finally, athletes within a challenge state experience less "reinvestment" (Moore, Wilson, et al. 2013), which is the attempt to consciously control a well-learned skill under pressure (Masters, Polman, and Hammond, 1993), similar to Beilock's execution focus (the concept of "dispositional reinvestment" is discussed in part 13); that is why they are thought to be less likely to focus on the explicit components of their skill and are less vulnerable to choking through self-focus (Masters and Maxwell 2008). However, studies have failed to find a consistent link between challenge/threat appraisal, attention control, and performance across groups (Moore, Wilson, et al. 2013), meaning further research is required before conclusions can be drawn.

Other mechanisms have been proposed to explain how challenge and threat appraisals affect performance, though they have received less research attention to date. They include the use of problem- and emotion-coping strategies during a challenge state (Allen, Frings, and Hunter 2012), which may be possible because of the associated cardiovascular changes enhancing the athlete's available energy resources, which can then sustain such effortful approach-coping. Additionally, an increased efficiency of kinematics has also been suggested as a mechanism through which appraisals can impact performance. As an example, Moore et al. (2012) observed efficient forearm muscle activity during a putting task for those athletes who were in a challenge state, when compared with their threat counterparts.

11 How Do Personality Characteristics Influence Proneness to Pressure? Choking and Self-Presentation Theory

The two dominant choking models as recounted earlier in the chapter differ substantially in the roles they attribute to attention and the nature of the shifts of attention that they envision to occur during performance under pressure. As we have described, there is evidence for both sets of processes and for interactions and changing relations between their effects as level of skill increases. Even more complex, however, is how personality characteristics may interact with these sets of cognitive processes and the processes and behaviors of self-presentation. These interactions can lead to increased pressure and decreased performance, and so should be integrated into models of performance under pressure.

Self-presentation is the process by which people attempt to monitor and control what they do in public and hence how they are perceived and evaluated by others (Schlenker 1980). Mesagno and colleagues (Mesagno 2009; Mesagno, Harvey, and Janelle

2011) proposed that concerns about self-presentation may be the origin of the increased state anxiety for choking-susceptible athletes (those more likely to experience choking). Mesagno's model was conceptualized from qualitative research and grounded in Leary's (1992) suggestion that competitive anxiety is a sport-specific class of social anxiety. While competitive anxiety might not be limited to sports—it might arise in many arenas of life where people compete with one another—sports provide a clear avenue for study. In an initial investigation of the self-presentation model of choking in sporting environments described earlier, Mesagno, Harvey, and Janelle (2011) found that self-presentation pressure manipulations (such as having an audience of knowledgeable and talented teammates, or knowing that performance would be evaluated by their coaches) increased anxiety and choking tendencies more than did a motivational pressure-comparison condition involving monetary reward, with cognitive state anxiety mediating the relationship between self-presentation and performance. These results provided initial support for a linkage among self-presentation, increased state anxiety (at least as measured by self-reports of the content of thoughts—rather than physiology—as discussed earlier), and choking.

Mesagno and colleagues (Mesagno 2009; Mesagno, Harvey, and Janelle 2011) argue that the interaction of high athletic identity (described below), choking susceptibility through certain personality characteristics, and situational factors that affect perceived pressure are likely to increase the likelihood of elevated perceived pressure and choking. Baumeister (1984) defines pressure as "any factor or combination of factors that increases the importance of performing well on a particular occasion" (610). Personality characteristics and situational factors can interact to influence the perception of pressure in the context. One epitome of being an elite athlete is showing publicly that you have the ability to perform successfully under pressure. One key facet of the self-presentation model is athletic identity. Athletic identity is the degree to which individuals define themselves as athletes, and, as argued by Brewer, Van Raalte, and Linder (1993), such definition is central to many athletes' self-concepts.

Brewer and colleagues divided athletic identity into three components: social identity, exclusivity, and negative affectivity. Social identity refers to the degree that individuals view others' perceptions of them as athletes. Exclusivity is how strongly people rely on their athletic identities and whether they identify themselves weakly (or strongly) with other important life roles. Negative affectivity refers to the degree individuals negatively respond as a result of being unable to participate in sport (Martin, Eklund, and Mushett 1997). Researchers have found that a stronger and more exclusive athletic identity may lead to negative psychological and social concerns including decreased self-esteem (Crook and Robertson 1991), emotional difficulties (Lavallee, Gordon, and

Grove 1997), and mood disturbances (Brewer 1993). Based on these findings, Mesagno and colleagues argue that a stronger athletic identity could be a factor that increases perceived pressure, especially if the athlete views himself or herself exclusively as an athlete; yet, empirical evidence on this link is still to be determined. Nevertheless, personality characteristics that lead to choking susceptibility may influence the perception of pressure. In some ways this notion maps onto the similarities Beilock et al. (2006) identified between stereotype threat and choking, given that stereotype threat is widely regarded as dependent on how important are the links between a task to be performed and one's sense of self, and the large impact of the presence of an audience on the magnitude of stereotype threat that might call one's sense of self to the fore or participate in evaluation of the task's performance.

12 What Personality Characteristics Might Make Someone Choking-Susceptible?

Just as a full and detailed consideration of the relations among emotions and choking was beyond the limits of this chapter, we can provide only a brief overview of how personality characteristics might relate to choking (but see Jackson, Beilock, and Kinrade 2013; Mesagno, Geukes, and Larkin 2015 for recent reviews). To date, researchers have found support that self-consciousness, trait anxiety, fear of negative evaluation, fear of failure, perfectionism, dispositional reinvestment, and narcissism are likely characteristics of choking-susceptible athletes.

Self-consciousness is defined as the tendency to direct attention either inward, focusing on covert aspects of self related to one's inner thoughts and feelings, or outward, focusing on aspects of self that are public to others (Fenigstein, Scheier, and Buss 1975; Scheier and Carver 1985). Initial investigations (e.g., Baumeister 1984) indicated that individuals low in self-consciousness perform poorly under pressure. However, other researchers (e.g., Masters, Polman, and Hammond 1993; Dandy, Brewer, and Tottman 2001; Wang et al. 2004) have provided evidence that highly self-conscious athletes are more likely to experience choking. Geukes et al. (2013) suggested that the mixed findings may be explained by the relevance of private versus public self-consciousness in a situational context. That is, Geukes and colleagues found that private self-consciousness is negatively associated with performance under pressure in laboratory-based high-pressure situations (i.e., one to seven spectators), while public self-consciousness is positively related to performance under public pressure (i.e., in front of a large audience of 1,500 to 2,000 spectators). Nevertheless, more evidence indicates that highly self-conscious individuals generally are more likely to experience choking.

Trait anxiety is the disposition to perceive a wide range of situations as threatening and to respond with state anxiety (Spielberger 1966), which appears, as discussed earlier, to play a major role in choking. Test/examination anxiety researchers have confirmed that individuals high in trait anxiety react to pressure situations with greater levels of state anxiety than individuals low in trait anxiety (Spielberger, Anton, and Bedell 1976). Furthermore, Calvo, Alamo, and Ramos (1990; Kurosawa and Harackiewicz 1995) found that high-trait-anxious individuals perform poorer under pressure than low-trait-anxious individuals. Sport anxiety researchers have also confirmed that trait anxiety is a strong predictor of state anxiety (e.g., Marchant, Morris, and Andersen 1998; Williams and Krane 1992). Baumeister and Showers (1986) posited that individuals high in trait anxiety would be more susceptible to choking than individuals low in trait anxiety, and Wang et al. (2004) found that trait anxiety (specifically, somatic trait anxiety) was negatively correlated with basketball free-throw performance under pressure. Thus, although a dearth of research has been focused on the effects of trait anxiety on performance, trait anxiety has links to choking effects, but further research is necessary to understand the underlying mechanisms regarding trait anxiety as a predictor of choking.

For many athletes, elite-level competition is a stressful and anxiety-provoking environment. When athletes experience pressure in sport, their ability to deal with being in the spotlight of competitive sport and achieve optimal performance may be substantially influenced by their coping skills. Two major classes of coping skills are discussed in the choking literature, and each may have a different effect on how performers deal with anxiety and pressure. Approach coping involves focusing on a particular concern by using direct cognitive effort (Crocker and Graham 1995), whereas avoidance coping typically entails directing cognitions away from the threat-related stimulus (Anshel and Weinberg 1999). Wang, Marchant, and Morris (2004) found that basketball players using approach coping were less accurate on a basketball free-throw shooting task under high pressure than those using avoidance coping. Based on a multiple regression analysis, Wang et al. (2004) found that approach coping accounted for 7 percent of the explained performance variance under pressure. From the resultant outcome and although largely speculative and without direct evidence, Wang et al. suggested that approach "copers" ruminate about anxiety-related cognitions during performance, which may increase perceived threat as they search for explanations for the increase in anxiety and actively seek to reduce the anxiety symptoms and experience. This irrelevant attentional focus minimizes task-relevant cognitions, which leads to poorer performance outcomes—at least in situations in which explicit task-relevant cognitions are needed (an issue already much-discussed in earlier parts of the chapter).

13 Fear of Negative Evaluation, Fear of Failure, Dispositional Reinvestment, Perfectionism, Narcissism

Since anxiety, impression management, and self-presentation seem to play important roles in performance under pressure, researchers have suggested that fear of negative evaluation may be a predictor of choking. Carleton et al. (2006) define fear of negative evaluation (FNE) as "apprehension and distress arising from concerns about being judged disparagingly or hostilely by others" (297). As a follow-up to the Mesagno, Harvey, and Janelle (2011) study of the impact of different kinds of pressure on professional field hockey players taking penalty shots, Mesagno, Harvey, and Janelle (2012) found that participants high in fear of negative evaluation increased anxiety and decreased basketball free-throw shooting percentage under high pressure, whereas participants low in fear of negative evaluation maintained similar anxiety levels and increased free-throw shooting percentage from the low- to high-pressure situation. Mesagno and colleagues suggested that athletes who rate high in FNE may be susceptible to choking, and as discussed earlier, this notion figures heavily in the self-presentation-related theoretical approach to choking.

Atkinson (1957) defined fear of failure (FOF) as a "disposition to avoid failure and/or a capacity for experiencing shame or humiliation as a consequence of failure" (13). Choking researchers (e.g., Jordet and Hartman 2008; Gucciardi et al. 2010; Hill et al. 2010b) have found both quantitative (i.e., behavioral indicators in World Cup soccer penalty shoot-outs) and qualitative evidence for the positive link between choking and FOF. In qualitative studies, Gucciardi et al. (2010) and Hill et al. (2010b) separately interviewed choking-susceptible golfers and found FOF as categories from their interviews. Apparently, fear (of negative evaluation or failure) may play a role in predicting choking. Nevertheless, only limited quantitative studies have focused on FNE, and primarily qualitative studies have identified that FOF is a theme, with minimal quantitative, laboratory-based studies having been conducted. To further develop this area, studies need to be conducted to tease out how these types of fear affect anxiety and performance under pressure.

Dispositional reinvestment is an athlete's overall tendency to attempt to consciously control a well-learned skill under pressure (Masters, Polman, and Hammond 1993). Reinvestment theory "argues that the propensity for consciousness to control movements on-line is a function of individual personality differences, specific contexts and a broad range of contingent events that can be psychological, physiological, environmental or even mechanical" (Masters and Maxwell 2008, 160). Sport psychology researchers (e.g., Masters, Polman, and Hammond 1993; Maxwell, Masters, and Eves 2000;

Masters and Maxwell 2004; Poolton, Maxwell, and Masters 2004; Jackson, Ashford, and Norsworthy 2006; Kinrade, Jackson, and Ashford 2010) have repeatedly confirmed that individuals high in dispositional reinvestment experience choking in sensorimotor skills, compared with those low, at least when the performers being tested are experienced rather than novices. To our knowledge, this measure has not been applied to non-sensorimotor working-memory-intensive skills, but the prediction is clear: reinvestment might benefit performance rather than hurt it (see Beilock, Bertenthal, et al. 2004; Carr 2015).

Perfectionism reflects a person's compulsive pursuit to set and attempt to reach excessively high standards and a tendency to engage in harsh, overly critical self-evaluation (Flett and Hewitt 2005). High standards are important and beneficial to sport performance, but when perfection is the only acceptable standard and non-perfection is common, a negative self-concept and fear of failure are increasingly likely to develop (e.g., Williams and Leffingwell 2002). Perfectionists, compared with non-perfectionists, rate task importance as significantly higher across different evaluative threats and tasks (e.g., Frost and Marten 1990) and have high social or trait anxiety (e.g., Alden, Ryder, and Melling 2002; Frost and Henderson 1991). Researchers (e.g., Clark and Wells 1995; Schlenker and Leary 1982) have also incorporated interpersonal and self-presentation components of perfectionism into their models of social anxiety. Recently, qualitative researchers (e.g., Gucciardi et al. 2010; Hill et al. 2010b) have identified perfectionism as a theme (or psychological attribute) associated with athletes who experience choking. Flett and Hewitt (2005) also illustrated the link between perfectionism and self-presentation by explaining that perfectionistic self-presentation (i.e., striving to create a flawless public image) may be common within sport and could be considered as an antecedent to increases in competitive anxiety. Thus, it appears that perfectionism may be linked to many of the other personality characteristics within the choking literature and could be an important predictor, but additional research is needed to determine how important.

Narcissism is characterized as an addiction to self-esteem and an obsession with demonstrating personal superiority or greatness over others (Baumeister and Vohs 2001). Only limited research has focused on narcissism and choking but, when it has been studied, researchers (e.g., Geukes et al. 2012, 2013; Wallace and Baumeister 2002) have found that narcissism decreases the likelihood of choking. For example, Wallace and Baumeister (2002, experiment 3) asked participants to perform a dart-throwing task in both a low-pressure (with only the researcher present) and a high-pressure condition (where the experimenter offered a monetary incentive) and found that individuals high in narcissism were more accurate under pressure than those low in narcissism.

However, the findings of Mesagno, Harvey, and Janelle (2011) that monetary reward may actually increase performance, whereas the presence of an audience and the prospect of evaluation decreases performance, make this finding difficult to interpret. A bit of light might be cast by the findings of Geukes et al. (2012, 2013), who also found empirical support for a positive relationship between narcissism and performance under pressure on a handball penalty-taking task. However, the narcissism results were found only when pressure was manipulated in a public manner in front of a large crowd of 1,500 to 2,000 spectators. Consistent with earlier discussions of comparisons between real-world and laboratory pressure situations, narcissism did not significantly correlate with high-pressure performance in a laboratory-based pressure manipulation (Geukes et al. 2012, 2013). Thus, further research should tease out the reasons for these contextual explanations of narcissistic tendencies on performance under pressure.

14 Situational Factors in Perception of Pressure and Occurrence of Choking

Situational factors of choking are often changing, and depend on environmental and psychological circumstances that differentially affect performance. Perceptions of these internal and external factors, however, can be easily modified to help individuals manage the situation. Baumeister and Showers (1986) provided an extensive explanation of these factors in their review of literature that relate (but are not limited) to: self- and others' expectations, the importance of performing well, audience and video camera presence, and monetary incentives.

If the situation is threatening and/or important to the athlete, then increases in perceived pressure occur, which usually result in higher state anxiety. The more an athlete is susceptible to increases in perceived pressure through personality characteristics, the more likely the athlete may develop self-presentation concerns. Sport provides a social situation where real and imagined self-presentation concerns are abundant and perceptions of threat increase competitive anxiety. This is especially true considering sport anxiety researchers (e.g., James and Collins 1997; Wilson and Eklund 1998; Williams, Hudson, and Lawson 1999; Bray, Martin and Widmeyer 2000; Hudson and Williams 2001; Lorimer 2006) have consistently found a positive relationship between state and trait anxiety and self-presentation concerns. For example, researchers (Wilson and Eklund 1998; Hudson and Williams 2001) have found that self-presentation concerns are more strongly related to cognitive than somatic trait anxiety. Furthermore, Bray et al. (2000) also found that evaluative concerns were significantly, albeit modestly, related to precompetitive state anxiety among athletes, with nonspecific and performance-specific evaluative concerns both related to cognitive anxiety. The link between competitive anxiety and self-presentation has also been identified in "choking-susceptible" athletes, with researchers (e.g., Gucciardi et al. 2010; Hill et al. 2010a) explaining that self-presentation concerns and social evaluation were themes that led to increased anxiety and choking experiences.

Leary (1992) argued that, during competition, athletes risk conveying a variety of negative images of themselves to an array of evaluative others including (but not limited to) spectators, teammates, coaches, and opposing team members. Those who are prone to choking susceptibility want others to view them in a desirable way; they attempt to control inferences made about them by others, often behaving or thinking in ways that might convey a positive image about themselves to others, to perhaps minimize social anxiety. In their self-presentation model of social anxiety, Schlenker and Leary (1982) explained how social anxiety increases when people are motivated to make a desired impression on others but doubt they will be successful. Leary (2001) expanded the original self-presentation theory by suggesting that social anxiety increases if there is potential for relational devaluation to occur; when people believe that the impressions made will lead others to devalue, avoid, or reject their relationships with them. For the choking-susceptible athlete, if the public self (the image of oneself that exists in the minds of others; Baumeister 1982) is discredited, a negative self-presentation and relational devaluation may occur. Particularly for the athlete who is high in athletic identity, being portrayed as an unsuccessful athlete under pressure or, more drastically, a "choker," can clearly lead to self- and relational devaluation. When athletes are concerned about what others think of them, their behaviors, cognitions, and emotions in competitive sport settings may change. Thus, during performance under pressure, choking-susceptible athletes may draw on cognitions within choking models (i.e., distraction and self-focus approaches) to help them (counterproductively) make a positive impression in the public setting so a negative image of them as an elite athlete does not occur. The effects of the audience-presence and evaluation-by-coaches conditions in Mesagno, Harvey, and Janelle's (2011) experimental study of performance under pressure in field hockey penalty shots are certainly consistent with this idea.

15 Conclusion

Our review of the scientific study of choking has specifically focused on the domain of sensorimotor skills. The research shows that when one is a novice at a new sport skill, concentration on the step-by-step performance of that skill is required in order to do one's best, while distracting thoughts about the audience, possible failure, or other irrelevant tasks imposed from the outside are heavily disruptive.

Highly practiced experts appear to be somewhat the opposite, when performing a very well-practiced task in their domain of expertise, as they benefit from letting go of conscious control. Their performance improves if they rely on what has been called "automaticity" from a skilled-performance perspective (e.g., Fitts and Posner 1967; Anderson 1982; Brown and Carr 1989; Beilock and Carr 2001; Beilock et al. 2002), "flow" from a more humanistic or "positive psychology" perspective (Jackson and Csíkszentmihályi 1999; Shernoff et al. 2003), or "enactive creativity" from a philosophical perspective (Rucińska 2014a, 2014b; Rucińska and Aggerholm, this volume).

However, there are limits. The benefits of a state of "flow" or "enactive creativity" that allows "automatic" procedures to govern performance can arise only if the performer possesses enough well-practiced knowledge and skill to support them, can control and use his or her emotions sufficiently and effectively, and can resist the pull to shift attention toward conscious control of particular steps of performance and/or particular body parts that carry out those steps.

What governs this shift of control? Increases in arousal accompany the experience of pressure. Moderate increases help performance by increasing available energy, increasing processing capacity, and focusing attention on task-relevant information, but larger increases in arousal eventually push performers over the top of the Yerkes-Dodson arousal-performance function, leading to decreases in performance as attention narrows, concentration falters, and reward processes shift from aiming for gains to avoiding losses.

At the highest levels of arousal in the Yerkes-Dodson function, panic may begin to set in, and withdrawal from performance altogether can be the outcome. This is the sort of end state that phenomenological reports using qualitative interview methods have obtained from high-level athletes talking about experiences of choking. Athletes say they could not do anything right and their only desire was to get off the field, to escape. This is of course an extreme response, but we must consider the extremes in order to figure out how "choking" arises, what it is like, and what it entails.

The entire human organism is involved in the processes we have described, from the earliest applications of attention for gaining perceptual information to the interpretative and judgmental processes by which that information is evaluated to the working memory processes by which explicit thoughts are entertained and portions of the goal structure of the task are activated for implementation to the implementation processes and the actions themselves, whose forms, trajectories, and outcomes are shaped as much by the physiognomy of the body as by the goals and operations of the mind. All of these rather cognitive- and kinesiological-sounding processes are governed by and integrated with emotional and motivational states and processes, which can vary significantly both with situational conditions and with measurable facets of personality.

All of the above simply repeats facts that have been reviewed in this chapter. But what remains to be determined? In our view, the important questions are what are all the various states and processes occurring in real time in athletes that change when "pressure" is felt, what states and processes change in the laboratory performer and is the lab experience anything like what an athlete experiences in moments of intense competition, and what sorts of internal and external conditions can create a feeling of "pressure"—witness the differences among conditions in the comparison of reward, presence of an audience, and evaluation by Mesagno, Harvey, and Janelle (2011).

This leads us to ask whether all the ways of creating what has been called a "pressure" situation (both real-world and laboratory) operate on states and processes in the same way—the answer at present appears to be no—and what if anything can be done to help sensorimotor-skilled performers avoid the negative effects of pressure while channeling the positive effects. To date, three answers to this question have been offered from a primarily cognitive perspective: (1) distract them while they are learning (Masters), (2) distract them while they are performing (Beilock, Masters), and (3) put them under pressure while they are learning, so they get used to it (Beilock).

Another set of answers has been offered from the phenomenological and clinical perspectives. These include (1) help performers view extremely demanding competitive situations as challenges rather than threats, and (2) help performers adopt avoidance strategies for ignoring or putting aside fearful and failure-oriented thoughts and feelings, rather than engaging and magnifying them. Each of these approaches has evidence to support it, so perhaps they are all true and their implications must be appreciated together. This recalls the old story about the blind men feeling the elephant—no one story was correct, but all together they had it right.

In some ways it may seem that the list of relevant factors considered in this chapter is so broad and disparate as to defy coherent integration or concerted investigation. Our belief is that new advances in both theoretical understanding of choking and clinical intervention in its management will require coherent integration and concerted investigation across the many factors and approaches we have raised and reviewed. This in turn will require a truly interdisciplinary approach in which philosophers, sport psychologists, cognitive scientists, personality researchers, and educational researchers learn one another's languages and techniques and collaborate together. The research undertaken so far in each of these fields has made considerable progress, as we have tried to show. The next task is to try to bring these fields together to make a sum that can be greater than its individual parts.

Acknowledgments

This research on choking and embodied cognition was partly sponsored by a UPAR grant by UAE National Research Foundation, "Sport and Brain Science: Technological Applications for Peaking Performances" (grant code: 31H087-UPAR (3) 2014).

Notes

1. Breivik (2007, 2013) and Birch, Fusche Moe, and Breivik (this volume) emphasize the need to overcome the stereotypical characterization of the expert performer as a mindless automata or consciousnessless zombie, incapable of deliberation or aware control during peak performance. Their accurate phenomenology of skillful action carefully reflects how self-awareness and attention are important components of peak performance. In dialogue with their proposal, Cappuccio (2017) suggests a nuanced account of consciousness in skillful performance that is informed by the concerns raised by Birch and colleagues, while recognizing that "flow" activities (Swann et al. 2012) and highly proceduralized execution routines are characterized by peculiar adumbrations of consciousness.

2. The internal/external distinction assumed by AFT has been criticized for its vagueness (for a review, see Montero, Toner, and Moran, this volume; a partial reply to some of these critical analyses is offered by Wulf 2016). A similar criticism might also be formulated against EFT, but it would not apply in the same way. The potential ambiguity of EFT, if any exists, concerns the proper analysis of the task's control structure (as task analysis is not a fully-agreed-upon exercise), not what is "near"/"far from" the performing subject.

3. While EFT claims that explicit control of one's own actions is detrimental only to peak performance of experts (not novices), AFT claims that internal focus universally undermines performance, regardless of skill level and expertise type (Wulf 2013, 2015), and that external foci, in turn, benefit both experienced professionals during competition and learning novices during training (Wulf, Lauterbach, and Toole 1999; Wulf, Shea, and Park 2001; Wulf et al. 2002).

4. While as described earlier, Mesagno, Harvey, and Janelle (2011) found no impact of physiologically expressed anxiety as measured by self-report, these results show that a direct measure of physiological state can predict performance-relevant responses to pressure.

References

Abreu, Ana Maria, E. Macaluso, R. T. Azevedo, Paola Cesari, Cosimo Urgesi, and Salvatore Maria Aglioti. 2012. "Action Anticipation beyond the Action Observation Network: A Functional Magnetic Resonance Imaging Study in Expert Basketball Players." *European Journal of Neuroscience* 35 (10): 1646–1654.

Aglioti, Salvatore M., Paola Cesari, Michela Romani, and Cosimo Urgesi. 2008. "Action Anticipation and Motor Resonance in Elite Basketball Players." *Nature Neuroscience* 11 (9): 1109–1116.

Alden, Lynn E., Andrew G. Ryder, and Tanna M. B. Mellings. 2002. "Perfectionism in the Context of Social Fears: Toward a Two-Component Model." In *Perfectionism: Theory, Research and Treatment*, edited by G. L. Flett and P. L. Hewitt, 373–391. Washington, DC: American Psychological Association.

Allen, Mark S., Daniel Frings, and Steve Hunter. 2012. "Personality, Coping, and Challenge and Threat States in Athletes." *International Journal of Sport and Exercise Psychology* 10 (4): 264–275.

Anderson, John R. 1982. "Acquisition of Cognitive Skill." *Psychological Review* 89 (4): 369.

Anshel, Mark H., and Robert S. Weinberg. 1999. "Re-Examining Coping among Basketball Referees Following Stressful Events: Implications for Coping Interventions." *Journal of Sport Behavior* 22 (2): 141–161.

Aspinwall, L. G., and S. E. Taylor. 1997. "A Stitch in Time: Self-Regulation and Proactive Coping." *Psychological Bulletin* 121 (3): 417–436.

Atkinson, John W. 1957. "Motivational Determinants of Risk-Taking Behavior." *Psychological Review* 64 (6): 359–372.

Baumeister, Roy F. 1982. "A Self-Presentational View of Social Phenomena." *Psychological Bulletin* 91 (1): 3–26.

Baumeister, Roy F. 1984. "Choking under Pressure: Self-Consciousness and Paradoxical Effects of Incentives on Skillful Performance." *Journal of Personality and Social Psychology* 46 (3): 610–620.

Baumeister, Roy F., and Todd F. Heatherton. 1996. "Self-Regulation Failure: An Overview." *Psychological Inquiry* 7 (1): 1–15.

Baumeister, Roy F., and Jill Lobbestael. 2011. "Emotions and Antisocial Behavior." *Journal of Forensic Psychiatry and Psychology* 22 (5): 635–649.

Baumeister, Roy F., and S. J. Scher. 1988. "Self-Defeating Behavior Patterns among Normal Individuals: Review and Analysis of Common Self-Destructive Tendencies." *Psychological Bulletin* 104 (1): 3–22.

Baumeister, Roy F., and Carolin J. Showers. 1986. "A Review of Paradoxical Performance Effects: Choking under Pressure in Sports and Mental Tests." *European Journal of Social Psychology* 16 (4): 361–383.

Baumeister, Roy F., and Kathleen D. Vohs. 2001. "Narcissism as Addiction to Esteem." *Psychological Inquiry* 12 (4): 206–210.

Baumeister, Roy F., Kathleen D. Vohs, C. Nathan DeWall, and Liqing Zhang. 2007. "How Emotion Shapes Behavior: Feedback, Anticipation, and Reflection, Rather than Direct Causation." *Personality and Social Psychology Review* 11 (2): 167–203.

Beilock, S. L., and R. Gray. 2012. "From Attentional Control to Attentional Spillover: A Skill-Level Investigation of Attention, Movement, and Performance Outcomes." *Human Movement Science* 31 (6): 1473–1499.

Beilock, Sian. 2015. *How The Body Knows Its Mind*. London: Hachette UK.

Beilock, Sian L. 2008a. "Beyond the Playing Field: Sport Psychology Meets Embodied Cognition." *International Review of Sport and Exercise Psychology* 1 (1): 19–30.

Beilock, Sian L. 2008b. "Math Performance in Stressful Situations." *Current Directions in Psychological Science* 17 (5): 339–343.

Beilock, Sian L. 2011. *Choke*. Boston: Little, Brown.

Beilock, Sian L., Bennett I. Bertenthal, Michael Hoerger, and Thomas H. Carr. 2008. "When Does Haste Make Waste? Speed-Accuracy Tradeoff, Skill Level, and the Tools of the Trade." *Journal of Experimental Psychology: Applied* 14 (4): 340–352.

Beilock, Sian L., Bennett I. Bertenthal, Annette M. McCoy, and Thomas H. Carr. 2004. "Haste Does Not Always Make Waste: Expertise, Direction of Attention, and Speed versus Accuracy in Performing Sensorimotor Skills." *Psychonomic Bulletin and Review* 11 (2): 373–379.

Beilock, Sian L., and Thomas H. Carr. 2001. "On the Fragility of Skilled Performance: What Governs Choking under Pressure?" *Journal of Experimental Psychology: General* 130 (4): 701–725.

Beilock, Sian L., Thomas H. Carr, Clare MacMahon, and Janet L. Starkes. 2002. "When Paying Attention Becomes Counterproductive: Impact of Divided versus Skill-Focused Attention on Novice and Experienced Performance of Sensorimotor Skills." *Journal of Experimental Psychology: Applied* 8 (1): 6–16.

Beilock, Sian L., and Marci S. Decaro. 2007. "From Poor Performance to Success under Stress: Working Memory, Strategy Selection, and Mathematical Problem Solving under Pressure." *Journal of Experimental Psychology: Learning, Memory, and Cognition* 33 (6): 983–998.

Beilock, Sian L., and Rob Gray. 2007. "Why Do Athletes Choke under Pressure?" In *Handbook of Sport Psychology*, 3rd ed., edited by Gershon Tenenbaum and Bob Eklund, 425–444. Hoboken, NJ: John Wiley.

Beilock, Sian L., William A. Jellison, Robert J. Rydell, Allen R. McConnell, and Thomas H. Carr. 2006. "On the Causal Mechanisms of Stereotype Threat: Can Skills That Don't Rely Heavily on Working Memory Still Be Threatened?" *Personality and Social Psychology Bulletin* 32 (8): 1059–1071.

Beilock, Sian L., Catherine A. Kulp, Lauren E. Holt, and Thomas H. Carr. 2004. "More on the Fragility of Performance: Choking under Pressure in Mathematical Problem Solving." *Journal of Experimental Psychology: General* 133 (4): 584–600.

Beilock, Sian L., Ian M. Lyons, Andrew Mattarella-Micke, Howard C. Nusbaum, and Steven L. Small. 2008b. "Sports Experience Changes the Neural Processing of Action Language." *Proceedings of the National Academy of Sciences of the United States of America* 105 (36): 13269–13273.

Bhalla, Mukul, and Dennis R. Proffitt. 1999. "Visual—Motor Recalibration in Geographical Slant Perception." *Journal of Experimental Psychology: Human Perception and Performance* 25 (4): 1076.

Blascovich, Jim. 2008. "Challenge, Threat, and Health." In *Handbook of Motivation Science*, edited by James Y. Shah and Wendi L. Gardner, 481–493. New York: Guilford Press.

Blascovich, Jim, and Wendy B. Mendes. 2000. "Challenge and Threat Appraisals: The Role of Affective Cues." In *Feeling and Thinking: The Role of Affect in Social Cognition,* edited by J. Forgas, 59–82. Cambridge: Cambridge University Press.

Blascovich, Jim, Wendy Berry Mendes, Sarah B. Hunter, and Brian Lickel. 2000. "Stigma, Threat, and Social Interactions." In *The Social Psychology of Stigma,* edited by T. Heatherton, R. Kleck, M. R. Hebl, and J. G. Hull, 307–333. New York: Guilford.

Blascovich, Jim, and Joe Tomaka. 1996. "The Biopsychosocial Model of Arousal Regulation." *Advances in Experimental Social Psychology* 28: 1–51.

Bradley, Jeff. 2003. "The Flash." *ESPN Magazine*, May 27. http://www.espn.com/magazine/vol5no11ichiro.html

Bray, S. R., K. A. Martin, and W. N. Widmeyer. 2000. "The Relationship between Evaluative Concerns and Sport Competition State Anxiety among Youth Skiers." *Journal of Sports Sciences* 18 (5): 353–361.

Breivik, Gunnar. 2007. "Skillful Coping in Everyday Life and in Sport: A Critical Examination of the Views of Heidegger and Dreyfus." *Journal of the Philosophy of Sport* 34 (2): 116–134.

Breivik, Gunnar. 2013. "Zombie-Like or Superconscious? A Phenomenological and Conceptual Analysis of Consciousness in Elite Sport." *Journal of the Philosophy of Sport* 40 (1): 85–106.

Brewer, Britton W. 1993. "Self-Identity and Specific Vulnerability to Depressed Mood." *Journal of Personality* 61 (3): 343–364.

Brewer, Britton W., Judy L. Van Raalte, and Darwyn E. Linder. 1993. "Athletic Identity: Hercules' Muscles or Achilles Heel?" *International Journal of Sport Psychology* 24 (2): 237–254.

Brown, Tracy L., and Thomas H. Carr. 1989. "Automaticity in Skill Acquisition: Mechanisms for Reducing Interference in Concurrent Performance." *Journal of Experimental Psychology: Human Perception and Performance* 15 (4): 686–700.

Bruner, Jerome S. 1957. "On Perceptual Readiness." *Psychological Review* 64 (2): 123–152.

Bruner, Jerome S. 1966. *Toward a Theory of Instruction*. Cambridge, MA: Harvard University Press.

Calvo, Manuel G., Leopoldo Alamo, and Pedro M. Ramos. 1990. "Test Anxiety, Motor Performance and Learning: Attentional and Somatic Interference." *Personality and Individual Differences* 11 (1): 29–38.

Cañal-Bruland, Rouwen, J. R. Pijpers, and Raôul R. D. Oudejans. 2010. "The Influence of Anxiety on Action-Specific Perception." *Anxiety, Stress, and Coping* 23 (3): 353–361.

Cañal-Bruland, Rouwen, and John van der Kamp. 2009. "Action Goals Influence Action-Specific Perception." *Psychonomic Bulletin and Review* 16 (6): 1100–1105.

Cañal-Bruland, Rouwen, Frank F. Zhu, John van der Kamp, and Rich S. W. Masters. 2011. "Target-Directed Visual Attention Is a Prerequisite for Action-Specific Perception." *Acta Psychologica* 136 (3): 285–289.

Cappuccio, Massimiliano L., ed. 2015. "Unreflective Action and the Choking Effect." *Phenomenology and the Cognitive Sciences* 14 (2): 213–225.

Cappuccio, Massimiliano L. 2016. "Mind-Upload. The Ultimate Challenge to the Embodied Mind Theory." *Phenomenology and the Cognitive Sciences* 16 (3): 1–24.

Cappuccio, Massimiliano L. 2017. "Flow, Choke, Skill: The Role of the Non-Conscious in Sport Performance." In *Before Consciousness: In Search of the Fundamentals of Mind,* edited by Zdravko Radman, 246–283. Exeter, UK: Imprint Academic.

Carleton, R. Nicholas, Donald R. McCreary, Peter J. Norton, and Gordon J. G. Asmundson. 2006. "Brief Fear of Negative Evaluation Scale-Revised." *Depression and Anxiety* 23 (5): 297–303.

Carr, Thomas H. 2015. "Strengths and Weaknesses of Reflection as a Guide to Action: Pressure Assails Performance in Multiple Ways." *Phenomenology and the Cognitive Sciences* 14 (2): 227–252.

Carver, Charles. 2003. "Pleasure as a Sign You Can Attend to Something Else: Placing Positive Feelings within a General Model of Affect." *Cognition and Emotion* 17 (2): 241–261.

Carver, Charles S., and Michael F. Scheier. 1981. *Attention and Self-Regulation: A Control-Theory Approach to Human Behavior.* Springer Series in Social Psychology. New York: Springer.

Castaneda, Brooke, and Rob Gray. 2007. "Effects of Focus of Attention on Baseball Batting Performance in Players of Differing Skill Levels." *Journal of Sport and Exercise Psychology* 29 (1): 60–77.

Christensen, Wayne, John Sutton, and Doris McIlwain. 2015. "Putting Pressure on Theories of Choking: Towards an Expanded Perspective on Breakdown in Skilled Performance." *Phenomenology and the Cognitive Sciences* 14 (2): 253–293.

Christensen, Wayne, John Sutton, and Doris J. F. McIlwain. 2016. "Cognition in Skilled Action: Meshed Control and the Varieties of Skill Experience." *Mind & Language* 31 (1): 37–66.

Clark, Andy. 2015. *Surfing Uncertainty: Prediction, Action, and the Embodied Mind.* Oxford: Oxford University Press.

Clark, David M., and Adrian Wells. 1995. "A Cognitive Model of Social Phobia." *Social Phobia: Diagnosis, Assessment, and Treatment* 41 (68): 00022–00023.

Coombes, Stephen A., Torrie Higgins, Kelly M. Gamble, James H. Cauraugh, and Christopher M. Janelle. 2009. "Attentional Control Theory: Anxiety, Emotion, and Motor Planning." *Journal of Anxiety Disorders* 23 (8): 1072–1079.

Cosmelli, Diego, and Evan Thompson. 2010. "Embodiment or Envatment? Reflections on the Bodily Basis of Consciousness." In *Enaction: Towards a New Paradigm for Cognitive Science,* edited by J. Stewart, O. Gapenne, and E. Di Paolo, 361–385. Cambridge, MA: MIT Press.

Crocker, Peter R. E., and Thomas R. Graham. 1995. "Emotion in Sport and Physical Activity: The Importance of Perceived Individual Goals." *International Journal of Sport Psychology* 26 (1): 117–137.

Crook, Jan M., and Sharon E. Robertson. 1991. "Transitions Out of Elite Sport." *International Journal of Sport Psychology* 22 (2): 115–127.

Csíkszentmihályi, Mihaly. 1996. *Flow and the Psychology of Discovery and Invention*. New York: HarperCollins.

Dandy, J., N. Brewer, and R. Tottman. 2001. "Self-Consciousness and Performance Decrements within a Sporting Context." *Journal of Social Psychology* 141 (1): 150–152.

Davids, Keith, Duarte Araújo, Robert Hristovski, Pedro Passos, and Jia Yi Chow. 2012. "Ecological Dynamics and Motor Learning Design in Sport." In *Skill Acquisition in Sport: Research, Theory and Practice*, 2nd ed., edited by M. Williams and N. Hodges, 112–130. London: Routledge.

DeCaro, Marci S., Robin D. Thomas, Neil B. Albert, and Sian L. Beilock. 2011. "Choking under Pressure: Multiple Routes to Skill Failure." *Journal of Experimental Psychology: General* 140 (3): 390–406.

Dreyfus, Hubert L. 1996. "The Current Relevance of Merleau-Ponty's Phenomenology of Embodiment." *Electronic Journal of Analytic Philosophy* 4 (Spring): 1–16.

Dreyfus, Hubert L. 2002. "Intelligence without Representation—Merleau-Ponty's Critique of Mental Representation, the Relevance of Phenomenology to Scientific Explanation." *Phenomenology and the Cognitive Sciences* 1 (4): 367–383.

Dreyfus, Hubert L. 2012. "Introductory Essay: The Mystery of the Background qua Background." In *Knowing without Thinking*, edited by Zdravko Radman, 1–10. New Directions in Philosophy and Cognitive Science. Basingstoke, UK: Palgrave Macmillan.

Dreyfus, Stuart E., and Hubert L. Dreyfus. 1980. "A Five-Stage Model of the Mental Activities Involved in Directed Skill Acquisition." Berkeley: University of California Operations Research Center.

Erez, Amir, and Alice M. Isen. 2002. "The Influence of Positive Affect on the Components of Expectancy Motivation." *Journal of Applied Psychology* 87 (6): 1055–1067.

Evans, Jonathan B. T., and Keith E. Stanovich. 2013. "Dual-Process Theories of Higher Cognition: Advancing the Debate." *Perspectives on Psychological Science: A Journal of the Association for Psychological Science* 8 (3): 223–241.

Eysenck, Michael W., and Manuel G. Calvo. 1992. "Anxiety and Performance: The Processing Efficiency Theory." *Cognition and Emotion* 6 (6): 409–434.

Eysenck, Michael W., Nazanin Derakshan, Rita Santos, and Manuel G. Calvo. 2007. "Anxiety and Cognitive Performance: Attentional Control Theory." *Emotion* 7 (2): 336–353.

Fenigstein, Allan, Michael F. Scheier, and Arnold H. Buss. 1975. "Public and Private Self-Consciousness: Assessment and Theory." *Journal of Consulting and Clinical Psychology* 43 (4): 522–527.

Ferrari, Pier Francesco, and Giacomo Rizzolatti. 2015. *New Frontiers in Mirror Neurons Research.* Oxford: Oxford University Press.

Fink, Philip W., Patrick S. Foo, and William H. Warren. 2009. "Catching Fly Balls in Virtual Reality: A Critical Test of the Outfielder Problem." *Journal of Vision* 9 (13): 14.1–8.

Fitts, P. M., and M. I. Posner. 1967. *Human Performance.* Pacific Grove, CA: Brooks/Cole.

Flett, Gordon L., and Paul L. Hewitt. 2005. "The Perils of Perfectionism in Sports and Exercise." *Current Directions in Psychological Science* 14 (1): 14–18.

Fredrickson, B. L. 2001. "The Role of Positive Emotion in Positive Psychology: The Broaden-and-Build Theory of Positive Emotion." *American Psychologist* 56:218–226.

Fredrickson, Barbara L. 2003. "The Value of Positive Emotions." *American Scientist* 91 (4): 330–335.

Frost, Randy O., and Katherine J. Henderson. 1991. "Perfectionism and Reactions to Athletic Competition." *Journal of Sport and Exercise Psychology* 13 (4): 323–335.

Frost, Randy O., and Patricia A. Marten. 1990. "Perfectionism and Evaluative Threat." *Cognitive Therapy and Research* 14 (6): 559–572.

Gallagher, Shaun. 2005. *How the Body Shapes the Mind.* New York: Oxford University Press.

Gallagher, Shaun. 2011. "Interpretations of Embodied Cognition." In *The Implications of Embodiment: Cognition and Communication,* edited by W. Tschacher and C. Bergomi, 59–70. Exeter, UK: Imprint Academic.

Gallese, Vittorio. 2007. "The Shared Manifold Hypothesis: Embodied Simulation and Its Role in Empathy and Social Cognition." In *Empathy in Mental Illness and Health,* edited by Tom F. D. Farrow and Peter W. R. Woodruff, 448–472. Cambridge: Cambridge University Press.

Geukes, Katharina, Jack T. Harvey, Alexandra Trezise, and Christopher Mesagno. 2017. "Personality and Performance in Real-World Competitions: Testing Trait Activation of Fear of Negative Evaluation, Dispositional Reinvestment, and Athletic Identity in the Field." *Psychology of Sport and Exercise* 30:101–109.

Geukes, Katharina, Christopher Mesagno, Stephanie J. Hanrahan, and Michael Kellmann. 2012. "Testing an Interactionist Perspective on the Relationship between Personality Traits and Performance under Public Pressure." *Psychology of Sport and Exercise* 13 (3): 243–250.

Geukes, Katharina, Christopher Mesagno, Stephanie J. Hanrahan, and Michael Kellmann. 2013. "Activation of Self-Focus and Self-Presentation Traits under Private, Mixed, and Public Pressure." *Journal of Sport and Exercise Psychology* 35 (1): 50–59.

Gibson, James J. 1977. "The Theory of Affordances." In *Perceiving, Acting, and Knowing: Toward an Ecological Psychology,* edited by Robert Shaw and John Bransford, 67–82. New York: Routledge.

Gibson, James J. 1979. *The Ecological Approach to Visual Perception.* Boston: Houghton Mifflin.

Gibson, James Jerome. 1966. *The Senses Considered as Perceptual Systems*. Boston, MA: Houghton Mifflin.

Gray, Rob. 2004. "Attending to the Execution of a Complex Sensorimotor Skill: Expertise Differences, Choking, and Slumps." *Journal of Experimental Psychology: Applied* 10 (1): 42–54.

Gray, Rob. 2011. "Links between Performance Outcomes, Attention and Movement in Skilled Motor Action." *Current Directions in Psychological Science* 20:301–306.

Gray, Rob. 2013. "Being Selective at the Plate: Processing Dependence between Perceptual Variables Relates to Hitting Goals and Performance." *Journal of Experimental Psychology: Human Perception and Performance* 39 (4): 1124–1142. doi:10.1037/a0030729.

Gray, Rob. 2014. "Embodied Perception in Sport." *International Review of Sport and Exercise Psychology* 7 (1): 72–86.

Gray, Rob, and Jonathan Allsop. 2013. "Interactions between Performance Pressure, Performance Streaks, and Attentional Focus." *Journal of Sport and Exercise Psychology* 35 (4): 368–386.

Gray, Rob, Jonathan Allsop, and Sarah Williams. 2013. "Changes in Putting Kinematics Associated with Choking and Excelling under Pressure." *International Journal of Sport Psychology* 44 (4): 387–407.

Gray, Rob, and Rouwen Cañal-Bruland. 2015. "Attentional Focus, Perceived Target Size, and Movement Kinematics under Performance Pressure." *Psychonomic Bulletin and Review* 22 (6): 1692–1700.

Gucciardi, Daniel F., Jay-Lee Longbottom, Ben Jackson, and James A. Dimmock. 2010. "Experienced Golfers' Perspectives on Choking under Pressure." *Journal of Sport and Exercise Psychology* 32 (1): 61–83.

Hanin, Yuri L. 2000. "Successful and Poor Performance and Emotions." In *Emotions in Sport*, edited by Yuri L. Hanin, 157–187. Champaign, IL: Human Kinetics.

Hanin, Yuri L. 2007. "Emotions in Sport: Current Issues and Perspectives." In *Handbook of Sport Psychology*, edited by Gershon Tenenbaum and Robert C. Eklund, 31–58. Hoboken, NJ: John Wiley.

Hill, Denise M., Sheldon Hanton, Scott Fleming, and Nic Matthews. 2009. "A Re-Examination of Choking in Sport." *European Journal of Sport Science* 9 (4): 203–212.

Hill, Denise M., Sheldon Hanton, Nic Matthews, and Scott Fleming. 2010a. "Choking in Sport: A Review." *International Review of Sport and Exercise Psychology* 3 (1): 24–39.

Hill, Denise M., Sheldon Hanton, Nic Matthews, and Scott Fleming. 2010b. "A Qualitative Exploration of Choking in Elite Golf." *Journal of Clinical Sport Psychology* 4 (3): 221–240.

Hill, Denise M., Sheldon Hanton, Nic Matthews, and Scott Fleming. 2011. "Alleviation of Choking under Pressure in Elite Golf: An Action Research Study." *Sport Psychologist* 25 (4): 465–488.

Hill, Denise M., and Brian Hemmings. 2015. "A Phenomenological Exploration of Coping Responses Associated with Choking in Sport." *Qualitative Research in Sport, Exercise and Health* 7 (4): 521–538. doi.org/10.1080/2159676X.2014.981573.

Hill, Denise M., and Gareth Shaw. 2013. "A Qualitative Examination of Choking under Pressure in Team Sport." *Psychology of Sport and Exercise* 14 (1): 103–110.

Hostetter, Autumn B., and Martha W. Alibali. 2008. "Visible Embodiment: Gestures as Simulated Action." *Psychonomic Bulletin and Review* 15 (3): 495–514.

Hudson, Joanne, and Matthew Williams. 2001. "Associations between Self-Presentation and Competitive A-Trait: A Preliminary Investigation." *Social Behavior and Personality: An International Journal* 29 (1): 1–10.

Jackson, Robin C., Kelly J. Ashford, and Glen Norsworthy. 2006. "Attentional Focus, Dispositional Reinvestment, and Skilled Motor Performance under Pressure." *Journal of Sport and Exercise Psychology* 28 (1): 49–68.

Jackson, Robin C., and Sian L. Beilock. 2008. "Performance Pressure and Paralysis by Analysis: Research and Implications." In *Developing Sports Expertise: Researchers and Coaches Put Theory into Practice,* edited by Damian Farrow, Joseph Baker, and Clare MacMahon, 104–118. London: Routledge.

Jackson, Robin C., Sian L. Beilock, and Noel P. Kinrade. 2013. "'Choking' in Sport: Research and Implications." In *Developing Sport Expertise: Researchers and Coaches Put Theory in to Practice,* 2nd ed., edited by Damian Farrow, Joseph Baker, and Clare MacMahon, 177–194. London: Routledge.

Jackson, Susan A., and Mihaly Csíkszentmihályi. 1999. *Flow in Sports*. Champaign, IL: Human Kinetics.

James, Benjamin, and David Collins. 1997. "Self-Presentational Sources of Competitive Stress during Performance." *Journal of Sport and Exercise Psychology* 19 (1): 17–35.

Jones, G. 1995. "More than Just a Game: Research Developments and Issues in Competitive Anxiety in Sport." *British Journal of Psychology* 86 (Pt 4) (November): 449–478.

Jones, Marc, Carla Meijen, Paul Joseph McCarthy, and David Sheffield. 2009. "A Theory of Challenge and Threat States in Athletes." *International Review of Sport and Exercise Psychology* 2 (2): 161–180.

Jordet, Geir. 2009. "Why Do English Players Fail in Soccer Penalty Shootouts? A Study of Team Status, Self-Regulation, and Choking under Pressure." *Journal of Sports Sciences* 27 (2): 97–106.

Jordet, Geir. 2010. "Choking under Pressure as Self-Destructive Behavior." In *Coping in Sport: Theory, Methods, and Related Constructs,* edited by Adam R. Nicholls, 239–259. New York: Nova Science.

Jordet, Geir, and Esther Hartman. 2008. "Avoidance Motivation and Choking under Pressure in Soccer Penalty Shootouts." *Journal of Sport and Exercise Psychology* 30 (4): 450–457.

Kerr, John H. 2014. *Motivation and Emotion in Sport: Reversal Theory*. London: Psychology Press.

Kinrade, Noel P., Robin C. Jackson, and Kelly J. Ashford. 2010. "Dispositional Reinvestment and Skill Failure in Cognitive and Motor Tasks." *Psychology of Sport and Exercise* 11 (4): 312–319.

Kirsh, David, and Paul Maglio. 1994. "On Distinguishing Epistemic from Pragmatic Action." *Cognitive Science* 18 (4): 513–549.

Kurosawa, Kaoru, and Judith M. Harackiewicz. 1995. "Test Anxiety, Self-Awareness, and Cognitive Interference: A Process Analysis." *Journal of Personality* 63 (4): 931–951.

Lane, A. M., C. J. Beedie, T. J. Devonport, and D. M. Stanley. 2011. "Instrumental Emotion Regulation in Sport: Relationships between Beliefs about Emotion and Emotion Regulation Strategies Used by Athletes." *Scandinavian Journal of Medicine and Science in Sports* 21 (6): e445–451.

Lavallee, David, Sandy Gordon, and J. Robert Grove. 1997. "Retirement from Sport and the Loss of Athletic Identity." *Journal of Personal and Interpersonal Loss* 2 (2): 129–147.

Lazarus, Richard S. 2000. "Cognitive-Motivational-Relational Theory of Emotion." In *Emotions in Sport,* edited by Yuri L. Hanin, 39–63. Champaign, IL: Human Kinetics.

Leary, Mark R. 1992. "Self-Presentational Processes in Exercise and Sport." *Journal of Sport and Exercise Psychology* 14 (4): 339–351.

Leary, Mark R. 2001. "Social Anxiety as an Early Warning System: A Refinement and Extension of the Self-Presentation Theory of Social Anxiety." In *From Social Anxiety to Social Phobia: Multiple Perspectives,* edited by Stefan G. Hoffman and Patricia Marten DiBartolo, 321–334. Needham Heights, MA: Allyn and Bacon.

Lorimer, Ross. 2006. "The Relationship between Self-Presentational Concerns and Competitive Anxiety: The Influence of Gender." *International Journal of Sport and Exercise Psychology* 37 (4): 317–329.

Marchant, Daryl B., Tony Morris, and Mark B. Andersen. 1998. "Perceived Importance of Outcome as a Contributing Factor in Competitive State Anxiety." *Journal of Sport Behavior* 21 (1): 71–91.

Martin, Jeffrey J., Robert C. Eklund, and Carol Adams Mushett. 1997. "Factor Structure of the Athletic Identity Measurement Scale with Athletes with Disabilities." *Adapted Physical Activity Quarterly* 14 (1): 74–82.

Masters, Richard S. W. 1992. "Knowledge, Knerves and Know-How: The Role of Explicit versus Implicit Knowledge in the Breakdown of a Complex Motor Skill under Pressure." *British Journal of Psychology* 83 (3): 343–358.

Masters, Richard S. W., and J. P. Maxwell. 2004. "Implicit Motor Learning, Reinvestment and Movement Disruption: What You Don't Know Won't Hurt You?" In *Skill Acquisition in Sport: Research, Theory and Practice,* edited by A. M. Williams and N. J. Hodges, 207–228. London: Routledge.

Masters, Richard S. W., and Jon P. Maxwell. 2008. "The Theory of Reinvestment." *International Review of Sport and Exercise Psychology* 1 (2): 160–183.

Masters, Richard S. W., R. C. J. Polman, and N. V. Hammond. 1993. "'Reinvestment': A Dimension of Personality Implicated in Skill Breakdown under Pressure." *Personality and Individual Differences* 14 (5): 655–666.

Maxwell, Jon P., Richard S. Masters, and F. F. Eves. 2000. "From Novice to No Know-How: A Longitudinal Study of Implicit Motor Learning." *Journal of Sports Sciences* 18 (2): 111–120.

McCarthy, Paul J. 2011. "Positive Emotion in Sport Performance: Current Status and Future Directions." *International Review of Sport and Exercise Psychology* 4 (1): 50–69.

McEnroe, John, and James Kaplan. 2002. *You Cannot Be Serious*. London: Penguin.

Meijen, Carla, Marc V. Jones, Paul J. McCarthy, David Sheffield, and Mark S. Allen. 2013. "Cognitive and Affective Components of Challenge and Threat States." *Journal of Sports Sciences* 31 (8): 847–855.

Mendes, Wendy Berry, Brenda Major, Shannon McCoy, and Jim Blascovich. 2008. "How Attributional Ambiguity Shapes Physiological and Emotional Responses to Social Rejection and Acceptance." *Journal of Personality and Social Psychology* 94 (2): 278–291.

Mesagno, C., and D. M. Hill. 2013. "Definition of Choking in Sport: Re-Conceptualization and Debate." *International Journal of Sport Psychology* 44 (4): 267–277.

Mesagno, Christopher. 2009. "Choking under Pressure: Toward a Self-Presentation Explanation of Why Athletes Use Self-Monitoring Techniques." Paper presented at the 12th World Congress of Sport Psychology. Marrakesh, Morocco.

Mesagno, Christopher, and Jürgen Beckmann. 2017. "Choking under Pressure: Theoretical Models and Interventions." *Current Opinions in Psychology* 16:170–175.

Mesagno, Christopher, Katharina Geukes, and Paul Larkin. 2015. "Choking under Pressure: A Review of Current Debates, Literature, and Interventions." In *Contemporary Advances in Sport Psychology*, edited by S. D. Mellalieu and S. Hanton, 148–174. Abingdon, UK: Routledge.

Mesagno Christopher, Jack T. Harvey, and Christopher M. Janelle. 2011. "Self-Presentation Origins of Choking: Evidence from Separate Pressure Manipulations." *Journal of Sport and Exercise Psychology* 33:441–459.

Mesagno Christopher, Jack T. Harvey, and Christopher M. Janelle. 2012. "Choking under Pressure: The Role of Fear of Negative Evaluation." *Psychology of Sport and Exercise* 13:60–68.

Mesagno, Christopher, Daryl Marchant, and Tony Morris. 2009. "Alleviating Choking: The Sounds of Distraction." *Journal of Applied Sport Psychology* 21 (2): 131–147.

Montero, Barbara G. 2010. "Does Bodily Awareness Interfere with Highly Skilled Movement?" *Inquiry: A Journal of Medical Care Organization, Provision and Financing* 53 (2): 105–122.

Montero, Barbara G. 2014. "Is Monitoring One's Actions Causally Relevant to Choking under Pressure?" *Phenomenology and the Cognitive Sciences* 14 (2): 379–395.

Montero, Barbara G. 2016. *Thought in Action: Expertise and the Conscious Mind.* Oxford: Oxford University Press.

Moore, Lee J., Samuel J. Vine, Paul Freeman, and Mark R. Wilson. 2013. "Quiet Eye Training Promotes Challenge Appraisals and Aids Performance under Elevated Anxiety." *International Journal of Sport and Exercise Psychology* 11 (2): 169–183.

Moore, Lee J., Samuel J. Vine, Mark R. Wilson, and Paul Freeman. 2012. "The Effect of Challenge and Threat States on Performance: An Examination of Potential Mechanisms." *Psychophysiology* 49 (10): 1417–1425.

Moore, Lee J., Samuel J. Vine, Mark R. Wilson, and Paul Freeman. 2015. "Reappraising Threat: How to Optimize Performance under Pressure." *Journal of Sport and Exercise Psychology* 37 (3): 339–343.

Moore, Lee J., Mark R. Wilson, Samuel J. Vine, Adam H. Coussens, and Paul Freeman. 2013. "Champ or Chump? Challenge and Threat States during Pressurized Competition." *Journal of Sport and Exercise Psychology* 35 (6): 551–562.

Neil, Rich, Sheldon Hanton, Stephen D. Mellalieu, and David Fletcher. 2011. "Competition Stress and Emotions in Sport Performers: The Role of Further Appraisals." *Psychology of Sport and Exercise* 12 (4): 460–470.

Nobles, Charlie. 1995. "Basketball: Scott Fires First Shots in Magic Arsenal." *New York Times*, Sports, May 25.

O'Connor, Ian. 2016. "Jordan Spieth's Collapse at the Masters the Most Shocking in Golf History." *ESPN Golf*, April 11. http://www.espn.co.uk/golf/masters16/story/_/id/15176844/jordan-spieth-collapse-masters-most-shocking-golf-history.

Otten, Mark. 2009. "Choking vs. Clutch Performance: A Study of Sport Performance under Pressure." *Journal of Sport and Exercise Psychology* 31 (5): 583–601.

Oudejans, Raôul R. D., Wilma Kuijpers, Chris C. Kooijman, and Frank C. Bakker. 2011. "Thoughts and Attention of Athletes under Pressure: Skill-Focus or Performance Worries?" *Anxiety, Stress, and Coping* 24 (1): 59–73.

Piaget, Jean. 1971. *The Theory of Stages in Cognitive Development.* New York: McGraw-Hill.

Piaget, Jean. 1977. "The Role of Action in the Development of Thinking." In *Knowledge and Development,* edited by Willis F. Overton and Jeanette McCarthy Gallagher, 17–42. New York: Springer.

Poolton, Jamie, Jon Maxwell, and Rich Masters. 2004. "Rules for Reinvestment." *Perceptual and Motor Skills* 99 (3 Pt 1): 771–774.

Posner, Michael I., and Charles R. Snyder. 1975. "Attention and Cognitive Control." In *Information Processing and Cognition: The Loyola Symposium*, edited by R. L. Solso, 55–82. Hillsdale, NJ: Erlbaum.

Proffitt, Dennis R. 2006. "Embodied Perception and the Economy of Action." *Perspectives on Psychological Science* 1 (2): 110–122.

Rizzolatti, Giacomo, and Corrado Sinigaglia. 2007. "Mirror Neurons and Motor Intentionality." *Functional Neurology* 22 (4): 205–210.

Rucińska, Zuzanna. 2014a. "Basic Pretending as Sensorimotor Engagement?" In *Contemporary Sensorimotor Theory* 15:175–187.

Rucińska, Zuzanna. 2014b. "Radically Enacted Creativity in Sports." First International Conference on Sport Psychology and Embodied Cognition. Al Ain UAE, February.

Scheier, Michael F., and Charles S. Carver. 1985. "The Self-Consciousness Scale: A Revised Version for Use with General Populations." *Journal of Applied Social Psychology* 15 (8): 687–699.

Schlenker, B. R., and M. R. Leary. 1982. "Social Anxiety and Self-Presentation: A Conceptualization and Model." *Psychological Bulletin* 92 (3): 641–669.

Schlenker, Barry R. 1980. *Impression Management: The Self-Concept, Social Identity, and Interpersonal Relations*. Pacific Grove, CA: Brooks/Cole.

Schnall, Simone, Jonathan R. Zadra, and Dennis R. Proffitt. 2010. "Direct Evidence for the Economy of Action: Glucose and the Perception of Geographical Slant." *Perception* 39 (4): 464–482.

Shernoff, David J., Mihaly Csíkszentmihályi, Barbara Shneider, and Elisa Steele Shernoff. 2003. "Student Engagement in High School Classrooms from the Perspective of Flow Theory." *School Psychology Quarterly* 18 (2): 158.

Skinner, Natalie, and Neil Brewer. 2004. "Adaptive Approaches to Competition: Challenge Appraisals and Positive Emotion." *Journal of Sport and Exercise Psychology* 26 (2): 283–305.

Spielberger, Charles D. 1966. "Theory and Research on Anxiety." In *Anxiety and Behavior,* edited by Charles D. Spielberger, 3–20. Amsterdam: Elsevier.

Spielberger, Charles D., William D. Anton, and Jeffrey Bedell. 1976. "The Nature and Treatment of Test Anxiety." In *Emotions and Anxiety: New Concepts, Methods, and Applications,* edited by C. D. Zuckerman and C. D. Spielberger, 317–345. New York: Erlbaum.

Sutton, John. 2007. "Batting, Habit and Memory: The Embodied Mind and the Nature of Skill." *Sport in Society* 10 (5): 763–786.

Sutton, John. 2008. "Material Agency, Skills and History: Distributed Cognition and the Archaeology of Memory." In *Material Agency,* edited by Carl Knappett and Lambros Malafouris, 37–55. New York: Springer.

Sutton, John, Doris McIlwain, Wayne Christensen, and Andrew Geeves. 2011. "Applying Intelligence to the Reflexes: Embodied Skills and Habits between Dreyfus and Descartes." *Journal of the British Society for Phenomenology* 42 (1): 78–103.

Swann, Christian, Richard Keegan, Lee Crust, and David Piggott. 2016. "Psychological States Underlying Excellent Performance in Professional Golfers: 'Letting It Happen' vs. 'Making It Happen.'" *Psychology of Sport and Exercise* 23 (March): 101–113.

Swann, Christian, Richard J. Keegan, David Piggott, and Lee Crust. 2012. "A Systematic Review of the Experience, Occurrence, and Controllability of Flow States in Elite Sport." *Psychology of Sport and Exercise* 13 (6): 807–819.

Tenenbaum, Gershon, and Michael Bar-Eli. 1993. "Decision Making in Sport: A Cognitive Perspective." In *Handbook of Research on Sport Psychology*, edited by R. N. Singer, 171–192. New York: Macmillan library reference.

Thomas, Owen, Ian Maynard, and Sheldon Hanton. 2007. "Intervening with Athletes during the Time Leading up to Competition: Theory to Practice II." *Journal of Applied Sport Psychology* 19 (4): 398–418.

Toner, John, Barbara Gail Montero, and Aidan Moran. 2014. "Considering the Role of Cognitive Control in Expert Performance." *Phenomenology and the Cognitive Sciences* 14 (4): 1127–1144.

Toner, John, Barbara Gail Montero, and Aidan Moran. 2015. "The Perils of Automaticity." *Review of General Psychology: Journal of Division 1, of the American Psychological Association* 19 (4): 431–442.

Toner, John, Barbara Gail Montero, and Aidan Moran. 2016. "Reflective and Prereflective Bodily Awareness in Skilled Action." *Psychology of Consciousness: Theory, Research, and Practice* 3 (4): 303–315. doi:10.1037/cns0000090.

Toner, John, and Aidan Moran. 2015. "Enhancing Performance Proficiency at the Expert Level: Considering the Role of 'Somaesthetic Awareness.'" *Psychology of Sport and Exercise* 16 (January): 110–117.

Totterdell, P. 2000. "Catching Moods and Hitting Runs: Mood Linkage and Subjective Performance in Professional Sport Teams." *Journal of Applied Psychology* 85 (6): 848–859.

Turing, Alan Mathison. 1937. "On Computable Numbers, with an Application to the Entscheidungsproblem." *Proceedings of the London Mathematical Society*, Third Series 2 (1): 230–265.

Turner, Martin J., Marc V. Jones, David Sheffield, and Sophie L. Cross. 2012. "Cardiovascular Indices of Challenge and Threat States Predict Competitive Performance." *International Journal of Psychophysiology* 86 (1): 48–57.

Uphill, Mark, Ryan Groom, and Marc Jones. 2014. "The Influence of In-Game Emotions on Basketball Performance." *European Journal of Sport Science: Official Journal of the European College of Sport Science* 14 (1): 76–83.

Vallerand, Robert J., and Celine M. Blanchard. 2000. "The Study of Emotion in Sport and Exercise: Historical, Definitional, and Conceptual Perspectives." In *Emotions in Sport*, edited by Yuri L. Hanin, 3–37. Champaign, IL: Human Kinetics.

Varela, Francisco J., Evan Thompson, and Eleanor Rosch. 1991. *The Embodied Mind: Cognitive Science and Human Experience*. Cambridge, MA: MIT Press.

Vickers, Joan N. 2007. *Perception, Cognition, and Decision Training: The Quiet Eye in Action*. Champaign, IL: Human Kinetics.

Vine, Samuel J., Paul Freeman, Lee J. Moore, Roy Chandra-Ramanan, and Mark R. Wilson. 2013. "Evaluating Stress as a Challenge Is Associated with Superior Attentional Control and Motor Skill Performance: Testing the Predictions of the Biopsychosocial Model of Challenge and Threat." *Journal of Experimental Psychology: Applied* 19 (3): 185–194.

Vine, Samuel James, Lee J. Moore, Andrew Cooke, Christopher Ring, Mark Robert Wilson, and Others. 2013. "Quiet Eye Training: A Means to Implicit Motor Learning." *International Journal of Sport Psychology* 44 (4): 367–386.

Wallace, Harry M., and Roy F. Baumeister. 2002. "The Performance of Narcissists Rises and Falls with Perceived Opportunity for Glory." *Journal of Personality and Social Psychology* 82 (5): 819–834.

Wang, Jin, Daryl Marchant, and Tony Morris. 2004. "Coping Style and Susceptibility to Choking." *Journal of Sport Behavior* 27 (1): 75–92.

Wang, Jin, Daryl Marchant, Tony Morris, and P. Gibbs. 2004. "Self-Consciousness and Trait Anxiety as Predictors of Choking in Sport." *Journal of Science and Medicine in Sport / Sports Medicine Australia* 7 (2): 174–185.

Will, George F. 1990. *Men at Work*. New York: Macmillan.

Williams, Jean M., and Vikki Krane. 1992. "Coping Styles and Self-Reported Measures of State Anxiety and Self-Confidence." *Journal of Applied Sport Psychology* 4 (2): 134–143.

Williams, Jean M., and Thad R. Leffingwell. 2002. "Cognitive Strategies in Sport and Exercise Psychology." In *Exploring Sport and Exercise Psychology*, 2nd ed., edited by Judy L. Van Raalte and Britton W. Brewer, 75–98. Washington, DC: American Psychological Association.

Williams, Matthew, Joanne Hudson, and Romy J. Lawson. 1999. "Self-Presentation in Sport: Initial Development of a Scale for Measuring Athletes' Competitive Self-Presentation Concerns." *Social Behavior and Personality: An International Journal* 27 (5): 487–502.

Williams, Sarah E., Jennifer Cumming, and George M. Balanos. 2010. "The Use of Imagery to Manipulate Challenge and Threat Appraisal States in Athletes." *Journal of Sport and Exercise Psychology* 32 (3): 339–358.

Wilson, Philip, and Robert C. Eklund. 1998. "The Relationship between Competitive Anxiety and Self-Presentational Concerns." *Journal of Sport and Exercise Psychology* 20 (1): 81–97.

Wine, Jeri D. 1971. "Test Anxiety and Direction of Attention." *Psychological Bulletin* 76 (2): 92–104. http://dx.doi.org/10.1037/h0031332.

Witt, Jessica K., Susan C. South, and Mila Sugovic. 2014. "A Perceiver's Own Abilities Influence Perception, Even When Observing Others." *Psychonomic Bulletin and Review* 21 (2): 384–389.

Woodman, Tim, Paul A. Davis, Lew Hardy, Nichola Callow, Ian Glasscock, and Jason Yuill-Proctor. 2009. "Emotions and Sport Performance: An Exploration of Happiness, Hope, and Anger." *Journal of Sport and Exercise Psychology* 31 (2): 169–188.

Wrosch, Carsten, Michael F. Scheier, Gregory E. Miller, Richard Schulz, and Charles S. Carver. 2003. "Adaptive Self-Regulation of Unattainable Goals: Goal Disengagement, Goal Reengagement, and Subjective Well-Being." *Personality and Social Psychology Bulletin* 29 (12): 1494–1508.

Wulf, Gabriele. 2013. "Attentional Focus and Motor Learning: A Review of 15 Years." *International Review of Sport and Exercise Psychology* 6 (1): 77–104.

Wulf, Gabriele. 2015. "An External Focus of Attention Is a Condition Sine qua Non for Athletes: A Response to Carson, Collins, and Toner (2015)." *Journal of Sports Sciences* 34 (13): 1293–1295.

Wulf, Gabriele. 2016. "Why Did Tiger Woods Shoot 82? A Commentary on Toner and Moran (2015)." *Psychology of Sport and Exercise* 22 (January): 337–338.

Wulf, Gabriele, B. Lauterbach, and T. Toole. 1999. "The Learning Advantages of an External Focus of Attention in Golf." *Research Quarterly for Exercise and Sport* 70 (2): 120–126.

Wulf, Gabriele, Nathan McConnel, Matthias Gärtner, and Andreas Schwarz. 2002. "Enhancing the Learning of Sport Skills through External-Focus Feedback." *Journal of Motor Behavior* 34 (2): 171–182.

Wulf, Gabriele, N. H. McNevin, T. Fuchs, F. Ritter, and T. Toole. 2000. "Attentional Focus in Complex Skill Learning." *Research Quarterly for Exercise and Sport* 71 (3): 229–239.

Wulf, Gabriele, and W. Prinz. 2001. "Directing Attention to Movement Effects Enhances Learning: A Review." *Psychonomic Bulletin and Review* 8 (4): 648–660.

Wulf, Gabriele, C. Shea, and J. H. Park. 2001. "Attention and Motor Performance: Preferences for and Advantages of an External Focus." *Research Quarterly for Exercise and Sport* 72 (4): 335–344.

Wulf, Gabriele, and Jiang Su. 2007. "An External Focus of Attention Enhances Golf Shot Accuracy in Beginners and Experts." *Research Quarterly for Exercise and Sport* 78 (4): 384–389.

Mesh: Cognition, Body, and Environment in Skilled Action[1]

A New Introduction to "Cognition in Skilled Action"

Wayne Christensen and John Sutton

A central theme of embodied cognition research is the idea that cognition is grounded in the rich interaction processes by which individuals navigate the world—interaction processes that are deeply shaped by the physical structure of bodies and the environment. It is, moreover, often suggested that traditional cognitive science has neglected these interaction processes, and that properly taking them into account has profound conceptual consequences. For obvious reasons skill research and sport psychology are areas of prime interest for embodied cognition theory—advanced skills exemplify highly tuned, richly interactive human abilities. Recently we have proposed a theory of skill called *Mesh* (Christensen, Sutton, and McIlwain 2016), and at the kind invitation of the editor, Max Cappuccio, the original paper is reprinted here. In this new introduction we expand on the issues that *Mesh* tries to address and discuss some of the connections between *Mesh* and broader issues in embodied cognition and sport psychology.

One of our objectives in developing *Mesh* has been to articulate key concepts and issues in a way that opens them up to further investigation. *Mesh* takes a particular stance on skill learning, but our feeling is that it is at least as important to further unpack the issues as it is to take a stance at this point. Skill theory must grapple with many of the most fundamental issues in cognitive science and in turn should be one of the primary arenas for theory in cognitive science, given that most human abilities involve skill to some degree. Yet skill theory has until recently been relatively neglected. The two most influential foundational theories remain Fitts and Posner (1967) and Dreyfus and Dreyfus (1986), with Ericsson (2006) providing an important alternative perspective. As valuable as these theories have been, given the complexity of the underlying issues and their importance there is surely scope for a broader and more elaborated body of theory. If we can enrich our conceptual resources, undertake a more critical analysis of intuitions and phenomenology, bring to bear recent developments in cognitive science, and develop a more comprehensive empirical picture, then new avenues of investigation should emerge and a much richer body of theory will become possible.

Intuitions and phenomenology are important sources of influence for theoretical and empirical researchers. This is especially clear in the case of the theories of Fitts and Posner and Dreyfus and Dreyfus, which present a qualitative picture of skill learning that is based primarily on intuitive phenomenology, but the influence can also manifest in less visible framing assumptions that shape experimental and theoretical work. The Fitts and Posner and Dreyfus theories depict skill learning as a progression from initial problem solving in the novice followed by a reduction in conscious cognitive control that culminates in full automaticity in the expert. A major reason for their appeal is that they resonate with common skill experiences and fit a widespread folk view of skill (Montero 2016). Intuitive folk wisdom deserves careful scrutiny, however, and the "mindless" view of skill phenomenology has in recent years been challenged by a number of authors—see, for example, Breivik (2007), Sutton (2007), Geeves et al. (2008), and Montero (2010).

The tension between "mindless" and "minded" interpretations of the phenomenology of skill played an important role in the development of *Mesh*, and we were in particular struck by inconsistencies in practitioners' lore and phenomenological reports. On the one hand, experts sometimes stress the way the body takes over as skill develops, and often express concern about overthinking on the basis of their experience of the disruptive effects of certain kinds of reflection and explicit thought. On the other hand, experts often underline the need to adapt rapidly and appropriately to novel or challenging conditions, thinking on their feet and on the fly. Our ideas about "applying intelligence to the reflexes" (Sutton et al. 2011, 78; see also McIlwain and Sutton 2014; Geeves et al. 2014) were a first attempt to resolve this apparent paradox, by shifting attention to the improvisatory roles of intelligent cognitive control in guiding and adjusting action, so that thinking itself is, for experts, rapid, fleet-footed, and context-sensitive, not effortful and lumbering. *Mesh* takes this further, systematically identifying forms of phenomenology associated with automaticity and cognitive control and developing a theory that can accommodate both. As we emphasize, however, this analysis is simply a preliminary step toward a systematic program of empirical investigation. For example, if we can reliably associate certain kinds of experience with automaticity or cognitive control, then we may be able to employ questionnaires and interviews, administered shortly after real-world performances, as a way of investigating skill in its ecological context. If applied at many levels of skill and to a wide variety of skills, this approach has the potential to yield a rich and nuanced empirical picture.

Such an approach could contribute to a broader program of ecological skill research that develops a clearer understanding of skill in its natural context.

One reason that a clearer ecological understanding of skill is important is because it can inform experimental research, including by providing a basis for assessing the ecological validity of experimental designs. Another of our goals in the development of *Mesh* was to articulate concerns that existing experimental research, which appears to show skill automaticity (e.g., Beilock and Carr 2001), suffers from problems of ecological validity. The nub of the issue is that this research has generally employed tasks that are easy for the expert participants. Skills in the real world are often difficult and performed in challenging conditions, especially at elite levels. This much is obvious—the contribution that *Mesh* makes in this regard is to provide an argument that this fact has significant implications. The nature of control may differ between easy and challenging conditions.

Our emphasis on the importance of studying cognition "in the wild" is in keeping with prevalent themes of embodied cognition (Hutchins 2010; Heft 2013). But some approaches, such as ecological psychology, see this as requiring a strong set of theoretical commitments, whereas we don't think that such strong commitments are needed as a starting point for naturalistic investigation. Indeed, it is important not to prejudge central issues—a robust theoretical understanding of cognition in its natural context will emerge only as the result of extensive empirical investigation. The overarching framework for ecological skill research should be relatively minimal in order to allow for a diversity of approaches to flourish.

More specifically, the question of whether skill automates bears strongly on a repeatedly invoked division between radical and moderate approaches to embodied cognition. On the standard view of the terrain, so-called radical approaches see a proper understanding of embodied, situated cognition as requiring a new conceptual framework that eschews the representational, information-processing framework of conventional cognitive science. Moderate approaches believe that standard cognitive science can be extended to accommodate the phenomena of interest to embodied cognition (Shapiro 2010). One of the key theoretical issues in this debate has centered on the idea that certain kinds of problems are "representation-hungry" (Clark 1997), and hence cannot be explained by nonrepresentational frameworks such as dynamical systems theory. The question of whether skill automates can be thought of as a question as to whether advanced skills are representation-hungry or, perhaps, hungry for the kinds of representations employed by higher cognition according to mainstream cognitive psychology.

With regard to this issue, our approach is decidedly moderate, and we have formulated *Mesh* so that it draws on recent cognitive science research on cognitive control and automaticity to the greatest extent possible. Critics of representationalist cognitive science often associate it with a Fodorian picture in which control is performed by a central executive operating on amodal language-like representations. But cognitive neuroscience presents a very different picture in which there are multiple levels of control, including lower-level, fast perception-action loops and higher-level loops that integrate more widely and process more abstract information, with the loops functioning in intimate interaction (Fuster 2004). Rather than there being a single, abstract language-like representational format, neuroscientific research points to progressive increases in abstraction in the flow from the sensory periphery (e.g., Binder and Desai 2011). In our view it is plausible that mental representations are often model-based rather than language-like. The significance of this distinctive picture has not been widely appreciated, and *Mesh* attempts to elaborate some of its theoretical implications. On a more traditional dual process view, cognitive processes are *either* automatic or controlled, but this hardly makes sense on the neuroscientific picture, since most cognitive processes involve brain-wide interactions that include both automatic and controlled executive components.

In this picture, overall control is distributed across higher and lower systems, which presents the challenge of understanding how they function in relation to each other. Anti-representationalists have often adopted the strong assumption that the problem of what to do can be resolved unambiguously based on immediate perceptual information—the expert just sees what to do (Dreyfus and Dreyfus 1986). In a follow-up paper we argue that this is not the case—the complex, variable problems confronted by practitioners of elite skills present ambiguity that can be resolved only by means of higher levels of integration. It is necessary to track the unfolding structure of the performance situation, anticipate how it might unfold, and draw on background knowledge to interpret the situation.

In addition, though, on our account the cognitive processes employed in action control are reshaped during skill acquisition and come to be highly tuned to the demands of control. This means both that they reflect in increasingly intimate ways the structure of bodily interaction and also that they incorporate increasingly rich representations *of* bodily interaction. Christensen, Bicknell, et al. (2015) explore these issues in relation to sense of agency and sense of control, proposing new conceptualizations of these forms of awareness in terms of awareness of control influences on a complex interaction process and awareness of performance state in relation to the limits of control (the performance envelope). This account is based on investigation of mountain biking performance and illustrates the way that attention to the nature of skilled action in complex, real-world conditions can inform conceptions of cognitive representations and processes.

However, we dispute the idea that questions about representation should be the primary basis for understanding the significance of embodied cognition. In the development of embodied and distributed approaches to cognitive science, arguments for and against representations are distinct from arguments for or against individualism or internalism, the idea that (the vehicles of) cognitive processes and cognitive control are entirely brain-bound (Sutton 2015). In our view, anti-individualism (in its different forms) is the most far-reaching and "radical" development in the recent cognitive sciences, though the language of revolution is perhaps not entirely appropriate (Sutton et al. 2010). *Mesh* is representationalist, but it tends to support anti-individualism and anti-internalism. By showing how cognition can be intimately structured for the demands of interaction, it can help illuminate the way that task control can be flexibly distributed across body and world, and between individuals, as well as across the brain.

To sum up, we want to reiterate that further opening up the issues that *Mesh* is trying to address is as important as the specific claims of the theory. There is a need for an enriched body of theory on skill that can (a) foster the development of a clearer picture of skill in its ecological context, (b) inform experimental work by contributing to ecologically valid designs and by filling out the theoretical space, (c) bring to bear related research in the cognitive sciences, and (d) furnish new conceptualizations of the context, experiences, and mechanisms of skilled action. In turn, skill theory has the potential to inform many areas of cognitive science, not least the foundational questions that have concerned embodied cognition researchers.

A more concrete concern, however, is the question of what *Mesh* can specifically contribute to research on sporting and related skills. The short answer is that it begins to develop a systematic basis for addressing the idea that skills may involve both automaticity and cognitive control, and this can encourage new lines of investigation into the possible contributions of cognitive control to the study of skills thought to be largely automatic. Toner, Montero, and Moran (2014) argue that the approach may help illuminate the nature and role of cognitive processes in training and online execution, such as the use of "instructional nudges" to adjust performance. Toner, Montero, and Moran (2015) argue that excessive automation of performance results in errors, and they develop a taxonomy of errors that can arise. Collins, Collins, and Carson (2016) found that high-level sport coaches showed metacognitive awareness of the advantages and disadvantages of intuitive versus more deliberative styles of decision making in a given context, allowing them to switch styles appropriately. The authors argue that this is consistent with *Mesh*, and in particular with the idea that the athlete maintains an appropriate balance between cognitive and automatic aspects of control. Demos, Lisboa, and Chaffin (2016) investigated flexibility of expression in classical concert piano performance, finding evidence that cognitive control was employed at phrase boundaries and suggestions that it may have operated more continuously through phrases. Using a golf-putting task, Arsal, Eccles, and Ericsson (2016) obtained results supporting three key claims made by both *Mesh* and Ericsson's theory, namely that experts should show greater awareness of performance than do those with less experience, that increasing task challenge should result in greater cognitive control, and that cognitive control is often concerned with strategic aspects of performance. If performance does involve both cognitive and automatic components, this has pedagogical implications, and Collins, Carson, and Collins (2016) suggest that *Mesh* aligns with an approach developed in coach education called Cognitive Apprenticeship. This method encourages the learner to consciously articulate processes associated with performing complex skills, such as decisions involved in placing an anchor while rock climbing.

In short, *Mesh* resonates with and can help to inform some promising lines of investigation into sporting and other skills.

References

Arsal, Güler, David W. Eccles, and K. Anders Ericsson. 2016. "Cognitive Mediation of Putting: Use of a Think-Aloud Measure and Implications for Studies of Golf-Putting in the Laboratory." *Psychology of Sport and Exercise* 27 (November): 18–27. doi:10.1016/j.psychsport.2016.07.008.

Beilock, Sian L., and Thomas H. Carr. 2001. "On the Fragility of Skilled Performance: What Governs Choking under Pressure?" *Journal of Experimental Psychology: General* 130 (4): 701–725. doi:10.1037/0096-3445.130.4.701.

Binder, Jeffrey R., and Rutvik H. Desai. 2011. "The Neurobiology of Semantic Memory." *Trends in Cognitive Sciences* 15 (11): 527–536. doi:10.1016/j.tics.2011.10.001.

Breivik, Gunnar. 2007. "Skillful Coping in Everyday Life and in Sport: A Critical Examination of the Views of Heidegger and Dreyfus." *Journal of the Philosophy of Sport* 34 (2): 116–134.

Christensen, Wayne, Kath Bicknell, Doris McIlwain, and John Sutton. 2015. "The Sense of Agency and Its Role in Strategic Control for Expert Mountain Bikers." *Psychology of Consciousness: Theory, Research, and Practice* 2 (3): 340–53. doi:10.1037/cns0000066.

Christensen, Wayne, John Sutton, and Doris J. F. McIlwain. 2016. "Cognition in Skilled Action: Meshed Control and the Varieties of Skill Experience." *Mind & Language* 31 (1): 37–66. doi:10.1111/mila.12094.

Clark, Andy. 1997. *Being There: Putting Brain, Body, and World Together Again.* Cambridge, MA: MIT Press.

Collins, Dave, Loel Collins, and Howie J. Carson. 2016. "'If It Feels Right, Do It': Intuitive Decision Making in a Sample of High-Level Sport Coaches." *Frontiers in Psychology* 7 (April): 504. doi:10.3389/fpsyg.2016.00504.

Collins, Loel, Howie J. Carson, and Dave Collins. 2016. "Metacognition and Professional Judgment and Decision Making in Coaching: Importance, Application and Evaluation." *International Journal of Sports Science and Coaching* 3 (3): 355–361.

Demos, Alexander P., Tânia Lisboa, and Roger Chaffin. 2016. "Flexibility of Expressive Timing in Repeated Musical Performances." *Frontiers in Psychology* 7 (October): 1490. doi:10.3389/fpsyg.2016.01490.

Dreyfus, Hubert L., and Stuart E. Dreyfus. 1986. *Mind Over Machine: The Power of Human Intuition and Expertise in the Era of the Computer.* New York: Free Press.

Ericsson, K. Anders. 2006. "The Influence of Experience and Deliberate Practice on the Development of Superior Expert Performance." In *The Cambridge Handbook of Expertise and Expert Performance*, edited by K. Anders Ericsson, Neil Charness, Paul J. Feltovich, and Robert R. Hoffman, 685–705. Cambridge: Cambridge University Press.

Fitts, Paul Morris, and Michael I. Posner. 1967. *Human Performance.* Pacific Grove, CA: Brooks/Cole.

Fuster, Joaquín M. 2004. "Upper Processing Stages of the Perception-Action Cycle." *Trends in Cognitive Sciences* 8 (4): 143–145. doi:10.1016/j.tics.2004.02.004.

Geeves, Andrew, Wayne D. Christensen, John Sutton, and Doris McIlwain. 2008. "Review: Roger Chaffin, Gabriela Imreh and Mary Crawford, Practicing Perfection: Memory and Piano Performance. New York: Laurence Erlbaum Associates, 2002." *Empirical Musicology Review* 3 (3): 163–172.

Geeves, Andrew, Doris J. F. McIlwain, John Sutton, and Wayne Christensen. 2014. "To Think or Not To Think: The Apparent Paradox of Expert Skill in Music Performance." *Educational Philosophy and Theory* 46 (6): 674–691. doi:10.1080/00131857.2013.779214.

Heft, Harry. 2013. "An Ecological Approach to Psychology: Review of General Psychology." *Educational Publishing Foundation* 17 (2): 162–167. doi:10.1037/a0032928.

Hutchins, Edwin. 2010. "Cognitive Ecology." *Topics in Cognitive Science* 2 (4): 705–715. doi:10.1111/j.1756-8765.2010.01089.x.

McIlwain, Doris, and John Sutton. 2014. "Yoga From the Mat Up: How Words Alight on Bodies." *Educational Philosophy and Theory* 46 (6): 655–673. doi:10.1080/00131857.2013.779216.

Montero, Barbara. 2010. "Does Bodily Awareness Interfere with Highly Skilled Movement?" *Inquiry: A Journal of Medical Care Organization, Provision and Financing* 53 (2): 105–122. doi:10.1080/00201741003612138.

Montero, Barbara Gail. 2016. *Thought in Action: Expertise and the Conscious Mind.* Oxford: Oxford University Press.

Shapiro, Lawrence. 2010. *Embodied Cognition.* London: Routledge.

Sutton, John. 2007. "Batting, Habit and Memory: The Embodied Mind and the Nature of Skill." *Sport in Society* 10 (5): 763–786. doi:10.1080/17430430701442462.

Sutton, John. 2015. "Remembering as Public Practice: Wittgenstein, Memory, and Distributed Cognitive Ecologies." In *Mind, Language, and Action: Proceedings of the 36th Wittgenstein Symposium,* edited by D. Moyal-Sharrock, A. Coliva, and V. Munz, 409–443. Berlin: Walter de Gruyter.

Sutton, John, Celia B. Harris, Paul G. Keil, and Amanda J. Barnier. 2010. "The Psychology of Memory, Extended Cognition, and Socially Distributed Remembering." *Phenomenology and the Cognitive Sciences* 9 (4): 521–560. doi:10.1007/s11097-010-9182-y.

Sutton, John, Doris McIlwain, Wayne Christensen, and Andrew Geeves. 2011. "Applying Intelligence to the Reflexes: Embodied Skills and Habits between Dreyfus and Descartes." *Journal of the British Society for Phenomenology* 42 (1): 78–103.

Toner, John, Barbara Gail Montero, and Aidan Moran. 2014. "Considering the Role of Cognitive Control in Expert Performance." *Phenomenology and the Cognitive Sciences* 14 (4): 1127–1144. doi:10.1007/s11097-014-9407-6.

Toner, John, Barbara Gail Montero, and Aidan Moran. 2015. "The Perils of Automaticity." *Review of General Psychology: Journal of Division 1, of the American Psychological Association* 19 (4): 431–442.

6 Cognition in Skilled Action: Meshed Control and the Varieties of Skill Experience

Wayne Christensen, John Sutton, and Doris McIlwain[2]

Introduction

Influential characterizations of skill acquisition in both psychology and philosophy depict it as a progression from an initial cognitive phase to an expert phase in which performance is largely automatic (Fitts and Posner 1967; Dreyfus and Dreyfus 1986). The enduring appeal of this picture is illustrated in Schmidt and Wrisberg's (2008) textbook account of motor skill learning, which describes skill learning as a progression to an autonomous stage in which learners "are able to produce their actions almost automatically with little or no attention" (202). This seems to suggest that higher cognition typically plays no role in skill control, and Dreyfus and Dreyfus are explicit on this point, saying that "*When things are proceeding normally, experts don't solve problems and don't make decisions; they do what normally works*" (30–31, italics original). The idea that advanced skills are noncognitive is also prevalent among sport practitioners and in popular culture. To give just one recent example, the elite Sri Lankan cricketer Kumar Sangakkara has said, "Basically in batting, you have to be mindless. You've done all the practice, you have your muscle memory and your reflexes are more than quick to deal with any kind of delivery. You've got to let your body do all those things by itself without letting your mind take control" (Sadikot 2014). Such claims have been taken by some philosophers as evidence that expert performance is automatic. Brownstein (2014), for instance, uses reports like this as a central component of an argument that much skilled action is unreflective, in the sense that it occurs with little conscious awareness of what is being done. Like Dreyfus (2013), Brownstein claims that this lack of awareness is sufficiently profound that experts will often be unable to explain their actions after the fact. Recently, though, a number of philosophers and psychologists have reacted against this kind of view: Sutton (2007), Montero (2010), Sutton et al. (2011), Stanley and Krakauer (2013), Papineau (2013), Fridland (2014), and Toner et al.

(2015) all criticize the mindless view of expert performance and begin to make the case that cognition does make some important contribution to skilled action.

Our intention here is to develop a broadly based, systematic theory of skill learning and control that clearly articulates the idea that cognitive and automatic processes both make a major contribution to skilled action. The basic idea on which this theory is based is that cognitive control is not eliminated in advanced skill, but is rather shifted, primarily to higher-level action control. This idea is not new—it can be found in varied forms in prior work. Thus, although Schmidt and Wrisberg (2008) characterize skill learning as a progression to increasingly automatic action production, they *also* say that increased automaticity in motor production and sensory analysis "frees the best performers to engage in higher-order cognitive activities, such as split-second shifts in strategy during a basketball game or spontaneous adjustments in the form or style of a movement in dance or in figure skating" (202). Suggestions of this kind of shift in the role of cognitive control can be found in Bryan and Harter's (1899) study of skill learning in telegraphers; they describe a series of stages in which the learner first "hustles for the letters," is then "after words," then phrases and sentences, and finally is able to focus on the meaning of the message (352). There is a hint that Fitts and Posner may have believed that it is primarily component processes that automate (1967, 14), and Logan (1985) and Jonides, Naveh-Benjamin, and Palmer (1985) explicitly argued that overall action control does not automate. Vallacher and Wegner (1987) gave an account of a shift in attentional focus during skill learning similar to that of Bryan and Harter. They argued that in the initial stages of learning, the difficulty of the actions results in a focus on low-level aspects of the actions, while improving mastery involves a "chunking" of actions into larger action units and a conscious focus on high-level aspects of the actions (1987, 7–8).

But if the basic idea is not uncommon, it has also not yet been systematically developed. In our view there are good reasons to think that higher cognition does make substantial contributions to advanced skills, and a theory of skill learning and control must clearly recognize this. Such a theory would address not only the automation of aspects of control but also the shift in the role of cognitive control, its main processes, and the relations between automatic and cognitive control in performance. This theory should be synthetic, framed at the same level of generality as the theories of Fitts and Posner and Dreyfus and Dreyfus, and draw on a wide range of evidence across multiple disciplines. In this paper we develop the basic structure of the account, show how it can accommodate several important strands of experimental skill research, and suggest avenues for further empirical investigation.

Our aim is to construct an inclusive and systematic framework. We begin by delineating the space of theoretical options in a way that is deliberately coarse-grained, identifying a basic set of theoretical possibilities and locating our account within this space. This leaves aside the fine-grained structure of extant positions but allows us to identify general issues that any skill theory should address. We next describe a range of types of skill experience that are suggestive of either automatic or cognitive control, and show that our account provides a better overall account of these types of experience than does an account that sees skill control as automatic. This analysis is not intended to provide definitive support—it rather helps to clarify our account and identify key issues and forms of evidence. We then show the value of the account by using it to interpret and evaluate several extant positions with respect to skill learning and control. Dreyfus (1997) defends his account against contrary evidence concerning expert decision making, and we use our analysis to highlight conceptual weaknesses in Dreyfus's position that undermine his attempt to downplay the significance of this evidence. An influential strand of research in complex motor skills has produced evidence that has been taken to show that skills like dribbling a hockey puck and putting a golf ball are automatic. We use our framework to argue that this interpretation relies on questionable assumptions about real-world skill performance and suggest an experimental approach that would provide a better test of the respective contributions of automatic and cognitive processes to skill performance.

1 Cognitive and Automatic Control: Dual Process versus System Views

Before discussing their respective roles in skill, we need an initial characterization of cognitive and automatic control. The term "cognitive control" comes from cognitive psychology and broadly refers to control associated with conscious awareness and intentionality. Posner and Snyder (1975) proposed that cognitive control is the product of a flexible, limited-capacity system that, through conscious attention, establishes a program or strategy for processing information. They operationally characterized automatic control as occurring without attention, without conscious awareness, and without producing interference with other ongoing mental activity (56).

Recent research has introduced a number of complexities, however, and we can distinguish between two broad conceptions of the nature of, and relations between, cognitive and automatic control. The differences between these conceptions have important consequences for skill theory. The first is relatively straightforward, and close to the classical view outlined by Posner and Snyder. For reference we'll call it the *dual process view*. According to this conception, there is a fairly robust contrast between processes that are rapid and autonomous, and tend to govern responses when there is no higher cognitive intervention, and effortful explicit (conscious) reasoning processes that are strongly dependent on working memory. This conception has been codified in dual-process accounts of cognitive architecture, recently defended by Evans and Stanovich (2013).

The second conception is discernible in a number of different strands of research on cognitive and automatic control. This view has two key elements: (1) a stronger emphasis on cognitive control as the product of an executive system, which involves a broader understanding of the processes involved in cognitive control, and (2) a more complex and nuanced understanding of automaticity. We'll call this the *systems view* to flag the fact that it involves a shift toward an understanding of cognitive and automatic control in terms of systemic interactions and away from a simple contrast between two kinds of processes.

As noted, Posner and Snyder associated cognitive control with the operation of a flexible executive system, and this is also a feature of contemporary dual process views (Evans and Stanovich 2013). But dual process views nevertheless frame the contrast between cognitive and automatic control in terms of two kinds of processes. Conscious reasoning is taken as the paradigmatic form of controlled cognitive process. This contrast breaks down for the systems view: cognitive control, understood in terms of the operation of the executive system, involves a broader range of processes than just conscious reasoning, and many of these processes can show a great deal of automaticity.

More specifically, cognitive neuroscience research on cognitive control has associated it with a neural system that includes the prefrontal and parietal cortices (Miller 2000; Fuster 2008). Some of the primary functions that have been associated with cognitive control in this tradition include controlling attention, actively maintaining and processing information (working memory), flexibly integrating information related to the current situation and activities, setting and switching between goals, establishing an action or task "set" (a processing configuration for the situation), inhibiting inappropriate responses, forming action plans, decision making, and problem solving (Miller 2000; Duncan 2010). Many of the processes involved in performing these functions are not conscious or only partly conscious. For instance, an individual focused on interpreting the situation may be only partly aware of adopting a particular action set for the situation and unaware of the inhibition of responses that are incompatible with the task set.

Research on automaticity has seen similar complexification, with greater recognition of rich systemic interactions. Moors and De Houwer (2006) distinguish four main feature clusters linked to automaticity concerning goal and intentions, consciousness, cognitive efficiency, and speed. With respect to goals and intentions, automaticity has been characterized in terms of processes that are uncontrolled, occurring independently of intentions and goals. A strongly automatic process, in this sense, is *autonomous*—roughly, it is not initiated by intentions and it runs to completion without regulation by goals (307–308). With respect to consciousness, automatic processes have been characterized as nonconscious or involving low awareness. With respect to efficiency, automatic processes have been characterized as attentionally undemanding and as being experienced as effortless (if they are experienced at all). With respect to speed, automatic processes are characterized as fast, in contrast with cognitive processes that are often assumed to be characteristically slow. Further complexity arises because these various attributes do not group together in a simple way. On some views, intentions and goals can be nonconscious (Bargh 1990); different aspects of a given process may be conscious or nonconscious, including the input, the process itself, the output, and the consequences; nonconscious processes can be influenced by cognitively controlled processes (and are then not truly autonomous); conscious processes may be fast and subjectively effortless; and so on.

The significance of the distinction between the dual process and systems views for skill theory is that the latter raises new possibilities. The dual process view is central to standard views of skill learning, which posit a qualitative transition from responses based on effortful reasoning to responses based on effortless, autonomous processes (Fitts and Posner 1967; Dreyfus and Dreyfus 1986; Schmidt and Wrisberg 2008). Given that background conception of cognitive and automatic control, this seems plausible. But we'll argue that the systems view lends itself to a more nuanced view of the changes in cognitive and automatic control during skill acquisition.

2 A Sketch of the Basic Options for Skill Theory

We can now delineate some basic options for theories of skill learning and control. Our initial set of contrasts takes the dual process view of cognitive control and automaticity as the conceptual framework, then we describe a different type of skill theory based on the systems view.

Starting with the dual process view, one possibility is that the control of skilled action in normal conditions is almost entirely automatic, a view that we call *Automatic*. According to *Automatic*, cognitive control reduces during skill learning and makes no positive contribution to performance with the attainment of advanced skill (figure 6.1a). Another possibility, which we call *Full Cognitive*, is that there is no reduction, and skilled action is under full step-by-step cognitive control, even at advanced levels of ability (figure 6.1b). A third possibility is that automatic processes and cognitive control both contribute to skilled action. We'll call this *Hybrid*. According to *Hybrid*, cognitive control reduces during skill learning as automatic control comes to play an increasing role, but cognitive control continues to make a substantial positive contribution at advanced levels of skill (figure 6.1c).

The skill theory presented by Dreyfus and Dreyfus (1986) is the clearest example of an *Automatic* account. Fitts and Posner's account of skill acquisition lends itself to an

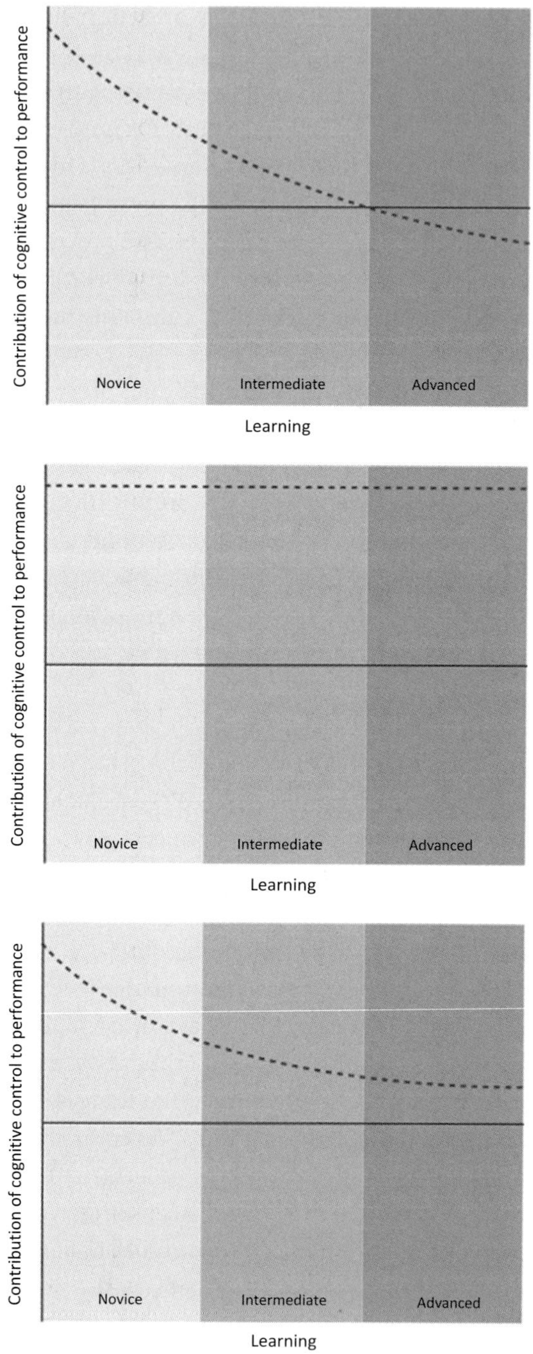

Figure 6.1

Cognitive control and experience. (a) Automatic, (b) Full cognitive, (c) Hybrid.

Automatic view of skill, but as we noted in the introduction, there is some ambiguity since they may have intended the account to apply to component processes rather than action control as a whole. Schmidt and Wrisberg (2008) focus on automaticity but make claims that align their position with *Hybrid*. From the other direction, Ericsson focuses primarily on the role of cognition in skill and claims that experts resist automation (Ericsson 2006). Viewed superficially, his position would seem to be a version of *Full Cognitive*, but he recognizes that automation plays a role in skill, so his position is properly a kind of *Hybrid* account. Despite Shiffrin and Schneider's (1977) influential contrast between controlled and automatic processes, they too recognized that hybrid control occurs. Thus, they say, "Particularly in complex processing situations, (such as reading), an ongoing mixture of controlled and automatic processing is utilized" (1977, 161).

But although many researchers have recognized hybrid control as a possibility, hybrid control hasn't been a focus of investigation in its own right. This leaves it unclear how hybrid control operates and in what circumstances it occurs. There are many possibilities, depending on specific assumptions concerning the nature of controlled and automatic processes, but as a first approximation we distinguish two major versions of *Hybrid*. The first, which we call *Autonomous*, is based on the dual process view, and associates cognitive control with conscious reasoning. In contrast with *Automatic*, *Autonomous* claims that abbreviated forms of reasoning occur in complex, temporally extended skilled action. For example, a soccer player at a particular point in a game may adopt a particular strategy, such as attacking up the left wing to exploit a hole in the defense. The player may also make fast decisions in pursuing this strategy, for instance whether to pass or go around a defender. But these conscious cognitive processes are fleeting, and based on underlying processes that are largely automatic ("intuition"). Moreover, while they produce intentions that guide action, these intentions are at a high level (such as pass to a teammate) and do not play a strong guiding role in the on-line execution of action, which is largely autonomous.

Such a view seems to be implied by the Schmidt and Wrisberg passage we quoted in the introduction, which associates cognitive control with strategic decisions and occasional adjustments to the overall form of movement in sports like figure skating. A hybrid view of this kind has also found support in philosophy (Papineau 2013). Beilock and Gray (2007) explicitly identify the role of cognition in performance as being concerned with strategizing, problem solving, and decision making, and further distinguish between skills that require these functions and skills that don't. In the latter group they include skills like golf putting and baseball batting (434). Thus, for *Autonomous*, some skills are performed largely automatically.

We argue for a different kind of hybrid theory, which we call *Mesh*. Like *Autonomous*, *Mesh* sees a broadly hierarchical division of control responsibilities, with cognitive control usually focused on strategic aspects of performance and automatic processes more concerned with implementation. But unlike *Autonomous*, *Mesh* proposes that controlled and automatic processes are closely integrated in skilled action, and that cognitive control directly influences motor execution in many cases. This difference is in part based on the systems view of cognitive and automatic control described above. One of the cognitive functions associated with cognitive control on the systems view is the flexible integration of information concerning the situation. In skills and expertise research this has been conceptualized as situation awareness, and can involve explicit inferences (Endsley 1995). But much of the information-integration that contributes to situation awareness is not based on explicit inferences (Miller 2000; Duncan 2010), and we assume that situation awareness often occurs without explicit inferential reasoning processes. On the other hand, situation awareness is typically constructed progressively and is closely linked to attentional control. As situation interpretation develops, attention is directed to relevant information that serves to elaborate or revise the interpretation. Situation awareness serves to establish a cognitive and motor configuration appropriate to the context (Duncan 2010).

These functions contribute to virtually all skilled action, according to *Mesh*, and directly influence action execution. In addition, we claim that skilled actions are often directed by a cognitive action "gist." *Autonomous* assumes that intentions are generated in the course of complex skilled action but views these as being relatively coarse-grained (e.g., pass the ball). A high-level action intention of this kind serves to cue motor processes, but the situational specificity of the execution is the product of largely autonomous lower-order processes. In contrast, an action gist is more detailed, specifying not just an action type but also a particular way of performing the action appropriate to the circumstances. For instance, the soccer player may form a gist in kicking a pass that aims to put the ball into a particular area with a particular weighting that will wrong-foot a defender and allow a teammate to run onto the ball. The action gist directly shapes execution and, when action is sufficiently extended, can contribute to the regulation of execution.

Given that *Mesh* employs a different conception of cognitive control than does *Autonomous*, a worry might arise that the difference between the two theories is largely terminological. Processes that *Mesh* treats as part of cognitive control count as automatic from the perspective of *Autonomous*. However, such terminological differences are based on substantive conceptual differences and give rise to major differences in empirical prediction. The contrast between *Autonomous* and *Mesh* is especially clear in the case of a skill like golf putting. Here, *Autonomous* sees cognitive control as potentially responsible for initial strategic choices about the type of shot but as playing no role in execution. In contrast, *Mesh* sees cognitive control as contributing directly to execution by way of the influence of situation awareness on the action set and action gist. Note here that the influence of cognitive control on execution is *not* through step-by-step control of the movement—it is through selection of action type, determination of the perceptual-motor configuration, and parameterization of the action. While there are terminological differences in the way the processes are described, the conceptual differences manifest in a critical difference in prediction. According to *Autonomous*, distraction should not impair the execution of the action, and may be beneficial by preventing harmful cognitive interference. According to *Mesh*, distraction should tend to hurt execution: poor situation awareness will tend to result in a poorly established action set and/or a mis-specified action gist, resulting in a poor shot.

There are some important qualifications, however. *Mesh* claims that virtually all skilled action depends on situation awareness and an action set, and much action is guided by an action gist. But the relative importance of these cognitive structures increases with the complexity and difficulty of the situation and task. Simple, easy performance conditions place light demands on situation awareness and the action set, permitting a significant degree of tolerance to distraction and giving the appearance of overall automaticity. But complex, difficult performance conditions impose strong demands on situation awareness and the action set, and because of this performance will be significantly impaired by distraction. We'll argue in part 5 that these points provide an alternative explanation for experiments purporting to show that the execution of skills like golf putting is automatic.

First, however, we compare *Mesh* with *Automatic* in more detail. Given that automation is clearly an important part of skill acquisition, *Full Cognitive* is implausible, so we won't consider it further. Some may consider *Automatic* to be implausible on the grounds that explicit strategic cognitive processes do appear to play a role in complex temporally extended skills like basketball and figure skating. It remains a vigorously defended position, however (Dreyfus 2013; Brownstein 2014), and an evaluation of its strengths and limitations helps clarify key issues. *Autonomous* shares many key assumptions with *Automatic*, and in part 5 we'll show that the advantages of *Mesh* in comparison with *Automatic* also apply to *Autonomous*.

3 The Varied Nature of Skill Experience

We now examine *Mesh* and *Automatic* with respect to their ability to explain a set of common forms of skill experience. This strategy requires explanation because many scientists and naturalistically oriented philosophers regard phenomenological evidence as a dubious basis for theory. First, we do not rely on phenomenological evidence as a privileged source of information for skill theory—it is part of a matrix that includes experimental evidence and theoretical reasoning. Second, the kinds of skill experience we describe play a pervasive role in intuitions about skill, and are an important source of influence on skill research. Third, the experimental tests used to probe the automaticity (or otherwise) of skill in experimental research can be related directly to some of these forms of skill experience: understanding how these skill experiences are related provides a conceptual basis for interpreting this research. Fourth, this analysis of skill experience serves as starting point for a qualitative empirical research program investigating skill performance in natural settings. Laboratory-based experimental research can suffer from problems of ecological validity (Christensen, Sutton, and McIlwain 2015), so it is important to pursue complementary research streams: experimental research that investigates key questions with high levels of control, and qualitative investigation that illuminates real-world skill performance. The systematic analysis of skill experience we present here helps to emphasize the complex nature of skill and reveals problems that arise from a narrow focus on select aspects of skill.

3.1 Nine Common Forms of Skill Experience

Automatic fits well with some everyday features of personal experience. In particular, (1) attention to performance can be reduced once a skill has been acquired (for later reference we label this *reduced attention*), (2) a well-learned skill can often be performed in conjunction with other tasks with little detriment (*multitask tolerance*), (3) attention to the performance of a highly learned skill can be disruptive (*disruptive attention*), (4) sense of cognitive effort can be low (*reduced cognitive effort*), and (5) memory for the performance of a highly learned skill can be reduced or absent (*reduced memory*).

It is easy to find instances of each of these phenomena. Experienced drivers who drive cars with a manual gear shift typically don't pay attention to the specific movements involved in changing gear, in contrast with beginner drivers—a simple example of reduced attention. And, unlike a novice, under normal conditions an experienced driver can easily have a conversation with a passenger while driving, showing multitask tolerance. Moreover, if the experienced driver does pay attention to the details of the movements involved in shifting gear, this can be disruptive. A novice driver experiences a strong degree of cognitive effort during the performance of many operations, such as reversing out of a driveway, whereas sense of cognitive effort can be low for an experienced driver during the same kinds of maneuvers. A commonly mentioned example of reduced memory is the case of driving a familiar route and having little memory of the drive afterward. Another example of reduced memory is being unable to remember afterward whether you locked the front door as you left your house.

However there are also aspects of common experience that are clearly suggestive of a role for cognitive control and, in particular, of *Mesh*. These include (6) enhanced attention to strategic features of a task—the situations, goals, and methods involved in performing the task (*strategic focus*). In the case of driving, not having to pay attention to the mechanics of changing gear allows an experienced driver to devote greater attention to the larger situation, such as proximity to other cars and upcoming tasks like changing lanes. Strategic focus is linked to another common skill experience: (7) when not enough attention is given to the task at hand, the individual can sometimes perform the wrong action, for instance turning as if to drive to work when the goal is to go shopping (an *action slip*). And (8), although awareness can be relatively low when driving a familiar route, it can also be very high in demanding conditions, such as driving at night on a busy highway (*increased attention in response to challenge*). Increased attention can be accompanied by increased sense of cognitive effort (9), as possibilities are evaluated and decisions made (*increased cognitive effort in response to challenge*).

3.2 *Mesh* versus *Automatic*

When described in an unqualified way, these various forms of skill experience seem to conflict: attention and cognitive effort are reduced in skilled action, but also sometimes increased; attention to performance is bad, disrupting automatic processes, but insufficient attention to performance is also bad, resulting in action slips. Some scheme of contextual qualifications is needed to reconcile these contradictions, and we can extract from *Automatic* and *Mesh* different candidate schemes, summarized in table 6.1.

The defining claim of *Automatic* is that there is a global reduction of cognitive control in the course of skill learning as automation occurs, with cognitive control making no positive contribution to performance in advanced skill (figure 6.1a). Reduced attention, reduced cognitive effort, multitask tolerance, disruptive attention, and reduced memory are all phenomena that can be readily expected to result from this. Reduced attention and cognitive effort can be expected because attention and cognitive effort are associated with cognitive control, which has been supplanted by automation. Multitask tolerance can be expected because automatic processes can operate in parallel and because cognitive resources are free if a second task is demanding. Disruptive attention can be expected because attention to automated processes is likely to generate control input that will disturb their normal operation. Reduced memory can be expected because attention is thought to be required for memory formation (Craik et al. 1996).

Strategic focus, action slips, increased attention in response to challenge, and increased cognitive effort in response to challenge are all suggestive of cognitive control, so *Automatic* must locate them outside the range of normal conditions of competent

Table 6.1
Skill phenomena: *Automatic* versus *Mesh*.

		Automatic Interpretation		*Mesh* Interpretation	
Skill Experience		Scope	Mechanism	Scope	Mechanism
(1)	*Reduced attention*	Advanced skill, normal conditions.	Automation reduces cognitive demand.	Implementation, easy conditions.	Attention focus shifted from automated aspects, low cognitive demand in easy conditions.
(2)	*Multitask tolerance*	Advanced skill, normal conditions.	Reduced cognitive demand frees cognitive capacity for other tasks.	Implementation, easy conditions.	Automation of component skills, low cognitive demand in easy conditions.
(3)	*Disruptive attention*	Advanced skill, normal conditions.	Attention interferes with automated processes.	Implementation.	Misdirected attention to automated aspects of skill control.
(4)	*Reduced cognitive effort*	Advanced skill, normal conditions.	Automation reduces cognitive demand.	Easy conditions.	Streamlined cognition, low cognitive demand in easy conditions.
(5)	*Reduced memory*	Advanced skill, normal conditions.	Reduced attention results in reduced memory.	Implementation, easy conditions.	Low cognitive demand in easy conditions, shifted attention focus.
(6)	*Strategic focus*	Pre-expert skill, unusual conditions.	Cognitive demand in unfamiliar conditions.	Primary skill control, challenging conditions.	Shifted attention focus, cognitive demand increases with task difficulty.
(7)	*Action slips*	Pre-expert skill, unusual conditions.	Insufficient learning.	Especially familiar conditions with low arousal.	Inadequate situation awareness.
(8)	*Increased attention in response to challenge*	Pre-expert skill, unusual conditions.	Cognitive demand in unfamiliar conditions.	Challenging and unusual conditions.	Cognitive demand increases with task difficulty.
(9)	*Increased cognitive effort in response to challenge*	Pre-expert skill, unusual conditions.	Cognitive demand in unfamiliar conditions.	Challenging and unusual conditions.	Cognitive demand increases with task difficulty.

performance. *Automatic* sees a positive role for cognitive control only in the stages of learning prior to advanced ability (figure 6.1a), and in unusual conditions, where responses haven't fully automated (figure 6.2a). Reduced memory suggests that attention to performance isn't required, so strategic focus should have no benefit in normal conditions. Indeed, since attention to performance is supposed to be disruptive, attention to the strategic features of performance should disrupt those aspects of control, at least in normal conditions. Action slips are difficult to accommodate within the range of normal skill competency for much the same reason: in normal conditions attention isn't required, so low attention should have no negative consequences. Likewise, increases in attention and cognitive effort in response to challenge should only be beneficial if the challenge lies outside the range of normal performance conditions. Again, attention is supposed to be disruptive in normal conditions (experience 3), so increased attention in challenging-but-normal conditions should have the unfortunate effect of degrading ability just as demand on ability increases. The same is true for cognitive effort.

In contrast, *Mesh* provides an integrated explanation for strategic focus, action slips, and increased attention and cognitive effort in response to challenge. According to *Mesh*, cognitive control participates in skilled action and tends to be focused on strategic aspects of task control. We noted above that Bryan and Harter (1899) described a progression in learning telegraphy from focusing on letters, then words, then phrases and sentences, and then meaning. This suggests a hierarchical organization to skilled action, with component skills contributing to higher-order abilities. Figure 6.3 illustrates a hierarchical structure of this kind for driving. We'll distinguish between *primary skills*, which are relatively integrated action units, and *component skills*, which are integrated activities that contribute to the performance of primary skills. Driving is a complex primary skill that involves a suite of coupled component skills (including navigating, steering, accelerating and braking, and changing gear).

In figure 6.3, the organization of the control of driving is depicted as involving three levels. *Higher strategic control* involves overall control of the primary skill in relation to its goals. In the case of driving this includes navigation to the destination. *Situation control* involves the control of action in relation to the immediate situation. In the case of driving this involves proximal control of the car in relation to features of the situation, including maneuvers like accelerating to traffic speed, maintaining lane position, maintaining a safe distance from other cars, changing lanes, and so on. *Implementation control* involves performing actions that achieve situation control, which in the case of driving includes steering, accelerating, braking, changing gears, and so on.[3]

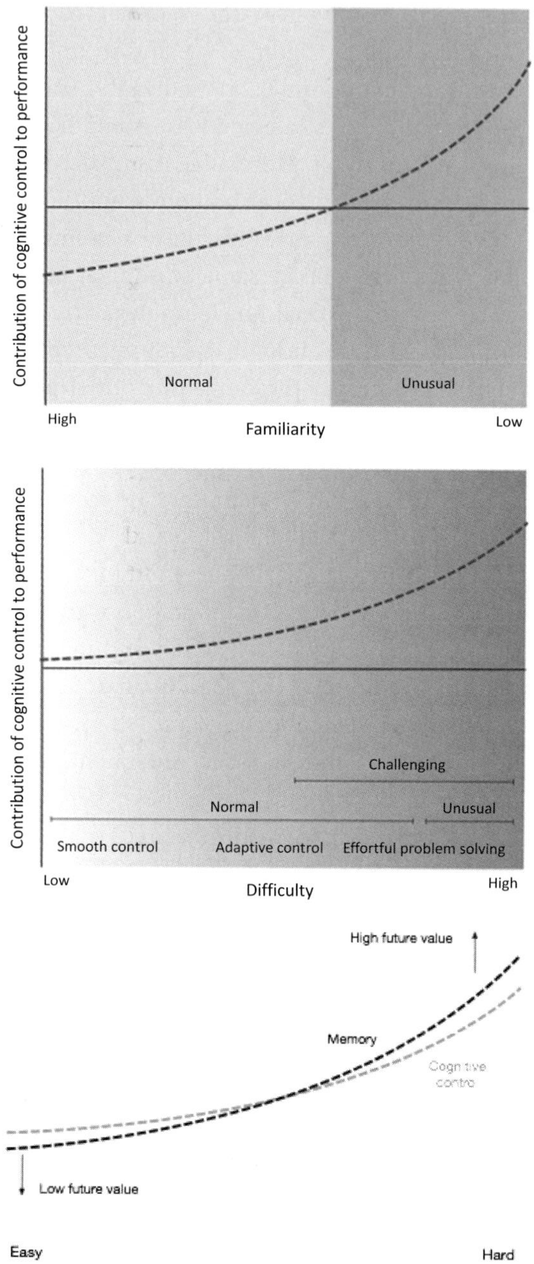

Figure 6.2
Cognitive control: familiarity and difficulty. (a) Automatic, (b) *Mesh*, (c) Memory and cognitive control.

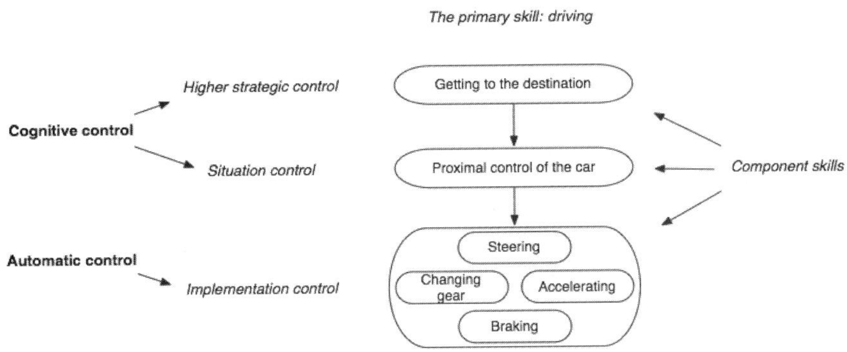

Figure 6.3
Control hierarchy: driving.

According to *Mesh*, automation tends to be strongest (though not complete) for implementation control, whereas situation control and higher strategic control do not tend to automate strongly (though learning will greatly improve the organization of control). The reason for this is that implementation control involves relatively stable relations (e.g., brake to slow down), while the relation of action to context is usually complex and variable (e.g., brake now to avoid the pedestrian on the crossing). In some cases some of the higher-order features of action have a high degree of constancy. For instance, navigation can become automated when a particular kind of journey almost always involves the same route, as in the case of driving to work in the morning. But in general, higher-order features of action will tend to show substantial variability.

In this account the role of cognitive control in skilled action is to manage the variable features of action, tracking the overall task and the structure of the situation and adjusting action appropriately. Thus, situation awareness in driving will include awareness of the destination and route and awareness of the immediate situation, including position on the road, speed, upcoming corners, other cars, and so on. Situation awareness will contribute to an action set, such as a pattern of attention and action appropriate for freeway driving in heavy traffic, or suburban driving at night. It can also contribute to the formation of an action gist, such as gentle early braking when approaching a corner in wet conditions.

Given this, action slips are readily explained as the result of weak higher-order control, resulting in misalignment of goals, situation, and action. Increased attention in response to challenge can be explained because in challenging conditions higher-order aspects of action control tend to be especially complex and variable (consider the routing and traffic problems facing a London cabby). Increased cognitive effort can be explained because in challenging conditions maintaining awareness often requires integrative interpretation, and because action selection is more complex.

Mesh recognizes a mixture of increased and reduced attention, so it can also accommodate the five kinds of skill experience we associated with *Automatic*. Enhanced strategic focus is compatible with reduced attention if the reduction of attention is to details of implementation. Thus, a driver can simultaneously have heightened awareness of nearby cars during a passing maneuver and low awareness of changing gears. Enhanced attention and cognitive effort in response to challenge is also compatible with reduced attention and cognitive effort when the conditions are unchallenging. When the strategic features of the task are simple and stable, then relatively little information is needed for effective control and there is little need for interpretation or planning. Reduced cognitive effort is also in part the result of cognitive streamlining, according to *Mesh*. As well as automating implementation, skill learning produces cognitive structures that are well organized for the demands of the task, reducing the cognitive effort needed for effective higher order action control.

Multitask tolerance can be explained if the conditions are such that relatively little higher order control is needed. Driving on a good road with moderate traffic and clear visibility is undemanding for an experienced driver; she does need to keep track of the relation of the car to the road and other cars, and turn at the appropriate places to reach the destination, but this is simple enough to afford spare cognitive capacity for other activities, such as conversation. Component skills must show some multitask tolerance because they are characteristically performed in conjunction with other component skills, and indeed, linkage between component skills can reduce cognitive demand. For instance, linkage between clutch control and shifting the gear lever reduces the need to directly attend to either. Disruptive attention can be explained as the misdirection of attention to the details of implementation when its proper focus is on higher-order aspects of performance.

Reduced memory is consistent with *Mesh* if the reduction is for details of implementation, or if conditions are easy. Some additional qualification is required here, however, because *Mesh* claims that there is always some cognitive control of action, even in easy conditions (figure 6.2b), yet memories for very routine actions can sometimes seem virtually nonexistent. To account for this, *Mesh* proposes that memory encoding is affected by more than just attention (figure 6.2c). In particular, memory encoding is affected by the relevance of information for future control. Information that is evaluated as likely to be important for future control is preferentially encoded, while information that is not likely to be important in the future is less likely to be encoded, even if this information is operative in immediate control (cf. Anderson and Schooler 2000; Michaelian

2011). Broadly speaking, it is more likely that there is something to be learned in challenging conditions compared with easy conditions, and so situational information in challenging conditions is more likely to be relevant in future. But we also think that experts have more fine-grained mechanisms for preferential memory encoding, based on memory structures organized for retrieval demands (Ericsson and Kintsch 1995). If the task demands are such that present information is needed in the future, then it is more likely to be encoded, even in easy conditions, whereas information not relevant to future control may not be encoded, even in challenging conditions.

The combined effect of these mechanisms is that experts will tend to encode large amounts of information *when the information is evaluated as relevant to future control*, but relatively little information when information about the current situation is unlikely to be important in future. Novices are constantly confronted with new tasks and will tend to have rich memories, but have less basis for predicting relevance in general, or relevance to future control. Their memories should therefore incorporate more incidental information than an expert's memories. Overall capacity to remember detail will be less than for an expert because situational information is much more meaningful for the expert. Thus, *Mesh* gives quite different predictions than does *Automatic* with respect to memory for performance.

The specificity of the scheme of qualifications given by *Mesh* is important. In general, *Mesh* would not expect reduced memory in challenging conditions (though this is modulated by future relevance), so cases of reduced memory in challenging conditions would be problematic. However the typical examples of reduced memory—like driving a familiar route—are cases where conditions are easy. And conversely, cases that illustrate enhanced attention to challenge—like driving at night on an icy road—are the kinds of situations that often produce vivid memories. Multitask tolerance in challenging conditions would not be consistent with *Mesh*, but again, typical cases of multitask tolerance involve easy conditions. Thus, it's not hard for a driver to hold a conversation when conditions are easy, but things are different in difficult conditions. Intuitively, conversation is more likely to impair driving ability when driving at night in icy conditions on a winding country road. Experimental evidence confirms that a secondary task can have a substantial detrimental effect on driving ability (Blanco et al. 2006).

Figure 6.2b represents the *Mesh* view of increasing cognitive demand as it contrasts with *Automatic* (figure 6.2a). The most basic difference is that the *x* axis in 6.2b shows difficulty rather than familiarity. *Automatic* effectively assumes that difficulty reduces to familiarity: tasks that are difficult for the novice (and hence cognitively demanding) become easy (and hence cognitively undemanding) with sufficient learning. Cognitive demand arises for the expert only in conditions that are unusual—conditions that haven't been experienced often enough for effective automatic responses to have been acquired. *Mesh,* on the other hand, treats difficulty and familiarity as distinct. While it's true that tasks generally become easier with learning, experts don't perform the same tasks as novices—they move on to tasks that are far more complex and challenging. And some tasks can have sufficient inherent complexity that no amount of learning makes them easy, or easy enough to be fully automated. More specifically, tasks that exhibit *strong control-relevant complexity* tend to be experienced as difficult even with extensive learning, and resist automation. A task has strong control-relevant complexity when (a) there are many task features, (b) there are strong interdependencies between task features, and (c) the success of particular actions is strongly sensitive to the specific state of these interdependencies on particular occasions. Accordingly, *Mesh* regards difficulty as the key parameter governing the degree of cognitive involvement in action control, rather than familiarity.

There is a temptation from an *Automatic* perspective to define cognitively involved performance as pre-expert (figures 6.1a and 6.2a). It might accordingly be claimed that putative experts who find their performances challenging (e.g., concert pianists) are for some reason stuck in a pre-expert mode. Given even more training, they might attain true expertise. But this is problematic. If individuals who have had a great deal of training and show an advanced level of ability find their performances challenging, we should reconsider our theoretical account of expertise, rather than stipulatively define their performance as sub-expert. Perhaps individuals with arbitrarily high capacity and training opportunity would eventually attain automaticity, but *Automatic* is not a very interesting position if it describes what skill would be like for gods.

In one respect, experts are often dealing with the unfamiliar, since their tasks are complex and frequently involve situations whose fine-grained structure hasn't been previously experienced. But we should nevertheless distinguish between normal variability and unusual performance conditions, where the latter is understood to mean that the general task parameters are different from the typical conditions of performance. A cab driver dealing with the vagaries of traffic in the city is experiencing normal variability, whereas a car driver attempting to drive a truck for the first time is experiencing unusual conditions.

Figure 6.2b associates with increasing difficulty three conceptualizations of performance: *smooth control* involves relatively effortless action in easy conditions, *adaptive control* involves greater attention and cognitive effort, and *effortful problem solving* involves relatively high degrees of attention and cognitive effort, and temporally extended cognitive processing to determine appropriate action.[4] In our view there is a high degree of continuity: smooth control shades into adaptive control, which shades into effortful problem solving. In terms of these conceptualizations, *Automatic* makes two key mistakes: it assumes that smooth control is normal, and it assumes that it involves no cognitive control (compare figure 6.2a with 6.2b, where "normal" in 6.2a corresponds to smooth control in 6.2b). Intuitively, conscious control is associated with effortful problem solving, and we think that the intuitive basis of *Automatic* involves a mistaken interpretation of the phenomenology of smooth control as indicating that control is noncognitive.

According to *Mesh*, normal performance conditions for most skills encompass all three modes of performance. Conditions are noticeably challenging at the high end of adaptive control, and many highly skilled individuals not infrequently need to engage in effortful problem solving. As noted, familiarity doesn't map into difficulty straightforwardly, but performance conditions that are both complex and unusual will be especially difficult. Figure 6.4 shows more directly the difference in expectations between *Automatic* and *Mesh* with respect to the frequency of the modes of performance that a highly skilled individual experiences. Some kinds of expertise are more challenging than others, and the skew of the distribution differs accordingly. Nevertheless, it is unlikely that many skills have a distribution as skewed as *Automatic* assumes (noting

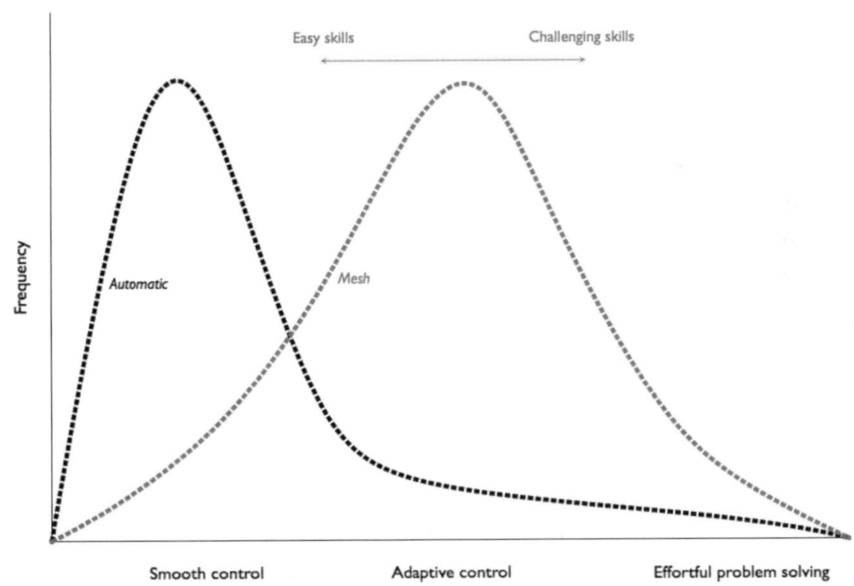

Figure 6.4
The distribution of performance conditions.

again that even if the distribution were this skewed, smooth control doesn't mean no cognitive control).

We're treating "normal" here as a simple matter of frequency, and this is a good first approximation: normal performance conditions are the conditions the individual usually experiences. But in many cases experts are expected to perform well in conditions that they experience relatively infrequently. Statistically speaking, performing in the Olympics is not normal for an Olympic athlete, but it would be odd to describe Olympic performance conditions as *unusual* for an Olympic athlete; they are at any rate not unusual in the way that driving a truck is unusual for a car driver. Similarly, engine failure is not a frequent occurrence for an airline pilot, but coping with an engine failure is expected of airline pilots and part of their normal training (Crespigny 2012). To clarify this, we distinguish a frequency-based conception of "normal conditions" from a normative conception of the conditions in which a particular kind of expert is expected to perform well, or the *conditions of expected skill*. What counts as normal, broadly understood, will be a complex mix of frequency of actual performance conditions, training, and expectations.

Summarizing, *Mesh* provides a more integrated explanation for the nine kinds of skill experience described above than does *Automatic*. *Automatic* provides a concise explanation for the first five kinds of experience, but the last four pose difficulties. They are suggestive of cognitive control, so *Automatic* must locate them outside the range of normal performance conditions (figure 6.2a). This takes no account of difficulty, however, and leads to rather implausible expectations about the kind of performance conditions that are normal (figure 6.4). *Mesh* is superficially more complicated, offering a more complicated set of qualifications (table 6.1), and making stronger claims about the nature of skilled action (it involves higher-order control of assemblages of component skills—figure 6.3) and skill domains (they often involve difficulty that can't be fully eliminated with learning). But these claims are well-founded, and they yield a more integrated explanation for the nine kinds of skill experience and a more integrated picture of skilled performance (figures 6.2b and 6.4).

4 Applying the Framework

Our analysis to this point has distinguished three broad possibilities for theories of skill (*Automatic, Full Cognitive*, and *Hybrid*) and two kinds of hybrid theory (*Autonomous* and *Mesh*). We have elaborated our preferred option, *Mesh*, in comparison with *Automatic*, by means of a careful comparative evaluation with respect to the ability to explain a set of diverse forms of skill experience. The next step is to apply the framework to extant skill theories. As a starting point, we use the framework to illuminate several key types of experimental research and the theoretical interpretations that have been given to the evidence.

4.1 Dreyfus and NDM Research on the Difficulty of Normal Conditions

As noted above, the theory of skill presented by Dreyfus and Dreyfus (1986) is the clearest example of *Automatic*. Dreyfus (1997) places this theory in the context of expertise research conducted within the naturalistic decision making (NDM) framework (Zsambok and Klein 1997). Like Dreyfus, NDM research has defined itself in contrast with formal decision-theoretic approaches to decision making, and NDM researchers share with Dreyfus the view that experts don't typically make decisions by generating and analyzing an extended list of options (Klein 1993). However, NDM research has arrived at a somewhat different picture of expert performance, indicating that experts often engage in quite extensive cognitive processes. For instance, in the context of battle command, Serfaty et al. (1997) propose a three-stage model of decision making in which an initial plan is formed on the basis of recognition of the nature of the situation, the plan is developed by exploring its structure, and the plan is then applied to the situation (235–238).

To explain this inconsistency between his account of expertise and the findings of NDM research, Dreyfus appeals to Heidegger's ([1927] 1962) tripartite distinction between *ready-to-hand* performance, in which the individual engages in intuitive smooth coping with ready-to-hand equipment; *unready-to-hand* performance, in which conditions are unusual and the individual must act deliberately; and *present-at-hand* performance, where the situation is highly unfamiliar and requires rational deliberation. Dreyfus claims that these are three kinds of skilled response to a situation "each with its own phenomenology and its own appropriate mode," and that his theory applies to ready-to-hand smooth coping, whereas NDM research has been examining unready-to-hand performance (1997, 27). His explanation for why the experts studied by NDM research are exhibiting unready-to-hand performance instead of ready-to-hand performance is that NDM researchers have been investigating "how decision-making works in complex, uncertain, unstable situations such as emergencies, where experts do not have enough experience to have an immediate, intuitive response" (1997, 28). He suggests that this complements the work that he and Stuart Dreyfus have done on transparent intuitive coping.

Several aspects of this attempted reconciliation are problematic. It is a mischaracterization to say that NDM researchers are studying the performance of experts in unusual conditions, as implied by classifying the performance as "unready-to-hand." Dreyfus explains unready-to-hand performance by saying that "when a piece of equipment is missing or when the situation is otherwise abnormal we have to stop and think" (1997, 27). But while the experimental conditions that NDM researchers have used are designed to be challenging, they are also intended to emulate real performance conditions. Studying battle commanders, for instance, Serfaty et al. say, "We designed an experiment that posed realistic, nontrivial problems, simulated the procedure and materials used in real-world tactical situations, and involved a significant number of military officers" (1997, 238). The conditions of performance being studied by NDM researchers are *uncertain,* as Dreyfus recognizes, but they are not *unusual.*

Rather than complementing Dreyfus's theory, NDM research looks like counterevidence. Dreyfus and Dreyfus (1986) described their theory as applying to expertise in domains with *unstructured problems:*

> As we examine in detail how a novice, if he possesses innate ability and has the opportunity to acquire sufficient experience, gradually becomes an expert, we shall focus upon the most common kind of problem area, sometimes called "unstructured." *Such areas contain a potentially unlimited number of possibly relevant facts and features, and the ways those elements interrelate and determine other events is unclear.* Management, nursing, economic forecasting, teaching, and all social interactions fall into that very large class. (20; emphasis added)

The theory is thus specifically intended to apply to expertise in problem situations that are complex and uncertain (economic forecasting!), and Dreyfus and Dreyfus see this as including many kinds of expertise. Examples they discuss include driving, aviation, nursing, medical diagnosis, air traffic control, chess, and marketing. NDM research defines its scope similarly: as expert decision making in situations where the problems are ill-structured, dynamic, and uncertain (Zsambok 1997, 5), and the fields it has investigated overlap with the fields discussed by Dreyfus and Dreyfus (1986) (see the various chapters in Zsambok and Klein 1997).

Dreyfus and Dreyfus (1986) say that experts deliberate "when time permits and much is at stake" (40). However, this must be relatively exceptional if it's true that experts "don't make decisions" in normal conditions. Dreyfus and Dreyfus also say that "few if any situations ... are seen as being of *exactly* the kind for which prior experience intuitively dictates what move or decision must be made," requiring the expert to evaluate possible actions and/or deliberatively adjust an action to the features of the current situation (37). This is an interesting claim, which anticipates in certain respects the model of Serfaty et al. (1997). But it raises for Dreyfus a problem of consistency: if "few if any" situations are close enough to past experience to be able to rely purely on intuition, then experts will *almost always* be using deliberative control. It is impossible to

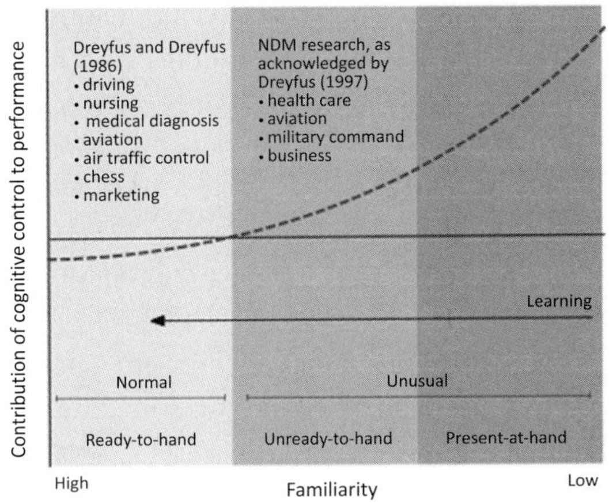

Figure 6.5
Dreyfus's account of skill control.

reconcile this with the claim quoted above that experts don't solve problems or make decisions when things are proceeding normally.

Thus, even if some of the claims that Dreyfus has made are broadly consistent with NDM research, they are not consistent with the main claims of his own theory. If Dreyfus is to fully embrace the findings of NDM research, he must make major changes to his theory.

Ready-to-hand, unready-to-hand, and present-at-hand forms of performance are characterized in terms of a spectrum of familiarity (figure 6.5), with ready-to-hand performance occurring in normal conditions (if we take seriously the claim that experts don't make decisions when things are normal). This accords with *Automatic*, as depicted in figure 6.2a. That ready-to-hand performance should be normal makes sense if the differences between these modes of performance are based on familiarity: increasing familiarity should drive a transition from present-at-hand to ready-to-hand performance. When we frame it in this way, it appears that the experts studied by NDM research get stuck partway along the progression, but why? An expert should be very familiar with the problems she deals with as a matter of course as part of her expertise. The obvious answer is that the problems are hard: but difficulty isn't taken into account by this conceptualization of performance. Difficult is not the same as unfamiliar.

In the part 4.2 we characterized a spectrum of forms of performance using the concepts of smooth control, adaptive control, and effortful problem solving (figure 6.2b). This is inspired by Dreyfus's Heideggerian conceptualization, but there are important differences. Understanding the spectrum in terms of difficulty rather than familiarity is one: whereas Dreyfus describes situations that induce unready-to-hand performance as abnormal, we don't think that a situation has to be abnormal for an expert to be using adaptive control—just mildly difficult. Nor does the situation have to be abnormal for effortful problem solving. Unready-to-hand performance would, in our terms, be one relatively strong form of effortful problem solving. We prefer "smooth control" to "smooth coping" because "coping" is too passive a concept. Experts don't simply cope with their environment—they are actively engaged with it. And we think that these forms of performance are highly continuous, whereas, in describing them as different modes, Dreyfus treats his categories as fairly distinct.

For these reasons figure 6.5 and figure 6.2b are not directly comparable, though we've designed them to make the comparison as close as possible. As a rough approximation, NDM research suggests that for the kinds of expertise investigated, the distribution of forms of performance is more like the *Mesh* curve than the *Automatic* curve in figure 6.4, skewed in these cases toward effortful problem solving, which is to be expected for challenging forms of expertise. We agree wholeheartedly with the claim that very few situations are so exactly like past experience that a prior solution can be applied without some evaluation or modification. But taking this claim seriously results in a theory different from that proposed by Dreyfus.

4.2 Tolerance to Distraction in Complex Motor Skills

The forms of expertise investigated by NDM research are ones that many would expect to involve explicit reasoning processes. As we discussed above, it is not uncommon to take the more restricted view that only lower-order aspects of performance tend to automate, with higher cognition continuing to play an important strategic role. In part 3 we distinguished *Automatic* and *Autonomous*, in which *Autonomous* holds that the execution of motor skills becomes automated but that decision making and other forms of conscious cognition still play a role in complex skills that have a substantial motor component, such as sporting skills like soccer. We further distinguished *Mesh* from *Autonomous* as two forms of hybrid theory, with *Mesh* proposing that cognitive control makes important contributions to virtually all skills, including those that *Autonomous* regards as largely automatic, such as golf putting. We now examine experimental research that bears on this issue, using the framework we've developed to reveal weaknesses in the framing of the experiments and the interpretation of the results.

Multitask tolerance is one form of skill experience that is suggestive of automaticity, and some experimental paradigms designed to test automaticity are based on multitask tolerance. Leavitt (1979) probed the automaticity of puck control in expert ice hockey players by measuring the effect on performance of a distracting second task. Leavitt compared the performances of ice hockey players of varying skill levels in skating through a slalom course while stickhandling a puck. In one condition the subjects performed a secondary task (identifying objects); Leavitt found that the speed and stickhandling performance of the experts was minimally affected by the secondary task, whereas the performance of players of lower skill levels was significantly impaired. Gray (2004) used baseball batting as the primary task and a secondary task that involved monitoring tones presented at random times during the batting task. Like Leavitt, Gray found that experts were not impaired by the distracting secondary task (compare Christensen, Sutton, and McIlwain, 2015).

These experiments do not take task difficulty into account, however: in each case the conditions are easy for the experts. The slalom course employed by Leavitt was a straight out-and-back course with five obstacles—easy compared with game conditions. The *Mesh* prediction is that expert performance would be impaired by a secondary task on a slalom course that players found challenging. Gray's (2004) experiments required baseball experts to hit a virtual ball, where there were only two kinds of pitches (fast and slow). Individuals completed between three hundred and five hundred trials. These conditions are again much easier than the conditions experts would experience during a game, and are also monotonous. *Mesh* predicts that performance would be impaired by the secondary task in conditions that are more realistic and have a degree of challenge commensurate with competition conditions.

4.3 Reduced Memory in Complex Motor Skills

In addition to multitask tolerance, other forms of evidence are used to infer automaticity. Reduced memory (experience 5 in table 6.1) is also associated with automaticity, and Beilock and Carr (2001) conducted experiments designed to assess reduced memory for performance. They compared novices and experts on a golf-putting task in the laboratory. Participants first performed twenty putts from a fixed location on a carpeted floor, attempting to place the ball as close as possible to a cross on the floor 1.5 meters away. After completing the putts, the subjects were asked to describe the steps involved in a typical putt. This was intended to assess generic knowledge of putting. Subjects then performed a second series of thirty putts, and were again asked to describe the steps involved in a typical putt. In the final phase of the experiment, a further twenty putts were performed, and subjects were then asked to describe the last putt they had taken. This was intended to gauge episodic memory for the putt (in contrast with generic knowledge of putting). The results were that, as expected, novices gave shorter generic descriptions than experts (experts have greater knowledge for the domain), whereas novices gave longer episodic descriptions than experts.

In 4.2 we argued that reduced memory can be consistent with both *Automatic* and *Mesh,* but that the two theories view the scope of the phenomenon differently. For skills like golf putting, *Autonomous* gives the same predictions as *Automatic*: reduced memory should occur in normal (but not unusual) conditions. In contrast, as a first approximation, *Mesh* expects reduced memory in easy conditions, but not in challenging-but-normal conditions or unusual conditions (figures 6.2b and 6.2c). This, however, is influenced by the specific memory demands of the task. In Beilock and Carr's experiments, the conditions for the experts were very easy: the subjects performed seventy identical putts indoors on carpet. The task had no informational dependencies over time, so current information had low relevance for future control once a reasonable standard of performance was obtained. Thus, although these results are consistent with *Autonomous,* they are also consistent with *Mesh.* Putting it another way, Beilock and Carr haven't shown expertise-induced amnesia for expert putting in general, only in easy conditions where information for control has no future relevance.

Beilock, Wierenga, and Carr (2002) conducted a study in which experts did have stronger memories than novices. They compared novices and experts using a "funny putter": a putter with an S-shape and unusual weighting. Experts using the funny putter had rich episodic memories for putts performed, suggesting high attention and cognitive involvement. This performance situation is clearly unusual, and like *Automatic, Autonomous* predicts cognitive control (figure 6.2a). But with respect to cognitive demand, it may be closer to the challenging conditions an expert golfer must cope with during competition than is performing seventy identical putts on carpet (figure 6.2b).

This further shows that our analysis illuminates—and reveals weakness in—extant skill research. Like Dreyfus, Beilock uses a simple distinction between normal and unusual conditions that doesn't recognize the possibility that there might be significant cognitive control in challenging-but-normal conditions. The key question for Beilock and Carr is whether expertise-induced amnesia will be found in challenging-but-normal conditions. *Mesh* predicts that expert golfers should show enhanced memory for performance in challenging conditions. There may be reduced memory for some implementation details, but there should be enhanced memory for important aspects of higher-order control, such as information involved in adjusting the putt for the specific features of the situation (situation control in figure 6.3).

Beilock (2011) suggests that, to avoid choking, "the best advice ... is to try to play 'outside your head' or at least outside your prefrontal cortex" (199). Again, *Mesh* supplies different expectations. In Beilock's account, distraction should reduce choking by preventing attention to automatic processes. She says, "Having a golfer count backward by threes, for example, or even having a golfer sing a song to himself uses up working memory that might otherwise fuel overthinking and a flubbed performance" (2011, 77). In contrast, on the basis of *Mesh*, we expect that achieving an effective strategic focus will be more beneficial than distraction. Distraction may be helpful in some circumstances, but it will also reduce the quality of the individual's situation awareness and higher-order control processes. Methods that improve focus should be especially valuable in challenging conditions, where situation awareness and higher-order control is most critical.

In sum, the problems of *Automatic* described in 4.2 also apply to *Autonomous* in the case of complex motor skills like golf putting. These problems are evident in Beilock's work: like Dreyfus, she fails to properly recognize the significance of difficulty, and she also fails to consider the possibility that some forms of attention to performance are disruptive and others are not.

5 Taking Stock: Understanding Complex Skills in Challenging Conditions

Mesh places greater emphasis on difficulty and complex action than does either *Automatic* or *Autonomous*. The preceding analysis shows the value of incorporating these aspects of skill into the picture more fully. Everyone knows that some tasks are difficult and that skilled action can be complex. But giving proper theoretical weight to these features of skill requires integrative theory to address multiple features of skill. The automated aspects of skill are, somewhat ironically, very salient, and it is easy to emphasize them at the expense of other aspects of skill. The positions we've critically examined do just this: they argue for skill automaticity based on select kinds of skill phenomena (experiences 1–5 in table 6.1) without properly considering the kinds of qualifications required or the broader range of phenomena that is relevant. In short, they overgeneralize.

Dreyfus and Dreyfus (1986) clearly expected that expertise in complex skill domains would be substantially automated, even though they noticed in passing what in our view is the basic reason why it isn't (performance conditions are usually too variable). Leavitt (1979) shows multitask tolerance in easy but not realistic conditions. Beilock and Carr (2001) assume that they can generalize from golf-putting performance in very easy conditions to putting in general—putting in "normal conditions." Beilock, Weirenga, and Carr (2002) examine putting performance in unusual conditions, but Beilock doesn't compare putting in easy, difficult, and unusual conditions, which would give a better overall picture of the nature of the control of putting.

In contrast, *Mesh* provides a more nuanced picture (figure 6.3b), which accommodates evidence for automaticity while highlighting the need to understand action complexity, demanding performance conditions, and the role of cognitive control. *Mesh* more specifically suggests three core issues that deserve systematic empirical investigation: (1) the range of performance conditions that experts experience, (2) possible changes in the nature of control across this performance range, and (3) complex patterns of attention in changing conditions.

With respect to the range of performance conditions experienced by experts, NDM experimental research, designed to be realistic, provides suggestive evidence for the *Mesh* curve in figure 6.4. But it would clearly be valuable to examine performance conditions more directly. Our phenomenological analysis can serve as the starting point for systematic qualitative investigation; an initial step toward this would be validation of the picture summarized in table 6.1 with systematic qualitative and cognitive ethnographic research—the investigation of skill experiences in varied real-world conditions across a range of skills. The skill experiences of interest for *Mesh* include sense of challenge, sense of cognitive effort, selective focus of attention, action slips, and poor or good memory for performance. Evidence for a range of ordinary and elite skills and performance circumstances would provide a much more detailed empirical basis for evaluating the contrasting theoretical claims depicted in figure 6.5.

With respect to changes in the nature of control across the performance range, experimental investigation can give a more detailed picture. Leavitt (1979) and Beilock and Carr (2001) compared novices and experts on tasks at a fixed level of difficulty. One way to probe whether cognitive control in experts varies with difficulty is to titrate the effect of changes in difficulty on measures of cognitive control, such as dual-task interference. Doing this for conditions that range from easy to highly challenging, and for a variety of kinds of skill, would provide a detailed test for the contrasting claims of figures 6.3a and 6.3b. Comparing increases in normal difficulty with changes that make a task progressively more unusual would help to further disambiguate difficulty and familiarity and might help identify differing patterns of control in challenging-but-normal conditions as compared with unusual conditions.

With respect to complex patterns of attention, the *Mesh* concept of strategic focus has some similarity to claims that we've associated with *Autonomous*, in particular the idea that attention shifts to higher-order cognitive processes, such as changes in strategy. Schmidt and Wrisberg make this claim, and Wulf (2007) similarly claims that, "As individuals gain experience with a certain skill, and the movement becomes more and more automated, the action is assumed to be monitored at progressively higher levels" (147). But according to *Mesh*, higher-order control plays a key role in virtually all skilled action—not just action that involves explicit reasoning. Moreover, as discussed above, we think that awareness can include information about body state and movement, so a shift to awareness at "higher levels" isn't necessarily a shift away from all lower-order detail. Rather, expert awareness should have shifted to focus on the *critical* information for performance; expert awareness will be selective, highly shaped to task demands, and may often "roam" or "float" as it flexibly and anticipatively seeks out important information. Attentional control will often include forms of self-regulation, as individuals induce in themselves cognitive, emotional, and bodily states appropriate for the situation. We noted in the introduction Kumar Sangakkara's claim that "in batting, you have to be mindless," but he clarifies this point immediately by noting that being "a thinking cricketer" is in fact "about deciding how and when to use your brain; when to think and when not to think" (Sadikot 2014). This in fact suggests that, rather than being generally mindless, expert cricketers are employing sophisticated forms of attentional control and self-regulation. We also note that, because cognitive control is broader than just conscious reasoning and decision making, and because many functions of cognitive control are not conscious or are only partly conscious, the state that Sangakkara calls "mindless" may involve significant cognitive control, including strong situation awareness and top-down regulation of the motor system. Investigating these kinds of higher-order cognition is challenging because detailed patterns of attention are task specific, vary across individuals, and may be disrupted by attentional instructions that induce "unnatural" attention patterns. Careful phenomenological investigation is required, together with experiments that are sensitive to the "natural" attention patterns of experts.

6 Conclusion

Automation has clear benefits for skill control: the integration and simplification of action control can make action production more efficient. But cognitive control nevertheless makes a vital contribution to skill control by determining the nature of the situation and configuring and adjusting lower-order sensorimotor processes appropriately. Cognitive and automatic processes thus characteristically operate together in an intimately meshed arrangement, with cognitive control typically focused on strategic task features and automatic control responsible for implementation. Experts often have to perform in complex, difficult conditions, and the interpretive and regulative functions of cognitive control gain increasing importance as difficulty increases.

In developing this account of skill learning and control, we've placed a strong emphasis on synthesis, and a sibling paper (in preparation) extends the synthesis presented here to encompass a number of key theories of skill learning and action control. Drawing on these theories, we can incorporate into *Mesh* an array of phenomena involved in skill, including proceduralization, dynamical constraints, nonanalytic pattern recognition, schematization, efficient memory organization, situation awareness, and action planning. The account also develops further a theoretical explanation for the persistence of cognitive control in advanced skill and characterizes a transformation in cognitive control to more efficient forms that involve substantial nonlinguistic structure. The importance of such synthesis for understanding skill should be emphasized: skill is complex, and it is difficult to integrate its many facets into a coherent picture. We've argued that a number of influential accounts of skill overemphasize automaticity at the expense of other aspects of skill control.

Notes

1. This chapter reproduces the contents of the article "Cognition in Skilled Action: Meshed Control and the Varieties of Skill Experience," originally published in 2016 by Wayne Christensen, John Sutton, and Doris J. F. McIlwain in *Mind & Language* 31 (1:37–66). The article is preceded by a new introduction ("Mesh: Cognition, Body and Environment in Skilled Action"), written for this volume by Wayne Christensen and John Sutton. I would like to thank the authors, the editors of *Mind & Language*, and the publishers of the journal for the permission to reproduce this paper (Massimiliano L. Cappuccio).

2. Our thanks to Kath Bicknell, Andrew Geeves, John Michael, and Kellie Williamson. We are also grateful for feedback from various audiences to whom we have presented earlier versions of this material, and from two anonymous reviewers. We note with sadness that since the acceptance of this paper Doris McIlwain has died, on April 26, 2015.

Address for correspondence: Professor John Sutton, Department of Cognitive Science, Macquarie University, Sydney, NSW 2109, Australia.

Email: john.sutton@mq.edu.au

3. Pacherie's (2008) similar hierarchical account of action control has influenced our account. Pacherie places greater emphasis on intentions and forward models. In a companion paper (Christensen et al. 2015) we discuss similarities and differences between the accounts.

4. These concepts correspond roughly to Dreyfus's Heideggerian conceptions of "ready-to-hand," "present-at-hand," and "unready-to-hand," modes of coping (Dreyfus 1997). We discuss some of the differences in the chapter.

References

Anderson, John R., and Lael J. Schooler. 2000. "The Adaptive Nature of Memory." In *The Oxford Handbook of Memory*, edited by E. Tulving and F. I. M. Craik, 557–570. New York: Oxford University Press.

Bargh, John A. 1990. "Auto-Motives: Preconscious Determinants of Social Interaction." In *Handbook of Motivation and Cognition: Foundations of Social Behavior*, 2nd ed., edited by E. T. Higgins and R. M. Sorrentino, 93–130. New York: Guilford Press.

Beilock, S. L., and T. H. Carr. 2001. "On the Fragility of Skilled Performance: What Governs Choking under Pressure?" *Journal of Experimental Psychology: General* 130 (4): 701–725. doi:10.1037/0096-3445.130.4.701.

Beilock, Sian. 2011. *Choke: What the Secrets of the Brain Reveal About Getting It Right When You Have To*. New York: Simon and Schuster.

Beilock, Sian L., and Rob Gray. 2007. "Why Do Athletes Choke under Pressure?" In *Handbook of Sport Psychology*, edited by Gershon Tenenbaum and Robert C. Eklund, 425–444. Hoboken, NJ: John Wiley and Sons.

Beilock, Sian L., Sarah A. Wierenga, and Thomas H. Carr. 2002. "Expertise, Attention, and Memory in Sensorimotor Skill Execution: Impact of Novel Task Constraints on Dual-Task Performance and Episodic Memory." *Quarterly Journal of Experimental Psychology A* 55 (4): 1211–1240. doi:10.1080/02724980244000170.

Blanco, Myra, Wayne J. Biever, John P. Gallagher, and Thomas A. Dingus. 2006. "The Impact of Secondary Task Cognitive Processing Demand on Driving Performance." *Accident: Analysis and Prevention* 38 (5): 895–906. doi:10.1016/j.aap.2006.02.015.

Brownstein, Michael. 2014. "Rationalizing Flow: Agency in Skilled Unreflective Action." *Philosophical Studies* 168 (2): 545–568. doi:10.1007/s11098-013-0143-5.

Bryan, William Lowe, and Noble Harter. 1899. "Studies on the Telegraphic Language: The Acquisition of a Hierarchy of Habits." *Psychological Review* 6 (4): 345–375. doi:10.1037/h0073117.

Christensen, Wayne, Kath Bicknell, Doris McIlwain, and John Sutton. 2015. "The Sense of Agency and Its Role in Strategic Control for Expert Mountain Bikers." *Psychology of Consciousness: Theory, Research, and Practice* 2 (3): 340–353. doi:10.1037/cns0000066.

Christensen, Wayne, John Sutton, and Doris McIlwain. 2015. "Putting Pressure on Theories of Choking: Towards an Expanded Perspective on Breakdown in Skilled Performance." *Phenomenology and the Cognitive Sciences* 14 (2): 253–293. doi:10.1007/s11097-014-9395-6.

Craik, Fergus, Richard Govoni, Moshe Naveh-Benjamin, and Nicole D. Anderson. 1996. "The Effects of Divided Attention on Encoding and Retrieval Processes in Human Memory." *Journal of Experimental Psychology: General* 125 (2): 159–180. doi:10.1037/0096-3445.125.2.159.

Crespigny, Richard de. 2012. *QF32*. Tuggerah, NSW: Macmillan.

Dreyfus, Hubert L. 1997. "Intuitive, Deliberative, and Calculative Models of Expert Performance." In *Naturalistic Decision Making*, edited by Caroline E. Zsambock and Gary A. Klein, 17–28. Mahwah, NJ: Lawrence Erlbaum.

Dreyfus, Hubert L. 2013. "The Myth of the Pervasiveness of the Mental." In *Mind, Reason, and Being-in-the-World: The McDowell-Dreyfus Debate*, edited by Joseph K. Schear, 15–38. New York: Routledge.

Dreyfus, Hubert L., and Stuart E. Dreyfus. 1986. *Mind over Machine: The Power of Human Intuition and Expertise in the Era of the Computer*. New York: Free Press.

Duncan, John. 2010. "The Multiple-Demand (MD) System of the Primate Brain: Mental Programs for Intelligent Behaviour." *Trends in Cognitive Sciences* 14 (4): 172–179. doi:10.1016/j.tics.2010.01.004.

Endsley, Mica R. 1995. "Toward a Theory of Situation Awareness in Dynamic Systems." *Human Factors* 37 (1): 32–64. doi:10.1518/001872095779049543.

Ericsson, Karl Anders. 2006. "The Influence of Experience and Deliberate Practice on the Development of Superior Expert Performance." In *The Cambridge Handbook of Expertise and Expert Performance*, edited by K. Anders Ericsson, Neil Charness, Paul J. Feltovich, and Robert R. Hoffman, 685–705. Cambridge: Cambridge University Press.

Ericsson, Karl Anders, and Walter Kintsch. 1995. "Long-Term Working Memory." *Psychological Review* 102 (2): 211–245. doi:10.1037/0033-295X.102.2.211.

Evans, Jonathan St. B. T., and Keith E. Stanovich. 2013. "Dual-Process Theories of Higher Cognition: Advancing the Debate." *Perspectives on Psychological Science* 8 (3): 223–241. doi:10.1177/1745691612460685.

Fitts, Paul Morris, and Michael I. Posner. 1967. *Human Performance*. Pacific Grove, CA: Brooks/Cole.

Fridland, Ellen. 2014. "They've Lost Control: Reflections on Skill." *Synthese* 191 (12): 2729–2750. doi:10.1007/s11229-014-0411-8.

Fuster, Joaquín M. 2008. *The Prefrontal Cortex*. 4th ed. London: Elsevier.

Gray, Rob. 2004. "Attending to the Execution of a Complex Sensorimotor Skill: Expertise Differences, Choking, and Slumps." *Journal of Experimental Psychology: Applied* 10 (1): 42–54. doi:10.1037/1076-898X.10.1.42.

Heidegger, Martin. [1927] 1962. *Being and Time*. Translated by John Macquarrie and Edward Robinson. New York: Harper and Row.

Jonides, John, Moshe Naveh-Benjamin, and John Palmer. 1985. "Assessing Automaticity." *Acta Psychologica* 60 (2/3): 157–171. doi:10.1016/0001-6918(85)90053-8.

Klein, Gary A. 1993. "A Recognition-Primed Decision (RPD) Model of Rapid Decision Making." In *Decision Making in Action: Models and Methods*, edited by A. Klein, J. Orasanu, R. Calderwood, and C. E. Zsambok, 138–146. Norwood, NJ: Ablex.

Leavitt, J. L. 1979. "Cognitive Demands of Skating and Stickhandling in Ice Hockey." *Canadian Journal of Applied Sport Sciences / Journal Canadien Des Sciences Appliquees Au Sport* 4 (1): 46–55.

Logan, Gordon D. 1985. "Skill and Automaticity: Relations, Implications, and Future Directions." *Canadian Journal of Psychology / Revue Canadienne de Psychologie* 39 (2): 367–386. doi:10.1037/h0080066.

Michaelian, Kourken. 2011. "The Epistemology of Forgetting." *Erkenntnis* 74: 399–424.

Miller, Earl K. 2000. "The Prefrontal Cortex and Cognitive Control." *Nature Reviews Neuroscience* 1: 59–65.

Montero, Barbara. 2010. "Does Bodily Awareness Interfere with Highly Skilled Movement?" *Inquiry* 53 (2): 105–122. doi:10.1080/00201741003612138.

Moors, Agnes, and Jan De Houwer. 2006. "Automaticity: A Theoretical and Conceptual Analysis." *Psychological Bulletin* 132 (2): 297–326. doi:10.1037/0033-2909.132.2.297.

Pacherie, Elisabeth. 2008. "The Phenomenology of Action: A Conceptual Framework." *Cognition* 107 (1): 179–217. doi:10.1016/j.cognition.2007.09.003.

Papineau, David. 2013. "In the Zone." *Royal Institute of Philosophy Supplement* 73:175–196. doi:10.1017/S1358246113000325.

Posner, Michael I., and Charles R. Snyder. 1975. "Attention and Cognitive Control." In *Information Processing and Cognition: The Loyola Symposium*, edited by R. L. Solso, 55–82. Hillsdale, NJ: Erlbaum.

Sadikot, Shirin. 2014. "Mindlessness Is Crucial in Batting: Sangakkara." BCCI: Board of Control for Cricket in India. November 9. http://www.bcci.tv/news/2014/features-and-interviews/8893/mindlessness-is-crucial-in-batting-sangakkara.

Schmidt, Richard A., and Craig A. Wrisberg. 2008. *Motor Learning and Performance: A Situation-Based Learning Approach*. Champaign, IL: Human Kinetics.

Serfaty, Daniel, Jean MacMillan, Elliot E. Entin, and Eileen B. Entin. 1997. "The Decision-Making Expertise of Battle Commanders." In *Naturalistic Decision Making*, edited by Caroline E. Zsambok and Gary A. Klein, 233–246. Hillsdale, NJ: Erlbaum.

Shiffrin, Richard M., and Walter Schneider. 1977. "Controlled and Automatic Human Information Processing: II. Perceptual Learning, Automatic Attending and a General Theory." *Psychological Review* 84 (2): 127–190.

Stanley, Jason, and John W. Krakauer. 2013. "Motor Skill Depends on Knowledge of Facts." *Frontiers in Human Neuroscience* 7 (August): 503. http://www.frontiersin.org/Human_Neuroscience/abstract/55476.

Sutton, John. 2007. "Batting, Habit and Memory: The Embodied Mind and the Nature of Skill." *Sport in Society* 10 (5): 763–786. doi:10.1080/17430430701442462.

Sutton, John, Doris McIlwain, Wayne Christensen, and Andrew Geeves. 2011. "Applying Intelligence to the Reflexes: Embodied Skills and Habits between Dreyfus and Descartes." *Journal of the British Society for Phenomenology* 42 (1): 78–103.

Toner, John, Barbara Gail Montero, and Aidan Moran. 2015. "Considering the Role of Cognitive Control in Expert Performance." *Phenomenology and the Cognitive Sciences* 14 (4): 1127–1144. doi:10.1007/s11097-014-9407-6.

Vallacher, Robin R., and Daniel M. Wegner. 1987. "What Do People Think They're Doing? Action Identification and Human Behavior." *Psychological Review* 94 (1): 3–15.

Wulf, Gabriele. 2007. *Attention and Motor Skill Learning*. Champaign, IL: Human Kinetics.

Zsambok, Caroline E. 1997. "Naturalistic Decision Making: Where Are We Now?" In *Naturalistic Decision Making*, edited by Caroline E Zsambok and Gary A. Klein, 3–16. Mahwah, NJ: Lawrence Erlbaum.

Zsambok, Caroline E., and Gary A. Klein. 1997. *Naturalistic Decision Making*. Mahwah, NJ: Lawrence Erlbaum.

7 Questioning the Breadth of the Attentional Focus Effect

Barbara Gail Montero, John Toner, and Aidan P. Moran

1 Introduction

According to the former Los Angeles Dodgers' pitcher Orel Hershiser, the key to playing at his best "is to forget about results and concentrate on execution" (Hershiser and Jenkins 1990, 21). One might interpret Hershiser's claim in various ways, but if what he means is that focusing on bodily positions and movements is conducive to optimal performance, then many coaches, athletes, and physical therapists would agree (Porter et al. 2010; Durham et al. 2009). A large body of experimental evidence, however, is commonly cited in support of a view called "the attentional focus effect," which is the hypothesis that focusing on the body (typically designated as an "internal" focus of attention) leads to suboptimal results relative to focusing on the consequences of bodily actions (commonly regarded as an "external" focus of attention) (see Wulf 2013 for a review). This effect is thought to apply to all skills at all levels of ability. As Reza Abdollahipour and colleagues (2015) put it, "It is now clear that the attentional focus effect is independent of the type of task … [and is] generaliz[able] across level of expertise, age, dis/ability, etc." (5–6). Or, in Gabriele Wulf's (2013) words, "[Fifteen years of research] demonstrate the broad generalizability of the attentional focus effect across tasks, populations, and performance measures" (95). However, in this chapter, after spending some time unfolding the nature and scope of the attentional focus effect, we look into the difficulty of eliminating confounds in experiments testing the effect and examine four situations in which an internal attentional focus appears to be preferable at times to an external one. These situations, we suggest, are worthy of further empirical investigation before we can accept that the attentional focus effect applies to *all* types of skills, *all* skill levels, and *all* measures of performance quality.

The sheer number of studies that claim to support the attentional focus effect is impressive (see details of such evidence in Wulf 2013). And we do not doubt that sometimes consequence-centered (external) foci lead to superior outcomes compared with body-centered (internal) foci. This is not merely because, for any given activity, it is likely that there is some consequence-centered focus that would generally lead to superior outcomes relative to some highly irrelevant body-centered focus (such as a focus on the right pinkie toe, or the left nostril). This is true, but trivial. Rather, we do not doubt the more significant claim that even with relevant body-centered foci, external foci often lead to superior results. What we question is the *universality* of the attentional focus effect, and by exploring the circumstances under which a body-centered attentional focus seems preferable to a consequence-centered one, we hope not only to sound a note of caution in this field but also to inspire further studies designed to explore the relative merits of different types of attentional foci for skill learning and skilled performance.

How does this relate to the topic of embodied cognition? In very general terms, the question of whether it is invariably preferable to adopt an external focus rather than an internal one is a question about which of two kinds of thinking—both of which are embodied, as they occur in concert with bodily action—skilled performers should adopt. In adopting either an external or an internal focus, athletes, as we see it, are thinking in and with the body; both types of foci facilitate thinking in action. All this will be implicit in the discussion that follows. However, in grappling with the difficulty of partitioning off a form of focus that is exclusively external, our discussion turns to a more explicit encounter with embodied cognition as we look into how adopting an enactive account of cognition (Maturana and Varela 1980; Varela, Thompson and Rosch 1991; O'Regan and Noë 2001; Thompson 2007; O'Regan 2011; Hutto and Myin 2012)—an account that posits that mental processes must be understood as interactions between the body and environment—highlights this difficulty.

2 The Distinction between External and Internal Foci of Attention

Wulf (2013), in summing up the support for the attentional focus effect, tells us that "empirical evidence has amassed for the benefits of adopting an external focus on the intended movement effect (e.g., on an implement) relative to an internal focus on body movements" (77). Above, we referred to the two kinds of foci at issue as being either "consequence-centered" or "body-centered." But this simple dichotomy may not fully capture the distinction as it is often employed. Wulf (2016) points out that the attentional focus effect has sometimes been misunderstood, and we suspect that some of this misunderstanding arises because the effect seems to take on different meanings in different contexts or, indeed, sometimes even in the same context, giving it a rather protean nature.[1]

Although most of the studies that directly test the attentional focusing hypothesis investigate the differential effects of certain kinds of cues (for example, whether the *instruction* to focus on pushing the water back results in a better outcome than the *instruction* to pull one's hands back), it seems that Wulf and others understand the hypothesis in terms of the differential effects of various attentional foci, or "what athletes direct their attention to" (Wulf 2016, 338). Accordingly, the results of the studies of the attentional focus effect are typically stated in terms of the kind of focus that is more beneficial: external or internal? (See Wulf 2013.) That much is clear. But how should we understand these two types of foci?

It is relatively straightforward to explain what counts as an internal focus of attention, since it typically involves targeting some isolated body part or parts such as hands, feet, knees, thighs, or fingers. "Bodily form" or physical configuration of the entire body (as opposed to isolated body parts) has occasionally been presented as an internal focus of attention (for example, Schücker et al. 2009; Perkins-Ceccato, Passmore, and Lee 2003). However, most studies on the attentional focus effect have sought to induce internal foci that are much more specific ("focus on your feet," Wulf, Höß, and Prinz 1998, or "focus on your fingers," Wulf and Dufek 2009, for example).

Identifying what counts as an external focus, however, is rather more challenging. Typically, it is defined as paying attention to something one's action affects: the movement of the golf club rather than the golfer's wrist movement, or, for a swimmer, the movement of the water rather than the movement of the swimmer's hands. The effect can be rather distant, such as in McKay and colleague's (2012) study of dart throwing wherein the bull's-eye counts as an object of external focus. Or it might be on something external but not necessarily affected by bodily movements at all, such as Zackry and colleague's (2005) study of basketball free-throwing, wherein focusing on the hoop counts as external.[2]

Also, a focus on qualities, such as smoothness—which, unless one believes in a world of Platonic forms, does not seem to be external to one's movement at all—is categorized as external, or at least the beneficial results of attention to such qualities are seen as supporting the attentional focus effect (see Neumann and Brown 2013). Similarly, the beneficial effects of focusing on more-metaphorically described qualities, such as "stretching like a star in all directions," are seen as counting in favor of the attentional focus effect. As Abdollahipour et al. (2015) put it, "[Since they do not direct] attention to body movements per se, … the external attentional focus created by those images is presumably responsible for their effectiveness" (1812). Thus, a rather motley collection of foci are counted as external. Indeed, although Stoate and Wulf (2011), do not identify "focusing on nothing" as external, when those results are summarized in Wulf (2013), data from subjects who reported that they focused on nothing are included, along with the data used to support the view that those with "more of an internal focus" had slower swim times than those with less of an internal focus (105).

A challenge to even posing the distinction between internal and external can be drawn from the theory of enactivism, according to which mind, body, and environment must all be understood reciprocally (Maturana and Varela 1980). For example, according to the enactivists Maturana and Varela (1980), mental processes are constituted by a coupling between agent and environment so that the one cannot be understood in isolation from the other. What this means is that the action of attending to the position of your wrists as you swing a golf club is, according to enactivism, in part constituted by the golf club itself; as such, so-called internal focus is necessarily also a focus on the environment. Similarly, because, on an enactivist account, our experience of our environment is in part constituted by our bodily interactions with the environment, so-called external focus encompasses the body as well. Thus, on an enactivist view it is impossible to identify a purely internal focus or a purely external focus. We remain neutral as to whether enactivism is a correct theory of the mind-body-world nexus in general; however, we shall return to specific examples of foci that are seen as external by defenders of the attentional focus effect yet seem to call for an enactivist interpretation.

Putting aside for now the question of enactivism, how shall we sum up the internal/external distinction? Since it is rare to loosen the definition of "internal" so as to include bodily form, let us reserve the phrase "internal focus" for a focus on body parts, such as hand, feet, knees, and so forth. (Besides, such a narrowing of the concept of internal can only make our goal of questioning the breadth of the attentional focus effect more challenging.) As for "external," since focusing on nothing is not explicitly identified as external, we shall say that an external focus is a focus on an effect of movement, or on an external object that is relevant to the movement, or on a quality or metaphorical description of movement. On this conception of the distinction between external and internal foci, focusing on the angle of one's wrist and focusing on one's wrist and hand taking the shape of a candy cane, for example, would both count as internal foci since they identify isolated bodily parts. In contrast, a focus on bending one's body like a candy cane would count as external, since it does not direct one's attention to an isolated body part.

3 The Scope of the Attentional Focus Effect

To what type of skills and what aspect of those skills is the attentional focus effect supposed to apply? Although the effect is thought to apply to all bodily skills (e.g., Wulf 2013; Abdollahipour et al. 2015), it is not clear whether all components of a task are thought to benefit from an external rather than an internal focus. Rather, Wulf (2016, 337) states that "adopting an external focus ... simply means the performer is focusing on the intended movement effect—while *preparing for the execution* of a ballistic skill (e.g., throwing or hitting a ball) or *during the execution* of a continuous skill (e.g., balancing, swimming, cross-country skilling)" (337, emphasis original). As such, the scope of the effect would seem limited to these two components of skill. However, the studies cited in support of the attentional focus effect not only, as we mentioned, sometimes investigate external foci other than movement effect, but also sometimes appear to test aspects of skill other than the preparatory phase of a ballistic skill or the ongoing action of a continuous skill. For example, in Abdollahipour and colleagues' (2015) study, gymnasts were asked to perform a 180-degree turning jump in the air and, while airborne, to focus on, for the external condition, which direction a tape marker on their chest was pointing after half the turn. For the internal condition, they were required to focus on which direction their hands were pointing after half the turn. Now, although it is not entirely trivial to identify precisely what ballistic skills are,[3] it would seem that turning midair is ballistic, if anything is. Thus, the attentional focus effect is sometimes seen as applying to more than merely the period of preparation for ballistic skills and continuous action (as turning midair presumably counts as neither preparation for a ballistic skill nor as a continuous skill). And we shall understand the attentional focusing hypothesis in this broad way as well. However, we also recognize that Wulf (2016) is perhaps most confident about the attentional focus effect as it applies to planning. As she says, "If movements are *not* planned in terms of the intended movement effect, but in terms of specific body movements, the outcome will always be less-than-optimal ... [and] learning/improving will be less-than-optimal" (338).

The attentional focus effect is also thought to apply to all levels of expertise and to be apparent in both training and performance. Accordingly, not only should the expert swimmer avoid focusing on any parts of her body, but the novice should not even be taught in terms that encourage focusing on body parts. This, as Wulf (2016) admits, might pose a challenge, yet she suggests that more-metaphorical instructions might solve this problem, trusting that coaches and instructors will be creative enough to divine good metaphors for the purpose. Proponents of the attentional focusing hypothesis, however, think that this extra effort on the part of coaches is worthwhile, since the benefits that external foci are thought to elicit include increased effectiveness (such as holding a balance longer, or hitting a target more accurately), increased efficiency (as measured, for example, by muscular activity, speed or endurance), increased learning speed, and even heightened artistry.

Given the various characterizations of the external-internal distinction as well as conflicting remarks about what part of a skill is under the scope of the attentional focus effect, it should not be surprising that, after evaluating the research literature on the relative benefits of external versus internal focus, one's head might begin to swim a bit (perhaps even to the degree that the question "What type of focus would identify a swimming head?" begins to swim through one's head). Nonetheless, the view we have arrived at is that the attentional focusing hypothesis asserts that, in preparation for a ballistic action or during a continuous action (as well as during other kinds of actions such as a jumping turn), focusing on a part of the body (internal) always produces suboptimal effects relative to focusing on any of the following: an effect of one's movement, a relevant external object, or a relevant quality or metaphorical description of movement (external). That said, because of the aforementioned protean nature of this hypothesis, we cannot be certain that our interpretation of it captures exactly what the researchers who support the hypothesis have in mind. Nonetheless, we shall use this conception of the attentional focus effect as our—to stay with the swimming metaphor—"diving-off" point as we proceed to indicate some reasons for why it might not be as well established as the results of the many years of research on this topic might lead one to believe.

4 The Difficulty of Distinguishing External from Internal Foci of Attention in Action

The attentional focus effect, as we have interpreted it, tells us that in preparation for a ballistic action or during continuous (and other types of) action, focusing on a part of the body (internal) always produces suboptimal effects relative to focusing on an effect of one's movement, a relevant external object, or a relevant quality or metaphorical description of movement (external). And this effect is postulated to hold for all skills at all levels. But do we have adequate support for such a strong claim? One reason to question whether we do is that it is not always clear that participants in studies in this field are adopting external foci, or at least exclusively external foci, when performing under so-called external foci conditions.

Consider Abdollahipour and colleagues' (2015) experiment on gymnasts in which the object of the external focus condition is a 2-by-5-centimeter piece of yellow tape attached to the participant's chest. This tape is considered "external" since it is not a part of the body and, inasmuch as it moves when the body moves, its movement is an effect of the relevant action. However, it is not entirely clear that the gymnasts, when focusing on tape on their chests, are not *also* focusing on their chests. For it seems that regardless of whether enactivism is true in general, regardless of whether it is impossible to partition the body from the environment, this particular case does invite a blurring of the distinction between the internal and external. To focus on the movements of a piece of tape on one's chest, in the enactivist account, is to have an experience of one's body affecting the movement of the tape. And it would seem at least difficult to exclude the possibility that external focus instructions elicit an amalgamated focus. As a matter of fact, athletes sometimes attach tape to parts of their bodies for, among other things, the purpose of helping them focus on those taped bodily parts (Williams et al. 2012).

In such a case, the focus on the tape is itself a focus on one's bodily movements and positions. To be sure, the tape in the experiment of Abdollahipour and colleagues might not be attached to the gymnast's skin, since "attached to the participant's chest" might simply be shorthand for "attached to the fabric on the participant's chest," and the tape may have been quite different from the type of tape typically used by athletes (Kinesio tape). Furthermore, there is some question as to the general effectiveness of such tape in facilitating proprioception (Halseth et al. 2004). Nonetheless, whether the tape was on the skin in the experiment of Abdollahipour and colleagues or on tight fabric that moved with the body, it seems possible that the attention to the marker and the attention to the body were inseparable; attention, in such a situation, might go right through to the skin and beyond.[4]

The potential inextricability of the external and internal is apparent in other studies as well. For example, in thinking about "pushing the water back" (Freudenheim et al. 2010), might one be thinking about pushing the water back *with one's hands* or *with one's arms and hands*? Experimental manipulation checks that require participants to report on what they were focusing on while executing the task could help weed out these (and other) possibilities. However, such checks are not always used; for example, although Freudenheim et al. (2010) asked participants whether they had followed instructions, they did not ask them to state their actual thoughts. Or consider Totsika and Wulf's (2003) study, in which, during the external focus condition, participants were told, while using a pedalo, to focus on pushing the board under their feet away.

Could they really focus on doing this without also focusing on the feet and legs that are doing the actual pushing? Of course, if what we are interested in is not so much *what type of focus* is conducive to optimal performance but rather *what instructions elicit the best outcome*, then the possibility that a cue to engage in an external focus may instead or in part elicit an internal focus is beside the point. If, for example, asking swimmers to focus on pushing the water back (whether or not this is strictly external) produces better results than asking them to focus on pushing their hands back (whether or not this is strictly internal), then swim coaches, in general, should frame their instructions in terms of moving the water back. However, as we shall argue, because of possible confounding factors in the experiments testing the attentional focus effect, it is not even clear that external cues are invariably preferable to internal ones.[5]

5 The Difficulty of Eliminating Possible Confounding Factors

In discussing the small number of experiments that have shown the beneficial effects of internal as compared with external foci, Wulf (2013) notes that "some claims of superiority of an internal relative to an external focus can be attributed to experimental manipulations that confounded the type of attentional focus with other variables" (91). And she goes on to present persuasive explanations of these various confounds. For example, she points out that if one set of instructions is more complicated than another or if one set of instructions encourages an additional focus while the other does not, this can skew the results.

Since Wulf made this claim, however, additional experimental data have emerged to support the relative superiority (or at least lack of inferiority) of an internal focus. Rienhoff et al. (2015), for example, found that for basketball players, an external focus on the ball led to a significant decrease in free-throw shooting performance and a significant reduction in "quiet-eye" duration, a prolonged final visual fixation on a target that is characteristic of expert athletes (Williams, Singer, and Frehlich 2002). And Querfurth et al. (2016) found no differences in dart-throwing performance with respect to attentional focus, while quiet-eye duration was found to be longest in the internal focus condition. It is likely one could identify possible confounds here as well, since eliminating such factors in experiments testing the attentional focus effect is challenging (Toner and Moran 2015; Carson, Collins, and Toner 2015; Peh, Chow, and Davids 2011). But our point is that confounding factors can creep in not only to the experiments that tell against that attentional focus effect; though less frequently noted, they can creep in to the experiments that claim to support it as well.

What types of confounds may have skewed the results in favor of the attentional focus effect? Ideally, one wants to set up experiments such that the internal and external foci are either both equally natural or equally unnatural for participants. Unfortunately, for many of the studies, it is not clear that this has been done adequately. Yet if the external target of focus is highly natural (in the sense that the athletes being tested

hands with the middle finger touching the thumb, while the other fingers are extend (as this approximates the desired position). Moreover, there may be some dancers who naturally hold their fingers in precisely the right way. However, if, as we suspect, not all dancers are able to attain the correct position automatically, attention to and conscious control over fingers would seem to be conducive to achieving the optimal aesthetic position for one's hands.

To further support our view that low-level focus can be beneficial to skill, we would like to also suggest that an internal focus can be in itself pleasurable and interesting and, as such, is conducive to longer practice sessions. The need to find one's activity enjoyable and interesting might also call for changing of the objects of one's attention over a lifetime of practice. As Masters and Maxwell (2008) point out, skilled individuals might resort to conscious control by tinkering with their technique because of boredom during practice. But although Masters and Maxwell see this as lamentable, we see it as a beneficial aspect of practice. The reason is that not only might the novelty motivate continued training but, in line with Anders Ericsson's theory of deliberate practice (Ericsson, Krampe, and Tesch-Römer 1993), according to which automaticity leads to aborted improvement, varying foci during a lifetime of practice by putting a wrench in the works may also jump-start an athlete, dancer, or other highly skilled individual's technical or artistic development.

6.4 Alleviating Anxiety

Fourth, an internal focus may alleviate anxiety. Excessive anxiety is capable of impeding skilled performance in sundry ways. And, arguably, one reason why it does so is because anxiety distracts one from one's optimal focus, turning one's mind to disturbing thoughts about such things as what others will think, about failure, about, indeed, how much the mind is racing and not focusing on what is important (Wine 1971). But what is the optimal focus? Although how to best cope with anxiety is very much an open question, there is some indication that athletes sometimes, or even frequently, cope with it by focusing on the details of their movements. For example, five out of the six golfers who choked in the study by Hill and colleagues (2010) claimed that self-focus *helped* prevent a more severe performance breakdown (228). Though we know of no studies of this, a similar process of directing attention to details of movement might prevent performance failure caused by anxiety in dance. For example, a ballet dancer who is nervous about whether a pirouette is going to be successful might block out detrimental distracting thoughts by focusing on the precise position of the heel of her foot positioned under her knee as she turns, or perhaps even on lifting the pelvic floor (a focus which is, presumably about as internal as it can get). There may be external foci that can do the trick as well. However, for some, a demanding internal focus might be just as, if not or more, beneficial in calming nerves.

To be sure, when intently focusing on the details of their movements, athletes and performing artists will likely need to resort to automatic control of myriad other aspects of their actions. So, although champions of the external focus effect advocate an external focus in part because it leads to greater automatic control, internal focus, we would like to suggest, may also lead to a greater degree of automatic control. And when anxiety is incapacitating, such automatic control may facilitate a better performance. This is not to say that performing automatically is, all other things being equal, the best way to attain excellence. We think it is not (Montero 2010, 2013, 2015, 2016; Toner, Montero and Moran (2015a, 2015b, 2016). However, in a situation where not everything else is equal, a situation where anxiety precludes high-level thought and threatens to thwart performance (because, for example, it leads to a loss of confidence), focusing on the details of movement can be a useful tool, since it can both help calm the flurry of anxious thoughts and, if this is not entirely successful, help one perform automatically so that the flurry need not get in the way.

Let us sum up our thoughts on when an internal focus may be preferable to an external one. We maintain that an internal focus is beneficial for activities whose success conditions are, at least in part, explicitly defined in terms of attaining a body-centered focus, such as the dance practice Gaga. We also suggest that internal attentional foci can promote conscious cognitive control, which may ultimately benefit performance, especially in the long run, and especially given that the long-term effects of adopting an internal focus during practice have not been tested. We additionally argue that an internal focus may be conducive to aesthetic awareness and enjoyment, both of which may facilitate optimal performance. And, finally, we suggest that an internal focus may alleviate anxiety. We think that before accepting the attentional focusing hypothesis in its full generality, these situations are worthy of further investigation.

7 Conclusion

Although a large body of experimental evidence is commonly cited in support of the attentional focus effect, we have argued, in this chapter, that there may be confounding factors in the experiments that purport to show the benefit of external over internal foci of attention, and because of such confounds, the results of these studies may depend, in some cases, more on whether the focus is natural or beneficial to performance (for reasons other than it being external) than on whether it is external or internal. In addition, because there are a number of reasons to think that an internal focus (and presumably the corresponding cues) may be useful, we questioned the universality of the attentional focus effect: Some activities have success conditions that are stated explicitly in terms of internal awareness; long-term improvement might sometimes depend on internal foci; an internal focus may be conducive to aesthetic awareness and enjoyment; and internal awareness might be called for to alleviate nerves or even to promote automaticity. For these reasons, we think that Wulf and her colleagues' claims that the attentional focus effect applies to all skills, all people, and all measures of performance is overstated. Thus, when Los Angeles Dodgers' pitcher Orel Hershiser tells us that the key to playing at his best "is to forget about results and concentrate on execution," he may be right.

Wulf (2016) criticizes Toner and Moran's (2015) proposal that bodily awareness plays a useful role in high-level athletic endeavors for, among other things, relying on case studies. However, case studies, since they are capable of providing in-depth analyses of individuals, have led to some major discoveries in psychology (e.g., see Rezlescu, Pitcher, and Duchaine's 2012 study of prosopagnosia or "face-blindness"). When it comes to investigating attentional focus in expert action, we see case studies and controlled experiment as standing in a mutually supportive relation. As mentioned, an especially challenging aspect of studying attentional focus is determining which particular focus to test. Presumably, one wants to test ecologically valid foci, that is, foci that athletes and performing artists normally employ. Case studies can help identify these. Looking at what coaches identify as beneficial targets of focus may be useful as well. Wulf, however, seems less than sanguine about the insights coaches might have into optimal attentional foci, for she seems to think that the reason coaches and physical therapists recommend internal foci is that, in the absence of familiarity with the literature on the relative merits of external versus internal foci, they adhered to "established or intuitive instructional methods" (2013, 98). But another explanation is that through trial and error they have hit on instructions that—in certain contexts—work.

Apart from being wary of Toner and Moran's (2015) use of case studies, Wulf (2016) is somewhat dismissive about their reliance on "philosophers' views" to bolster their claims (337). We believe, however, along with Thagard (2009) and others, that philosophers play an important role in the interdisciplinary enterprise that is cognitive science. And although it is beyond the scope of this chapter to defend that view, we can say this: we think that it is always worthwhile (whether one is a philosopher or not) to step back from the experimental findings and clarify the nature of the claims being made and question the degree to which the available data support the conclusions being drawn. Such clarifications and evaluations can only improve the quality of research probing the attentional focus effect.

Notes

1. One example of this, which we relegate to this footnote, as we are unsure how to interpret it, is that in close succession Wulf (2015) claims that "adopting an external focus does not mean that the performer is not aware of her or his body movements" (337), and that an external focus is "related to the *planning* of the movement, but *has nothing to do with the processing of intrinsic feedback or bodily awareness*" (337, latter italics ours). These two claims could be interpreted as contradictory: external focus both allows and excludes an internal focus (bodily awareness). However, when she says that adopting an external focus "has nothing to do with" bodily awareness, Wulf might very well mean that it has no implications for whether one is adopting an internal focus. As such, the two statements are no longer contradictory, however, one is left wondering how to distinguish an external focus from an internal one since being aware of bodily movements sounds very much like an internal focus. Perhaps her point is that that a conscious or central external focus can occur simultaneously with a nonconscious or peripheral internal focus and that it is merely the conscious or central internal focus that thwarts movement success. If so, our arguments are intended to question the universality of that claim as well.

2. To be sure, one's movement affects such things as basketball hoops and bulls-eye's indirectly via basketballs and darts respectively. Alternatively, someone with idealist inclinations might claim that since hoops and bulls-eyes are (at least in part) the way they are because we perceive them and since our eyes are in constant motion during vision (Engbert and Kliegl 2003), the bull's-eye and the hoop are a direct effect of one's movement. Furthermore, if one thinks that the collapse of the wave function in quantum mechanics requires observation and that observation is a form of movement, one might go so far as to say that in some sense the entire world is an effect of one's movement. But we assume that defenders of the attentional focus effect would not go that far. (Thanks to Alejandro Louro for suggesting these considerations.)

3. Roughly, one might say that they are skills that once started are not able to be stopped. However, when one recalls the time Tiger Woods was able to stop his swing midair at height of his backswing because he was distracted by the click of a camera, one might think that this definition is too exclusive. In any event, we shall take the meaning of ballistic skill to be clear enough from the examples Wulf provides ("throwing or hitting a ball").

4. What are we to say about the fact that the external focus cues here and in some other studies (Munzert, Maurer, and Reiser 2014; Rienhoff et al. 2015) produce better results than the control condition in which participants are cued to perform how they normally would. One possibility is that the researchers happened upon a useful external focus, which would not imply that there are no internal focus cues that would have helped performance more than normal. Moreover, studies with highly trained individuals do not always reveal the same pattern presumably because

such individuals normally perform their skills with the optimal focus (Wulf 2013). Of course, Stoate and Wulf (2011) did find that participants who claimed to employ external foci ("going fast," "getting to the other side" for example) swam faster than those who did not. And, whether this supports the view that an *external* focus to an internal (see note 3 above), it might seem to support the idea that internal foci lead to suboptimal performance relative to non-internal foci. However, before one makes this inference it would useful to know whether adopting the external focus was causally relevant to their faster performance (for it might have been that the faster swimmers did not need to think about the details of their technique) as well as whether focusing on going fast or on getting to the other side, for example, are foci that also target the body.

5. Regarding the difficulty of distinguishing external from internal foci, one might want to consider how sometimes a tool that one is highly familiar with apparently gets mapped onto one's bodily image (Obayashi et al. 2001). And thus, in a sense, focusing on the tool is focusing on the body. And, of course, with a prosthetic device, the mapping is even tighter.

6. For further discussion of this experiment see (Toner, Montero, and Moran 2016).

7. For experts, the distinction between familiar versus unfamiliar and productive versus counterproductive might often amount to the same thing since, presumably, the focus experts are familiar with is typically the one that is most productive. However, as most of the studies testing the attentional focus effect are not on experts, it is worth considering this distinction separately.

8. And likely, as the schematic of the jump shows the hands, not crossed but pointed towards one another on a horizontal line, it is was a horizontal bar. A "v" or an "x" shape might be better approximate the location of the hands during the turn, if the hands were crossed, as they were described. However, the marker is described as a single piece of tape (2 cm by 5 cm). Other orientations, such as a slanted marker, though possible, would seem unlikely choices.

References

Abdollahipour, Reza, Gabriele Wulf, Rudolf Psotta, and Miriam Palomo Nieto. 2015. "Performance of Gymnastics Skills Benefits from an External Focus of Attention." *Journal of Sports Sciences* 33 (17): 1807–1813.

An, J., G. Wulf, and S. Kim. 2013. "Increased Carry Distance and X-Factor Stretch in Golf through an External Focus of Attention." *Journal of Motor Learning and Development* 1:2–11.

Carson, H. J., D. Collins, and J. Toner. 2015. Letter to the editor concerning the article, "Performance of Gymnastics Skill Benefits from an External Focus of Attention," by Abdollahipour, Wulf, Psotta, and Nieto (2015). *Journal of Sports Sciences*. Advance online publication. doi:10.1080/02640414.2015.1098782.

Chiviacowsky, S., G. Wulf, and L. T. G. Avila. 2013. "An External Focus of Attention Enhances Motor Learning in Children with Intellectual Disabilities." *Journal of Intellectual Disability Research* 57 (7): 627–634. doi:10.1111/j.1365-2788.2012.01569.x.

Durham, K., P. M. Van Vliet, F. Badger, and C. Sackley. 2009. "Use of Information Feedback and Attentional Focus of Feedback in Treating the Person with a Hemiplegic Arm." *Physiotherapy Research International* 14:77–90. doi:10.1002/pri.431.

Engbert, Ralf, and Reinhold Kliegl. 2003. "Microsaccades Uncover the Orientation of Covert Attention." *Vision Research* 43 (9): 1035–1045.

Ericsson, K. Anders, Ralf T. Krampe, and Clemens Tesch-Römer. 1993. "The Role of Deliberate Practice in the Acquisition of Expert Performance." *Psychological Review* 100 (3): 363–406.

Frawley, David. 2008. *Yoga: The Greater Tradition*. San Rafael, CA: Mandala Publishing.

Freudenheim, A. M., G. Wulf., F. Madureira, S. C. Pasetto, U. C. Corrêa, S. C. P. Corrêa, B. U. Ried. 2010. An External Focus of Attention Results in Greater Swimming Speed. *International Journal of Sport Science and Coaching* 5:533–542

Galili, Deborah Friedes. 2015. "Gaga: Moving beyond Technique with Ohad Naharin in the Twenty-First Century." *Dance Chronicle* 38 (3): 360–392.

Granados, C. 2010. "Effects of Observation, Dialogue, and Attentional Focus in Dyadic Training Protocol." Unpublished master's thesis, University of Nevada, Las Vegas.

Halseth, Travis, John W. McChesney, Mark DeBeliso, Ross Vaughn, and Jeff Lien. 2004. "The Effects of Kinesio Taping on Proprioception at the Ankle." *Journal of Sports Science and Medicine* 3 (1): 1–7.

Hershiser, Orel, and Jerry B. Jenkins. 1990. *Out of the Blue*. New York: Jove Books.

Hill, Denise, S. Hanton, N. Matthews, and S. Fleming. 2010. "A Qualitative Exploration of Choking in Elite Golf." *Journal of Clinical Sport Psychology* 4:221–240.

Hutto, Daniel D., and Erik Myin. 2012. *Radicalizing Enactivism: Basic Minds without Content*. Cambridge, MA: MIT Press.

Katan-Schmid, Einav. 2016. *Embodied Philosophy in Dance: Gaga and Ohad Naharin's Movement Research*. New York: Springer.

Masters, R. S. W., and J. Maxwell. 2008. "The Theory of Reinvestment." *International Journal of Sport and Exercise Psychology* 1:160–183.

Maturana, H. R., and F. J. Varela. 1980. *Autopoiesis: The Organization of the Living Autopoiesis and Cognition; The Realization of the Living*. Dordrecht, Holland: Kluwer Academic.

Maurer, Heiko, and Jörn Munzert. 2013. "Influence of Attentional Focus on Skilled Motor Performance: Performance Decrement under Unfamiliar Focus Conditions." *Human Movement Science* 32 (4): 730–740.

McKay, Brad, and Gabriele Wulf. 2012. "A Distal External Focus Enhances Novice Dart Throwing Performance." *International Journal of Sport and Exercise Psychology* 10 (2): 149–156.

Montero, B. 2010. "Does Bodily Awareness Interfere with Highly Skilled Movement?" *Inquiry* 53:105–122.

Montero, B. G. 2013. "A Dancer Reflects: Deliberation in Action," in *Mind, Reason and Being-in-the-World: The McDowell-Dreyfus Debate*, edited by J. Schear, 303–319. London: Routledge.

Montero, Barbara G. 2015. "Thinking in the Zone: Reflection and Attention in Expert Action." *Southern Journal of Philosophy* 53 (S1): 126–140.

Montero, Barbara G. 2016. *Thought in Action: Expertise and the Conscious Mind.* Oxford: Oxford University Press.

Montero, Barbara G. 2018. "Aesthetics from an Embodied Point of View." In *The Oxford Handbook of Cognition: Embodied, Embedded, Enactive and Extended*, edited by A. Newen, L. de Bruin, and S. Gallagher.

Munzert, Jörn, Heiko Maurer, and Mathias Reiser. 2014. "Verbal-Motor Attention-Focusing Instructions Influence Kinematics and Performance on a Golf-Putting Task." *Journal of Motor Behavior* 46 (5): 309–318.

Neumann, D. L., and J. Brown. 2013. "The Effect of Attentional Focus Strategy and Motor Performance during a Sit-Up Exercise." *Journal of Psychophysiology*.

Obayashi, S., T. Suhara, K. Kawabe, T. Okauchi, J. Maeda, Y. Akine, H. Onoe, and A. Iriki. 2001. "Functional Brain Mapping of Monkey Tool Use." *NeuroImage* 14 (4): 853–861.

O'Regan, J. Kevin. 2011. *Why Red Doesn't Sound Like a Bell: Understanding the Feel of Consciousness.* Oxford: Oxford University Press.

O'Regan, J. Kevin, and Alva Noë. 2001. "A Sensorimotor Account of Vision and Visual Consciousness." *Behavioral and Brain Sciences* 24 (5): 939–973; discussion 973–1031.

Oudejans, Raoul R. D., Wilma Kuijpers, Chris C. Kooijman, and Frank C. Bakker. 2011. "Thoughts and Attention of Athletes under Pressure: Skill-Focus or Performance Worries?" *Anxiety, Stress, and Coping* 24 (1): 59–73.

Peh, Shawn Yi-Ching, Jia Yi Chow, and Keith Davids. 2011. "Focus of Attention and Its Impact on Movement Behaviour." *Journal of Science and Medicine in Sport / Sports Medicine Australia* 14 (1): 70–78.

Perkins-Ceccato, N., S. R. Passmore, and T. D. Lee. 2003. Effects of Focus of Attention Depend on Golfers' Skill. *Journal of Sport Sciences* 21:593–600.

Porter, J. M., R. P. Nolan, E. J. Ostrowski, and G. Wulf. 2010. "Directing Attention Externally Enhances Agility Performance: A Qualitative and Quantitative Analysis of the Efficacy of Using Verbal Instructions to Focus Attention." *Frontiers in Psychology* 1. doi:10.3389/fpsyg.2010.00216.

Querfurth, Sydney, Linda Schücker, Marc H. E. de Lussanet, and Karen Zentgraf. 2016. "An Internal Focus Leads to Longer Quiet Eye Durations in Novice Dart Players." *Frontiers in Psychology* 7 (May): 633.

Ravn, Susanne, and Mette Krogh Christensen. 2014. "Listening to the Body? How Phenomenological Insights Can Be Used to Explore a Golfer's Experience of the Physicality of Her Body." *Qualitative Research in Sport, Exercise and Health* 6 (4): 462–477.

Rezlescu, Constantin, David Pitcher, and Brad Duchaine. 2012. "Acquired Prosopagnosia with Spared Within-Class Object Recognition but Impaired Recognition of Degraded Basic-Level Objects." *Cognitive Neuropsychology* 29 (4): 325–347.

Rienhoff, R., L. Fischer, B. Strauss, J. Baker, and J. Schorer. 2015. "Focus of Attention Influences Quiet-Eye Behavior: An Exploratory Investigation of Different Skill Levels in Female Basketball Players." *Sport, Exercise, and Performance Psychology* 4 (1): 62.

Schucker, L., N. Hagemann, B. Strauss, and K. Völker. 2009. "The Effect of Attentional Focus on Running Economy." *Journal of Sport Sciences* 12:1242–1248.

Stoate, I., and G. Wulf. 2011. "Does the Attentional Focus Adopted by Swimmers Affect Their Performance?" *International Journal of Sports Science and Coaching* 6:99–108.

Thagard, Paul. 2009. "Why Cognitive Science Needs Philosophy and Vice Versa." *Topics in Cognitive Science* 1 (2): 237–254.

Thompson, Evan. 2007. *Mind in Life: Biology, Phenomenology, and the Sciences of Mind*. Cambridge, MA: Harvard University Press.

Toner, J., and A. Moran. 2015. "Enhancing Performance Proficiency at the Expert Level: Considering the Role of Somaesthetic Awareness." *Psychology of Sport and Exercise* 16:110–117.

Toner, John, Barbara Gail Montero, and Aidan Moran. 2015a. "Considering the Role of Cognitive Control in Expert Performance." *Phenomenology and the Cognitive Sciences* 14 (4): 1127–1144.

Toner, John, Barbara Gail Montero, and Aidan Moran. 2015b. "The Perils of Automaticity." *Review of General Psychology: Journal of Division 1, of the American Psychological Association* 19 (4): 431–442.

Toner, John, Barbara Gail Montero, and Aidan Moran. 2016. "Reflective and Prereflective Bodily Awareness in Skilled Action." *Psychology of Consciousness: Theory, Research, and Practice* 3 (4): 303–315.

Toner, John, and Aidan Moran. 2016. "On the Importance of Critical Thinking: A Response to Wulf's (2015) Commentary." *Psychology of Sport and Exercise* 22 (January): 339–340.

Totsika, V., and G. Wulf. 2003. The Influence of External and Internal Foci of Attention on Transfer to Novel Situations and Skills. *Research Quarterly Exercise and Sport* 74:220–225.

Varela, Francisco J., Evan Thompson, and Eleanor Rosch. 1991. *The Embodied Mind: Cognitive Science and Human Experience*. Cambridge, MA: MIT Press.

Williams, A. M., R. A. Singer, and S. Frehlich. 2002. "Quiet Eye Duration, Expertise, and Task Complexity in a Near and Far Aiming Task." *Journal of Motor Behavior* 34:197–207.

Williams, Sean, Chris Whatman, Patria A. Hume, and Kelly Sheerin. 2012. "Kinesio Taping in Treatment and Prevention of Sports Injuries: A Meta-Analysis of the Evidence for Its Effectiveness." *Sports Medicine* 42 (2): 153–164.

Wine, Jeri. 1971. "Test Anxiety and Direction of Attention." *Psychological Bulletin* 76 (2): 92–104.

Wulf, G., M. Höß, and W. Prinz. 1998. "Instructions for Motor Learning: Differential Effects of Internal Versus External Focus of Attention." *Journal of Motor Behavior* 30 (2): 169–179.

Wulf, Gabriele. 2013. "Attentional Focus and Motor Learning: A Review of 15 Years." *International Review of Sport and Exercise Psychology* 6 (1): 77–104.

Wulf, Gabriele. 2016. "Why Did Tiger Woods Shoot 82? A Commentary On." *Psychology of Sport and Exercise* 22:337–338.

Wulf, Gabriele. 2008. "Attentional Focus Effects in Balance Acrobats." *Research Quarterly for Exercise and Sport* 79 (3): 319–325.

Wulf, Gabriele, and J. S. Dufek. 2009. "Increased Jump Height with an External Focus due to Enhanced Lower Extremity Joint Kinetics." *Journal of Motor Behavior* 41 (5): 401–409. doi:10.1080/00222890903228421.

Wulf, Gabriele, Matthias Weigelt, Damian Poulter, and Nancy McNevin. 2003. "Attentional Focus on Suprapostural Tasks Affects Balance Learning." *Quarterly Journal of Experimental Psychology A: Human Experimental Psychology* 56 (7): 1191–1211.

Zachry, T., G. Wulf, J. Mercer, and N. Bezodis. 2005. "Increased Movement Accuracy and Reduced EMG Activity as the Result of Adopting an External Focus of Attention." *Brain Research Bulletin* 67:304–309.

Zarghami, M., E. Saemi, and I. Fathi. 2012. "External Focus of Attention Enhances Discus Throwing Performance." *Kinesiology*. Citeseer. http://citeseerx.ist.psu.edu/viewdoc/download?doi=10.1.1.899.2473&rep=rep1&type=pdf.

8 Knowledge, Consciousness, and Sporting Skills

Jens E. Birch, Vegard Fusche Moe, and Gunnar Breivik

1 Introduction

Why does it seem to be popular opinion that sport is not a cognitive activity?[1] A dogmatic answer must be that sport is something we do with our arms or legs, while cognition is something that goes on in our brains. Nowadays we should all know that mechanisms involved in learning and performing basketball, piano, writing, arithmetic, or controlling fear all go on in the brain. The idea that playing basketball is not something cognitive still seems to persist. In this chapter, we inquire into two beliefs that underlie the view that sporting skills are not cognitive. The first is the belief that sporting skills are not knowledge. The other is that sporting skills go on (or should go on) without consciousness.

The aim of this chapter is to undermine both these beliefs, which usually appear in standard cognitive science and information-processing theories. Knowledge and consciousness must be said to be hallmarks of cognition, and activities without apparent signs of them are easily dismissed as not cognitive. We argue that the view of sporting skill as something lacking knowledge and consciousness is flawed. We claim that skilled athletes have knowledge, and that they are indeed conscious while performing. Hence, they are cognitive persons. If there are sound reasons to consider skillful athletes knowledgeable, conscious, and cognitive, even if we cannot find or describe algorithmic processes and/or representations in these states, then embodied cognition has something to offer sport psychology as a research program.

2 The Track and Field Ahead

First we look at the philosophical ideas behind the view that skills are not, or do not contain, knowledge. We take a brief look at memory research, before we describe different types of sports along two continuums of opposition and participation. Different types of sports suggest different or *several* types of skills. Different skills also suggest different degrees of automation according to the degree of closed-ended or open-ended sports.[2]

We, second, argue that the type of sport, skills, and situation involves different states of knowledge, consciousness, and, hence, cognition. We apply David Chalmers's (1996) concepts of *phenomenal consciousness* and *psychological consciousness* to sporting skills, and argue that psychological and phenomenal consciousness is always present during athletic performance.

Third, we draw on the neuroscientific discovery of mirror neurons. The mirror neuron theory of action understanding (Rizzolatti and Sinigaglia 2008) implies there can be intentional, goal-directed, and cognitive behavior even without reportable access to psychological states of desires and beliefs.[3]

Fourth, we provide a phenomenological description of motor intentionality. Our description, if plausible, may complement the mirror neuron theory of action understanding. Here, we also emphasize certain characteristics of embodied cognition. Before summing up, we finish with some thoughts on phenomenology and knowledge, and suggest sport psychology and the research program of embodied cognition should use phenomenology as a methodological tool.

3 Sport, Knowledge, and Memory

Philosophical epistemology inquires into what knowledge is and what conditions are needed to have knowledge proper. According to the standard analysis, justified, true belief is necessary and sufficient for knowledge (see, e.g., Dancy 1985). During the last forty years, debates in the philosophy of sport have questioned what kind of knowledge is involved in sport. Discussions have usually departed from the viewpoint that sport is a skill, and then analyzed what kind of knowledge a skill is.[4] Following Gilbert Ryle's (1949) distinction between "knowing that" and "knowing how," skills have been identified with knowing how. *Knowing that* is so-called propositional knowledge: a relation between the content of a proposition and the state of the world. *Knowing how* is a matter of knowing how *to do* something. According to what Ryle called intellectualism, only propositions can be true and justified and hence only "knowing that" is knowledge. A problem arises: if skills are knowing how and only propositional knowledge is knowledge proper, then knowing how/skills are not knowledge proper. These fundamental epistemological issues have great bearings on standard cognitive science, sport psychology, and on the central themes of embodied cognition: if something is not considered (or does not contain) knowledge, it can hardly be an interesting target for research programs dealing with cognition. Like Stanley and Krakauer (2013), we argue that skills are not solely the execution of (motor) movements, but knowledge in itself. Stanley and Krakauer claim that motor skills depend on propositional knowledge. It may be argued that they follow the picture Churchland (1989, 68–69) paints of standard cognitive science's skill characterization: there are two representations in the brain, one motor and one discursive. The latter is knowledge, it is a description (knowing that) of skillful movements. The other is the ability and acuity of following the trajectory outlined in the discursive representation.[5] If one agrees with Stanley and Krakauer that skills contain knowledge, but only propositional knowledge, then standard cognitive science seems to have all the tools for analyzing skill. If one does not, then one must claim there exists knowledge outside the domain of the propositional. That is our path. We claim that the program of embodied cognition can present either different or better perspectives on matters regarding sporting skills. We start with what lies at the heart of standard cognitive science's skill characterization: long-term memory.

4 Learning, Memory, and Knowledge

The traditional way of describing long-term memory is to make a distinction between declarative (explicit) and nondeclarative (implicit) long-term memory, both being independent of each other (see, e.g., Gazzaniga, Ivry, and Mangun 2014, ch. 9). Declarative memory is divided into semantic memory (the capital of France is Paris) and episodic memory (I visited the Eiffel Tower in 1987). Both semantic and episodic long-term memory are instances of declaring something linguistically. Nondeclarative long-term memory is not linguistic in this sense. If we have learned to hit a free throw, we do not have to declare linguistically something before or parallel to such an action. Skills (and learning them) are therefore considered instances of procedural long-term memory, a subdivision of nondeclarative memory, just like a learned contingent reflex movement in a sea slug.[6]

According to the analysis of skill in memory research, skills are just like reflexes: they are *nonconscious* since they are seemingly not guided by linguistic thought prior or parallel to the (motor) action, and they are *automatic* since the (motor) actions are produced instantly to some external stimuli. Playing tennis, for example, is a nonconscious automated skill, accordingly (see, e.g., Kandel's 2006 description of Andre Agassi's ground strokes, 279). Kandel (132–133) identifies implicit memory with knowing how, and declarative memory with knowing that. Summing up: categorizing sporting skills as procedural long-term memory leads to the idea that skills are nondeclarative and not knowledge-based, automatic, and nonconscious. We find this to be a too-simple and un-nuanced view of sporting skills.[7] We undermine this view by asking, what do sporting skills consist of? To answer such a question, we must at least look at different types of sport.

5 Types of Sport, Types of Skills

In the philosophy of sport, considerable effort has been made to describe what we mean by "sport."[8] Suggestions for sufficient and/or necessary conditions have been the presence of goals, means, rules, competition, and, last but not least, some kind of motor action. The kind of game sport seems to be must not be one of mere chance; sport must be *trainable*. So much so, that a lot of effort and time would or should increase motor action performance so it becomes a *skill*. If we agree that sport comes in numerous varieties, then it would also seem that sporting skill is not a skill at all, but a vast range of sporting *skills*. Yet, we are often inclined to talk about sporting skill as essentially one same thing.[9] Such a view—we may call it folk psychology—might also make us talk about *the* skill of the sport, as if there is one basketball skill underlying all instances of playing basketball. We try to show that sports and sporting skills come in so many nuances that we must also put forward a revised view of automation, the role of consciousness, and the cognitive status of sport. We present a way of classifying sports developed by Breivik (1998), which has implications for our discussion.

Breivik's classificatory model builds on a phenomenological description of how humans interact with the environment in existentially different ways. The single

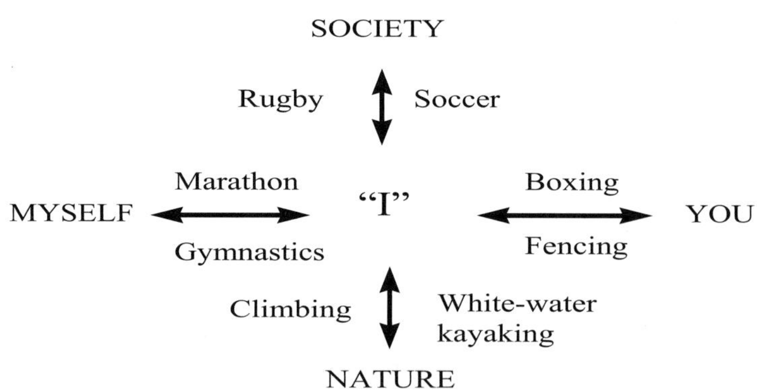

Figure 8.1
The existential dimensions and examples of sports.
Source: Breivik (1998).

existential subject stands in four ontological dimensions. As a human being, I have a fundamental relation to *myself*. This relation is different from the relation I have to the person I directly interact with in an I-*You* situation. The way I interact with other people in groups or a *society* is existentially different from the single You, or the reflective Myself. I may interact in various ways with *nature*. Sports reflect these various interactions in the ontologically different dimensions. What does this mean?

In climbing or white-water kayaking, the interaction with nature's elements is what it's all about. One has to *know* the ontological logic, the mode of being in certain natural elements, to be able to play and move on vertical walls or wild rivers. In sports like rugby or football, it is an ability to take the perspective of the other (teammates and the other team) to understand, foresee, and contribute to human interaction. In the I-You interaction as we experience it in boxing and tennis, the unique experience is of a You that is there face-to-face, and with whom I interact directly. In marathon and gymnastics, I am performing with and through the body certain possible movements that express the I-Myself and the body's unique capacities. This is the logic of the different types of sport as they are in their fundamental nature, according to their constitutive rules. Secondarily all these sports can be organized as competitions, whether parallel (running), serial (gymnastics), or interactive (football). In competitions, the goal is to beat opponents, and in this sense, all sports are social events. The four dimensions represent ideal structures. We can now make up four major types of sports, with rather clear-cut examples at opposite ends of the vertical and horizontal axis:

1. sports that interact with *nature* and its elements alone: noncompetitive parachuting
2. *team sports* with no nature: football
3. *one-on-one sports*, I-You: single tennis
4. *individual sports*, I: single diving

We now have the more difficult task of placing not-so-clear-cut examples. Take cycling: at the velodrome, cycling may be individual, one-on-one, and a team sport without nature. Tour de France is an individual team sport, and interacts with nature. Trial and MTB cycling are not team sports, but the interaction with nature is much more defining. This categorization, which is not exhaustive, puts the finger on at least one important aspect of skill: the type of skill (or types of skills) is widespread, varies, and changes. Trial cycling must certainly involve other skills than would winning Tour de France or one-on-one velodrome cycling.

Let us add one further component of sport. Along a continuum it is customary to classify sports as open-ended or closed-ended (Knapp 1963). Open-ended sports do not have fixed patterns, while closed-ended sports do. It's typical of closed-ended sports to repeat exact movement patterns. Competitive diving is illustrative: you try to move in a defined way, and even the judges know beforehand what you are going to do. Team sports vary from closed-ended sports like troop gymnastics to very open-ended sports like football (soccer) and ice hockey. In tennis, the opposition cannot directly interfere with your movements, so it is classified as a half open-ended sport. In running, like cycling, it depends. A marathon is different from sprinting the 100-meter dash, since what the competitors do has significant causal effects on strategy. One may also have to adjust to terrain and weather conditions. Even running consists of a wide variety of types, situations, and perhaps skills.

It is not the goal of this chapter to come up with clear categorizations and answers for what kind of sport each sport is. The goal is to make us better equipped to handle questions on the role of consciousness and knowledge in sporting skills. Hopefully, the above discussion makes it clearer that the role of automation and consciousness differs in these different types of sport, and in different situations. These considerations are related to the cognitive status of sporting skills. Let us elaborate on these matters, then.

6 Automation in Sport

That something is automatic is to say that it happens by itself, like triggering an alarm.[10] Automation is defined by an exact response to a specific stimulus, or standard solutions to standard situations. This is automation in the *strong* sense: responses that could not have been otherwise—responses that are programmed, genetically (a motor reflex) or *possibly* by contingent learning (withdrawal from a hot plate). These types of automatic movements must be said to be nonconscious. Are sporting skills like this? Should the purpose of training be to become an automaton?[11]

Think about a great goalie. Commentators often exclaim, "That save was a reflex movement!" This is obviously not the case, since there are no muscular reflexes for saving a ball or puck. What we *should* say is that the goalie acted so fast that it *seemed* like a reflex movement, but was in fact a case of short reaction time (and a number of other things, like action understanding and motor intentionality). Perhaps we should also say that the goalie acted just *like* it was automatic, but actually it was not, since it was not an exact response to a specific stimulus. Such a save is automatic in the *weak* sense. Contrast these descriptions of an open-ended sport with a diver doing a triple somersault. In this case, the diver *wants* the action to be automated, although in the strong sense it is not. If indeed it was, the diver could perform identical jumps every time. Competitions would be dull. What we are closing in on is that closed-ended sports have a greater degree of automation, or a *different* degree of automation. In these sports, the purpose of training is to increase the ability to do some complex movement, and then be able to repeat it as close as possible to the highest standard of evaluation. It is the essence of some of the skills involved in such sports.

Isn't that essential also in (half) open-ended sports? Well, yes and no. Take tennis. We have classified tennis as a one-on-one (I-You) sport which is half open-ended. A tennis player that actually wanted to do everything automatically would be like the tennis ball machine: hitting hard and long, but very predictable. In addition, automatic hits would work only for a narrow range of counter shots. The tennis serve is the most closed-ended situation, except that it must vary depending on wind, opposition, surface, and variation in itself if not to become too predictable. Choice and decision making are essential to some skills involved in tennis. So is action *understanding*, which we will return to later. Could tennis players actually be conscious and cognitive?[12] To answer this we need to inquire into consciousness.

7 Sporting Skills and Consciousness

As we have seen, motor skills are usually categorized as instances of nondeclarative procedural long-term memory in cognitive science. In the tradition of motor control learning, nondeclarative procedural skills and automation often go hand in hand (see, e.g., Schmidt and Lee 2011): behavior might start from declarative rule following, but gradually and eventually becomes procedural, nondeclarative, and automated. This easily leads to the idea that consciousness does not play a part in skillful performance (see, e.g., Dreyfus and Dreyfus 1986) and that sporting skills are not cognitive in their essence (or at all). Athletes are more like mindless zombies than cognitive persons, accordingly.[13] Philosopher David Armstrong (1981) has a famous example of the long-distance driver: driving for a long time, not thinking, everything going on autopilot. Armstrong calls this driving without consciousness. Driving on cruise control may *seem* automatic and nonconscious, but the driver is monitoring and (one hopes) prepared to act if a deer leaps out from the dark. Several (open-ended) sports and skills are more similar to driving in chaotic Bangkok than in the desert.

In neuroscientific terms, nonconscious means that the neural networks involved in (motor) actions do not involve neural networks or parts of the brain that are defined as a neural correlate of consciousness (NCC).[14] Candidates for NCC range from global distribution in the brain (Edelman and Tononi 2000b; Baars 1997), to minimum requirements in neurotransmitter uptake or release (LeDoux 2003; Koch 2004).[15] Either way, consciousness is described as being *aware of* (having access to) *the content* of consciousness.

There is a difference in the content of consciousness between "shoot a three-pointer just like that," seemingly without doing some thinking, and pre-reflexively declaring, "I must bend my knees, aim at the backboard, and roll the ball through my fingers." In the latter case, neuroscientific and cognitive accounts are inclined to say that the shot is guided by *conscious thought*, while the former is not.

Such interpretation states that in the heat of the moment, shooting the ball is not a conscious action, and perhaps not cognitive either. We need to *think* this through. Do we accept a theory wherein the novice who must pre-reflexively go through every step of some basketball movement is *more* conscious and cognitive than Michael Jordan? According to Edelman's (1992) *theory of neuronal group selection* (TNGS), the aim of training is to select, prune, and myelinate neural networks causing actions so they are as cost-efficient as possible. This means that the fewer neurons involved in performing action *Y*, the better. The evolutionary benefit is clear. The less energy spent to perform *Y*, the more energy left to do other things. Efficient neural pathways typifies skillful experts: in standard situations they have less brain-area and neural activation than novices (Milton et al. 2007; Ross et al. 2003).

In novel situations, brain activation is widely distributed (Edelman and Tononi 2000b, 142). To be able to solve novel situations (which typify half and open-ended sports), one must use minimum neural activity on standard tasks. We might say that a side effect of gaining cost-efficient neural networks is that pre-reflexive/parallel declarative thought is lost on the way. If we claim that we also lose consciousness and cognition, then we are claiming that we are only conscious and cognitive when we are not skillful. Should we rather claim that consciousness (and hence cognition) works in *different* or even several ways for the skilled and the novice?

So far we have described *conscious* as a reflective thought where the content of consciousness can be declared.[16] If actions are not guided by pre-reflexive or parallel declarative thoughts (or an athlete cannot report how she did that move), then motor actions are easily deemed nonconscious. To consider if this is a sound idea, we must go to the philosophy of mind and present a short view of what is called *psychological* and *phenomenal* consciousness (Chalmers 1996). In this now-standard way of classifying consciousness, psychological consciousness is a mental state that plays a causal/functional role in the production of behavior. Psychological consciousness is characterized by what it *does*; typical examples are awakeness, introspection, reportability, self-consciousness, attention, voluntary control, awareness, and knowledge (we return to knowledge in part 10). Phenomenal consciousness is characterized by how it *feels*, and in the tradition of Thomas Nagel (1974) described as "what is it like." Chalmers uses phenomenal consciousness to distinguish humans from zombies/robots because they might show all varieties of the causal/functional roles of psychological consciousness. Phenomenal consciousness is *the* sufficient and necessary criteria of consciousness: if there is something it is like to be that creature for that creature, it has consciousness. The cognitive sciences might be said to be mostly interested in aspects of psychological consciousness (what consciousness does) described above. We first look at aspects of psychological consciousness: are they present in skillful sport performance? We then turn to phenomenal consciousness.

Awakeness is often held to be the demarcation of consciousness, at least outside philosophy (see, e.g., Edelman and Tononi 2000a, 3). We may say that awakeness seems to be a necessary state of consciousness for *other* states of psychological consciousness. That athletes are awake while performing is unquestionable.

Athletes also *introspect* while performing: they use the process of introspection to become aware of the content of conscious states.[17] Athletes monitor the angles of joints, that breathing is relaxed, and so on. Athletes use these kinds of cues to check themselves constantly, whether it's alpine skiing or 200-meter running. Michael Johnson was asked whether he thinks during a race. He answered, "You are making a lot of decisions during the race based on what just happened—whether it happened right or happened wrong—you make a lot of adjustments and decisions—you need to make adjustments you know—and so on. It looks like the gun goes off and we just run is what happens, but internally in order to execute that race right, you know, there are a lot of things going on."[18] Monitoring, or proprioception, enables one to stop a golf swing, abort a serve, or adjust to terrain. Monitoring may neuronally be connected to Damasio's (1994) somatic marker hypothesis. Damasio claims that the brain constantly maps the body's states as influenced by internal and external causes. If a creature has a feeling of these changes and can act accordingly, it has consciousness. The brain's mapping of the body is automatic and nonconscious; we cannot choose to stop an evolutionary trait securing homeostasis and survival. But skillful actions performed as a result of these mappings are not automatic or nonconscious.

Athletes may and may not use *reportability* as a state of psychological consciousness. We may report the content of our states after performance, but trying to do so while performing often chokes the performance.[19] Reportability is central in all aspects of declarative—but not procedural—long-term memory. It is lack of reportability that often leads to the idea that athletes are nonconscious and noncognitive: "I just did it, but I don't know how."[20] What they "don't know" seems to be certain processes that accompany the performance, because they certainly *know how* to do (something) when they repeat actions, and/or act efficiently from internal and external causes.

Self-consciousness is usually taken to mean awareness of our existence distinct from others. Even though athletes may connect with objects and others to such a degree that they seem totally intertwined, it might be argued that self-consciousness is central to the skill of extending oneself.

Attention works differently in different sports. In closed-ended sport, attention may be narrow, on small parts, like the friction of one's grip. In open-ended (team) sports, it surely is beneficial for attention to work wide, so one does not miss the gorilla of attentional blindness (Simons and Chabris 1999). No matter how attention is described (focused, selective, spotlight, integrated, divided, alternating, etc.), it would be ridiculous to claim that attention is not a main feature of sporting skills.[21]

It must also be reasonable to say that athletes have *voluntary control*. Indeed, the more skilled an athlete is, the more voluntary control he or she has. Here again, it must be considered wrong to claim that athletes are not psychologically conscious of motor control even if they do not reflectively think/declare before or during actions. Andre Agassi's backhands are certainly not random or lucky (although that might occur); they are the product of voluntary control.

We have now claimed that skillful athletes show all signs of psychological consciousness. We could have ended here, but we finish this section with a discussion of phenomenal consciousness. Phenomenal consciousness has been treated as the key feature of consciousness in the philosophy of mind to distinguish humans (and hence athletes) from (automated and nonconscious) robots/zombies that also may show all the signs of psychological consciousness. We believe that research on phenomenal consciousness is where the program of embodied cognition has something to bring to the table.

Phenomenal consciousness is typified by subjective experience: there is something it is like to experience *X*, and it is something it is like for me. The private character of phenomenal consciousness has an excluding effect on scientific research. What skydiving feels like might be different to you (fun) and me (frightening), and the same declared "fear" might feel different to two individuals. Nevertheless, if we agree that there is something it is like to perform a sport, then performance is phenomenally conscious. Whether athletes are aware (psychological consciousness) of the phenomenal feel of experience is another question. If they are not, it might be argued that phenomenality in sport is often subliminal, so that athletes are not able to report the content of the phenomenal state. That does not mean that they are not phenomenally conscious. We should not define conscious *only* when humans declare, report, or reflect on something. Edelman (1992, 135–136) argues that so-called *qualia* (the qualitative and phenomenal feel of subjective experience) have causal impact on discriminating sensory perceptions. How something feels has an effect on action and behavior, whether we are able to report it or not. Maybe research into phenomenal consciousness could be useful in solving the mysteries of home court advantage? There is something it is like to climb a rock, shoot and kick a ball, stand on your hands, or play in front of twenty thousand spectators.[22] There is something this is like, whether you reflect on it, declare it, or not. Athletes are not automatic or nonconscious robots; they are phenomenally conscious.

In this discussion, we have argued that treating skillful athletes as automatic and nonconscious is flawed. We now continue with some other aspects of sporting skills that are also signs of consciousness and cognition. We do this by a brief discussion on the mirror neuron theory of action *understanding*, and the concept of motor *intentionality*. Finally, we end this chapter with some ideas as to what phenomenology could do to enhance our views about sporting skills, consciousness, and cognition.

8 Mirror Neurons and Action Understanding

The discovery of mirror neurons by Rizzolatti and colleagues (Rizzolatti et al. 1996) is just as astonishing as a game-tying three-pointer at the buzzer. During a single-cell recording of a macaque monkey, they accidently found that the same neurons fired when the monkey observed an experimenter grasping a cup as when the monkey did the grasping itself. This means that action observation causes in the observer the activation of the same neural mechanism triggered by action execution. A hypothesis presented itself: the motor system is not a purely executive system; there are neurons (in the motor area F5, among others) that have both visual and motor properties working in parallel. Some of these have been known as *mirror neurons*.[23] The best way for evolution to make things happen fast and fluidly is to evolve neurons with more than one property. Picking up an object is a combination of two processes, reaching and grasping. It may seem that reaching precedes grasping but neuronal recordings show that grasping starts simultaneously as the arm moves to reach (Rizzolatti and Sinigaglia 2008, 21). The hand assumes the shape needed to grasp instantly. Other single-cell recordings have shown that bending a finger to scratch activates different neurons than bending a finger to grasp. Although the mechanical movements are identical, they have different *meaning*. Rizzolatti and Sinigaglia's (35–47) interpretation is that F5 contains a vocabulary of motor acts so that we have a repertoire that is at the basis of cognitive functions usually associated with the visual system.

What are the mirror neurons for then? Rizzolatti and Sinigaglia (94–97) argue that the mirror neuron system is not an evolutionary mechanism for learning, but primarily for *action understanding*. The mirror neuron system provides the mechanism wherein we combine visual input with motor *knowledge* to understand the actions of others. Thanks to this mechanism we do not have to reflect on what others are doing, but understand directly and can make quick and adequate responses. There simply isn't time to first calculate a 200 km/h sliced tennis serve, then make some considerations, and finally respond with a top-spin forehand (see, e.g., Milton, Solodkin, and Small 2008). Having motor knowledge is necessary and sufficient to understand sensory information involved in the action of others.

According to Rizzolatti and Sinigaglia (2008), motor knowledge is "of fundamental importance for building a basic intentional cognition" (106). Having motor knowledge in this sense means that we must first *learn* motor responses, and *then* the mirror neuron system kicks in when observing others perform movements. Motor knowledge in Rizzolatti's sense is connected to long-term *memory*. The mirror neuron system is established in a way similar to Edelman's theory of neuronal group selection—the mirror neuron system is *trainable* (see Aglioti et al. 2008; Calvo-Merino et al. 2005). Before we move on to the final discussion of motor intentionality and phenomenology, I hope we have a rather clear view of the connection between skill and the mirror neuron system. The mirror neuron system is not primarily involved in learning motor skills, but when these are learned the mirror neuron system makes it possible to respond quickly and efficiently. In (half) open-ended sports this is essential.

In one-on-one sports and team sports, the mirror neuron system seems to be a fundamental neuronal mechanism accompanying prolific performance. This mechanism is automatic in the sense that we can neither turn it off nor be consciously aware of it in a reflective or declarative way. But it is not automatic in the sense that we are nonconscious robots. If the theory is sound, it shows us that we can be cognitive, intentional, and understand while not thinking reflectively.[24] We are, as Bermúdez (2003) puts it, thinking without words.

9 Phenomenology and Motor Intentionality

Our account of sporting skill has wandered between a higher-order psychological and philosophical level and a lower-order neuroscientific level. We have attempted to show that skills that are well rehearsed and seem automatic (weak automation) are still performed consciously, in both the psychological and phenomenal senses. Skillfullness often displays declarative knowledge in the sense that athletes know the rules of the game and remember episodes that are important for their performance. Since this kind of propositional knowledge often remains in the background and is hard to declare linguistically in action, we will search for another way to describe sporting skills by a phenomenological attitude.

We first look into what Merleau-Ponty calls a movement project—a motor intentionality—to see if it can provide us with a complementary understanding of the mirror neuron mechanism that enables an athlete's quick and efficient responses to a changing environment. Second, we look to Heidegger for a phenomenological treatment of knowledge. Merleau-Ponty's concept of "motor intentionality" draws our attention to the body in movement. With motor intentionality, "we are brought to the recognition of something between movement as a third person process and thought as a representation of movement—something which is an anticipation of, or arrival at, the objective and is ensured by the body itself as a motor power, a 'motor project,' a 'motor intentionality'" (Merleau-Ponty 2002, 126–127).

According to Heidegger (see below), we are first of all active and engaged agents in the world. With Merleau-Ponty, we learn that this active engagement is enabled by our lived, perceiving body. In a basic understanding of the term, motor intentionality marks our "normal unity and integration of bodily movement and our intuitive awareness of a given, stable environment" (Carman 2008, 117). Thus, bodily movement is laden with intentionality and provides us with a directedness, a bodily grip, on the world. Furthermore, we can use the concept to understand concrete motor action in sport. Let us first look into the distinction between a cognitive understanding of intentionality and a bodily/motor understanding of intentionality.

Cognitive intentional states are characterized by an intentional content and a psychological mode (Searle 1983) that can be logically separated. For instance, I can have the belief that eye-to-hand-coordination practice is efficient for improving my dribbling skills. The content of my intentional state is "eye-to-hand-coordination practice is efficient for improving my dribbling skills," and the psychological attitude is a belief. I can also know that this is a fact, and I can hope that it is. We see that the content and the attitude can be logically separated from each other. However, the logical structure of motor intentionality is different. According to Kelly (2003), "For motor-intentional activities, there is no independently specifiable content toward which the subject can have an attitude. This is because motor-intentional activity identifies its object in such a highly specific and context-sensitive way that any attempt to take up that specification of the object as such changes it into something other than it was at the time it was had" (133).

Kelly's point is that a movement project is ingrained with a bodily intentionality, which display a direct, fine-grained and context-sensitive understanding through a person's doings when she or he moves in a meaningful situation. Think about grasping a ball that someone throws you. Grasping an object is a basic skill in sports like basketball, and it is also a skill that most people can adapt to quickly and adequately. Suppose we observe two athletes passing the ball to each other. We see that they grasp the ball quickly and efficiently. We can say that the athletes simply grasp the ball, "just like that!" How can we as phenomenologically inspired observers/coaches describe this situation?

First, when a pass is made, and the ball is approaching the athlete, we can see how his or her body is directed toward the ball. This seems to mark an essentially bodily and object-directed understanding of the task. Merleau-Ponty (2002) describes it as "knowledge in the hands which is forthcoming only when bodily effort is made, and cannot be formulated in detachment of that effort" (166). We see that "knowledge in the hands" is articulated through the athlete's movement project. This marks a bodily *understanding* of the situation that simply would not have been displayed in the absence of this particular movement project. As Kelly (2003) emphasizes, "My bodily activity with respect to the object is my way of understanding it" (132). Hence, motor intentionality illuminates our *embodied* and object-directed consciousness. It is knowledge *extended* into the world beyond the subject itself.

Second, this is a very context-sensitive and precise understanding. When athletes pass and move in a game of basketball, they are moving around in a highly complex, dynamic, and constantly changing environment. In short, the athlete will grip the ball and pass it farther at a certain place, time, and way. If the situation had been otherwise, the athlete would have moved differently. For instance, if a pass was made quickly instead of slowly, we will see that the athlete who attempts to grip the ball moves equivalently quickly. Furthermore, the athlete's understanding is very precise and fine-grained. For instance, when an athlete's arm goes up in order to grip the ball, it happens in one particular way. The arm reaches some sort of "an adequate position." If the arm had reached "an adequate position" that was slightly different, its understanding would have been "slightly different," as instantiated by the fact that the arm was a little more extended.

Third, a contextual understanding is a nonreducible understanding. When the athlete grips the ball and passes it, his or her movement is always part of a larger meaningful situation. For instance, the athlete moves and passes the ball in an area that is restricted by the rules of the game in an attempt to participate or to score points. In this sense we can see how a passing movement emerges as a figure on the game's background. Another way of describing this is to say that motor intentionality *embeds* an athlete's movement project into a complex game environment and its further horizons.

Furthermore, the bodily understanding of grasping the ball has success conditions. It marks thus a normative understanding of the object. Normally, an athlete gets an immediate feeling in the fingertips whether the ball has been grasped successfully or not. When everything is going well, the athlete grasps the ball and passes it farther "just like that!" But once in a while the ball will hit the fingertips in such a way that it hurts. Then, another (conscious) awareness of the situation emerges that underlines that there are several ways to understand the activity in question. In either case, motor intentionality is present in the athlete's doings. Thus, motor intentionality marks our doings and is in this sense *enacted* on to the world.[25]

Of course, this normative understanding is always present in our bodily way of dealing with objects in the sense that it provides us with a "here and a now." Thus, it is our bodily engagement with the world that gives us a perspective on it, or to describe it as Merleau-Ponty (2002) did, "The body is the general medium of having a world" (169). So when I play basketball, I will always experience this activity from a particular point of view, which is something that will be determined by how I move around and alter my bodily view of the field in accordance with the affordances or what shows up as important to me.[26]

If the descriptions above are plausible, then our motor intentionality seems like the kind of activity that provides us with a bodily understanding of the world that resembles a mirror neuron system's capacity to respond adequately to a constantly changing environment. We think that these characteristics of motor intentionality provide us with the tools we need to understand why motor intentionality is at the core of embodied cognition. Because we have indicated that motor intentionality is embodied, embedded, extended, and enacted knowledge and consciousness, it marks central features of embodied cognition (Rowlands 2010).

10 Phenomenology and Knowledge in Sport

The analytic tradition in philosophy has typically focused on knowing that and knowing how. Philosophers in the phenomenological tradition have also discussed problems of knowledge in relation to activities like sports.[27] As we have seen above, Merleau-Ponty's work has implications for understanding consciousness. We will now look at Heidegger, since Heidegger's early philosophy laid out the foundation for many of the recent approaches to knowledge in sport.

Heidegger (1962) defined the human mode of being (*Dasein*) as *being-in-the-world*, thereby indicating the strong bond between humans and the environing world. Heidegger's goal in his early philosophy was to reach an understanding of the basic ontological structures of the human being-in-the-world. One of these basic structures is *understanding* (*verstehen*), since humans always have an understanding of their situation in the world. Understanding is directed toward the future, since the goal is to take care of oneself in relation to what comes. By looking into the future, being aware of the past, and relating to the present, the human being carries his or her life project toward death.

We can call this *existential knowledge,* since it means that we understand our own existence in the world as "being toward death." This type of existential knowledge is especially relevant in sports where a risk of death may be a possible reality. According to Heidegger, there are two other types of knowledge, one theoretical and the other practical. Whereas theoretical knowledge has a high prestige, this type of knowledge is, according to Heidegger, *not* the primary one. Our primary mode of understanding the world is not to describe the things we encounter but to use them as pieces of equipment. Most of the time, entities in the world are discovered in their functionality, which is taken in a very wide sense by Heidegger (1962): "In our dealings we come across equipment for writing, sewing, working, transportation, measurement" (97). That which makes things suitable for such uses is what he called "equipmentality" (*zeughaftigkeit*). The carpenter thus has a practical grip on the world. A hammer is a piece of equipment: it is used in an equipmental context of hammer, nails, planks, walls, house. To *describe* the hammer as an object with a certain form, weight, color is a secondary way of relating to it. According to Heidegger, we thus have at least three forms of knowledge: existential, practical, and theoretical knowledge.

From a phenomenological viewpoint, we are not individual human beings secondarily relating to the world around us. We are immersed in the world and directly from early childhood on we know how the world operates and how we can interact with it, not least in play and sports. Whereas analytic philosophy tends to study knowing how related to the individual athlete, phenomenologists look at the individual-environment interaction. They focus on how sporting skill is about not only what/how an athlete can do, but also how the world operates and how things work—how knowledge is embedded and extended. Heidegger's notion of a fundamental "equipmentality" of the world is close to Gibson's idea of the fundamental "affordances" of our environing world.

Gibson uses the concept of "affordance" to characterize our environment in its ability to present (afford) possibilities for use or exploration (Gibson 1986). A stone invites to be thrown; a tree invites to be climbed. Several recent approaches, like the so-called radical embodied cognitive neuroscience (REC), combine phenomenology with theories of embodied cognition, ecological psychology, dynamical systems theory, and neurodynamics to better understand the human-environment interaction and interactions in and between teams (Bruineberg and Rietveld 2014; Hutto and Sánchez-García 2015; Araújo and Bourbousson 2016).

Heidegger's idea of being-in-the-world has thus strongly influenced how we perceive and understand human action in sports. Humans have an immediate understanding of the environment that is developed early in childhood and onward. Play in children selects and prunes neural networks that underlie answers to questions like "What can I do?" (Fagen 1981). This bodily relation to the world is explored in extreme forms in some sports. Building on Heidegger, Breivik (2011) studied how climbers explore vertical cliff, skydivers play with wind resistance in empty space, and kayakers dance with, and on, white water.

Dangerous play with the elements presupposes a knowledge of "what I can do" and of "how I can do it" in relation to specific natural elements. Based on long experience, some people simply understand how water behaves, how air resistance builds up in free fall, and how a rock allows for finger holds. Similarly, people in one-on-one open-ended sports like wrestling or boxing have an immediate understanding of their opponents based on interaction with other people from early infancy.

This immediate understanding may be based on the mirror neuron system. Phenomenology thus transcends the focus on the individual athlete's declarative cognitive content (knowing that) in standard cognitive science (and analytic philosophy). Phenomenology might therefore be a tool to investigate knowledge and consciousness as something embedded, extended, enacted, and embodied in sporting skills.

11 Conclusion

In this chapter, we have tried to undermine the view that skillful athletes are like automatic and nonconscious robots and that sport is not a cognitive activity. Such views are to be found in philosophy, treating solely "knowing that" as knowledge proper; psychological memory research, seeing procedural skills as independent from declarative memory; or neuroscience, searching for NCC in the declarative domain. We have tried to show that there are many types of sport and skill. How automation, consciousness, and cognition is instantiated is just as diverse. Athletes rely on propositional knowledge during performance. They must know the rules (semantic memory), and they know about failures and successful actions in the past (episodic memory).

This knowledge has effects on the skill performed. If you know that Roger's backhand is weak and you have played against him before, then you may skillfully turn this propositional fact of episodic memory to an advantage. Football players constantly act on the offside rule; it is embodied in both the defensive and offensive skill, *and* embedded in the sport itself. Athletes are phenomenologically conscious of and display such knowledge all the time, but only rarely do they make the content of psychological consciousness declarative and reportable.

Unlike Libet (2004), we have argued that humans and athletes act consciously even if reflective thought occurs after a specific action, or not at all. We have also argued that, although there are several automatic and nonconscious processes underlying skillful actions, that does not necessarily mean that skillful actions are automatic and nonconscious. We have done this by distinguishing between strong and weak automation, connecting the mirror neuron theory of action understanding to skill, and trying to apply the concept of motor intentionality to a sporting context. We have argued that coming up with a novel solution or handling a novel situation are not acts of automation, but typical conscious and cognitive acts.

We might also want to argue that the so-called automated act of moving your feet is also conscious (unlike the blink reflex). Moving your feet is automation in a *weak* sense: automatic in the sense that it goes on without declarative reflective thought, but not in the sense that it goes on without control and intention. So-called automated acts of moving your feet are also signs of understanding: it's an answer to a question posed by the context-dependent situation. In some sports, mirror neurons may be essential to coming up with efficient answers to such questions. Moving your feet is what we have called a motor project; it is an intentional act extending consciousness to the ground and world. The seemingly simple act of moving your feet is what Heidegger called existential knowledge—enactive and skillfully bringing us forward in our lifeworld. Moving your feet is thus conscious and cognitive action.

To complement or enhance our understanding of sporting skills, the research program of embodied cognition should dismiss the distinction between knowing that and knowing how, and between the declarative and the procedural. Furthermore, consciousness should not be investigated only through linguistic content of psychological consciousness. What it is like to skillfully handle complex and context-dependent motor projects like sports may be better left to phenomenological and embodied research than to standard cognitive science and its methods.

Notes

1. See, e.g., Wallace (2006).

2. One could say, with Shapiro (2011), that the world (sport) or the body (skill) play a *constitutive* role in cognition.

3. One could say (again with Shapiro 2011) that a body's interaction with others *replaces* the need for representational processes.

4. For a review, see Breivik (2014).

5. This account claims knowing how simply *is* knowing that (see also Stanley and Williamson 2001), and that skill is knowing that *and* the ability and acuity of performing knowing that.

6. Kandel's original work was on *Aplysia californica*.

7. For a more detailed discussion on skill and memory, see Birch (2011).

8. See, e.g., Suits (1995) and Meier (1988).

9. See, e.g., Speelman and Kirsner (2005, ch. 2).

10. Merriam-Webster's full definition: 1: largely or wholly involuntary; *especially*: reflex, 2: having a self-acting or self-regulating mechanism, 3: *of a firearm*: firing repeatedly until the trigger is released

11. See, e.g., Milton, Small, and Solodkin (2004).

12. For a review of cognitive and automatic processes, see Christensen, Sutton and McIlwain (2016). They propose a systematic theory where both automatic and cognitive processes contribute in skillful action. Their main idea is that cognition is not lost, but rather shifted to higher-level action control.

13. See also Bargh and Chartrand (1999).

14. Block (2005) argues there may be two sets of NCC: one for psychological consciousness and one for phenomenal consciousness. Investigations have focused on NCC for psychological (access) consciousness because they can be correlated with declarative reports.

15. Other candidates are, for example, Damasio's theory (1994; 1999) of a higher-order representation (a conscious feeling) of a lower-level state (an emotion) and Crick's (1994) 40 hz hypothesis.

16. We may call this a Cartesian legacy.

17. Introspection is what Armstrong argues lacks when driving for a long time.

18. http://www.nrk.no/nett-tv-klipp/228005.

19. See, e.g., Beilock and Carr (2001); and Beilock, Wierenga, and Carr (2003).

20. See, e.g., Thagard (2014) for an account treating explicit awareness as the primary mode of cognitive function.

21. See, e.g., Sánchez-García and Sebastián (2015) for an overview of attention in sport.

22. For a more in-depth inquiry into sport and consciousness, see Birch (2009).

23. Others are *canonical neurons*, which will not be discussed here.

24. For a critique of the theory, see, e.g., Hickok (2009).

25. For work on enaction, see Varela, Thompson, and Rosch (1991). For enaction in sport, see Laurent and Ripoll (2009), and Bourbousson et al. (2010). See also Noë's (2004) view that our ability to perceive is constituted by our possession of "sensorimotor knowledge."

26. See Gibson (1986) and chapter text for an elaboration of the concept of "affordances," and Bruineberg and Rietveld's (2014) view on affordances in relation to skilled intentionality and its underlying neurodynamics.

27. See Martínková and Parry (2013).

References

Aglioti, Salvatore, Paola Cesari, Michela Romani, and Cosimo Urgesi. 2008. "Action Anticipation and Motor Resonance in Elite Basketball Players." *Nature Neuroscience* 11 (9): 1109–1106.

Araújo, Duarte, and Jerome Bourbousson. 2016. "Theoretical Perspectives on Interpersonal Coordination for Team Behaviour." In *Interpersonal Coordination and Performance*, edited by Pedro Passos, Keith Davids, and Jia Yi Chow, 126–139. London: Routledge.

Armstrong, David M. 1981. "What Is Consciousness?" *The Nature of Mind, and Other Essays*, edited by John Heil, 55–67. Brisbane: University of Queensland Press.

Baars, Bernard. 1997. *In the Theater of Consciousness: The Workspace of the Mind*. New York: Oxford University Press.

Bargh, John A., and Tanya L. Chartrand. 1999. "The Unbearable Automaticity of Being." *American Psychologist* 54 (7): 462–479.

Beilock, Sian, and Thomas Carr. 2001. "On the Fragility of Skilled Performance: What Governs Choking under Pressure?" *Journal of Experimental Psychology: General* 130 (4): 701–725.

Beilock, Sian L., Sarah A. Wierenga, and Thomas H. Carr. 2003. "Memory and Expertise: What Do Experienced Athletes Remember." In *Expert Performance in Sports: Advances in Research on Sport Expertise*, edited by Janet Starkes and Anders Ericsson, 295–320. Champaign, IL: Human Kinetics.

Bermúdez, José Luis. 2003. *Thinking without Words*. Philosophy of Mind Series. New York: Oxford University Press.

Birch, Jens E. 2009. "A Phenomenal Case for Sport." *Sport, Ethics and Philosophy* 3 (1): 30–48.

Birch, Jens Erling. 2011. "Skills and Knowledge—Nothing but Memory?" *Sport, Ethics and Philosophy* 5 (4): 362–378.

Block, Ned. 2005. "Two Neural Correlates of Consciousness." *Trends in Cognitive Sciences* 9 (2): 46–52.

Bourbousson, Jerome, Germain Poizat, Jacques Saury, and Carole Seve. 2010. "Team Coordination in Basketball: Description of the Cognitive Connections among Teammates." *Journal of Applied Sport Psychology* 22 (2): 150–166.

Breivik, Gunnar. 1998. "Sport in High Modernity: Sport as a Carrier of Social Values." *Journal of the Philosophy of Sport* 25 (1): 103–118.

Breivik, Gunnar. 2011. "Dangerous Play with the Elements: Towards a Phenomenology of Risk Sports." *Sport, Ethics and Philosophy* 5 (3): 314–330.

Breivik, Gunnar. 2014. "Sporting Knowledge and the Problem of Knowing How." *Journal of the Philosophy of Sport* 41 (2): 143–162.

Bruineberg, Jelle, and Erik Rietveld. 2014. "Self-Organization, Free Energy Minimization, and Optimal Grip on a Field of Affordances." *Frontiers in Human Neuroscience* 8 (599): 1–14.

Calvo-Merino, Beatriz, Daniel Glaser, Julie Grèzes, Richard Passingham, and Patrick Haggard. 2005. "Action Observation and Acquired Motor Skills: An fMRI Study with Expert Dancers." *Cerebral Cortex* 15 (8): 1243–1249.

Carman, Taylor. 2008. *Merleau-Ponty*. Oxfordshire, UK: Routledge.

Chalmers, David J. 1996. *The Conscious Mind: In Search of a Fundamental Theory*. Oxford: Oxford University Press.

Christensen, Wayne, John Sutton, and Doris J. F. McIlwain. 2016. "Cognition in Skilled Action: Meshed Control and the Varieties of Skill Experience." *Mind & Language* 31 (1): 37–66.

Churchland, Paul. 1989. *A Neurocomputational Perspective: The Nature of Mind and the Structure of Science*. Cambridge, MA: MIT Press.

Crick, Francis. 1994. *The Astonishing Hypothesis: The Scientific Search for the Soul*. New York: Scribner.

Damasio, Antonio R. 1994. *Descartes' Error: Emotion, Reason and the Human Brain*. Fort Mill, SC: Quill House.

Damasio, Antonio R. 1999. *The Feeling of What Happens: Body, Emotion and the Making of Consciousness*. New York: Harcourt Brace.

Dancy, Jonathan. 1985. *An Introduction to Contemporary Epistemology*. Oxford: Blackwell.

Dreyfus, Hubert, and Stuart Dreyfus. 1986. *Mind over Matter: The Power of Human Intuition and Expertise in the Era of the Computer*. New York: Free Press.

Edelman, Gerald. 1992. *Bright Air, Brilliant Fire: On the Matter of the Mind*. New York: Basic Books.

Edelman, Gerald, and Giulio Tononi. 2000a. *A Universe Of Consciousness: How Matter Becomes Imagination*. New York: Basic Books.

Edelman, Gerald M., and Giulio Tononi. 2000b. "Reentry and the Dynamic Core: Neural Correlates of Conscious Experience." In *Neural Correlates of Consciousness: Empirical and Conceptual Questions,* edited by Thomas Metzinger, 139–151. Cambridge, MA: MIT Press.

Fagen, Robert. 1981. *Animal Play Behavior*. Oxford: Oxford University Press.

Gazzaniga, Michael, Richard Ivry, and George Mangun. 2014. *Cognitive Neuroscience: The Biology of the Mind*. 4th ed. New York: W.W. Norton.

Gibson, James. 1986. *The Ecological Approach to Visual Perception*. Hillsdale: Lawrence Erlbaum.

Heidegger, Martin. 1962. *Being and Time*. Translated from the German by John Macquarrie and Edward Robinson. New York: Harper and Row.

Hickok, Gregory. 2009. "Eight Problems for the Mirror Neuron Theory of Action Understanding in Monkeys and Humans." *Journal of Cognitive Neuroscience* 21 (7): 1229–1243.

Hutto, Daniel D., and Raúl Sánchez-García. 2015. "Choking RECtified: Embodied Expertise beyond Dreyfus." *Phenomenology and the Cognitive Sciences* 14 (2): 309–331.

Kandel, Eric. 2006. *In Search of Memory: The Emergence of a New Science of Mind*. New York: W.W. Norton.

Kelly, Sean. 2003. "Edmund Husserl and Phenomenology." In *The Blackwell Guide to Continental Philosophy*, edited by Robert Solomon and David Sherman, 112–136. Oxford: Blackwell.

Knapp, Barbara. 1963. *Skill in Sport: The Attainment of Proficiency*. London: Routledge and Kegan Paul.

Koch, Christof. 2004. *The Quest for Consciousness: A Neuroscientific Approach*. Englewood: Roberts and Company.

Laurent, Eric, and Hubert Ripoll. 2009. "Extending the Rather Unnoticed Gibsonian View That 'Perception Is Cognitive': Development of the Enactive Approach to Perceptual-Cognitive Expertise." In *Perspectives on Cognition and Action in Sport*, edited by Duarte Araújo, Hubert Ripoll, and Markus Raab, 133–146. New York: Nova Science.

LeDoux, Joseph E. 2003. *Synaptic Self: How Our Brains Become Who We Are*. London: Penguin Books.

Libet, Benjamin. 2004. *Mind Time: The Temporal Factor in Consciousness*. Cambridge, MA: Harvard University Press.

Martínková, Irena, and Jim Parry. 2013. *Phenomenological Approaches to Sport*. London: Routledge.

Meier, Klaus V. 1988. "Triad Trickery: Playing With Sport and Games." *Journal of the Philosophy of Sport* 15 (1): 11–30.

Merleau-Ponty, Maurice. 2002. *Phenomenology of Perception*. Translated by Colin Smith. London: Routledge Classics.

Milton, John, Ana Solodkin, Petr Hlustík, and Steven L. Small. 2007. "The Mind of Expert Motor Performance Is Cool and Focused." *NeuroImage* 35 (2): 804–813.

Milton, John, Ana Solodkin, and Steven Small. 2008. "Why Did Casey Strike Out? The Neuroscience of Hitting." In *Your Brain on Cubs: Inside the Heads of Players and Fans*, edited by Dan Gordon, 43–57. New York: Dana Press.

Milton, John G., Steven S. Small, and Ana Solodkin. 2004. "On the Road to Automatic: Dynamic Aspects in the Development of Expertise." *Journal of Clinical Neurophysiology* 21 (3): 134–143.

Nagel, Thomas. 1974. "What Is It Like to Be a Bat?" *Philosophical Review* 83 (4): 435–450.

Noë, Alva. 2004. *Action in Perception*. Cambridge, MA: MIT Press.

Rizzolatti, Giacomo, Luciano Fadiga, Vittorio Gallese, and Leonardo Fogassi. 1996. "Premotor Cortex and the Recognition of Motor Actions." *Brain Research: Cognitive Brain Research* 3 (2): 131–141.

Rizzolatti, Giacomo, and Corrado Sinigaglia. 2008. *Mirrors in the Brain: How Our Minds Share Actions and Emotions*. Oxford: Oxford University Press.

Ross, Jeffrey S., Jean Tkach, Paul M. Ruggieri, Michael Lieber, and Eric Lapresto. 2003. "The Mind's Eye: Functional MR Imaging Evaluation of Golf Motor Imagery." *American Journal of Neuroradiology* 24 (6): 1036–1044.

Rowlands, Mark. 2010. *The New Sciences of the Mind: From Extended Mind to Embodied Phenomenology*. Cambridge, MA: MIT Press.

Ryle, Gilbert. 1949. *The Concept of Mind*. Chicago: University of Chicago Press.

Sánchez-García, Raúl, and Miguel Ángel Sebastián. 2015. "Attention Alters Appearances and Solves the 'Many-Many Problem': Implications for Research in Skill Acquisition and Execution." *European Journal of Human Movement* 34:156–179.

Schmidt, Richard A., and Timothy Donald Lee. 2011. *Motor Control and Learning: A Behavioral Emphasis*. 5th ed. Champaign IL: Human Kinetics.

Searle, John R. 1983. *Intentionality: An Essay in the Philosophy of Mind*. Cambridge: Cambridge University Press.

Shapiro, Lawrence. 2011. *Embodied Cognition*. London: Routledge.

Simons, Daniel, and Christopher Chabris. 1999. "Gorillas in Our Midst: Sustained Inattentional Blindness for Dynamic Events." *Perception* 28 (9): 1059–1074.

Speelman, Craig P., and Kim Kirsner. 2005. *Beyond the Learning Curve: The Construction of Mind*. Oxford: Oxford University Press.

Stanley, Jason, and John W. Krakauer. 2013. "Motor Skill Depends on Knowledge of Facts." *Frontiers in Human Neuroscience* 7 (503): 1–11.

Stanley, Jason, and Timothy Williamson. 2001. "Knowing How." *Journal of Philosophy* 98 (8): 411–444.

Suits, Bernard. 1995. "The Elements of Sport." In *Philosophic Inquiry in Sport*, 2nd ed., edited by William Morgan and Klaus Meier, 8–15. Leeds, UK: Human Kinetics.

Thagard, Paul. 2014. "Cognitive Science." *Stanford Encyclopedia of Philosophy*. http://plato.stanford.edu/entries/cognitive-science/.

Varela, Francisco, Evan Thompson, and Eleanor Rosch. 1991. *The Embodied Mind: Cognitive Science and Human Experience*. Cambridge, MA: MIT Press.

Wallace, David Foster. 2006. "How Tracy Austin Broke My Heart." In *Consider the Lobster and Other Essays*, 142–143. New York: Black Bay Books.

III Learning by Moving: Skill Development through Physical Education and Sport Pedagogy

9 Embodied Cognition and Sport Pedagogy

Denis Francesconi and Shaun Gallagher

1 Introduction

The concept of embodied cognition (EC) includes a variety of approaches involving embedded, extended, ecological, and enactive cognition (sometimes referred to as the 4Es). The increased emphasis on EC in theoretical and empirical research in recent years has also found its way into a number of disciplines outside of mainstream cognitive science, including education and sport education. Although notable advances have been made in EC research, there is still a general uncertainty about what exactly "embodiment" means, and little consensus about the exact role it plays over and above more traditional approaches that focus on neurocentric explanations (Shapiro 2011). Moreover, recent developments have highlighted a growing set of theoretical differences among embodiment theorists (Kiverstein and Clark 2009). To clarify these issues, and to show the relevance of EC to sport pedagogy, we start by outlining two of the recent approaches to embodied cognition, focusing on the contrasts between conceptions of extended or distributed cognition, and the enactivist approach, in contrast to approaches that focus just on brain-based processes.

We then present a brief examination of two concepts from the psychological and phenomenological literatures, namely "body image" and "body schema," in order to help clarify the notion of embodiment. Body image refers to a system of perceptions, attitudes, and beliefs pertaining to one's own body, while body schema refers to a system of sensorimotor processes that function without awareness or the necessity for perceptual monitoring (Gallagher 2005a). Clarifying these concepts will be helpful not only because they have a strong connection to embodiment research, but also because of their widespread use in the sport science literature. Their widespread use notwithstanding, and as with approaches to embodied cognition, a large amount of confusion remains as to what they entail, and some uncertainty about how they should guide theoretical, empirical, and practical projects.

We conclude with a reflection on contemplative practices as exemplificative activities for the integration of EC in sport pedagogy, and to avoid purely brain-based or motoric-based conceptions of sport pedagogy. The epistemological definition and taxonomy of sport pedagogy is still fuzzy and animated (Tinning 2008, 2011; Thorburn and Stolz 2017) and we do not discuss it here. However, we take sport pedagogy to be an intertwined field composed by sport sciences and educational sciences, wherein the word "sport" relies on its etymological meaning as leisure and entertainment, and not only that of professional sport and athleticism. We consider sport pedagogy a theory and practice devoted to human flourishing (Stolz 2013) through bodily activities and leisure. Teaching and learning motor competences or rule-governed individual or group physical activities should be considered a subset of it. In this way, contemplative practices can help support an embodied conception of sport pedagogy and physical education.

In order to see how EC and sport pedagogy could converge, we must first consider that sport pedagogy and all its variants—physical education, movement education, exercise education, kinesthetic education, psychomotricity, and a few others—have never been central in educational debates. Historically this is due to a more general acceptance of a type of disembodiment of the mind promoted by Western philosophy and philosophy of education, which, in turn, has shaped the modern educational system, included the school system. The relative exclusion of the body from the scientific and social discourse has had and still has clear implications in the underestimation of the academic disciplines related to it and its practical applications. In a typical school, we can easily see the lack of importance of the role of the body in learning process by simply looking at the ergonomics of the classroom: physical space, desks, chairs, and their orthogonal disposition, everything is designed to reduce the degree of physical freedom of students for a supposed gain in cognitive performance. The normal school practice, indeed, is often sedentary. If we look at physical education as a school subject, we see that the hourly amount devoted to physical movement is outstandingly low, around 5 percent of British formal curriculum in an academic year, approximately seventy-six hours (Standal 2016). Lastly, vocational schools and apprenticeship training, where practical knowledge is promoted as *praxis* and *praktognosia*, are often believed to be second-class schools.

Besides the poor consideration of body-related activity in the school system, there is also the risk of what critical theorists have pointed out as "the panopticon of physical education": from this perspective, physical education is seen as a Foucauldian technology for stereotype propagation, gender, and race discrimination, and social power legitimation (Azzarito 2009). A few pedagogical models capable of challenging the dominant disembodied model of mind in education can be found in the history of education, for instance the well-known Montessori Method. In recent times, we have been witnessing an increasing number of new proposals in this direction, which are still in need of careful empirical investigation and evaluation, such as "nonlinear pedagogy" (Chow et al. 2007), "flipped classroom" methods, and the "whole school approach" (Weare 2002). However, these proposals don't formulate an articulated analysis of the bodily dimension of learning experience. We intend to promote a discussion about the support that EC as a theoretical framework and scientific program can offer to sport pedagogy's theory and practice.

2 Embodied Cognition

What exactly counts as an "embodied" theory of cognition? If we take this in a broad sense, all theorists would agree that the body plays some role in cognition and the development of expertise. Yet traditional cognitivist approaches are primarily computational and internalist in nature; cognition is what happens in the brain, which is simply served by sensory input and sometimes results in motor output. Embodied approaches, in contrast, foreground the various ways that brain, body, and world dynamics non-trivially interact to form and sustain cognitive processes. When we look closer at how embodied theories have been conceived in the literature, however, we can distinguish several different approaches. Here we focus on two of the most recently developed approaches, the extended (or distributed) mind hypothesis and the enactivist approach.

2.1 Extended Mind

Extended and distributed cognition theorists emphasize the ways in which our grounding within particular artifactual and sociohistorical conditions not only sets the limits of cognition, but gives rise to various cognitive capacities and practices (Clark and Chalmers 1998; Clark 2008). The extended mind hypothesis defends the notion that the body plays an important role as part of the extended mechanisms of cognition. Not only the physical body, but also objects and instruments in the environment, can function as nonneural vehicles for cognitive processes, performing a function similar to the processes of neurons, the primary vehicles of cognition in the classic view. As Clark puts it, "The larger systemic wholes, incorporating brains, bodies, the motion of sense organs, and (under some conditions) the information-bearing states of non-biological props and aids, may sometimes constitute the *mechanistic supervenience base* for mental states and processes" (2008, 38; emphasis original).

For extended mind theorists, then, retaining a computational and functionalist conception, part of the computing mechanism can include the body or the environment. In accomplishing certain tasks, for example, we could store task-relevant information in our brain-based memory system and consult the information in that store; alternatively, we could leave the information in the environment where it already is (or where we put it) and simply use our bodies to perceptually consult it when needed. In the latter case, consistent with Rob Wilson's (1994) notion of "exploitative representation" and "wide computing," the perceiving body is playing a certain computational role that under some circumstances could be done fully "in the head"—the body does this sort of thing frequently, and in effect operates as an "external" vehicle for cognition.

Clark and Chalmers (1998) define the parity principle as follows: "If, as we confront some task, a part of the world functions as a process which, *were it done in the head*, we would have no hesitation in recognizing as part of the cognitive process, then that part of the world *is* (so we claim) part of the cognitive process" (Clark and Chalmers 1998, 8; emphasis original). A good example can be found in the context of team cognition (Salas, Fiore, and Letsky 2013). For example, use of diagrams (on paper, in playbooks, or on chalkboard), or the use of videos, in order to work out the detailed strategies of different plays in preparation for a football game is a case of using objects or processes in the external environment to accomplish a cognitive task. The understanding achieved by the full team using such methods puts everyone on the same page and constitutes a shared representation. According to the parity principle, there is no principled difference between trying to imagine different plays in one's head and using different external media to represent such plays.

A number of extended mind theorists, such as John Sutton (2010) and Richard Menary (2007, 2010), have suggested that the parity principle remains too narrow to capture the potential of the extended mind idea. The standard should not be based on similarities across different cognitive processes. It should rather be about the integration of neural and embodied capacities interacting with each other, involving differences between internal and external processes that complement and augment cognitive capacities. The use of various communication mediums—for example, gestures or writing—is not similar to what we can do "in our heads" but can still be part of a process that extends our cognitive abilities. Language itself can be treated as an extended part of cognition, and communicative practices may in fact shape our individual or group intention formation. All of this, in obvious ways, is directly relevant to team sports and to instruction and learning in such contexts. Sutton notes the importance of "instructional nudges" in the case of sports, that is, when not just beginners, but also experts "in open ball sports, for example, mutter 'watch the ball'" (2007, 50). Such nudges are not always cases of self-instruction;[1] they sometimes function as maxims or material symbols that embody, in a condensed form, previous lessons and that effect a positive adjustment of body posture.

> These embodied cognitive capacities are interwoven in complex ways with our use of the technological, natural, and social resources mentioned above. Although analytically distinguishable, we can also include here the kinds of thinking-in-action apparent in the exercise of learned skills in sport, music, and dance .... In these cases occurrent cognitive activity can—in the right circumstances—be distributed across whole patterned sequences of allowable bodily response repertoires, coupling and coalescing dynamically in real time with complex and simultaneous changing physical, technological, and social parameters. For these reasons, expert embodied performance in these domains, and the interactions between kinaesthetic and episodic memory, is a rich and barely-tapped domain of investigation. (Sutton 2006, 239)

Building on the extended mind hypothesis, material engagement theory (MET) has pointed to the importance of cultural artifacts and practices in cognitive processes and, specifically, to the materiality of the artifacts that we use in such contexts (Malafouris 2013; Sutton 2007). In sport contexts, for example, differences in the weight of a baseball bat, the texture of the playing surface, the shape of a rowing scull, may impact the dynamical timing of our perceptual and decision processes and have a direct effect on performance.

The promotion of student interaction with objects and environments is at the core of some practical pedagogies based on psychomotor assumptions that combine kinesthetic-physical movement dimensions and cognitive tasks. Such approaches can be based on interactive school furniture that can be used for both physical activity and standard school subject learning. An example can be found in the iMo Learn project (http://imolearn.dk/). Here a cube with rounded edges, for instance, functions as a chair allowing moderate swinging so that basal micro-kinematic activity is possible, as well as more complicated motor activities such as balancing if standing on the cube. Moreover, it can be used like a joystick to be controlled by body movements to select answers in multiple-choice questions posed by the teachers. Finally, with numbers on the walls, it can be used for elementary numeracy.

Another example of the relevance of the codependence of body-cognition-object-environment can be found in "nonlinear pedagogy" (Chow et al. 2007; Chow et al. 2009; Lee et al. 2014). As Lee and colleagues (2014) say,

> Traditionally, practitioners (e.g., coaches, teachers, etc.) have adopted approaches which are prescriptive and repetitive, utilizing technical demonstrations that provide learners with a "visual template or criterion model" for the desired skill. The underlying assumption that has fuelled such pedagogies is that an ideal movement pattern exists for a task and that the practitioner's role is to help learners to recreate that pattern. Furthermore, some theorists have

> suggested that learning is a gradual, linear process.... An increasing amount of evidence from the Dynamical Systems Theory (DST) perspective challenge these traditional assumptions about skill acquisition. From the DST viewpoint, the learning process does not generally follow continuous linear progressions of behaviour but rather involves sudden discontinuous changes over time. Learners should be conceived as nonlinear dynamical systems, comprising numerous component parts that interact and self-organize to form stable patterns. The emergence of self-organized functional movement solutions is facilitated through the interaction of performer, task and environment constraints which act as boundaries to shape goal-directed behaviours. (1)

The authors found out that a four-week intervention involving a nonlinear pedagogy (i.e., manipulation of task constraints including equipment and rules) compared with a linear pedagogy (i.e., prescriptive, repetitive skills) approach to learning a tennis forehand stroke increases not only performance accuracy scores over time, as for the linear pedagogy group, but also improves the number of movement clusters at posttest (Lee et al, 2014). The authors suggest that this indicates the acquisition and availability of a larger range of motor patterns to achieve the same motor outcome.

2.2 Enactivism

Enactivist accounts (Gallagher 2005a, 2017; Noë 2004; Thompson 2007; Varela, Thompson, and Rosch 1991) foreground the fact that cognition is primarily action oriented in a dynamically changing environment. These are similar to concepts of extended mind or distributed cognition in arguing that cognition is distributed across brain, body, and environment and therefore is not entirely "in the head." In contrast to the functionalist view of extended mind, however, enactivists claim that bodily processes shape and contribute to the constitution of consciousness and cognition in an irreducible and irreplaceable way.

In the enactivist view, biological aspects of bodily life have a permeating effect on cognition, as do processes of sensorimotor coupling between organism and environment. An enactivist account of perception highlights the integration of a variety of bodily factors into perception. First, perception depends on sensorimotor contingencies (O'Regan and Noë 2001; Noë 2004). This means that perception is a pragmatic, exploratory activity, mediated by movement or action and constrained by contingency relations between sensory and motor processes. One can think of this in terms of ecological psychology, wherein one's perception of the environment includes information about one's own posture and movement, and one's posture and movement will determine how one experiences the environment. In terms of body-schematic processes, agentive control over movement, our capacities and skills for moving around the environment, and for reaching and grabbing things introduces specific biases into what we perceive. We see things in terms of what we can do with them and how we can reach and manipulate them.

Embodiment, however, involves more than sensorimotor processes. An account that would focus only on sensorimotor contingencies would be incomplete, since it would neglect the relevance of affective aspects of embodiment. These include factors that pertain to mood and emotion, bodily states such as hunger, fatigue, and pain, as well as a complex motivational dimension that animates body-world interaction (Stapleton 2013; Colombetti 2013). Likewise, biological (hormonal and chemical) processes having to do with homeostasis modulate body-environment coupling and become part of the reciprocal causal relations that shape cognitive processes. Moreover, in the enactivist view, to fully understand cognition, one has to consider the effects of intersubjective interaction in social and socially organized environments (Gallagher 2013). In explaining intersubjective contexts, enactivists invoke fully embodied dynamical interactions that rely on facial expression, posture, movement, gestures, and distinct forms of sensory-motor couplings (Gallagher 2001, 2005a; Thompson and Varela 2001). Context and social environment, including normative factors, also contribute to "secondary intersubjective" practices starting at nine–twelve months of age (Trevarthen and Hubley 1978). Perception, in such contexts, is often for *inter*-action with others.

Accordingly, in the enactivist view, the body's influence on cognition is, at least, three-dimensional, including the influence of sensorimotor contingencies, affective factors, and intersubjective processes. The mind is enacted by the whole system of brain-body-environment, in virtue of its specific structure and organization.

Enactivists argue for a nonrepresentationalist account of basic action-perception processes. One of the most commonly discussed examples concerns fielding (trying to catch) a ball (McBeath, Shaffer, and Kaiser 1995). We won't repeat the frequently repeated analysis (see Shapiro and Spaulding, this volume, for a good account), except to point out that in both the linear optical trajectory (LOT) account—where the outfielder runs in a way so as to make the ball appear to follow a straight line—and the enactivist-favored optical acceleration cancellation (OAC) account—where the outfielder aligns herself with the flight path of ball and runs forward to make the ball appear to move with constant velocity—what is important is bodily movement. Vision and bodily movement solve the problem without the need to invoke internal mental representations.

Enactivism argues that perception, movement, and context are dynamically related. To see what this means, let's switch games and consider the kind of joint attention and coordination required when playing team sports like football. Merleau-Ponty offers the following account.

> For the player in action the football field is not an "object," that is, the ideal term which can give rise to an indefinite multiplicity of perspectival views and remain equivalent under its apparent transformations. It is pervaded with lines of force (the "yard line"; those lines that demarcate the "penalty area") and is articulated in sectors (for example, the "openings" between the adversaries) which call for a certain mode of action and which initiate and guide the action as if the player were unaware of it. The field is not given to him, but present as the immanent term of his practical intentions; the player becomes one with it and feels the direction of the "goal," for example, just as immediately as the vertical and the horizontal planes of his own body. (Merleau-Ponty 1983, 168–169)

The player's intentions and actions are shaped by the physical environment and by the nature and rules of the game he is playing. Controlling the ball on this field and what some might consider strategizing to reach the goal are not things accomplished purely in the player's head; they are enmeshed with the affordances offered by position on the field and the position of other players. As Merleau-Ponty acknowledges, this field is not empty of others. And many of these others are clearly in relations of joint attention with the one who controls the ball. John Campbell puts it this way: "A team playing football are continuously monitoring one another's attention. But this does not require them to be engaged in conceptual thought, or to have even iterated knowledge of the direction of each other's attention" (2005, 245). This, of course, does not rule out conceptual thought or a tactical decision making that involves declarative knowledge, but that kind of process is fully embedded in the ongoing situation and depends on the action that is played out on the field, just as a foreground depends on a background. That the players are engaged in a complex joint action (playing the game) means that much of their cognitive processes are intertwined in the dynamical relations established along the parameters of the field and are shaped by the material conditions imposed by artifacts, tools, media, and the like, as well as by intersubjective, normative, and institutional practices (including the rules of the game) (Gallagher and Ransom 2016).

Bringing enactivism into sport pedagogy means bringing in more than motor skills or even sensorimotor process; it means taking seriously the idea that a bodily experience is phenomenologically more than a motor experience and valuing its affective dimension. The inclusion of the affective dimension of bodily experiences, indeed, can be a key factor in extending the range of sport pedagogy and facilitating its connection with EC. The promotion of self-awareness or the agent-environment entanglement, for instance, has been rarely considered in physical education, and an embodied-oriented sport pedagogy can offer the necessary framework for designing curricula and activities in line with that. The phenomenological approach to sport pedagogy (Standal 2016) emphasizes the nonreductionist view of the body (*versus* instrumental, functional, or merely operative conceptions of the body) supporting an enactivist view that includes affective and reflective skills. How does one do that? By using either established activities with different goals, or different and relatively new activities. For instance, even the most common and standard activities and sports usually implemented in physical education hours in secondary school, such as athletics, soccer, or basketball, can be usefully applied to reach phenomenological goals—for example, differentiating between body schema and body image, developing self-awareness skills, and emphasizing social and affective dimensions of such sports—if the teacher is aware of this approach and discourse and is able to implement it in the field. Otherwise, specifically planned activities such as contemplative practices—meditation, tai chi, yoga, and so on—which are already "phenomenologically loaded" (Francesconi 2018; Francesconi and Tarozzi 2012), can be used to intentionally intervene on affective and reflective skills. A short indication in this respect is proposed below; however, scientific and applicative literature on contemplative education is growing fast, while its connection with sport pedagogy is still missing or rarely elaborated (Martin and Ergas 2016).

The risk of reductionism in sport pedagogy, however, is always close by. If standard school-system conceptions of education have emphasized the transmission of high-order cognitive skills by treating students as what philosophers call *brains-in-vats*—that is, totally ignoring the bodily dimension of students' life—in sport pedagogy there might be the opposite risk: an emphasis on a sort of *body-with-no-mind*, wherein the body is understood in a purely reductionist and utilitarian way, like a body-as-an-object rather than as-an-agent. This risk often goes hand in hand with an emphasis on sport performance, prodromal to athleticism (Kirk 2002 Kirk and Gorely 2000). The dichotomy that exists in education between utilitarian aspects of education (which we should better name "instruction") and the holistic dimension of education (which derives from the ancient Greek and Roman concepts of *Paideia* and *Humanitas* on one side, and the Classic German concept of *Bildung* on the other) seems to find its way into sport pedagogy as well.

In the sport pedagogy literature, some authors call for attention to the global dimension of human experience in sport pedagogy research and practice, even though an explicit reference to EC seems to be missing. As indicated by Bailey and colleagues (2009), empirical research in physical education and sport pedagogy usually falls into the areas of physical benefits, social benefits, affective benefits, and cognitive benefits. Alexander and Luckman (2001) affirm that research in sport education is mainly done using the five common content standards: motor skill development, tactical knowledge and performance, fitness, personal and social development, and student attitudes and values. Similarly, Stolz (2003) suggests that a whole-person approach to physical education should include the psychomotor, the cognitive, and the affective domains. In other words, these various theorists advocate for a kind of holism consistent with enactivist approaches, without explicitly citing the enactivist arguments. It is in this regard that we believe that the enactive approach may provide a useful theoretical background to justify these practices, for instance through the clarification of concepts such as body image and body schema.

3 Body Image and Body Schema

The concepts of *body image* and *body schema* have a long history and continued applications in a number of disciplines, including psychology, psychiatry, philosophy, and sport science. Unfortunately, the use of these terms has been plagued with conceptual confusions (Gallagher 2005a). Not only do different authors operate with divergent and occasionally conflicting definitions, it is not uncommon that what clearly counts as body schema for one researcher will be defined as body image by another.

We offer the following conceptual clarification (see Gallagher 2005a, 2005b). *Body image* is constituted by a set of intentional states that are sometimes conscious (or for the most part can be made conscious). It consists of a system of perceptions, (emotional) attitudes, and beliefs that pertain to one's own body. Although all of these features are in principle accessible by consciousness, not all of them are consciously accessed at every given moment. Accordingly, there are instances in which we have no occurrent conscious body image: when, for example, immersed in some worldly task or a game, we are not explicitly conscious of or attending to our body as an intentional object.

Studies involving body image (e.g., Cash and Brown 1987; Gardner and Moncrieff 1988; Powers et al. 1987) distinguish among three intentional elements:

a subject's perceptual experience of his/her own body;

a subject's conceptual understanding (including folk and/or scientific knowledge) of the body in general; and

a subject's emotional attitude toward his or her own body.

In contrast to body image, the *body schema* is the system of sensorimotor processes that function without necessarily involving conscious perceptual monitoring or awareness. The body schema controls posture and motor performance during action, much of which occurs automatically and nonconsciously. In contrast to the body image, which may involve focusing on one's body-as-object, the body schema involves the activity of the body-as-agent.

In typical everyday action, body image and body schema are not easily distinguished. Empirical studies, however, suggest a double dissociation between body image and body schema. In some cases of unilateral body neglect (following stroke) one finds an intact body schema (which permits the subject to walk or to use the neglected limb to complete a task such as dressing) but a problematic body image that does not perceptually register the left side of their body (Denny-Brown, Meyer, and Horenstein 1952). The other side of the dissociation is to be found in cases of deafferentation, wherein subjects have lost touch and proprioception below the neck (Cole 1995). In such cases, the subject is perfectly aware of his body primarily through vision (having an intact visual body image) but is unable to control bodily movement in the typical way. In this case, there is a loss of body schema that is compensated for by a strong use of the body image (visual monitoring and cognitive effort) to control movement (Gallagher and Cole 1995).

In learning a new movement, in the context of athletic practice, for example, one may start by self-consciously attending to one's physical body parts as one attempts to move them properly to the task. One's attention might also be directed to such bodily movement by the instructions of a trainer. In such cases one is relying on one's perceptual body image to guide action. With practice, however—the formation of motor habits—and with gains in expertise in movement, one's attention is typically directed elsewhere, away from the specifics of bodily movement and more toward elements of the world, including other agents. In such cases, body-schematic processes take over and at least some aspects of movement and action become trained or automatic (Pereira, Abreu, and Castro-Caldas 2013).

Some theorists, citing the historical confusions about these concepts, suggest that we simply abandon the concepts altogether, or that we reduce the body schema or body image to a strictly neuronal representation or body map in the brain (e.g., Holmes and Spence 2006). Berlucchi and Aglioti (2010), for example, look in the brain for two partly divided anatomical and functional neural systems: one responsible for the immediate and automatic guidance of action, centered in the posterior parietal cortex (correlating to body schema), and the other responsible for conscious body perception, centered in the insula (corresponding to body image). This "body-in-the-brain" strategy, however, runs into problems that derive in part from the complex ambiguities involved when it comes to mapping out brain function. Berlucchi and Aglioti, who turned to strictly neuroscientific accounts to escape the conceptual ambiguity associated with behavioral characterizations of body image and body schema, admit that what they propose is not an absolutely clean neurological independence between body schema and body image, since there are various ways in which these systems integrate. Processes in the posterior parietal cortex, for instance, different from those that guide action, may also be involved in high-level visuospatial and semantic consciousness of the body. Other studies show that the insula is involved in sensory integration and motor control processes that purportedly involve the body schema (e.g., Farrer and Frith 2002; Farrer et al. 2003). The fact that both behavioral and neuroscientific explanations encounter ambiguities, however, may not be due to conceptual confusion, but may reflect an actual ambiguity existing in the phenomena under study. Even if a clear conceptual distinction can be maintained between body image and body schema, to insist that such phenomena be reduced to clean neurological distinctions or else abandoned on the claim they are explanatory unhelpful, when they are in fact behaviorally and phenomenologically integrated and indicative of the complexity of the system under study, seems unscientific.

In a more dynamical-embodied conception, body-schematic processes involve extensive peripheral and extra-neural factors, including proprioceptors, joints, and muscles. In this respect, body-schematic processes are not equivalent to simple motor programs (as characterized, e.g., by Schmidt 1976; see Shapiro and Spaulding, this issue), which would be equivalent to a computational preprogramming of movement that is automatically and inflexibly exercised in a certain behavioral context. More recent conceptions of motor programs recognize the importance of feedback processes (see, e.g., Schmidt and Wrisberg 2008). In terms of dynamical systems theory, body schema processes involve ongoing adjustments made in response to environmental changes, in which parts of the environment, including clothes, tools, and instruments, modulate and are incorporated into the body schema (Gallagher 2005b).[2] One finds the examples of the blind man's cane or the feather in the woman's hat mentioned frequently (Head 1920; Merleau-Ponty 2012). Empirical studies have shown that various tools are incorporated into the body schema (Maravita and Iriki 2004; Maravita et al. 2002). In this regard, body-schematic processes also relate to defining peripersonal space, which extends to encompass the reach of the tool during use. There is also evidence for the formation of a "joint body schema" during a cooperative action scenario; this involves the extension of peripersonal space to include the reachable space of one's nearby action partner (Soliman et al. 2015; Soliman and Glenberg 2014).

Such processes are directly relevant to performance in sports that require one to use a bat, tennis racquet, or other instrument during play. Such instruments, through habitual use, become extensions of one's body, and any modification in the instrument involves a modulation in the body schema. The notion of a joint body schema may be possible in noncompetitive relations—perhaps with other team members. This would require further empirical testing, but one could hypothesize that a joint body schema (or extension of peripersonal space) might occur, for example, between partners on the same side of the net during a tennis match.

The attunement of the body schema to specialized movements in athletics is an important aspect of training and self-training. The body schema begins to develop early in fetal development and is functional at birth in a way that may explain phenomena such as early hand-mouth coordination, and the possibility of neonate imitation (Gallagher and Meltzoff 1996). Even if present at birth, it continues to develop, along with body growth and development, throughout childhood. One may raise questions here about the proper time frame for training of specific bodily performances (dance, music, sports)—during what phase of development training in specific sports works best, or, in some cases, has adverse effects (Schubring and Thiel 2014).

Aspects of body image and body schema are clearly affected by various cultural and interpersonal factors. There have been many studies investigating perceptions and attitudes of athletes toward their bodies (Hausenblas and Downs 2001). Athletes may devote too much attention to their bodies in the context of competitive sports in which weight requirements are important, or where body shape is an issue—for example, dancers, boxers, wrestlers, weight lifters, jockeys, and the like. Body image problems may lead to a variety of problems, including anorexia nervosa and other eating disorders. Wrestlers, compared with swimmers and cross-country skiers, have higher levels of eating disturbances (Enns, Drenowski, and Grinker 1987). There are also various gender differences in college-age athletes with respect to body image attitudes (Casper and Reed 1998; Kosteli et al. 2014; Smith 2014; Stewar et al. 2003; Stuart et al. 2015). A significant percentage of professional ballet students develop anorexia nervosa or bulimia nervosa (Garner et al. 1987; Pickard 2013). One should note, however, that the practice of ballet dance may be therapeutic for conditions such as cerebellar ataxia—that is, specifically with respect to improving body-schematic function and movement (Garcez et al. 2016).

The usefulness of the concepts of body image and body schema in sport pedagogy, then, depends on the specific area one is operating in and the goals one wants to reach. The concept of body image in sport pedagogy, for instance, has a prominent role in health and sociocultural aspects such as health education, eating disorder prevention, and socio-emotional learning (O'Dea 2005). Body schema, on the other side, is certainly more relevant in motor learning and the acquisition of motor skills.

However, both body image and body schema can be usefully employed in sport pedagogy to promote "bodily and kinematic literacy," that is, basic knowledge of concepts such as peripersonal space, bodily blurring and merging, multisensory integration, and bodily awareness. For example, activities requiring synchronous movements can be applied in sport pedagogy settings to introduce the topic of bodily perception and the difference between physical and perceptual borders of the body. Paladino and colleagues (2010) found that synchronous multisensory stimulation leads to self-other merging. In this study, researchers were brushing the cheek of each participant as he or she watched a stranger's cheek being brushed in the same way, either in synchrony or in asynchrony. This study shows how multisensory integration and synchronous movement can affect body and social perception and how it can create a sense of self-other similarity. Synchronous bodily movement activities can also be fostered in order to promote group social cohesion, as suggested by Wiltermuth and Heath (2009). Here authors show how acting in synchrony with others can increase cooperation by strengthening social attachment among group members. Moreover, as indicated below, bodily and kinematic literacy can include bodily awareness and psychophysical wellbeing as primary goals of ad hoc activities such as meditation and yoga.

The notion of peripersonal space, mentioned above, and the fact that peripersonal space is modified depending on tool use or movement can be introduced in many different ways in educational settings. For instance, as indicated by Noel and colleagues (2015), walking can trigger peripersonal space extension, suggesting that kinematics and proprioceptive cues, rather than visual cues, are critical in activating the effect. This study remarks that peripersonal space constitutes a dynamic sensory-motor interface between the individual and the environment. Remapping of peripersonal space is also action-specific, which means that there is a functional link between voluntary object-oriented actions and the multisensory coding of the space around us; thus, performing different actions toward the same object implies differential modulations of peripersonal space (Brozzoli et al. 2010). These studies show how our interaction with the space around us is shaped and modified by movement, actions, and tools. This can lead to numerous practical activities, from sport teaching to social-skills promotion in sport pedagogy contexts. These are topics that require further scientific investigation.

4 Meditation as Enactive Practice in Sport Pedagogy

Bodily perception, bodily experience, awareness, and other similar concepts, as said, don't seem to be on top of the sport pedagogy and physical education agenda. Here we briefly present training in contemplative practices—specifically, mindfulness meditation, but also including tai chi, yoga, and other practices, as a possible way to introduce such concepts into sport pedagogy and to open the debate about their applicability in sport pedagogy. Meditation certainly is a good example of embodied and enactive practices, as already pointed out in the seminal book *The Embodied Mind* by Varela, Rosch, and Thompson, and it may be useful in sport pedagogy given its double aspect of physical activity and affective-cognitive experience.

Although the relevance of contemplative practices to sport pedagogy is open to debate (Martin and Ergas 2016), it is clear that such practices could be easily integrated within the realm of sport pedagogy for at least three reasons:

Contemplative practices are based on the bodily dimension of experience, which certainly pertains to the competences of sport and physical educators and teachers.

Contemplative practices are educational and leisure activities.

Physical education settings are suitable for contemplative practices in schools.

Among the many effects that contemplative practices have been shown to promote, we can cite here improved sport performance (Gardner and Moore 2012) as well as improved cognitive performance: from focused and open attention (Lutz et al. 2008), to greater ability to sustain attention (Zeidan et al. 2010), better attentional functions and cognitive flexibility (Moore and Malinovski 2009), and emotion regulation (Gregucci et al. 2015). It is also important to mention the positive outcomes on stress reduction and prevention (Baer 2015; Gu et al. 2015). On a more metacognitive level, long-term meditators have been found to develop an attitude of reflective thought about their ongoing experience. According to Shapiro et al. (2006), mindfulness practice can accompany a perspectival shift that allows a person to step back and "re-perceive" his or her own experience in a less reactive and judgmental way. Contemporary research on meditation has also shown structural changes in the brain in long- and short-term meditators. Specifically, Lazar and colleagues (2005) discovered that meditation is associated with increased cortical thickness, which suggests a positive effect of meditation in reducing natural brain deterioration in aging. Finally, somatosensory enhancement can be promoted through relaxation and self-perception exercises. Specific studies on meditative practices and tai chi support these results (Kerr et al. 2011; Kerr et al. 2013). Yoga can also play a role in promoting positive body image. A recent study (Mahlo and Tiggemann 2016) shows that yoga practitioners score higher in test measuring positive body image and embodiment and lower in self-objectification than non-yoga participants. The authors conclude that yoga is an embodying activity able to support the cultivation of a positive body image.

From the educational point of view, we can ask what we learn when we meditate. In connection with the embodied approach, as indicated since the very beginning by Varela, Thompson, and Rosch (1991), meditation represents the very best concrete example of training awareness: the first step of mindfulness training, is the discovery of the wandering/disconnected mind:

> Eventually, it begins to dawn on the meditators that there is an actual difference between being present and not being present. In daily life they also begin to have instants of waking up to the realization that they are not present and of flashing back for a moment to be present—not to the breath, in this case, but to whatever is going on. Thus the first great discovery of mindfulness meditation tends to be not some encompassing insight into the nature of mind but the piercing realization of just how disconnected humans normally are from their very experience. (25)

According to Langer, who proposes a model of mindful learning (1989), when we learn mindfulness we learn "to implicitly or explicitly 1) view a situation from several perspectives, 2) see information presented in the situation as novel, 3) attend to the context in which we are perceiving the information, and eventually 4) create new categories through which this information may be understood" (111). For Langer these features of multiple perspectives, novelty, context, and new categories are the essence of mindful learning. Baer and colleagues (2006) offer a rather similar model, wherein mindfulness training has been operationalized as (1) nonreactivity to inner experience; (2) observing/noticing/attending to sensations, perceptions, thoughts, feelings; (3) acting with awareness/not on automatic pilot/concentration/nondistraction; (4) describing/labeling with words; (5) being nonjudgmental of experience.

From the perspective of EC, Varela, Thompson, and Rosch (1991, 26) suggest that mindfulness should be considered one skill among others, like reading and writing, and its development has to be treated in the same way the others are developed. The relevance of mindfulness training to sport pedagogy and physical education is clear. Through repetitive meditative sessions one starts to get acquainted with bodily sitting posture—or other postures usually taken in meditative practices—integrating them into the body schema and enriching the agency of the subject. Mindfulness involves a strengthening of the embodied mind, like the training of a muscle that can then perform more difficult work for a longer time without getting tired easily. The specific aim of mindfulness meditation, according to Varela and colleagues, lies in the ability to develop "presence in the moment," that is the ability to be aware of the dynamic flow of embodied experience without necessarily getting stuck in it. As they write (37), "Mindfulness means that the mind is present in embodied everyday experience; mindfulness techniques are designed to lead the mind back from its theories and preoccupations, back from the abstract attitude, to the situation of one's experience itself."

Contemplative practices lead us back to the I-world entanglement, which too often remains tacit in the background, within a naïve, unreflected, unquestioned cognitive posture that takes the appearance of the world as given. The ability to throw light on the structure of intentional consciousness—the co-determination and coupling of the perceiving subject and the perceived world—through meditation is one of the goals among others that sport pedagogy should consider more carefully and that an embodied sport pedagogy should start to define.

5 Conclusion

As indicated by Bailey and colleagues (2009), the nature of physical education and school sport "have shifted over time, moving from an initial health-related rationale in the first half of the twentieth century to more performance-related consideration following the Second World War, to concerns about the health impact of sedentary behaviors more recently" (7). The heated debate between those holding a narrowly scientific motor learning understanding of sport and physical education and those following the broader cognitive and expressive movement education approach is still valid today.

As suggested by Martin and Ergas (2016), the attempts in the tradition of analytic philosophy of education to offer a justification of physical activity and sport have not been sufficiently grounded in the most distinctive feature of those activities—the body. In their own words, "As many theorists of physical education curricula have rightly complained, today, physical education is preoccupied with the transmission of academic knowledge about the body and 'fitness.' … As these critics have pointed out, this completely decouples physical education from any kind of meaningful relationship with physical activity. It sees the body simply as an instrumental vehicle through which propositional content can be transmitted to the student" (3–4).

Embodied approaches that recognize principles of extended mind and enactivism, phenomenological approaches that foster an understanding of body image and body schema, as well as approaches that incorporate contemplative practices, can support the proposal of an embodied sport pedagogy. The legitimacy and value of the application of this approach to sport pedagogy requires further discussion and investigation within the sport pedagogy community.

Notes

1. As one reviewer points out, in the example discussed by Sutton, despite saying to themselves "keep your eye on the ball," many batsmen do not in fact keep their eye on the ball. Such cases support the idea that instructional nudges do not always function as instructions.

2. See the discussion of Thelen, Ulrich, and Wolff's (1991) analysis in Shapiro and Spaulding (this volume).

References

Alexander, Ken, and Jan Luckman. 2001. "Australian Teacher's Perceptions and Uses of the Sport Education Curriculum Model." *European Physical Education Review* 7 (3): 243–267. doi:10.1177/1356336X010073002.

Azzarito, Laura. 2009. "The Panopticon of Physical Education: Pretty, Active and Ideally White." *Physical Education and Sport Pedagogy* 14 (1): 19–39.

Baer, Ruth A. 2015. *Mindfulness-Based Treatment Approaches: Clinician's Guide to Evidence Base and Applications*. Burlington, VT: Elsevier.

Baer, Ruth A., Gregory T. Smith, Jaclyn Hopkins, Jennifer Krietemeyer, and Leslie Toney. 2006. "Using Self-Report Assessment Methods to Explore Facets of Mindfulness." *Assessment* 13 (1): 27–45.

Bailey, Richard, Kathleen Armour, David Kirk, Mike Jess, Ian Pickup, and Rachel Sandford. 2009. "The Educational Benefits Claimed for Physical Education and School Sport: Academic Review." *Research Papers in Education* 24 (1): 1–27. doi:10.1080/02671520701809817.

Berlucchi, Giovanni, and Salvatore M. Aglioti. 2010. "The Body in the Brain Revisited." *Experimental Brain Research* 200:25–35. doi:10.1007/s00221-009-1970-7.

Brozzoli, Claudio, Lucilla Cardinali, Francesco Pavani, and Alessandro Farnè. 2010. "Action-Specific Remapping of Peripersonal Space." *Neuropsychologia* 48 (3): 796–802. doi.org/10.1016/j.neuropsychologia.2009.10.009.

Campbell, John. 2005. "Joint Attention and Common Knowledge." In *Joint Attention: Communication and Other Minds*, edited by Naomi M. Eilan, Christoph Hoerl, Teresa McCormack, and Johannes Roessler, 287–297. Oxford: Oxford University Press.

Cash, Thomas F., and Timothy A. Brown. 1987. "Body Image in Anorexia Nervosa and Bulimia Nervosa: A Review of the Literature." *Behavior Modification* 11:487–521. doi:10.1177/01454455870114005.

Casper, Regina C., and Ellen Reed. 1998. "Body and Self-Image in College Athletes." *Stanford Humanities Review* 6 (2). https://web.stanford.edu/group/SHR/6-2/html/casper.html#10.

Chow, Jia Y., Keith W. Davids, Chris Button, Ian Renshaw, Rick Shuttleworth, and Luiz Antonio Uehara. 2009. "Nonlinear Pedagogy: Implications for Teaching Games for Understanding (TGfU)." In *TGfU: Simply Good Pedagogy: Understanding a Complex Challenge*, edited by Tim Hopper, Joy Butler, and Brian Storey, 131–143. Vancouver: QUT/Physical and Health Education.

Chow, Jia Y., Keith Davids, Chris Button, Rick Shuttleworth, Ian Renshaw, and Duarte Araújo. 2007. "The Role of Nonlinear Pedagogy in Physical Education." *Review of Educational Research* 77 (3): 251–278. doi:10.3102/003465430305615.

Clark, Andy. 2008. *Supersizing the Mind*. Oxford: Oxford University Press.

Clark, Andy, and David Chalmers. 1998. "The Extended Mind." *Analysis* 58 (1): 7–19.

Cole, Jonathan. 1995. *Pride and a Daily Marathon*. Cambridge, MA: MIT Press.

Colombetti, Giovanna. 2013. *The Feeling Body: Affective Science Meets the Enactive Mind*. Cambridge, MA: MIT Press.

Denny-Brown D., John S. Meyer, and Simon Horenstein. 1952. "The Significance of Perceptual Rivalry Resulting from Parietal Lesion." *Brain: A Journal of Neurology* 75 (4): 596–601. doi.org/10.1093/brain/75.4.432.

Enns, Melvin P., Adam Drewnowski, and Joel A. Grinker. 1987. "Body Composition, Body Size Estimation and Attitudes towards Eating in Male College Athletes." *Psychosomatic Medicine* 49 (1): 56–64.

Farrer, Chloe, Nicolas Franck, Nicolas Georgieff, Chris D. Frith, Jean Decety, and Marc Jeannerod. 2003. "Modulating the Experience of Agency: A Positron Emission Tomography Study." *NeuroImage* 18 (2): 324–333. doi:10.1016/S1053-8119(02)00041-1.

Farrer, Chloe, and C. D. Frith. 2002. "Experiencing Oneself vs Another Person as Being the Cause of an Action: The Neural Correlates of the Experience of Agency." *NeuroImage* 15 (3): 596–603. doi:10.1006/nimg.2001.1009.

Francesconi, Denis. 2018. "Eudaimonic Wellbeing in Education." In *Routledge Handbook on Well-Being*, edited by Kathleen Galvin. Oxon, UK: Routledge.

Francesconi, Denis, and Massimiliano Tarozzi. 2012. "Embodied Education: A Convergence of Phenomenological Pedagogy and Embodiment." *Studia Phaenomenologica. Societatea Română de Fenomenologie* 12 (12): 263–288. doi:10.7761/SP.12.263.

Gallagher, Shaun. 2001. "The Practice of Mind: Theory, Simulation, or Primary Interaction?" *Journal of Consciousness Studies* 8 (5–7): 83–107.

Gallagher, Shaun. 2005a. *How the Body Shapes the Mind*. Oxford: Oxford University Press.

Gallagher, Shaun. 2005b. "Dynamic Models of Body Schematic Processes." In *Body Image and Body Schema*, edited by Helena De Preester and Veroniek Knockaert, 233–250. Amsterdam: John Benjamins.

Gallagher, Shaun. 2013. "The Socially Extended Mind." *Cognitive Systems Research* 25/26:4–12. http://dx.doi.org/10.1016/j.cogsys.2013.03.008.

Gallagher, Shaun. 2017. *Enactivist Interventions: Rethinking the Mind*. Oxford: Oxford University Press.

Gallagher, Shaun, and Jonathan Cole. 1995. "Body Image and Body Schema in a Deafferented Subject." *Journal of Mind and Behaviour* 16 (4): 369–389.

Gallagher, Shaun, and Denis Francesconi. 2012. "Teaching Phenomenology to Qualitative Researchers, Cognitive Scientists, and Phenomenologists." *Indo-Pacific Journal of Phenomenology* 12 (3): 1–10. doi: 10.2989/IPJP.2012.12.3.4.1112.

Gallagher, Shaun, and Andrew N. Meltzoff. 1996. "The Earliest Sense of Self and Others: Merleau-Ponty and Recent Developmental Studies." *Philosophical Psychology* 9 (2): 211–233. doi: 10.1080/09515089608573181.

Gallagher, Shaun, and Tailer G. Ransom. 2016. "Artifacting Minds: Material Engagement Theory and Joint Action." In *Embodiment in Evolution and Culture*, edited by Gregor Etzelmuller and Christian Tewes, 337–351. Berlin: de Gruyter.

Garcez, Priscila A., Lavinia Teixeira-Machado, and Josimari M. Desantana. 2016. "Ballet Dance Portrays the Balance and Coordination Duality in Cerebellar Ataxia: A Case Report." *International Journal of Scientific Engineering and Applied Science* 2 (5): 246–254.

Gardner, Frank L., and Zella E. Moore. 2012. "Mindfulness and Acceptance Models in Sport Psychology: A Decade of Basic and Applied Scientific Advancements." *Canadian Psychology* 53 (4): 309–318.

Gardner, Rick M., and Cathy Moncrieff. 1988. "Body Image Distortion in Anorexics as a Non-Sensory Phenomenon: A Signal Detection Approach." *Journal of Clinical Psychology* 44:101–107.

Garner, David M., Paul E. Garfinkel, Wendy Rockert, and Marion P. Olmsted. 1987. "A Prospective Study of Eating Disturbances in the Ballet." *Psychotherapy and Psychosomatics* 48 (1–4): 170–175.

Gregucci, Alessandro, Edoardo Pappaianni, Roma Siugzdaite, Anthony Theuninck, and Remo Job. 2015. "Mindful Emotion Regulation: Exploring the Neurocognitive Mechanisms behind Mindfulness." *BioMed Research International* (June): 670724. doi:10.1155/2015/670724.

Gu, Jenny, Clara Strauss, Rod Bond, and Kate Cavanagh. 2015. "How Do Mindfulness-Based Cognitive Therapy and Mindfulness-Based Stress Reduction Improve Mental Health and Wellbeing? A Systematic Review and Meta-Analysis of Mediation Studies." *Clinical Psychology Review* 37 (April): 1–12. doi.org/10.1016/j.cpr.2015.01.006.

Hausenblas, Heather A., and Danielle S. Downs. 2001. "Comparison of Body Image between Athletes and Nonathletes: A Meta-Analytic Review." *Journal of Applied Sport Psychology* 13 (3): 323–339.

Head, Henry. 1920. *Studies in Neurology* 2. London: Oxford University Press.

Holmes, Nicholas P., and Charles Spence. 2006. "Beyond the Body Schema: Visual, Prosthetic, and Technological Contributions to Bodily Perception and Awareness." In *Human Body Perception from the Inside Out*, edited by G. Knoblich, I. Thornton, M. Grosjean, and M. Shiffrar, 15–64. Oxford: Oxford University Press.

Kerr, Catherine E., Stephanie R. Jones, Qian Wan, Dominique L. Pritchett, Rachel H. Wasserman, Anna Wexler, Joel J. Villanueva, et al. 2011. "Effects of Mindfulness Meditation Training on Anticipatory Alpha Modulation in Primary Somatosensory Cortex." *Brain Research Bulletin* 85 (3/4): 96–103. doi:10.1016/j.brainresbull.2011.03.026.

Kerr, Catherine E., Matthew D. Sacchet, Sara W. Lazar, Christopher I. Moore, and Stephanie R. Jones. 2013. "Mindfulness Starts with the Body: Somatosensory Attention and Top-Down Modulation of Cortical Alpha Rhythms in Mindfulness Meditation." *Frontiers in Human Neuroscience* 7 (12): 1–15. doi:10.3389/fnhum.2013.00012.

Kirk, David. 2002. "The Social Construction of the Body in Physical Education and Sport." In *The Sociology of Sport and Physical Education: An Introduction*, edited by Anthony Laker, 79–91. London: Routledge.

Kirk, David, and Trish Gorely. 2000. "Challenging Thinking about the Relationship between School Physical Education and Sport Performance." *European Physical Education Review* 6 (2): 119–134. doi:10.1177/1356336X030093002.

Kiverstein, Julian, and Andy Clark. 2009. "Introduction: Mind Embodied, Embedded, Enacted: One Church or Many?" *Topoi: An International Review of Philosophy* 28 (1): 1–7. doi:10.1007/s11245-008-9041-4.

Kosteli, Maria-Christina, Judy L. Vanraalte, Britton W. Brewer, and Allen E. Cornelius. 2014. "Relationship between Sport Type and Body Image of Female Athletes." *Trends in Sport Sciences* 21 (2): 65–71.

Langer, Ellen J. 1989. *Mindfulness*. Reading, MA: Addison-Wesley.

Lazar, Sara W., Catherine E. Kerr, Rachel H. Wasserman, Jeremy R. Gray, Douglas N. Greve, Michael T. Tredway, Metta McGarvey, et al. 2005. "Meditation Experience Is Associated with Increased Cortical Thickness." *NeuroReport* 16 (17): 1893–1897.

Lee, Miriam C. Y., Jia Y. Chow, John Komar, Clara W. K. Tan, and Chris Button. 2014. "Nonlinear Pedagogy: An Effective Approach to Cater for Individual Differences in Learning a Sport Skill." *PLoS ONE* 9 (8): e104744. doi:10.1371/journal.pone.0104744.

Lutz, Antoine, Heleen A. Slagter, John D. Dunne, and Richard J. Davidson. 2008. "Attention Regulation and Monitoring in Meditation." *Trends in Cognitive Sciences* 12 (4): 163–169. doi:10.1016/j.tics.2008.01.005.

Mahlo, Leeann, and Marika Tiggemann. 2016. "Yoga and Positive Body Image: A Test of the Embodiment Model." *Body Image* 18 (September): 135–142. doi.org/10.1016/j.bodyim.2016.06.008.

Malafouris, Lambros. 2013. *How Things Shape the Mind*. Cambridge, MA: MIT Press.

Maravita, Angelo, and Atsushi Iriki. 2004. "Tools for the Body (Schema)." *Trends in Cognitive Sciences* 8 (2): 79–86. doi:10.1016/j.tics.2003.12.008.

Maravita, Angelo, Charles Spence, Steffan Kennett, and Jon Driver. 2002. "Tool-Use Changes Multimodal Spatial Interactions between Vision and Touch in Normal Humans." *Cognition* 83 (2): B25–B34.

Martin, Christopher, and Oren Ergas. 2016. "Mindfulness, Sport and the Body: The Justification of Physical Education Revisited." *Sport, Ethics and Philosophy* 10 (2): 161–174. doi:10.1080/17511321.2016.1166151.

McBeath, Michael K., Dennis M. Shaffer, and Mary K. Kaiser. 1995. "How Baseball Outfielders Determine Where to Run to Catch Fly Balls." *Science* 268 (5210): 569–573.

Menary, Richard. 2007. *Cognitive Integration: Attacking the Bounds of Cognition*. London: Palgrave Macmillan.

Menary, Richard. 2010. *The Extended Mind*. Cambridge, MA: MIT Press.

Merleau-Ponty, Maurice. 1983. *The Structure of Behavior*. Translated by Alden L. Fischer. Pittsburgh: Duquesne University Press.

Merleau-Ponty, Maurice. 2012. *Phenomenology of Perception*. Translated by Donald A. Landes. London: Routledge.

Moore, Adam, and Peter Malinovski. 2009. "Meditation, Mindfulness and Cognitive Flexibility." *Consciousness and Cognition* 18 (1): 176–186. doi:10.1016/j.concog.2008.12.008.

Noë, Alva. 2004. *Action in Perception*. Cambridge, MA: MIT Press.

Noel, Jean-Paul, Petr Grivaz, Patrick Marmaroli, Herve Lissek, Olaf Blanke, and Andrea Serino. 2015. "Full Body Action Remapping of Peripersonal Space: The Case of Walking." *Neuropsychologia* 70 (April): 375–384. doi.org/10.1016/j.neuropsychologia.2014.08.030.

O'Dea, Jennifer A. 2005. "School-Based Health Education Strategies for the Improvement of Body Image and Prevention of Eating Problems: An Overview of Safe and Successful Interventions." *Health Education* 105 (1): 11–33. doi:10.1108/09654280510572277.

O'Regan, Kevin J., and Alva Noë. 2001. "A Sensorimotor Account of Vision and Visual Consciousness." *Behavioral and Brain Sciences* 24 (5): 939–973. doi:10.1017/S0140525X01000115.

Paladino, Maria P., Mara Mazzurega, Francesco Pavani, and Thomas W. Schubert. 2010. "Synchronous Multisensory Stimulation Blurs Self-Other Boundaries." *Psychological Science* 21 (9): 1202–1207. doi:10.1177/0956797610379234.

Pereira, Tiago, Ana M. Abreu, and Alexandre Castro-Caldas. 2013. "Understanding Task- and Expertise-Specific Motor Acquisition and Motor Memory Formation and Consolidation." *Perceptual and Motor Skills: Learning and Memory* 117 (1): 1–22. doi:10.2466/23.25.PMS.117x14z0.

Pickard, Angela. 2013. "Ballet Body Belief: Perceptions of an Ideal Ballet Body from Young Ballet Dancers." *Research in Dance Education* 14 (1): 3–19. doi:10.1080/14647893.2012.712106.

Powers, P. S., R. G. Schulman, A. A. Gleghorn, and M. E. Prange. 1987. "Perceptual and Cognitive Abnormalities in Bulimia." *American Journal of Psychiatry* 144 (11): 1456–1460.

Salas, Eduardo, Stephen M. Fiore, and Michael P. Letsky. 2013. *Theories of Team Cognition: Cross-Disciplinary Perspectives*. New York: Routledge.

Schmidt, R. 1976. "Control Processes in Motor Skills." *Exercise and Sport Sciences Reviews* 4 (1): 229–262.

Schmidt, R. A., and Craig A. Wrisberg. 2008. *Motor Learning and Performance: A Situation-Based Learning Approach*. Champaign, IL: Human Kinetics.

Schubring, Astrid, and Ansgar Thiel. 2014. "Growth Problems in Youth Elite Sports: Social Conditions, Athletes' Experiences and Sustainability Consequences." *Reflective Practice* 15 (1): 78–91. doi:10.1080/14623943.2013.868793.

Shapiro, Lawrence. 2011. *Embodied Cognition*. London: Routledge.

Shapiro, Shauna L., Linda E. Carlson, John A. Astin, and Benedict Freedman. 2006. "Mechanisms of Mindfulness." *Journal of Clinical Psychology* 62 (3): 373–386. doi:10.1002/jclp.20237.

Smith, Katherine. 2014. Comparison of Energy Availability and Body Image between Female and Male Runners. PhD diss., Ohio State University, Columbus.

Soliman, Tamer M., Ryan Ferguson, M. Scott Dexheimer, and Arthur M. Glenberg. 2015. "Consequences of Joint Action: Entanglement with your Partner." *Journal of Experimental Psychology: General* 144 (4): 873–888. doi:10.1037/xge0000089.

Soliman, Tamer M., and Arthur M. Glenberg. 2014. "The Embodiment of Culture." In *The Routledge Handbook of Embodied Cognition*, edited by Lawrence Shapiro, 207–220. London: Routledge.

Standal, Oyvind F. 2016. *Phenomenology and Pedagogy in Physical Education*. New York: Routledge.

Stapleton, Mog. 2013. "Steps to a 'Properly Embodied' Cognitive Science." *Cognitive Systems Research* 22–23:1–11.

Stewar, Arthur D., Philip J. Benson, Evangelia G. Michanikou, Dimitra G. Tsiota, and Margarita K. Narli. 2003. "Body Image Perception, Satisfaction and Somatotype in Male and Female Athletes and Non-athletes: Results Using a Novel Morphing Technique." *Journal of Sports Sciences* 21(10): 815–823. doi:10.1080/0264041031000140338.

Stolz, Steven A. 2013. "Phenomenology and Physical Education." *Educational Philosophy and Theory* 45 (9): 949–962.

Stuart, Aami R., Britta F. Trepp, Rosalyn Kuhle, Brandon Slaugh, and Maureen A. Murtaugh. 2015. "Eating Disorders, Exercise Dependence and Body Image Dissatisfaction in Female Age Group Ironman Triathletes." *Journal of Food and Nutritional Disorders* 4 (4): 2. doi:10.4172/2324-9323.1000176.

Sutton, John. 2006. "Distributed Cognition: Domains and Dimensions." *Pragmatics and Cognition* 14 (2): 235–247. doi:10.1075/pc.14.2.05sut.

Sutton, John. 2007. "Batting, Habit and Memory: The Embodied Mind and the Nature of Skill." *Sport in Society* 10 (5): 763–786. doi:10.1080/17430430701442462.

Sutton, John. 2008. "Material Agency, Skills and History: Distributed Cognition and the Archaeology of Memory." In *Material Agency: Towards a Non-anthropocentric Approach*, edited by Carl Knappett and Lambros Malafouris, 37–55. New York: Springer Science and Business Media.

Sutton, John. 2010. "Exograms and Interdisciplinarity: History, the Extended Mind and the Civilizing Process." In *The Extended Mind*, edited by Richard Menary, 189–225. Cambridge, MA: MIT Press.

Sutton, John, Celia B. Harris, Paul G. Keil, and Amanda J. Barnier. 2010. "The Psychology of Memory, Extended Cognition, and Socially Distributed Remembering." *Phenomenology and the Cognitive Sciences* 9 (4): 521–560. doi:10.1007/s11097-010-9182-y.

Thelen, Ester, Beverly D. Ulrich, and Peter H. Wolff. 1991. "Hidden Skills: A Dynamic Systems Analysis of Treadmill Stepping during the First Year." *Monographs of the Society for Research in Child Development* 56 (1): i–103. doi:10.2307/1166099.

Thompson, Evan. 2007. *Mind in Life: Biology, Phenomenology, and the Sciences of Mind.* Cambridge, MA: Harvard University Press.

Thompson, Evan, and Francisco J. Varela. 2001. "Radical Embodiment: Neural Dynamics and Consciousness." *Trends in Cognitive Science* 5 (10): 418–425.

Thorburn, Malcolm, and Steven Stolz. 2017. "Embodied Learning and School-Based Physical Culture: Implications for Professionalism and Practice in Physical Education." *Sport, Education and Society* 22 (6): 721–731. doi:10.1080/13573322.2015.1063993.

Tinning, Richard. 2008. "Pedagogy, Sport Pedagogy, and the Field of Kinesiology." *Quest* 60 (3): 405–424.

Tinning, Richard. 2011. *Pedagogy and Human Movement: Theory, Practice, Research.* London: Routledge.

Trevarthen, Colwyn, and Penelope Hubley. 1978. "Secondary Intersubjectivity: Confidence, Confiding and Acts of Meaning in the First Year." In *Action, Gesture and Symbol: The Emergence of Language*, edited by Andrew Lock, 183–229. London: Academic Press.

Varela, Francisco J., Evan Thompson, and Eleanor Rosch. 1991. *The Embodied Mind: Cognitive Science and Human Experience.* Cambridge, MA: MIT Press.

Weare, Katherine. 2002. *Promoting Mental, Emotional and Social Health: A Whole School Approach.* London: Routledge.

Wilson, Robert A. 1994. "Wide Computationalism." *Mind* 103 (411): 351–372.

Wiltermuth, Scott S., and Chip Heath. 2009. "Synchrony and Cooperation." *Psychological Science* 20 (1): 1–5. doi:10.1111/j.1467-9280.2008.02253.x.

Zeidan, Fadel, Susan K. Johnson, Bruce J. Diamond, Zhanna David, and Paula Goolkasian. 2010. "Mindfulness Meditation Improves Cognition: Evidence of Brief Mental Training." *Consciousness and Cognition* 19 (2): 597–605. doi:10.1016/j.concog.2010.03.014.

10 Complex Motor Activities to Enhance Cognition

David Moreau and Phillip D. Tomporowski

1 Introduction

Decades of research have shown that training on a task typically leads to enhanced performance, provided certain task parameters remain consistent across training (for an example in the motor domain, see Schmidt and Wrisberg 2008). This line of work has paved the way for entire programs of research focusing on task-specific improvements and their neural correlates (e.g., Ericsson, Krampe, and Tesch-Römer 1993). When considering cognitive enhancement, however, a more exciting prospect is for training to elicit improvements on a *different* task (i.e., transfer). Finding effective means of transfer could have tremendous implications both in refining theoretical models of cognition and in terms of applications to clinical fields (e.g., Hertzog et al. 2008).

With this in mind, it is not surprising that brain training programs have flourished in the past few years. Often compared with physical exercise regimens, the idea of enhancing brain function through cognitive training is appealing, and has the potential to impact a wide range of real-life activities. Yet, as attractive as the premise is, findings have remained mixed so far (Au et al. 2014; Harrison et al. 2013; Hovik et al. 2013; Jaeggi et al. 2008; Jaeggi et al. 2011; Lampit, Hallock, and Valenzuela 2014; Redick et al. 2013; Rudebeck et al. 2012; Shipstead, Redick, and Engle 2012; Thompson et al. 2013), and have yet to demonstrate meaningful transfer. In line with mixed evidence, one consideration that has gained traction in recent discussions is the idea of opportunity costs (e.g., Moreau and Conway 2014): Is time spent playing training games wisely invested?

Here, we provide a tentative answer to this legitimate question, with a discussion of cognitive training regimens based on physical activity. Specifically designed to be challenging at the cognitive and physical levels, such regimens have the potential to elicit core improvements. Before presenting the rationale for this approach, we briefly discuss the mechanisms underlying the effect of physical exercise on cognition, as well as the fundamental aspects of effective learning. We conclude with a broader discussion of the impact of this line of research to cognitive training paradigms.

2 Physical Exercise, Neurogenesis, and Cognition

Physical exercise has been related to changes in neurobiological components, brain structure, brain function, and behavior. These have been documented for decades, both via animal and human experiments. Here, we provide a description of each of these, going from lower to higher levels (i.e., from neurobiology to behavior).

2.1 Neurobiological Mechanisms

Physical exercise is associated with myriad of benefits, some of which can be measured at the neurobiological level. For instance, exercise facilitates cerebral vascularization (Black et al. 1990) and brain insult resistance (Stummer et al. 1994) and increases concentrations of specific proteins and neurotransmitters (Mora, Segovia, and del Arco 2007). Exercise also affects neurogenesis and angiogenesis (Black et al. 1990; Praag et al. 2002; Praag, Kempermann, and Gage 1999) and contributes to neuronal survival and enhanced synaptic metabolism (Vaynman et al. 2006). Together, these processes suggest that exercise directly contributes to the maintenance of healthier, more efficient neural systems.

More specifically, brain-derived neurotrophic factor (BDNF) is thought to mediate many of the benefits of exercise on cognition. Evidence for the role of BDNF in this process originated in animal models (Neeper et al. 1995). BDNF concentration is typically increased after exercise (Ferris, Williams, and Shen 2007; Griffin et al. 2011; Schmolesky, Webb, and Hansen 2013), from within minutes to days, and can last up to several weeks (Berchtold et al. 2001). This effect appears to be most notable in the hippocampus, the caudal neocortex, and the dentate gyrus (Neeper et al. 1996). Importantly, Neeper and colleagues note that these regions are not primarily involved in motor control, and thus that increases in BDNF concentrations directly influence areas involved in cognitive function (Neeper et al. 1996).

It has been suggested that the increase in BDNF concentrations post-exercise is itself triggered by the release of insulin-like growth factor-1 (IGF-1; Cotman and Berchtold 2002), a growth factor involved in neuronal development (Arsenijevic and Weiss 1998). Because IGF-1 plays a role in cell proliferation and survival (Huat et al. 2014), it is also thought to be a very important contributor to memory consolidation and enhancement (Chen et al. 2011). Similarly, fibronectin type III domain-containing protein 5 (FNDC5) is suspected to mediate some of the effects of BDNF on brain function, particularly on hippocampal cell proliferation, via an effect on the activation of the BDNF gene (Boström et al. 2012). A detailed account of the neurobiological mechanisms underlying exercise is beyond the scope of this chapter, yet overall these findings suggest that physical exercise triggers a cascade of complex molecular processes via direct and indirect pathways, with significant impact on brain function and thus on cognition.

Beside direct positive effects, physical exercise also leads to benefits through downregulation of harmful factors. For example, exercise counteracts some of the deleterious effects of stress. When unaddressed, prolonged stress leads to the release of corticosteroids, hormones that negatively affect BDNF levels in the brain and can lead to neuronal degradation and dendritic atrophy (Gould et al. 1990). Exercise acts as a protective mechanism, an effect particularly pronounced in the hippocampus (Russo-Neustadt et al. 2001). The benefit of physical exercise on the concentration of several neurotransmitters has also been documented; in particular, monoamine (e.g., dopamine, epinephrine, norepinephrine) and tryptamine neurotransmitters (e.g., serotonin, melatonin) play a critical role in a wide range of neural processes. These neurobiological effects are thought to be associated with many of the observed effects on cognition (Praag et al. 1999; Winter et al. 2007), although pinpointing the exact mechanisms and interactions between neurotransmitters remains particularly difficult. Regardless, this body of work clearly underlines the importance of neurobiological factors in mediating the relationship between physical exercise and cognition.

2.2 Functional and Structural Changes

Additional exercise-induced changes at the structural and functional levels further demonstrate the potency of the neurobiological mechanisms aforementioned. Several randomized-controlled experiments have shown that physical exercise engenders wide benefits on brain function, often demonstrated with EEG or fMRI techniques (Chaddock-Heyman et al. 2013; Davis et al. 2011; Hillman et al. 2014; Kamijo et al. 2011). For example, Chaddock-Heyman and colleagues (2013) reported that children who engaged in sixty minutes of physical activity every week day for a school year showed decreases in BOLD signal in areas of the right anterior prefrontal cortex when performing a cognitive control task. Importantly, these changes in fMRI activation were also associated with behavioral improvements on this particular task. Davis and colleagues, on the other hand, found that thirteen weeks of exercise, half an hour a day, led to improved executive functions but increased bilateral prefrontal activity (Davis et al. 2011). Apparently disparate, these results suggest that complex factors are associated with cortical activity and enhanced performance on behavioral tasks, mirroring corroborating findings in more general literatures (e.g., Xu, Calhoun, and Potenza 2015).

Other, coarser brain changes have also been documented. For example, diffusion tensor imaging (DTI) studies in children suggest that physical exercise interventions leads to greater white-matter integrity, especially in the uncinate fasciculus (Schaeffer et al. 2014) and the superior longitudinal fasciculus (Krafft et al. 2014). These two tracts are fundamental networks involved in connecting the limbic system and the prefrontal cortex, and the temporal and parietal lobes, respectively. Observational evidence corroborates these findings, with noticeable white-matter integrity differences among children of various fitness levels (Chaddock-Heyman et al. 2014).

Further dramatic neural changes can typically be observed in older populations. For example, exercise regimens can potentially alleviate age-related brain atrophy and loss of brain tissue density (Colcombe et al. 2003), and it has been suggested that such direct relationship might explain the correlation between indices of reported aerobic fitness and cognitive function, especially executive processes (Weinstein et al. 2012). This potential for exercise to counteract the effects of aging on the brain is particularly significant when considering that brain atrophy is associated with both normal cognitive decline (Kooistra et al. 2014) and dementia (Bilello et al. 2015). Higher fitness is also correlated with larger hippocampus (Weinstein et al. 2012) and cortical areas (Erickson et al. 2009; Makizako et al. 2015), findings that are consistent with experimental evidence based on training designs (Colcombe et al. 2006; Erickson et al. 2011; Ruscheweyh et al. 2011). Finally, physical fitness also correlates with long-term potentiation (LTP), assessed through changes in the N1b component of visual-evoked potentials (Smallwood et al. 2015), suggesting that physical exercise may have a direct impact on human LTP.

2.3 Cognitive and Behavioral Improvements

Directly in line with the functional and structural changes previously described, individuals showing better self-reported fitness also tend to outperform less fit individuals on measures of executive functions and of spatial reasoning (Colcombe and Kramer 2003; Hillman, Erickson, and Kramer 2008). Some studies have suggested that the relationship between physical exercise and cognitive performance may be restricted to executive function tasks, at least in older adults (e.g., Kramer, Hahn, and Gopher 1999), yet broader literature would suggest that this link goes well beyond executive functions, with a wide range of cognitive abilities being associated with physical exercise habits and fitness indices. These include perceptual and spatial abilities, both fundamental to many of our day-to-day activities (see, for a review, Moreau and Conway 2013).

Adding to this line of research, complementary studies have sought to identify causal relationships between exercising and cognitive outcomes. For example, exercise interventions have been shown to improve attention in children with developmental coordination disorders (Tsai, Wang, and Tseng 2012) and in individuals with attention-deficit/hyperactivity disorder (ADHD, Archer and Kostrzewa 2012). Perhaps even more remarkable, a training intervention by Davis and colleagues found dose-response benefits of exercise on executive functions and mathematics achievement (2007). This finding is corroborated by other studies, which have found an association between physical fitness and both mathematics and reading achievement (Castelli et al. 2007), as well as between physical activity and overall academic grades (Coe et al. 2006). These studies reflect a general trend showing consistent associations between physical exercise, physical activity, fitness indices, and academic achievement (Donnelly et al. 2016; Keeley and Fox 2009).

Physical exercise is also associated with lower risks for mental and neurological conditions. A review by Penedo and Dahn (2005) found that many conditions, among them autism, ADHD, schizophrenia, dementia, and Alzheimer's disease, appear to benefit from exercise interventions, and poor physical fitness tends to exacerbates their associated symptoms. Consistent with the findings reported in this review, studies of older populations have found that exercise is linked to emotional stability (Blumenthal et al. 1991), better associative learning (Fabre et al. 2002), and improved cognition (Cancela Carral and Ayán Pérez 2007). We should point out, however, that the direct influence of exercise interventions in older people without cognitive impairment was recently questioned in a meta-analysis by the Cochrane Collaboration, which found "no evidence in the available data from RCTs that aerobic physical activities, including those which successfully improve cardiorespiratory fitness, have any cognitive benefit in cognitively healthy older adults" (Young et al. 2015, abstract). Because physical exercise interventions encompass a wide, often disparate range of training regimens, this finding highlights the need to further specify which interventions are the most effective to elicit robust and meaningful cognitive changes.

3 Learning and Synaptogenesis

One aspect that is often left out when seeking cognitive enhancement via physical exercise is the role of learning. As we have alluded to in the previous section, the human brain can produce up to tens of thousands of new cells every day, a process facilitated by physical exercise. Many of these, however, die out within a few weeks (Gould et al. 1999). This process may seem wasteful, yet it ensures that new cells are available when needed. Undoubtedly, physical exercise is a critical factor in the genesis of neural cells, but these are different from functional neurons. Many of these new cells may never mature into functional neurons, unless the right conditions are in place for their development. In particular, cell survival requires neurons to make contact with one another, a process called synaptogenesis, which is largely enhanced when physical exercise is accompanied by learning (Gould et al. 1999; Leuner et al. 2004). Thus, targeting cognitive enhancement based solely on physical exercise appears to be insufficient. An optimal solution may reside in combination with effortful learning, as we discuss hereafter.

3.1 Core Mechanisms and Function

In the adult human brain, many of the new neurons are generated in the hippocampus, a brain structure associated with various components of learning. Such localized process suggests that certain aspects of hippocampal-dependent learning can greatly benefit from a pool of continuously renewed neurons. Interestingly, the beneficial aspect of hippocampal neurogenesis was questioned a few decades ago by Pasko Rakic, who hypothesized that adult neurogenesis was not found in the primate brain for the purpose of network stability (Rakic 1985). Known as the stability-plasticity dilemma, his postulate was based on the assumption that systems that emphasize plasticity will learn easily, but storage will be compromised. At the other end of what can be thought of as a continuum, systems that favor stability can maintain information for a long time, but at the detriment of novel learning. Therefore, it follows that different systems may favor different positions on the stability-plasticity continuum, and Rakic's argument against adult neurogenesis was based on the idea that new neurons would be too disruptive to network stability in humans. Although plausible, this hypothesis has since been discarded, and neurogenesis is now thought of as part of the solution to the stability-plasticity dilemma, rather than as a fundamental problem irreconcilable with the notion of neurogenesis (Kempermann, Wiskott, and Gage 2004).

Provided that, over time, evolution has favored a plentiful supply of neurons in the hippocampus to facilitate learning (Amrein and Lipp 2009), it seems plausible that the act of learning itself would favor neuron survival. Note that these two processes operate on substantially different timescales, and therefore that the direct effect of learning on neuron survival needed experimental validation. More than fifteen years ago, Gould and colleagues provided that missing link. They reported that new neurons in the hippocampus of adult rodents could be rescued from death by learning and that new hippocampal neurons were involved in memory formation (Gould et al. 1999). Subsequent experiments have consistently demonstrated that not all types of learning are created equal when it comes to neuron survival (Curlik and Shors 2011; Waddell, Anderson, and Shors 2011): specific components appear to be critical in this complex process.

3.2 Enhancing Cell Survival via Effortful Learning

Research with animal models indicates that learning that depends on the hippocampus, such as conditioning or spatial navigation tasks, tend to increase neuron survival (Anderson et al. 2011). This is consistent with the idea that most new neurons originate in the hippocampus (Praag et al. 2002), although additional findings indicate that neuron survival can sometimes be dissociated from hippocampal involvement (Shors 2014). Together, this line of work suggests that effort might be the common feature in all tasks that favor neuron survival—difficulty forces neural adaptations in order to cope with new demands. The underlying rationale is that the neural system needs to be stressed up to a point where it needs additional resources (e.g., new neurons) to perform adequately. Interestingly, this rationale is also consistent with behavioral studies in humans, which have found that training on complex tasks offering sustained difficulty induces greater cognitive improvements than less complex regimens (e.g., Moreau, Morrison, and Conway 2015).

Moreover, individuals who find tasks more difficult and therefore need more time to reach a given level of performance rescue more neurons from death than those who reach that same level of performance easily (Nokia et al. 2012). Importantly, this is predicated on the fact that the individual is continuously learning (Curlik and Shors 2011). This is interesting because it suggests that effortful learning might mitigate initial disparities, by reducing gaps and differences. Once new neurons have been rescued from death, they can remain in the hippocampus several months (Curlik and Shors 2013). These neurons are also functional, which means that they have made contact with other neurons and can produce action potentials (Praag et al. 2002). The idea that learning can favor neuron survival has influenced research in many areas, including in the recent field of cognitive training.

3.3 Cognitive Training

Stemming from studies in the field of neurogenesis, the rationale for cognitive training is rather straightforward. Generally, training cognition involves focused, often repetitive, practice of a single or a set of cognitive tasks. What differentiates this form of training from typical learning following deliberate practice (Ericsson et al. 1993) is that in the case of cognitive training the regimen is designed to elicit improvements in other, different tasks (i.e., transfer). That this form of training leads to improvements in the ability or abilities targeted (near-transfer) is commonly accepted, even by skeptics of this approach (e.g., Harrison et al. 2013), provided adequate training design. Such improvements have also been correlated with functional and structural changes in the brain, for example regarding connectivity in the frontoparietal network (Caeyenberghs et al. 2016). What remains a matter of discussion, however, is the potential for such regimens to elicit substantial improvements outside of the trained abilities, particularly in ecological situations. Early findings of transfer (Jaeggi et al. 2008, 2014; Rudebeck et al. 2012) have failed to replicate in several subsequent studies (Redick et al. 2013; Thompson et al. 2013), resulting in some degree of skepticism over the validity of the rationale (Melby-Lervåg and Hulme 2013; Moreau and Conway 2014). In this context, more recent studies have emphasized the need to understand the underlying mechanisms of such discrepancies (Jaeggi et al. 2014; Moreau, Kirk, and Waldie 2016; Moreau 2014), so as to offer better, more potent interventions (Moreau and Waldie 2016).

4 Movement, Learning, and Cognition across the Lifespan

One particular approach that has shown promise is based on movement. Arguably, the recent surge of studies in the field of cognitive training has largely left out decades of research linking physical exercise and cognitive enhancement. Based on the current understanding of the underlying mechanisms mediating this relationship, such segregation seems unwise. Beyond a mere juxtaposition of research paradigms, and in order to understand the added value of situations involving complex motor coordination, it is helpful to describe the role of movement across the lifespan. We illustrate the relevance of this line of research to cognitive training in the following discussion.

4.1 Movement and Early Learning

Three long-standing lines of research and inquiry have focused on cognitive development: psychologists have concentrated on children's mental development, physical educators have observed and assessed the development and maturation of fundamental movement skills, and teachers have created pedagogical approaches to maximize learning. For over a century, considerable theoretical advances have been made within each of these areas; however, until recently, relatively little cross-disciplinary discussions have emerged. Currently, several researchers have emphasized the importance of understanding how cognitive development may be explained in terms of the interplay among these three lines of inquiry (Pesce et al. 2016).

The mental world of the infant has long intrigued parents and scientists alike. William James, who influenced the emergence of modern psychology, considered infancy to be a situation in which the baby's impression of the world was "one great blooming, buzzing confusion" (James [1890] 1981, 462). Modern research has revealed that James's view of infancy may not be entirely accurate; rather, as expressed by the influential developmental psychologist Esther Thelen, "The foundations of complex human thought and behavior have their origins in action and are always embedded in a history of acting" (Thelen 2004, 49). Infant learning is grounded in action that provides information concerning the infant's movements in space. Sensory experiences that occur with movement provide the bases of learning via action and perception.

During reaching movements, the infant's neural networks develop that later provide the basis for self-generated arm movements that provide viable solutions to task demands. Self-initiated responses reflect the biomechanics of the body, speed, and force of the action, and of environmental conditions presented at a particular point in time (Spencer et al. 2006). The contraction and lengthening of skeletal muscle build and refine neural networks that serve as the building blocks of skilled movement. These emerging networks also receive input from multiple sensory systems that provide information concerning the location of objects in the infant's world. Early research by Thelen and her colleagues demonstrated that the integration of sensory information from skeletal muscles and other systems is critical for infants' normal cognitive development (Thelen 1995). Indeed, children who lack sufficient interactions with their environment may fail to acquire the predictive control of actions that is vital for meeting the challenges faced during the first few years of life. For example, children with pervasive developmental delay (e.g., the autism spectrum) often show deficits in many areas of daily-life functioning (clumsiness, poor language, inappropriate social behavior). For these children, mental development may be supported by engaging in physical activities that lead to the generation of novel physical actions, thus favoring successful problem solving.

4.2 Movement and Executive Functions

The observation that young children diagnosed with autism and other developmental disorders often show poor motor coordination, high movement variability, and difficulty in predicting the sensory consequences of actions led several researchers in the fields of psychology (Diamond 2000) and motor development (Ben-Soussan, Glicksohn, and Berkovich-Ohana 2015) to consider the neurological development of the central nervous system: in particular, the emerging relation between the cerebellum and prefrontal cortex. Diamond's influential paper summarized existing neurophysiological evidence for a close interrelationship between the developing prefrontal cortex and the cerebellum (Diamond 2000). The cerebellum, because of its role in the control of discrete, rapid movements, was long considered to be involved primarily in motor skills. Similarly, the prefrontal cortex was viewed to be involved primarily in complex cognitive processes. Developmental neurophysiological evidence, however, suggests that bidirectional communication between the dorsolateral cortex and cerebellum via connection in the basal ganglia is critical for both executive processing and motor control. While the specific role of the relationship between cerebellum and prefrontal cortex has been debated (Leiner, Leiner, and Dow 1986, 1989, 1993), contemporary research in motor development tends to substantiate bidirectional views (Ben-Soussan et al. 2015).

The emergence of executive functions during early childhood has received considerable study and debate (Diamond 2013). During early childhood, children evidence changes in the ability to keep information in working memory, inhibit behaviors when appropriate, and to alternate actions when environmental conditions change. These behaviors are taken to reflect the emergence of the basic components of executive functions: updating, inhibition, and switching (Miyake et al. 2000). As addressed above, brain imaging studies reveal that specific neural prefrontal networks in the prefrontal cortex are established and circuitry with other brain structures is developed during childhood. Given the nature of executive functions, the cognitive-motor linkages between the dorsolateral prefrontal cortex and the cerebellum are essential. Executive control requires timed motor coordination and movement control when a child is faced with the need to allocate attention to a new task, when task conditions change, and when rapid actions are needed (Diamond 2000). Executive functions are particularly important when children encounter novel conditions that promote learning. Through planned actions, children experience and store the memories of their actions, the consequences of the actions, and the context in which the actions occurred. For these reasons, play, games, and sports provide unique contexts to promote mental development and learning.

4.3 Movement and Cognition beyond Development

Beside its impact on cognitive development, movement also has important implications across the lifespan. In particular, recent research in the field of embodied cognition has underlined the fundamental aspect our bodies, actions, and movements play in shaping cognition, and how action and cognition are inherently intertwined (Barsalou 2008; Gallese and Sinigaglia 2011; Glenberg 2010).

This interrelation has been studied in various contexts. For example, it has been demonstrated that expertise in a particular motor skill is typically associated with enhanced performance on a range of motor processing tasks (Güldenpenning et al. 2011), but also with other abilities outside the motor domain. These include cognitive abilities such as working memory capacity and spatial ability (Lehmann and Jansen 2012; Moreau 2012a, 2013), but also language (Holt and Beilock 2006), a skill thought to be removed from so-called lower-order motor mechanisms until recently.

The notion that the motor system is involved in many cognitive processes is further supported by research on the mirror system. Mirror neurons fire both when one performs an action and when one observes the same action being performed (Rizzolatti and Craighero 2004). This bidirectional neural mechanism has been put forward to explain our capacity to learn by observation and imitation (Oztop, Kawato, and Arbib 2006), and has been proposed as a central component mediating the influence of motor simulation to shape representations in the motor system (Jeannerod 2001). Indeed, motor simulation allows control over malleable motor representations, in the absence of overt movement (Jeannerod and Decety 1995), and motor actions allows alterations in the mental representations of movement (de Lange, Roelofs, and Toni 2008), therefore emphasizing the interdependent relationship between imagery and movement.

In addition, the mirror system has been established as a fundamental pillar of our ability to understand others' actions (Gallese 1998), and thus of our ability to navigate in social contexts (Schulkin 2000). Although it should be mentioned that the influence of the mirror system might have been exaggerated in some instances (Hickok 2009), the basic mechanisms underlying the relationship between action and cognition remain largely informative, especially for understanding the consequences of movement on human cognitive abilities. Together, this body of work supports the idea that motor actions ground mental representation in action (Beilock and Goldin-Meadow 2010), and therefore that movement itself is central to cognition. That is not to say that all cognition is embodied, as it cannot be excluded that some forms of thinking have evolved to be disembodied (Dove 2010), but it suggests that the role of movement in shaping and maintaining cognitive abilities cannot be dismissed and, more importantly, should be capitalized on.

5 Movement-Based Interventions to Enhance Cognition

Several researchers have proposed that optimal enhancement could be achieved through a form of exercise that incorporates difficult and challenging tasks. Possibilities are numerous, but results have been particularly promising when complex motor learning is combined with exercise (Curlik et al. 2013; Moreau, Morrison, and Conway 2015; Tomporowski, Lambourne, and Okumura 2011). In this section, we describe the findings of intervention studies that have coupled physical and cognitive demands.

5.1 In Children

Two explanations for the relationship between exercise and children's mental functioning have been offered: one focused on a quantitative approach, with exercise interventions based primarily on considerations of intensity and duration, and another, more qualitative, approach that manipulates physical activity in terms of the type of exercise and the cognitive abilities involved during movement (Pesce 2012). Based on the assumption that exercise directly affects brain health (Hillman et al. 2008), the majority of randomized controlled trials have focused on the manipulation of "dosage" (i.e., frequency, duration, and intensity). In these studies, various forms of aerobic exercise have been utilized to bring about changes in physical fitness as measured by cardiorespiratory capacity. Central to the quantitative approach is the notion that gains in cognitive function obtained from chronic exercise training would decay with reductions of the level of exercise activities.

From a qualitative perspective, it has been argued that interventions should focus on physical activities that include planning and problem solving, such as those involved in games or sport (Pesce 2012; Tomporowski et al. 2015). Through movement, it is hypothesized, individuals acquire knowledge about the actions that were performed, the consequences of those actions, and their context. Central to the qualitative approach is the assumption that executive functions can be enhanced with practice and experience, and that gains obtained from physical activity performed in complex environments will be maintained even as physical activity levels decline. Support for the benefits of mentally engaging physical activity interventions on cognitive function and learning has emerged over the past decade (Best 2010; Diamond and Lee 2011; Tomporowski et al. 2015). Drawing from contemporary motor-learning and rehabilitation research, greatest gains are achieved when tasks are based on the "optimal challenge point" hypothesis (Guadagnoli and Lee 2004), which posits that skill learning is facilitated when the skill level of the performer, the complexity of the task, and the task environment are taken into consideration. Convergent support comes from research that has examined the phenomena of contextual interference, which demonstrates superior motor and verbal learning when the order of training conditions are manipulated in ways that require an individual to vary the selection and execution of actions or mental processing from trial to trial (Tomporowski, McCullick, and Horvat 2010).

Maximizing the effects of physical activity interventions requires developing specific activities that are developmentally appropriate and cognitively and physically challenging, with target-specific outcome measures (Pesce 2012; Tomporowski et al. 2015). For example, younger children typically benefit from activities that are playful (Bjorklund and Brown 1998). Play includes activities that are freely chosen and intrinsically motivating and pleasurable. Children can engage in solitary play, parallel play, or cooperative play. During play, children are often engaged in make-believe and distortions of reality. As there are no exterior rules of play, children are provided the freedom to construct their own forms of reality. Play provides the opportunity to exercise and practice ways of physically and mentally altering the world. Children can construct, deconstruct, and reconstruct goal-directed activities (Scibinetti, Tocci, and Pesce 2011). Older children may benefit from game activities that are more structured and skill-based. As such, physical activity games are forms of competitive play characterized by established rules and set goals. Central to every game are challenges and obstacles to overcome. Indeed, successful games, whether they are video games, chess, or tag, are hallmarked by challenges that require very specific actions to be successful (Moreau 2015a; Tomporowski, McCullick, and Pesce 2015). As children's fundamental movement skills emerge, many children are introduced to sports, which are forms of competitive physical activity. Regardless of children's age, developmental level, and maturation, however, gains in cognitive outcomes hinge on involvement in sport or game conditions that place challenging, but manageable, problem-solving demands.

Successful interventions are characterized not only by the developmentally appropriate physical activity and exercise programs but also by the selection of outcome measures that are also developmentally appropriate and sensitive to change (Tomporowski 2009). The consensus drawn from recent comprehensive reviews of studies conducted with children, which examine the effects of chronic exercise and physical activity interventions on cognition and academic achievement, is that interventions influence specific mental process as opposed to exerting global widespread effects, such as general intelligence (Tomporowski, Naglieri, and Lambourne 2012).

5.2 In Young Adults

In contrast with early developmental stages, the potential for meaningful changes in the cognitive abilities of young adult populations was not fully recognized until recently. Young adults are usually thought to be at a cognitive peak (Salthouse and Davis 2006), thus leaving little room for improvement. Yet in recent years novel findings have shown that, although subtle, cognitive gains are still possible in adulthood. This line of work is rooted in decades of research showing the interrelation between motor processes and both spatial ability (Amorim, Isableu, and Jarraya 2006; Janczyk et al. 2012; Moreau 2012a; Steggemann, Engbert, and Weigelt 2011; Wraga et al. 2003) and working memory capacity (Moreau 2013), but also with language (Beilock et al. 2008), problem solving (Broaders et al. 2007), and reasoning (Beilock and Goldin-Meadow 2010; Cook, Mitchell, and Goldin-Meadow 2008). Corroborating evidence comes from studies of motor expertise, in which experts have been found to perform above average in assessments of perception (Wright et al. 2011), working memory capacity (Furley and Memmert 2010), attention (Memmert and Furley 2007), long-term memory (Dijkstra, MacMahon, and Misirlisoy 2008), and decision making (Raab and Johnson 2007).

Importantly, the implied directionality of these correlational findings has been confirmed by training studies, some of which have shown that forms of complex physical exercise trump more impoverished exercise workouts. Various approaches have been documented, including physical exercise, cognitive training, and hybrid forms of training (see, for a review, Moreau and Conway 2013). For example, wrestling, a sport that involves complex, unusual motor coordination, appears to elicit greater improvements in measures of spatial ability and working memory capacity than running, an activity largely automatized in adults (Moreau et al. 2012). We further replicated and extended these findings, with a training study that directly compared aerobic exercise, computerized cognitive training, and a hybrid condition we labeled *designed sport*, which combined high physical and cognitive demands in a single activity (Moreau, Morrison, and Conway 2015). Echoing the findings we described in the literature on children, we hypothesized that typical neurophysiological changes induced by exercise could be complemented by direct cognitive demands to maximize benefits. Not only did designed sport lead to larger cognitive gains in spatial ability and working memory capacity constructs, it also favored significant health improvements as measured by physiological markers such as resting heart rate and blood pressure. The holistic nature of these improvements confirmed our initial assumption: that is, complex motor activities are a potent way to elicit cognitive gains, with additional health benefits.

Crucially, one of the central points of this line of work is that designed sport can be adapted to individual affinities and demands, so that motivation and pleasure remain part of the equation. For example, there is extensive evidence that dance can be particularly well-adapted to cognitive training design, given the tremendous cognitive demands associated with the activity (Bläsing et al. 2012; Cross et al. 2013). Similarly, training simpler motor skills such as juggling has shown to induce gains in mental rotation performance (Lehmann and Jansen 2012), as does practicing sports or musical instruments, two types of activities including complex motor coordination (Moreau 2012b; Pietsch and Jansen 2012). Altogether, this body of evidence suggests that cognitive enhancement based on ecological activities might be preferable to so-called brain training programs, in the size and range of the effects (Moreau and Conway 2014).

5.3 In Older Adults

Because of the natural cognitive decline associated with age, older adult populations offer additional possibilities for enhancement. A large body of literature has looked at the impact of aerobic exercise interventions (Hertzog et al. 2008), for obvious reasons:

moderate-intensity exercise allows reducing risks of injury or cardiovascular complications, and such regimens are therefore more likely to obtain approval from medical and ethics boards. It is important to note, however, that the greater health safety of aerobic exercise interventions does not mean that they are the most suitable or the most optimal for everyone. When suitable, research to find alternative forms of exercise should be encouraged, so as to refine theoretical models of exercise-induced cognitive enhancement and to diversify the range of possibilities for consumers. Such studies are less common, but this body of work has been steadily growing over the past few years, and is expected to increase in the future.

Oftentimes, physical and cognitive components have been isolated and targeted in a sequential manner (Fabre et al. 2002; Legault et al. 2011; Oswald et al. 1996), with the advantages that implementation is typically easier, risks are restricted, and direct comparison of experimental conditions is more straightforward. Other forms of intervention have aimed at combining the two simultaneously (Eggenberger et al. 2015; Forte et al. 2013; Theill et al. 2013), with potential added improvements due to increased competition for cognitive resources. For example, a study by Eggenberger and colleagues found greater attention and working memory improvements after an intervention combining cognitive and physical components via distinct means than with physical exercise alone (Eggenberger et al. 2015).

Beyond the combination of separate tasks or activities, interventions that include adaptations of some form of complex motor activities have also been trialed, with encouraging results. For example, virtual reality videogames have been used to combine physical and cognitive training in single activities, setting the stage for a promising line of research (Pichierri et al. 2012; Pichierri, Murer, and de Bruin 2012).

Perhaps in a more ecological manner, a six-month dance intervention was found to enhance the cognitive performance of older adults, while no change was found in physiological markers of general health, thus suggesting that improvements were induced by motor demands, social engagement, or both, rather than by neurophysiological changes (Kattenstroth et al. 2013). Altogether, these findings are remarkably consistent with work in children (Pesce et al. 2016) and in young adults (Moreau, Morrison, and Conway 2015), further validating the rationale for a combined approach to maximize training outcomes (Moreau 2015a, 2015b).

6 Conclusion

The use of complex motor activities to enhance cognition is an exciting field of research with encouraging new developments. We have highlighted, throughout this chapter, some of the areas that have shown promising findings and applications. Although not exhaustive, the literature discussed herein provides solid grounds for understanding the mechanisms and the potential of this line of work.

We would like to leave the reader with a few thoughts, in the hope that these can stir the field in what we believe are interesting directions. First, it should be noted that blending training contents has potent implications, but also comes with challenges—it typically blurs the respective contribution of a given factor in an experimental design (Moreau, Kirk, and Waldie 2016). This in itself is not a valid argument against combinations of training regimens, but it emphasizes the need for additional research to correctly identify the underlying mechanisms and interactions of training-induced improvements. Research in this area will benefit from both tightly controlled but impoverished laboratory experiments and more-ecological but noisy interventions.

Second, whenever considering the implications of this line of research to society, one needs to consider opportunity costs, that is, what could I have done, as an individual, instead of training on a particular regimen. Not unlike current practices in pharmaceutical trials, where novel treatments need to demonstrate superiority over a placebo and over current drugs, if a given cognitive training program appears to be less effective than an existing regimen, its relevance should be questioned. The point is not to discourage novel interventions, as variety is critical to offer approaches suited to a wide range of individuals.

Yet one of the problems associated with computerized forms of cognitive training is that, despite dismissive attitudes toward potential risks of non-pharmaceutical or non-invasive interventions, the cost of ineffectiveness is high—if training improvements do not transfer to real-life abilities, time spent on the training regimen is wasted, and no useful skill or physiological by-product can be noted. The use of complex motor activities as a means of enhancing cognition is therefore appealing in that side effects are rewarding in and of themselves—improved physiological markers, general health, self-esteem, or stress reduction are hardly minimal outcomes (see, for a review, Moreau and Conway 2013). From there, risks are extremely mitigated, as time and effort invested in a program or an activity are more likely to be rewarded.

A challenge that remains, nevertheless, concerns the personalization of cognitive interventions. We now understand that not everyone will benefit equally from a given regimen, if at all, and therefore that finding the right intervention for an individual requires precise knowledge of the underlying mechanisms of improvement. Once cognitive training is based on sound and testable theoretical grounds, one can then envision apprehending enhancement probabilistically, with transparent information available to each individual regarding the likelihood and projected size of improvement. This is possibly the next frontier in the field of cognitive enhancement—individualized, dynamic, and information-rich content, so as to offer optimal interventions for everyone, at all times, in light of all the evidence available.

References

Amorim, Michel-Ange, Brice Isableu, and Mohamed Jarraya. 2006. "Embodied Spatial Transformations: 'Body Analogy' for the Mental Rotation of Objects." *Journal of Experimental Psychology: General* 135 (3): 327–347. doi:10.1037/0096-3445.135.3.327.

Amrein, Irmgard, and Hans-Peter Lipp. 2009. "Adult Hippocampal Neurogenesis of Mammals: Evolution and Life History." *Biology Letters* 5 (1): 141–144. doi:10.1098/rsbl.2008.0511.

Anderson, Megan L., Helene M. Sisti, Daniel M. Curlik II, and Tracey J. Shors. 2011. "Associative Learning Increases Adult Neurogenesis during a Critical Period." *European Journal of Neuroscience* 33 (1): 175–181. doi:10.1111/j.1460-9568.2010.07486.x.

Archer, Trevor, and Richard M. Kostrzewa. 2012. "Physical Exercise Alleviates ADHD Symptoms: Regional Deficits and Development Trajectory." *Neurotoxicity Research* 21 (2): 195–209. doi:10.1007/s12640-011-9260-0.

Arsenijevic, Yvan, and Samuel Weiss. 1998. "Insulin-Like Growth Factor-I Is a Differentiation Factor for Postmitotic CNS Stem Cell-Derived Neuronal Precursors: Distinct Actions from Those of Brain-Derived Neurotrophic Factor." *Journal of Neuroscience* 18 (6): 2118–2128.

Au, J., E. Sheehan, N. Tsai, G. J. Duncan, M. Buschkuehl, and S. M. Jaeggi. 2014. "Improving Fluid Intelligence with Training on Working Memory: A Meta-analysis." *Psychonomic Bulletin & Review* 22 (2): 366–377. http://doi.org/10.3758/s13423-014-0699-x.

Barsalou, Lawrence W. 2008. "Grounded Cognition." *Annual Review of Psychology* 59:617–645. doi:10.1146/annurev.psych.59.103006.093639.

Beilock, S. L., and S. Goldin-Meadow. 2010. "Gesture Changes Thought by Grounding It in Action." *Psychological Science* 21 (11): 1605–1610. doi:10.1177/0956797610385353.

Beilock, Sian L., Ian M. Lyons, Andrew Mattarella-Micke, Howard C. Nusbaum, and Steven L. Small. 2008. "Sports Experience Changes the Neural Processing of Action Language." *Proceedings of the National Academy of Sciences of the United States of America* 105 (36): 13269–13273. doi:10.1073/pnas.0803424105.

Ben-Soussan, Tal Dotan, Joseph Glicksohn, and Aviva Berkovich-Ohana. 2015. "From Cerebellar Activation and Connectivity to Cognition: A Review of the Quadrato Motor Training." *BioMed Research International* 2015 (October): 954901. doi:10.1155/2015/954901.

Berchtold, Nicole C., J. Patrick Kesslak, Christian J. Pike, Paul A. Adlard, and Carl W. Cotman. 2001. "Estrogen and Exercise Interact to Regulate Brain-Derived Neurotrophic Factor mRNA and Protein Expression in the Hippocampus." *European Journal of Neuroscience* 14 (12): 1992–2002.

Best, John R. 2010. "Effects of Physical Activity on Children's Executive Function: Contributions of Experimental Research on Aerobic Exercise." *Developmental Review* 30 (4): 331–551.

Bilello, Michel, Jimit Doshi, S. Ali Nabavizadeh, Jon B. Toledo, Guray Erus, Sharon X. Xie, John Q. Trojanowski, Xiaoyan Han, and Christos Davatzikos. 2015. "Correlating Cognitive Decline with White Matter Lesion and Brain Atrophy Magnetic Resonance Imaging Measurements in Alzheimer's Disease." *Journal of Alzheimer's Disease* 48 (4): 987–994. doi:10.3233/JAD-150400.

Bjorklund, D. F., and R. D. Brown. 1998. "Physical Play and Cognitive Development: Integrating Activity, Cognition, and Education." *Child Development* 69 (3): 604–606.

Black, J. E., K. R. Isaacs, B. J. Anderson, A. A. Alcantara, and W. T. Greenough. 1990. "Learning Causes Synaptogenesis, Whereas Motor Activity Causes Angiogenesis, in Cerebellar Cortex of Adult Rats." *Proceedings of the National Academy of Sciences of the United States of America* 87 (14): 5568–5572.

Bläsing, Bettina, Beatriz Calvo-Merino, Emily S. Cross, Corinne Jola, Juliane Honisch, and Catherine J. Stevens. 2012. "Neurocognitive Control in Dance Perception and Performance." *Acta Psychologica* 139 (2): 300–308. doi:10.1016/j.actpsy.2011.12.005.

Blumenthal, J. A., C. F. Emery, D. J. Madden, S. Schniebolk, M. Walsh-Riddle, L. K. George, D. C. McKee, M. B. Higginbotham, F. R. Cobb, and R. E. Coleman. 1991. "Long-Term Effects of Exercise on Psychological Functioning in Older Men and Women." *Journal of Gerontology* 46 (6): P352–361.

Boström, Pontus, Jun Wu, Mark P. Jedrychowski, Anisha Korde, Li Ye, James C. Lo, Kyle A. Rasbach, et al. 2012. "A PGC1-α-Dependent Myokine That Drives Brown-Fat-like Development of White Fat and Thermogenesis." *Nature* 481 (7382): 463–468. doi:10.1038/nature10777.

Broaders, Sara C., Susan Wagner Cook, Zachary Mitchell, and Susan Goldin-Meadow. 2007. "Making Children Gesture Brings out Implicit Knowledge and Leads to Learning." *Journal of Experimental Psychology: General* 136 (4): 539–550. doi:10.1037/0096-3445.136.4.539.

Caeyenberghs, Karen, Claudia Metzler-Baddeley, Sonya Foley, and Derek K. Jones. 2016. "Dynamics of the Human Structural Connectome Underlying Working Memory Training." *Journal of Neuroscience* 36 (14): 4056–4066. doi:10.1523/JNEUROSCI.1973-15.2016.

Cancela Carral, J. M., and Carlos Ayán Pérez. 2007. "Effects of High-Intensity Combined Training on Women over 65." *Gerontology* 53 (6): 340–346.

Castelli, Darla M., Charles H. Hillman, Sarah M. Buck, and Heather E. Erwin. 2007. "Physical Fitness and Academic Achievement in Third- and Fifth-Grade Students." *Journal of Sport and Exercise Psychology* 29 (2): 239–252.

Chaddock-Heyman, Laura, Kirk I. Erickson, Joseph L. Holtrop, Michelle W. Voss, Matthew B. Pontifex, Lauren B. Raine, Charles H. Hillman, and Arthur F. Kramer. 2014. "Aerobic Fitness Is Associated with Greater White Matter Integrity in Children." *Frontiers in Human Neuroscience* 8 (August): 584. doi:10.3389/fnhum.2014.00584.

Chaddock-Heyman, Laura, Kirk I. Erickson, Michelle W. Voss, Anya M. Knecht, Matthew B. Pontifex, Darla M. Castelli, Charles H. Hillman, and Arthur F. Kramer. 2013. "The Effects of Physical

Activity on Functional MRI Activation Associated with Cognitive Control in Children: A Randomized Controlled Intervention." *Frontiers in Human Neuroscience* 7 (March): 72. doi:10.3389/fnhum.2013.00072.

Chen, Dillon Y., Sarah A. Stern, Ana Garcia-Osta, Bernadette Saunier-Rebori, Gabriella Pollonini, Dhananjay Bambah-Mukku, Robert D. Blitzer, and Cristina M. Alberini. 2011. "A Critical Role for IGF-II in Memory Consolidation and Enhancement." *Nature* 469 (7331): 491–497. doi:10.1038/nature09667.

Coe, Dawn Podulka, James M. Pivarnik, Christopher J. Womack, Mathew J. Reeves, and Robert M. Malina. 2006. "Effect of Physical Education and Activity Levels on Academic Achievement in Children." *Medicine and Science in Sports and Exercise* 38 (8): 1515–1519. doi:10.1249/01.mss.0000227537.13175.1b.

Colcombe, Stanley, and Arthur F. Kramer. 2003. "Fitness Effects on the Cognitive Function of Older Adults: A Meta-Analytic Study." *Psychological Science* 14 (2): 125–130.

Colcombe, Stanley J., Kirk I. Erickson, Naftali Raz, Andrew G. Webb, Neal J. Cohen, Edward McAuley, and Arthur F. Kramer. 2003. "Aerobic Fitness Reduces Brain Tissue Loss in Aging Humans." *Journals of Gerontology A: Biological Sciences and Medical Sciences* 58 (2): 176–180.

Colcombe, Stanley J., Kirk I. Erickson, Paige E. Scalf, Jenny S. Kim, Ruchika Prakash, Edward McAuley, Steriani Elavsky, David X. Marquez, Liang Hu, and Arthur F. Kramer. 2006. "Aerobic Exercise Training Increases Brain Volume in Aging Humans." *Journals of Gerontology A: Biological Sciences and Medical Sciences* 61 (11): 1166–1170.

Cook, Susan Wagner, Zachary Mitchell, and Susan Goldin-Meadow. 2008. "Gesturing Makes Learning Last." *Cognition* 106 (2): 1047–1058. doi:10.1016/j.cognition.2007.04.010.

Cotman, Carl W., and Nicole C. Berchtold. 2002. "Exercise: A Behavioral Intervention to Enhance Brain Health and Plasticity." *Trends in Neurosciences* 25 (6): 295–301.

Cross, Emily S., Waltraud Stadler, Jim Parkinson, Simone Schütz-Bosbach, and Wolfgang Prinz. 2013. "The Influence of Visual Training on Predicting Complex Action Sequences." *Human Brain Mapping* 34 (2): 467–486. doi:10.1002/hbm.21450.

Curlik, D. M. II, and T. J. Shors. 2013. "Training Your Brain: Do Mental and Physical (MAP) Training Enhance Cognition through the Process of Neurogenesis in the Hippocampus?" *Neuropharmacology* 64 (January): 506–514. doi:10.1016/j.neuropharm.2012.07.027.

Curlik, Daniel M. II, Lisa Y. Maeng, Prateek R. Agarwal, and Tracey J. Shors. 2013. "Physical Skill Training Increases the Number of Surviving New Cells in the Adult Hippocampus." *PLoS ONE* 8 (2): e55850. doi:10.1371/journal.pone.0055850.

Curlik, Daniel M. II, and Tracey J. Shors. 2011. "Learning Increases the Survival of Newborn Neurons Provided That Learning Is Difficult to Achieve and Successful." *Journal of Cognitive Neuroscience* 23 (9): 2159–2170. doi:10.1162/jocn.2010.21597.

Davis, Catherine L., Phillip D. Tomporowski, Colleen A. Boyle, Jennifer L. Waller, Patricia H. Miller, Jack A. Naglieri, and Mathew Gregoski. 2007. "Effects of Aerobic Exercise on Overweight

Children's Cognitive Functioning: A Randomized Controlled Trial." *Research Quarterly for Exercise and Sport* 78 (5): 510–519. doi:10.1080/02701367.2007.10599450.

Davis, Catherine L., Phillip D. Tomporowski, Jennifer E. McDowell, Benjamin P. Austin, Patricia H. Miller, Nathan E. Yanasak, Jerry D. Allison, and Jack A. Naglieri. 2011. "Exercise Improves Executive Function and Achievement and Alters Brain Activation in Overweight Children: A Randomized, Controlled Trial." *Health Psychology* 30 (1): 91–98. doi:10.1037/a0021766.

de Lange, Floris P., Karin Roelofs, and Ivan Toni. 2008. "Motor Imagery: A Window into the Mechanisms and Alterations of the Motor System." *Cortex: A Journal Devoted to the Study of the Nervous System and Behavior* 44 (5): 494–506. doi:10.1016/j.cortex.2007.09.002.

Diamond, A. 2000. "Close Interrelation of Motor Development and Cognitive Development and of the Cerebellum and Prefrontal Cortex." *Child Development* 71 (1): 44–56.

Diamond, Adele. 2013. "Executive Functions." *Annual Review of Psychology* 64: 135–168. doi:10.1146/annurev-psych-113011-143750.

Diamond, Adele, and Kathleen Lee. 2011. "Interventions Shown to Aid Executive Function Development in Children 4 to 12 Years Old." *Science* 333 (6045): 959–964. doi:10.1126/science.1204529.

Dijkstra, Katinka, Clare MacMahon, and Mine Misirlisoy. 2008. "The Effects of Golf Expertise and Presentation Modality on Memory for Golf and Everyday Items." *Acta Psychologica* 128 (2): 298–303. doi:10.1016/j.actpsy.2008.03.001.

Donnelly, Joseph E., Charles H. Hillman, Darla Castelli, Jennifer L. Etnier, Sarah Lee, Phillip Tomporowski, Kate Lambourne, and Amanda N. Szabo-Reed. 2016. "Physical Activity, Fitness, Cognitive Function, and Academic Achievement in Children: A Systematic Review." *Medicine and Science in Sports and Exercise* 48 (6): 1197–1222.

Dove, Guy. 2010. "On the Need for Embodied and Dis-Embodied Cognition." *Frontiers in Psychology* 1:242. doi:10.3389/fpsyg.2010.00242.

Eggenberger, Patrick, Vera Schumacher, Marius Angst, Nathan Theill, and Eling D. de Bruin. 2015. "Does Multicomponent Physical Exercise with Simultaneous Cognitive Training Boost Cognitive Performance in Older Adults? A 6-Month Randomized Controlled Trial with a 1-Year Follow-Up." *Clinical Interventions in Aging* 10 (August): 1335–1349. doi:10.2147/CIA.S87732.

Erickson, Kirk I., Ruchika S. Prakash, Michelle W. Voss, Laura Chaddock, Liang Hu, Katherine S. Morris, Siobhan M. White, Thomas R. Wójcicki, Edward McAuley, and Arthur F. Kramer. 2009. "Aerobic Fitness Is Associated with Hippocampal Volume in Elderly Humans." *Hippocampus* 19 (10): 1030–1039. doi:10.1002/hipo.20547.

Erickson, Kirk I., Michelle W. Voss, Ruchika Shaurya Prakash, Chandramallika Basak, Amanda Szabo, Laura Chaddock, Jennifer S. Kim, et al. 2011. "Exercise Training Increases Size of Hippocampus and Improves Memory." *Proceedings of the National Academy of Sciences of the United States of America* 108 (7): 3017–3022. doi:10.1073/pnas.1015950108.

Ericsson, K. Anders, Ralf T. Krampe, and Clemens Tesch-Römer. 1993. "The Role of Deliberate Practice in the Acquisition of Expert Performance." *Psychological Review* 100 (3): 363–406.

Fabre, C., K. Chamari, P. Mucci, J. Massé-Biron, and C. Préfaut. 2002. "Improvement of Cognitive Function by Mental and/or Individualized Aerobic Training in Healthy Elderly Subjects." *International Journal of Sports Medicine* 23 (6): 415–421. doi:10.1055/s-2002-33735.

Ferris, Lee T., James S. Williams, and Chwan-Li Shen. 2007. "The Effect of Acute Exercise on Serum Brain-Derived Neurotrophic Factor Levels and Cognitive Function." *Medicine and Science in Sports and Exercise* 39 (4): 728–734. doi:10.1249/mss.0b013e31802f04c7.

Forte, Roberta, Colin A. G. Boreham, João Costa Leite, Giuseppe De Vito, Lorraine Brennan, Eileen R. Gibney, and Caterina Pesce. 2013. "Enhancing Cognitive Functioning in the Elderly: Multicomponent vs Resistance Training." *Clinical Interventions in Aging* 8 (January): 19–27. doi:10.2147/CIA.S36514.

Furley, Philip, and Daniel Memmert. 2010. "Differences in Spatial Working Memory as a Function of Team Sports Expertise: The Corsi Block-Tapping Task in Sport Psychological Assessment." *Perceptual and Motor Skills* 110 (3 Pt 1): 801–808. doi:10.2466/PMS.110.3.801-808.

Gallese, V. 1998. "Mirror Neurons and the Simulation Theory of Mind-Reading." *Trends in Cognitive Sciences* 2 (12): 493–501. doi:10.1016/S1364-6613(98)01262-5.

Gallese, Vittorio, and Corrado Sinigaglia. 2011. "What Is So Special about Embodied Simulation?" *Trends in Cognitive Sciences* 15 (11): 512–519. doi:10.1016/j.tics.2011.09.003.

Glenberg, Arthur M. 2010. "Embodiment as a Unifying Perspective for Psychology." *Wiley Interdisciplinary Reviews: Cognitive Science* 1 (4): 586–596. doi:10.1002/wcs.55.

Gould, E., A. Beylin, P. Tanapat, A. Reeves, and T. J. Shors. 1999. "Learning Enhances Adult Neurogenesis in the Hippocampal Formation." *Nature Neuroscience* 2 (3): 260–265. doi:10.1038/6365.

Gould, E., C. S. Woolley, M. Frankfurt, and B. S. McEwen. 1990. "Gonadal Steroids Regulate Dendritic Spine Density in Hippocampal Pyramidal Cells in Adulthood." *Journal of Neuroscience* 10 (4): 1286–1291.

Griffin, Éadaoin W., Sinéad Mullally, Carole Foley, Stuart A. Warmington, Shane M. O'Mara, and Aine M. Kelly. 2011. "Aerobic Exercise Improves Hippocampal Function and Increases BDNF in the Serum of Young Adult Males." *Physiology and Behavior* 104 (5): 934–941. doi:10.1016/j.physbeh.2011.06.005.

Guadagnoli, Mark A., and Timothy D. Lee. 2004. "Challenge Point: A Framework for Conceptualizing the Effects of Various Practice Conditions in Motor Learning." *Journal of Motor Behavior* 36 (2): 212–224. doi:10.3200/JMBR.36.2.212-224.

Güldenpenning, Iris, Dirk Koester, Wilfried Kunde, Matthias Weigelt, and Thomas Schack. 2011. "Motor Expertise Modulates the Unconscious Processing of Human Body Postures." *Experimental Brain Research* 213 (4): 383–391. doi:10.1007/s00221-011-2788-7.

Harrison, Tyler L., Zach Shipstead, Kenny L. Hicks, David Z. Hambrick, Thomas S. Redick, and Randall W. Engle. 2013. "Working Memory Training May Increase Working Memory Capacity but Not Fluid Intelligence." *Psychological Science* 24 (12): 2409–2419. doi:10.1177/0956797613492984.

Hertzog, Christopher, Arthur F. Kramer, Robert S. Wilson, and Ulman Lindenberger. 2008. "Enrichment Effects on Adult Cognitive Development: Can the Functional Capacity of Older Adults Be Preserved and Enhanced?" *Psychological Science in the Public Interest* 9 (1): 1–65. doi:10.1111/j.1539-6053.2009.01034.x.

Hickok, G. 2009. "Eight Problems for the Mirror Neuron Theory of Action Understanding in Monkeys and Humans." *Journal of Cognitive Neuroscience* 21 (7): 1229–1243. doi:10.1162/jocn.2009.21189.

Hillman, Charles H., Kirk I. Erickson, and Arthur F. Kramer. 2008. "Be Smart, Exercise Your Heart: Exercise Effects on Brain and Cognition." *Nature Reviews: Neuroscience* 9 (1): 58–65. doi:10.1038/nrn2298.

Hillman, Charles H., Matthew B. Pontifex, Darla M. Castelli, Naiman A. Khan, Lauren B. Raine, Mark R. Scudder, Eric S. Drollette, Robert D. Moore, Chien-Ting Wu, and Keita Kamijo. 2014. "Effects of the FITKids Randomized Controlled Trial on Executive Control and Brain Function." *Pediatrics* 134 (4): e1063–1071. doi:10.1542/peds.2013-3219.

Holt, Lauren E., and Sian L. Beilock. 2006. "Expertise and Its Embodiment: Examining the Impact of Sensorimotor Skill Expertise on the Representation of Action-Related Text." *Psychonomic Bulletin and Review* 13 (4): 694–701.

Hovik, Kjell Tore, Brit-Kari Saunes, Anne Kristine Aarlien, and Jens Egeland. 2013. "RCT of Working Memory Training in ADHD: Long-Term Near-Transfer Effects." *PLoS ONE* 8 (12): e80561. doi:10.1371/journal.pone.0080561.

Huat, Tee Jong, Amir Ali Khan, Soumya Pati, Zulkifli Mustafa, Jafri Malin Abdullah, and Hasnan Jaafar. 2014. "IGF-1 Enhances Cell Proliferation and Survival during Early Differentiation of Mesenchymal Stem Cells to Neural Progenitor-like Cells." *BMC Neuroscience* 15 (July): 91. doi:10.1186/1471-2202-15-91.

Jaeggi, Susanne M., Martin Buschkuehl, John Jonides, and Walter J. Perrig. 2008. "Improving Fluid Intelligence with Training on Working Memory." *Proceedings of the National Academy of Sciences of the United States of America* 105 (19): 6829–6833. doi:10.1073/pnas.0801268105.

Jaeggi, Susanne M., Martin Buschkuehl, John Jonides, and Priti Shah. 2011. "Short- and Long-Term Benefits of Cognitive Training." *Proceedings of the National Academy of Sciences of the United States of America* 108 (25): 10081–10086. doi:10.1073/pnas.1103228108.

Jaeggi, Susanne M., Martin Buschkuehl, Priti Shah, and John Jonides. 2014. "The Role of Individual Differences in Cognitive Training and Transfer." *Memory and Cognition* 42 (3): 464–480. doi:10.3758/s13421-013-0364-z.

James, W. [1890] 1981. *The Principles of Psychology*. Cambridge, MA: Harvard University Press.

Janczyk, Markus, Roland Pfister, Michael A. Crognale, and Wilfried Kunde. 2012. "Effective Rotations: Action Effects Determine the Interplay of Mental and Manual Rotations." *Journal of Experimental Psychology: General* 141 (3): 489–501.

Jeannerod, M. 2001. "Neural Simulation of Action: A Unifying Mechanism for Motor Cognition." *NeuroImage* 14 (1 Pt 2): S103–109. doi:10.1006/nimg.2001.0832.

Jeannerod, M., and J. Decety. 1995. "Mental Motor Imagery: A Window into the Representational Stages of Action." *Current Opinion in Neurobiology* 5 (6): 727–732.

Kamijo, Keita, Matthew B. Pontifex, Kevin C. O'Leary, Mark R. Scudder, Chien-Ting Wu, Darla M. Castelli, and Charles H. Hillman. 2011. "The Effects of an Afterschool Physical Activity Program on Working Memory in Preadolescent Children." *Developmental Science* 14 (5): 1046–1058. doi:10.1111/j.1467-7687.2011.01054.x.

Kattenstroth, Jan-Christoph, Tobias Kalisch, Stephan Holt, Martin Tegenthoff, and Hubert R. Dinse. 2013. "Six Months of Dance Intervention Enhances Postural, Sensorimotor, and Cognitive Performance in Elderly without Affecting Cardio-Respiratory Functions." *Frontiers in Aging Neuroscience* 5 (February): 5. doi:10.3389/fnagi.2013.00005.

Keeley, Thomas J. H., and Kenneth R. Fox. 2009. "The Impact of Physical Activity and Fitness on Academic Achievement and Cognitive Performance in Children." *International Review of Sport and Exercise Psychology* 2 (2): 198–214. doi:10.1080/17509840903233822.

Kempermann, Gerd, Laurenz Wiskott, and Fred H. Gage. 2004. "Functional Significance of Adult Neurogenesis." *Current Opinion in Neurobiology* 14 (2): 186–191. doi:10.1016/j.conb.2004.03.001.

Kooistra, Minke, Mirjam I. Geerlings, Yolanda van der Graaf, Willem P. T. M. Mali, Koen L. Vincken, L. Jaap Kappelle, Majon Muller, Geert Jan Biessels, and SMART-MR Study Group. 2014. "Vascular Brain Lesions, Brain Atrophy, and Cognitive Decline. The Second Manifestations of ARTerial Disease—Magnetic Resonance (SMART-MR) Study." *Neurobiology of Aging* 35 (1): 35–41. doi:10.1016/j.neurobiolaging.2013.07.004.

Krafft, Cynthia E., Nicolette F. Schwarz, Lingxi Chi, Abby L. Weinberger, David J. Schaeffer, Jordan E. Pierce, Amanda L. Rodrigue, et al. 2014. "An 8-Month Randomized Controlled Exercise Trial Alters Brain Activation during Cognitive Tasks in Overweight Children." *Obesity* 22 (1): 232–242. doi:10.1002/oby.20518.

Kramer, A. F., S. Hahn, and D. Gopher. 1999. "Task Coordination and Aging: Explorations of Executive Control Processes in the Task Switching Paradigm." *Acta Psychologica* 101 (2/3): 339–378.

Lampit, Amit, Harry Hallock, and Michael Valenzuela. 2014. "Computerized Cognitive Training in Cognitively Healthy Older Adults: A Systematic Review and Meta-Analysis of Effect Modifiers." *PLoS Medicine* 11 (11): e1001756. doi:10.1371/journal.pmed.1001756.

Legault, Claudine, Janine M. Jennings, Jeffrey A. Katula, Dale Dagenbach, Sarah A. Gaussoin, Kaycee M. Sink, Stephen R. Rapp, et al. 2011. "Designing Clinical Trials for Assessing the Effects of Cognitive Training and Physical Activity Interventions on Cognitive Outcomes: The Seniors

Health and Activity Research Program Pilot (SHARP-P) Study, a Randomized Controlled Trial." *BMC Geriatrics* 11 (May): 27. doi:10.1186/1471-2318-11-27.

Lehmann, Jennifer, and Petra Jansen. 2012. "The Influence of Juggling on Mental Rotation Performance in Children with Spina Bifida." *Brain and Cognition* 80 (2): 223–229. doi:10.1016/j.bandc.2012.07.004.

Leiner, H. C., A. L. Leiner, and R. S. Dow. 1986. "Does the Cerebellum Contribute to Mental Skills?" *Behavioral Neuroscience* 100 (4): 443–454.

Leiner, H. C., A. L. Leiner, and R. S. Dow. 1989. "Reappraising the Cerebellum: What Does the Hindbrain Contribute to the Forebrain?" *Behavioral Neuroscience* 103 (5): 998–1008.

Leiner, H. C., A. L. Leiner, and R. S. Dow. 1993. "The Role of the Cerebellum in the Human Brain." *Trends in Neurosciences* 16 (11): 453–454. doi:10.1016/0166-2236(93)90076-X.

Leuner, Bendetta, Sabrina Mendolia-Loffredo, Yevgenia Kozorovitskiy, Deanna Samburg, Elizabeth Gould, and Tracey J. Shors. 2004. "Learning Enhances the Survival of New Neurons beyond the Time When the Hippocampus Is Required for Memory." *Journal of Neuroscience* 24 (34): 7477–7481. doi:10.1523/JNEUROSCI.0204-04.2004.

Makizako, Hyuma, Teresa Liu-Ambrose, Hiroyuki Shimada, Takehiko Doi, Hyuntae Park, Kota Tsutsumimoto, Kazuki Uemura, and Takao Suzuki. 2015. "Moderate-Intensity Physical Activity, Hippocampal Volume, and Memory in Older Adults with Mild Cognitive Impairment." *Journals of Gerontology A: Biological Sciences and Medical Sciences* 70 (4): 480–486. doi:10.1093/gerona/glu136.

Melby-Lervåg, Monica, and Charles Hulme. 2013. "Is Working Memory Training Effective? A Meta-Analytic Review." *Developmental Psychology* 49 (2): 270–291. doi:10.1037/a0028228.

Memmert, Daniel, and Philip Furley. 2007. "'I Spy with My Little Eye!': Breadth of Attention, Inattentional Blindness, and Tactical Decision Making in Team Sports." *Journal of Sport and Exercise Psychology* 29 (3): 365–381.

Miyake, Akira, Naomi P. Friedman, Michael J. Emerson, Alexander H. Witzki, Amy Howerter, and Tor D. Wager. 2000. "The Unity and Diversity of Executive Functions and Their Contributions to Complex 'Frontal Lobe' Tasks: A Latent Variable Analysis." *Cognitive Psychology* 41 (1): 49–100. doi:10.1006/cogp.1999.0734.

Mora, Francisco, Gregorio Segovia, and Alberto del Arco. 2007. "Aging, Plasticity and Environmental Enrichment: Structural Changes and Neurotransmitter Dynamics in Several Areas of the Brain." *Brain Research Reviews* 55 (1): 78–88. doi:10.1016/j.brainresrev.2007.03.011.

Moreau, David. 2012a. "The Role of Motor Processes in Three-Dimensional Mental Rotation: Shaping Cognitive Processing via Sensorimotor Experience." *Learning and Individual Differences* 22 (3): 354–359.

Moreau, David. 2012b. "Training Spatial Ability: Comment on Pietsch and Jansen (2012) and Prospective Research Trends." *Learning and Individual Differences* 22 (6): 882–883. doi:10.1016/j.lindif.2012.07.006.

Moreau, David. 2013. "Motor Expertise Modulates Movement Processing in Working Memory." *Acta Psychologica* 142 (3): 356–361.

Moreau, David. 2014. "Making Sense of Discrepancies in Working Memory Training Experiments: A Monte Carlo Simulation." *Frontiers in Systems Neuroscience* 8 (September): 161. doi:10.3389/fnsys.2014.00161.

Moreau, David. 2015a. "Unreflective Actions? Complex Motor Skill Acquisition to Enhance Spatial Cognition." *Phenomenology and the Cognitive Sciences* 14 (2): 349–359. doi:10.1007/s11097-014-9376-9.

Moreau, David. 2015b. "Brains and Brawn: Complex Motor Activities to Maximize Cognitive Enhancement." *Educational Psychology Review* 27 (3): 475–482. doi:10.1007/s10648-015-9323-5.

Moreau, David, Jérome Clerc, Annie Mansy-Dannay, and Alain Guerrien. 2012. "Enhancing Spatial Ability through Sport Practice: Evidence for an Effect of Motor Training on Mental Rotation Performance." *Journal of Individual Differences* 33 (2): 83–88. doi:10.1027/1614-0001/a000075.

Moreau, David, and Andrew R. A. Conway. 2013. "Cognitive Enhancement: A Comparative Review of Computerized and Athletic Training Programs." *International Review of Sport and Exercise Psychology* 6 (1): 155–183. doi:10.1080/1750984X.2012.758763.

Moreau, David, and Andrew R. A. Conway. 2014. "The Case for an Ecological Approach to Cognitive Training." *Trends in Cognitive Sciences* 18 (7): 334–336. doi:10.1016/j.tics.2014.03.009.

Moreau, David, Ian J. Kirk, and Karen E. Waldie. 2016. "Seven Pervasive Statistical Flaws in Cognitive Training Interventions." *Frontiers in Human Neuroscience* 10 (April): 153.

Moreau, David, Alexandra B. Morrison, and Andrew R. A. Conway. 2015. "An Ecological Approach to Cognitive Enhancement: Complex Motor Training." *Acta Psychologica* 157 (May): 44–55. doi:10.1016/j.actpsy.2015.02.007.

Moreau, David, and Karen E. Waldie. 2016. "Developmental Learning Disorders: From Generic Interventions to Individualized Remediation." *Frontiers in Psychology* 6:2053. doi:10.3389/fpsyg.2015.02053.

Neeper, S. A., F. Gómez-Pinilla, J. Choi, and C. Cotman. 1995. "Exercise and Brain Neurotrophins." *Nature* 373 (6510): 109. doi:10.1038/373109a0.

Neeper, S. A., F. Gómez-Pinilla, J. Choi, and C. W. Cotman. 1996. "Physical Activity Increases mRNA for Brain-Derived Neurotrophic Factor and Nerve Growth Factor in Rat Brain." *Brain Research* 726 (1/2): 49–56.

Nokia, Miriam S., Helene M. Sisti, Monica R. Choksi, and Tracey J. Shors. 2012. "Learning to Learn: Theta Oscillations Predict New Learning, Which Enhances Related Learning and Neurogenesis." *PLoS ONE* 7 (2): e31375. doi:10.1371/journal.pone.0031375.

Oswald, W. D., R. Rupprecht, T. Gunzelmann, and K. Tritt. 1996. "The SIMA-Project: Effects of 1 Year Cognitive and Psychomotor Training on Cognitive Abilities of the Elderly." *Behavioural Brain Research* 78 (1): 67–72.

Oztop, Erhan, Mitsuo Kawato, and Michael Arbib. 2006. "Mirror Neurons and Imitation: A Computationally Guided Review." *Neural Networks* 19 (3): 254–271. doi:10.1016/j.neunet.2006.02.002.

Penedo, Frank J., and Jason R. Dahn. 2005. "Exercise and Well-Being: A Review of Mental and Physical Health Benefits Associated with Physical Activity." *Current Opinion in Psychiatry* 18 (2): 189–193.

Pesce, Caterina. 2012. "Shifting the Focus from Quantitative to Qualitative Exercise Characteristics in Exercise and Cognition Research." *Journal of Sport and Exercise Psychology* 34 (6): 766–786.

Pesce, Caterina, Ilaria Masci, Rosalba Marchetti, Spyridoula Vazou, Arja Sääkslahti, and Phillip D. Tomporowski. 2016. "Deliberate Play and Preparation Jointly Benefit Motor and Cognitive Development: Mediated and Moderated Effects." *Frontiers in Psychology* 7 (March): 349. doi:10.3389/fpsyg.2016.00349.

Pichierri, Giuseppe, Amos Coppe, Silvio Lorenzetti, Kurt Murer, and Eling D. de Bruin. 2012. "The Effect of a Cognitive-Motor Intervention on Voluntary Step Execution under Single and Dual Task Conditions in Older Adults: A Randomized Controlled Pilot Study." *Clinical Interventions in Aging* 7 (July): 175–184. doi:10.2147/CIA.S32558.

Pichierri, Giuseppe, Kurt Murer, and Eling D. de Bruin. 2012. "A Cognitive-Motor Intervention Using a Dance Video Game to Enhance Foot Placement Accuracy and Gait under Dual Task Conditions in Older Adults: A Randomized Controlled Trial." *BMC Geriatrics* 12 (December): 74. doi:10.1186/1471-2318-12-74.

Pietsch, Stefanie, and Petra Jansen. 2012/2. "Different Mental Rotation Performance in Students of Music, Sport and Education." *Learning and Individual Differences* 22 (1): 159–163. doi:10.1016/j.lindif.2011.11.012.

Praag, H., G. Kempermann, and F. H. Gage. 1999. "Running Increases Cell Proliferation and Neurogenesis in the Adult Mouse Dentate Gyrus." *Nature Neuroscience* 2 (3): 266–270. doi:10.1038/6368.

Praag, Henriette, Alejandro F. Schinder, Brian R. Christie, Nicolas Toni, Theo D. Palmer, and Fred H. Gage. 2002. "Functional Neurogenesis in the Adult Hippocampus." *Nature* 415 (6875): 1030–1034. doi:10.1038/4151030a.

Raab, Markus, and Joseph G. Johnson. 2007. "Expertise-Based Differences in Search and Option-Generation Strategies." *Journal of Experimental Psychology: Applied* 13 (3): 158–170. doi:10.1037/1076-898X.13.3.158.

Rakic, P. 1985. "Limits of Neurogenesis in Primates." *Science* 227 (4690): 1054–1056.

Redick, Thomas S., Zach Shipstead, Tyler L. Harrison, Kenny L. Hicks, David E. Fried, David Z. Hambrick, Michael J. Kane, and Randall W. Engle. 2013. "No Evidence of Intelligence Improvement after Working Memory Training: A Randomized, Placebo-Controlled Study." *Journal of Experimental Psychology: General* 142 (2): 359–379. doi:10.1037/a0029082.

Rizzolatti, Giacomo, and Laila Craighero. 2004. "The Mirror-Neuron System." *Annual Review of Neuroscience* 27:169–192. doi:10.1146/annurev.neuro.27.070203.144230.

Rudebeck, Sarah R., Daniel Bor, Angharad Ormond, Jill X. O'Reilly, and Andy C. H. Lee. 2012. "A Potential Spatial Working Memory Training Task to Improve Both Episodic Memory and Fluid Intelligence." *PLoS ONE* 7 (11): e50431. doi:10.1371/journal.pone.0050431.

Ruscheweyh, R., C. Willemer, K. Krüger, T. Duning, T. Warnecke, J. Sommer, K. Völker, et al. 2011. "Physical Activity and Memory Functions: An Interventional Study." *Neurobiology of Aging* 32 (7): 1304–1319. doi:10.1016/j.neurobiolaging.2009.08.001.

Russo-Neustadt, Amelia, Tony Ha, Ronald Ramirez, and J. Patrick Kesslak. 2001. "Physical Activity–Antidepressant Treatment Combination: Impact on Brain-Derived Neurotrophic Factor and Behavior in an Animal Model." *Behavioural Brain Research* 120 (1): 87–95.

Salthouse, Timothy A., and Hasker P. Davis. 2006. "Organization of Cognitive Abilities and Neuropsychological Variables across the Lifespan." *Developmental Review* 26 (1): 31–54. doi:10.1016/j.dr.2005.09.001.

Schaeffer, David J., Cynthia E. Krafft, Nicolette F. Schwarz, Lingxi Chi, Amanda L. Rodrigue, Jordan E. Pierce, Jerry D. Allison, et al. 2014. "An 8-Month Exercise Intervention Alters Frontotemporal White Matter Integrity in Overweight Children." *Psychophysiology* 51 (8): 728–733. doi:10.1111/psyp.12227.

Schmidt, Richard A., and Craig A. Wrisberg. 2008. *Motor Learning and Performance: A Situation-Based Learning Approach*. Champaign, IL: Human Kinetics.

Schmolesky, Matthew T., David L. Webb, and Rodney A. Hansen. 2013. "The Effects of Aerobic Exercise Intensity and Duration on Levels of Brain-Derived Neurotrophic Factor in Healthy Men." *Journal of Sports Science and Medicine* 12 (3): 502–511.

Schulkin, J. 2000. "Theory of Mind and Mirroring Neurons." *Trends in Cognitive Sciences* 4 (7): 252–254. doi:10.1016/S1364-6613(00)01500-X.

Scibinetti, Patrizia, Nicoletta Tocci, and Caterina Pesce. 2011. "Motor Creativity and Creative Thinking in Children: The Diverging Role of Inhibition." *Creativity Research Journal* 23 (3): 262–272.

Shipstead, Zach, Thomas S. Redick, and Randall W. Engle. 2012. "Is Working Memory Training Effective?" *Psychological Bulletin* 138 (4): 628–654. doi:10.1037/a0027473.

Shors, Tracey J. 2014. "The Adult Brain Makes New Neurons, and Effortful Learning Keeps Them Alive." *Current Directions in Psychological Science* 23 (5): 311–318. doi:10.1177/0963721414540167.

Smallwood, Nicola, Meg J. Spriggs, Christopher S. Thompson, Carolyn C. Wu, Jeff P. Hamm, David Moreau, and Ian J. Kirk. 2015. "Influence of Physical Activity on Human Sensory Long-Term Potentiation." *Journal of the International Neuropsychological Society* 21 (10): 831–840. doi:10.1017/S1355617715001095.

Spencer, John P., Melissa Clearfield, Daniela Corbetta, Beverly Ulrich, Patricia Buchanan, and Gregor Schöner. 2006. "Moving Toward a Grand Theory of Development: In Memory of Esther Thelen." *Child Development* 77 (6): 1521–1538. doi:10.1111/j.1467-8624.2006.00955.x.

Steggemann, Yvonne, Kai Engbert, and Matthias Weigelt. 2011. "Selective Effects of Motor Expertise in Mental Body Rotation Tasks: Comparing Object-Based and Perspective Transformations." *Brain and Cognition* 76 (1): 97–105. doi:10.1016/j.bandc.2011.02.013.

Stummer, W., K. Weber, B. Tranmer, A. Baethmann, and O. Kempski. 1994. "Reduced Mortality and Brain Damage after Locomotor Activity in Gerbil Forebrain Ischemia." *Stroke: A Journal of Cerebral Circulation* 25 (9): 1862–1869.

Theill, Nathan, Vera Schumacher, Rolf Adelsberger, Mike Martin, and Lutz Jäncke. 2013. "Effects of Simultaneously Performed Cognitive and Physical Training in Older Adults." *BMC Neuroscience* 14 (September): 103. doi:10.1186/1471-2202-14-103.

Thelen, E. 1995. "Motor Development: A New Synthesis." *American Psychologist* 50 (2): 79–95.

Thelen, Esther. 2004. "The Central Role of Action in Typical and Atypical Development." In *Movement and Action in Learning and Development*, 49–73. Amsterdam: Elsevier.

Thompson, Todd W., Michael L. Waskom, Keri-Lee A. Garel, Carlos Cardenas-Iniguez, Gretchen O. Reynolds, Rebecca Winter, Patricia Chang, et al. 2013. "Failure of Working Memory Training to Enhance Cognition or Intelligence." *PLoS ONE* 8 (5): e63614. doi:10.1371/journal.pone.0063614.

Tomporowski, Phillip D. 2009. "Methodological Issues: Research Approaches, Research Design, and Task Selection." In *Exercise and Cognitive Function*, 91–113. Hoboken, NJ: John Wiley and Sons.

Tomporowski, Phillip D., Kate Lambourne, and Michelle S. Okumura. 2011. "Physical Activity Interventions and Children's Mental Function: An Introduction and Overview." *Preventive Medicine* 52 (Suppl 1, June): S3–S9. doi:10.1016/j.ypmed.2011.01.028.

Tomporowski, Phillip D., Bryan A. McCullick, and Michael A. Horvat. 2010. "Role of Contextual Interference and Mental Engagement on Learning." In *Educational Games: Design, Learning, and Applications,* edited by F. Edvardsen and H. Kulle, 127–155. Hauppauge, NY: Nova Science.

Tomporowski, Phillip D., Bryan McCullick, Daniel M. Pendleton, and Caterina Pesce. 2015. "Exercise and Children's Cognition: The Role of Exercise Characteristics and a Place for Metacognition." *Journal of Sport and Health Science* 4 (1): 47–55. doi:10.1016/j.jshs.2014.09.003.

Tomporowski, Phillip, Bryan McCullick, and Catherine Pesce. 2015. *Enhancing Children's Cognition with Physical Activity Games*. Champaign. IL: Human Kinetics.

Tomporowski, Phillip D., Jack A. Naglieri, and Kate Lambourne. 2012. "20 Exercise Psychology and Children's Intelligence." In *The Oxford Handbook of Exercise Psychology*, edited by Edmund O. Acevedo, 409. Oxford: Oxford University Press.

Tsai, Chia-Liang, Chun-Hao Wang, and Yu-Ting Tseng. 2012. "Effects of Exercise Intervention on Event-Related Potential and Task Performance Indices of Attention Networks in Children with Developmental Coordination Disorder." *Brain and Cognition* 79 (1): 12–22. doi:10.1016/j.bandc.2012.02.004.

Vaynman, Shoshanna S., Zhe Ying, Dali Yin, and Fernando Gomez-Pinilla. 2006. "Exercise Differentially Regulates Synaptic Proteins Associated to the Function of BDNF." *Brain Research* 1070 (1): 124–130. doi:10.1016/j.brainres.2005.11.062.

Waddell, Jaylyn, Megan L. Anderson, and Tracey J. Shors. 2011. "Changing the Rate and Hippocampal Dependence of Trace Eyeblink Conditioning: Slow Learning Enhances Survival of New Neurons." *Neurobiology of Learning and Memory* 95 (2): 159–165. doi:10.1016/j.nlm.2010.09.012.

Weinstein, Andrea M., Michelle W. Voss, Ruchika Shaurya Prakash, Laura Chaddock, Amanda Szabo, Siobhan M. White, Thomas R. Wojcicki, et al. 2012. "The Association between Aerobic Fitness and Executive Function Is Mediated by Prefrontal Cortex Volume." *Brain, Behavior, and Immunity* 26 (5): 811–819. doi:10.1016/j.bbi.2011.11.008.

Winter, Bernward, Caterina Breitenstein, Frank C. Mooren, Klaus Voelker, Manfred Fobker, Anja Lechtermann, Karsten Krueger, et al. 2007. "High Impact Running Improves Learning." *Neurobiology of Learning and Memory* 87 (4): 597–609. doi:10.1016/j.nlm.2006.11.003.

Wraga, Maryjane, William L. Thompson, Nathaniel M. Alpert, and Stephen M. Kosslyn. 2003. "Implicit Transfer of Motor Strategies in Mental Rotation." *Brain and Cognition* 52 (2): 135–143.

Wright, M. J., D. T. Bishop, R. C. Jackson, and B. Abernethy. 2011. "Cortical fMRI Activation to Opponents' Body Kinematics in Sport-Related Anticipation: Expert-Novice Differences with Normal and Point-Light Video." *Neuroscience Letters* 500 (3): 216–221. doi:10.1016/j.neulet.2011.06.045.

Xu, Jiansong, Vince D. Calhoun, and Marc N. Potenza. 2015. "The Absence of Task-Related Increases in BOLD Signal Does Not Equate to Absence of Task-Related Brain Activation." *Journal of Neuroscience Methods* 240 (January): 125–127. doi:10.1016/j.jneumeth.2014.11.002.

Young, Jeremy, Maaike Angevaren, Jennifer Rusted, and Naji Tabet. 2015. "Aerobic Exercise to Improve Cognitive Function in Older People without Known Cognitive Impairment." *Cochrane Database of Systematic Reviews* 4 (April): CD005381. doi:10.1002/14651858.CD005381.pub4.

11 Neither Genes nor Deliberate Practice: An Embodied and Multidimensional Approach to Talent

Mirko Farina and Alberto Cei

1 Introduction

Since Francis Galton (1865) published his seminal papers on hereditary genius, which he subsequently expanded into the first book in the field of behavioral genetics, *Hereditary Genius: An Inquiry into Its Laws and Consequences* (Galton [1869] 1992), the issue of whether talent has any genetic basis has fascinated scholars, being at the forefront of discussions in many academic circles.

Galton (1865) famously argued that talent (both intellectual and physical) is an endowment that runs in families. His thesis was that "ability will out" regardless of the environment or, better, that heredity produces excellence in a certain area and that the environment may subsequently specify what that area shall be. In other words, Galton claimed that practice and training could improve performance, but believed that a ceiling to such performance existed for each person and that ceiling was determined—or at least very heavily influenced—by heritable characteristics. During the 150 years since Galton's first papers, his controversial ideas have thrived and inspired researchers in sport performance (for instance), who have looked at how genes and the environment interact in an attempt to answer the question of whether talent is born or made.

Our aim in this chapter is to analyze and discuss current understanding of the role of genes and environment in talent identification and acquisition of skill and expertise. In part 2, we review evidence for gene-centered approaches (Bouchard and Hoffman 2011; Montgomery and Safari 2007; Maes et al. 1996; Fox, Hershberger, and Bouchard Jr. 1996, among others) and subsequently point out a number of shortcomings affecting these research programs. These shortcomings lead us to explore (part 3) alternative ecological or environmentalist models (Ericsson, Krampe, and Tesch-Römer 1993; Ericsson 2006; Howe, Davidson, and Sloboda 1998) that have suggested that sport performance is constrained not by genetic factors but by engagement in deliberate practice and training during optimal periods of development.

We link this work in sport psychology with current research carried out on embodiment[1] in the philosophy of cognition (e.g., Clark 2008; Gallagher 2013; Christensen, Sutton, and McIlwain 2016) and show the profitable relations between these two research paradigms. After reviewing supporting evidence for ecological/environmentalist models, we point out a number of issues affecting radical environmentalist research (Tucker and Collins 2012; Hambrick et al. 2014; Duffy, Baluch, and Ericsson 2004) and reflect on the merits of these objections.

We then note (part 4) the need to develop a multidimensional model of talent identification (Baker et al. 2003, Baker 2007; Phillips et al. 2010; Vaeygens et al. 2008) and argue that this integrative account should fuse the best of both genetic and environmentalist research, while retaining a fully embodied perspective. We present two case studies (involving chess playing and Kenyan runners) to support our ideas. We conclude (part 7) by suggesting future research directions.

2 Talent and Skill: A Gene-Centered Perspective

Here we present a review of the contribution of genetic factors to sport performance and skill acquisition. One of the first and most comprehensive volumes aimed at investigating and explaining the contribution of genetic factors to fitness and physical performance was *Genetics of Fitness and Physical Performance* (Bouchard, Malina, and Pérusse 1997). This volume presented both the methods and the technologies available at the time for measuring the genetic basis of sophisticated human behaviors and summarized the evidence accumulated in the literature for the idea that fitness and performance traits are genetically determined.

Several other papers since the publication of that book have extended those results and provided more specific measures of heritability for different phenotypes related to sport performance. These include aerobic and anaerobic performance (Pérusse et al. 2000; Calvo et al. 2002), muscular endurance and strength (Beunen and Thomis 2004; Peeters et al. 2009), motor control and motor learning (Missitzi et al. 2013), and morphological (Silventoinen 2003), cardiac (Hong et al. 2001), and musculoskeletal characteristics (Collins and Raleigh 2009; Abney, McPeek, and Obner 2001).

Some researchers also investigated whether the process of transmission of phenotypic traits from parents to their offspring can determine a variation in response to training, thus testing the idea that inherited differences observed in performance do not arise uniquely from an inherited drive to train. Bouchard et al. (2011), for instance, put 473 sedentary volunteers through five months of training and measured their cardiorespiratory fitness levels before and after. As expected, most people improved their fitness level by average amounts. Specifically, 38 percent of the subjects involved in the testing improved it by between 300 and 500 ml/min. On both sides of this average response, however, extremes were found ("low responders," typically 7 percent, improved their fitness level by less than 100 ml/min, whereas "high responders," about 4 percent, improved by 800 ml/min to over 1,000 ml/min). Thus, while low responders improved their fitness level, on average, by 4 percent, high responders improved it by 40 percent. This means that researchers observed a maximum tenfold difference in adaptation to training in the pool of volunteers tested. This is a huge difference, which raises the obvious question of why, if we take a random sample of individuals and train them all the same way, we do not end up with everyone on the same level of performance: Why do we observe such a huge variation in human adaptive capacity relative to training?

To answer this question, Bouchard et al. (2011) performed a genome-wide association study and were able to isolate twenty-one genetic DNA variations that account for 49 percent of the differences observed in training responses. On the grounds of these results, Bouchard and colleagues claimed that the huge variation in training responses observed in their experiment had to be explained by virtue of those very genetic DNA variations they found among the subjects tested. This experiment is important for proponents of the gene-centered approach to talent identification because it provides solid evidence for the idea that athletes are individuals that also inherit a capacity to respond well to training.

For completeness we should note that there are studies arguing that exposure to training stimulus (i.e., the desire to exercise) is itself a trait that is very strongly genetically determined (Thorburn and Proietto 2000; Rowland 1998). In this regard, researchers have found that genetic factors may explain up to 63 percent of the variation in leisure-time physical activity (Maia, Thomis, and Beunen 2002). Furthermore, as noted by Montgomery and Safari (2007) in their state-of-the-art review of genetic bases of physical fitness, social exertion may also be heavily influenced by genetics, with such an effect displayed, for instance, in choosing to climb stairs after a meal rather than using an elevator (Lauderdale et al. 1997). Other studies (e.g., Aarnio et al. 1997) went on to further prove the validity of these ideas by showing that when both parents were active, the children were 5.8 times more likely to be active than children of two inactive parents. Thus, these results have shown that physical activity–related traits may be very strongly influenced (maximal heritability between 30 and 60 percent) by genetic factors. This points to a very minor role for embodied activities, sociocultural practices, and environmental influences in determining physical activity and instead reinforces the thought that biological control (in the form of heritable genes) is paramount to it.

Heritability, however, plays an important role not only in sport performance; it is also crucial, according to advocates of the gene-centered approach, in the acquisition of general skills and other capacities. To illustrate this point, consider next the following examples (involving motor skills and reading). Fox, Hershberger, and Bouchard Jr. (1996) engineered a training study on a motor skill that involved a sample of monozygotic and dizygotic twins who had been reared apart. The subjects involved in the testing had to learn to track a rotating target with a stylus. Researchers found out that more than half the variation in the initial ability to track the rotating object was inherited and that the contribution of heredity increased with practice, which led the authors to conclude that "the effect of practice is to decrease the effect of environmental variation (previous learning) and increase the relative strength of genetic influences on motor performance" (356).

Plomin et al. (2014) more recently investigated the genetic and environmental origins of exceptional performance in reading. He and his colleagues selected a pool of expert readers (top 5 percent from a sample of 10,000 twelve-year-old twins), conducted their experiment, and observed that (1) genetic factors account for more than half of the difference in performance between expert and normal readers, while (2) environmental factors (such as growing up in the same family or attending the same schools) account for less than one-fifth of the difference between them.

Over the years, many other researchers have emphasized the importance of heritability in skill acquisition (e.g., Maes et al. 1996) and explored the extent through which genetic influence may vary over the individual's lifespan, claiming that it is generally stronger before the end of puberty (Tiainen et al. 2005).[2] The research presented later in this discussion complements, betters, and expands on work discussed at the beginning, which shows that superior performance traits (such as aerobic or motor capacity and morphological, cardiac, and skeletal characteristics) can be largely inherited. Taken together, these findings point to a crucial role of genetics in influencing superior sport performance and in favoring the achievement of sophisticated expertise. Thus, these models provide support for the idea that talent, at least in part, is genetically transmitted and that success in any given domain may be innately contributed. However, there are a number of technical/methodological problems and even ethical issues potentially threatening this type of research. Next we summarize some of these problems.

Genetic testing is still largely restricted to the investigation of basic traits such as endurance or strength performance (Lippi, Longo, and Maffulli 2010). The study of these traits alone, however, will never allow gene-centered models to characterize the rich contributions of embodied, sociocultural, developmental, and environmental factors to talent (more on this in part 3 below). Using the newest and rapidly evolving laboratory technologies will certainly offer novel understandings of molecular and morphological aspects of exercise performance (consider the work previously discussed by Bouchard and colleagues on cardiorespiratory fitness in response to aerobic training). However, it seems unlikely that these approaches will shed light on individual differences in the complex and coordinated movement patterns of sports like football or rugby.

Genome-wide association studies (GWAS) are largely useless unless coupled with and complemented by epigenetics, that is, by the study of gene-gene and gene-environment interactions throughout the lifetime (Ehlert and Simon 2012). For example, GWAS investigating type 2 diabetes from eighteen genomic intervals associated with an increased risk of this disease account for less than 4 percent of the total heritability. Although genome-wide studies have provided new biological data, they have identified a very limited quantity of heritable component of any complex trait, and it remains a challenge to elucidate the functional link between associated variants and phenotypic traits (Frazer et al. 2009).

It has been shown that the probability of existence of an optimal genetic makeup is extremely low (0.0005 percent; see Williams and Folland 2008). This means that talent cannot be related only to genes, because if it were, the proportion of talented people would be extremely low (close to zero), coinciding with those possessing optimal genetic makeup.

Besides these technical and methodological problems, there are also important ethical issues limiting the application of gene-centered paradigms for talent search. There is a risk that genetic testing, especially as recently promoted in the media, can be seen as the ultimate tool for parents to guide and orient their children into a future professional career, whether the children like it or not (Camporesi 2013). Another issue may arise if children test negatively for their favorite sports. Would those children be discriminated against compared with children that test positively? And would it be warranted to exclude children who test negatively from further promotion, even if there are signs that they are willing to train hard? A further problem may arise if children were to be genetically tested without full understanding or approval (McNamee et al. 2009). Imagine that tests discover disease risks (e.g., cardiovascular disease); to whom should the results of these tests be communicated? (Roth 2012).

According to shared ethical standards (Miah and Rich 2006), all these ethical issues reflect a significant violation of a person's autonomy and should be carefully acknowledged. Unfortunately, several firms and many scientists working for them seldom consider these important issues and push ahead with their own agendas, not caring too much about the ethical downsides. Examples include Atlas Sports Genetics, a gene technology firm located in Boulder, Colorado, which marketed to parents a test to predict which sport would be best for their children, and the Shanghai Biochip Corporation, in Chongqinq, China, where scientists claimed to be able to isolate many different genetic traits including intelligence, memory, focus, emotional quotient, and entrepreneurship.

Despite these unethical behaviors, which are driven mostly by the prospect of immediate economic returns, genetic research is often welcomed by governing bodies and professional clubs. Why? The reason is that genetic testing is seen to allow a better utilization of economic resources. Our genetic endowment remains pretty much the same throughout our entire lifespan. Findings obtained from genetics can (the argument goes) be used irrespective of time and place, and independent of an athlete's age, training cycle, daily physical state, or health (Breitbach, Tug, and Simon 2014).

To balance out this claim, however, we must note that in recent years an increasing number of researchers and practitioners have attempted to demonstrate that extragenetic factors (such as practice, quality coaching, time spent learning, etc.) are more fundamental and important to talent and skill acquisition than genetic ones. Next we review evidence for this idea.

3 Performance and Skill: The Environmentalist Perspective

Here we review evidence for the idea that talent and superior performances are dynamically acquired through development (hence not genetically prespecified). Howe, Davidson, and Sloboda (1998) were among the first to provide a clear definition of "talent." Prior to their research, talent was defined in operational terms and largely identified with the idea that outstanding results were determined by gifts or genetic endowments, which were typically observed only in very few children. Instead, according to Howe, Davidson, and Sloboda (1998),

> Exceptional level of expertise may not be entirely inherited, as its full effects are often not entirely expressed in children (Michael Jordan is a famous example).
>
> There are certainly initial indicators, which allow individuals specifically trained to identify the presence of talent before children express exceptional performances, but these initial parameters only provide a very general basis to predict who can excel in the future.
>
> Only a minority of the population has talent, as if all people were talented, there would not be the opportunity to predict and explain the differences between their performances.
>
> Hence, talent is largely developed, environmentally or culturally driven, and specific to an area of competence.

Howe and colleagues' seminal definition filled an important gap in the literature and offered new insights for the idea that talent is largely related to embodied practices[3] and therefore not the exclusive fruit of inborn abilities. In short, Howe, Davidson, and Sloboda (1998) provided the conceptual palette necessary for understanding superior performance as dynamic in character. This is the idea that the same performance could be achieved through a combination of a wide range of skills, abilities, and attributes (competence phenomenon), with the importance of each varying in accordance with the level of development of the young.

It is possible to illustrate this point with a simple example: high stature is usually considered a determinant[4] attribute for success in certain disciplines (e.g., basketball); yet, there are some athletes of world-class level that do not possess that particular trait. How can this be explained? Certainly there must be other traits, possibly practice-related, hence embodied, that influence superior performance in basketball, and therefore stature cannot be taken as the only determinant attribute for success in that discipline.

The consequences of this idea were more effectively explored in a longitudinal study of one hundred tennis players (Bartmus, Neumann, and Demarees 1987), which investigated the importance of the compensation phenomenon in sport performance. The absence of stable predictive data found in this study demonstrated that shortage in one area (such as a player's speed) could be filled by a high level of expertise in another area (such as optimal game tactics). In a similar vein, Salmela, Petiot, and Hoshizaki (1987) showed that the predominance of factors that allow successful performances vary according to age and in relation to crucial phases of development, while Régnier (1987) proposed an approach called sliding population, which was based on the assumption that the reliability of the prediction on athletes' future achievements was inversely correlated to the length of the period for which it was considered valid.

All these results demonstrated the need to overcome gene-centrism and develop a multidimensional model of talent. Martens (1987), for instance, advocated the use of experiential knowledge (which is rich in useful information and could be investigated through idiographic systems and field studies) to complement and integrate data coming from traditional approaches. This avenue of research was pursued by Bloom (1985), who produced a study on a group of individuals involved in different activities and showed that talent develops in stages.

4 The Stages of Bloom's Talent Development

In his groundbreaking study aimed at clarifying how talent could be developed, Bloom conducted a four-year longitudinal study on the career development of 120 talented sculptors, concert pianists, mathematicians, neurologists, Olympic swimmers, and tennis champions. He asked them, through structured interviews, how they had developed their talent from the very first experiences they could remember all the way up through to the peak of their career. The interviews were done to get a retrospective picture of the talent-development process. Bloom believed that interviewing samples of twenty to twenty-five talented individuals in each specific field of expertise would allow him to have a clear picture of what is really needed to reach a high level of talent development.

Bloom concluded that it takes years of dedicated effort and training to become talented and that the amount of support received from parents and coaches and teachers is absolutely central to this process. In addition, he identified the presence of three stages of talent development, providing important insights into how these talented individuals had become high performers.

In the initial stage, children play the sport or activity for which they have a passion (drawing, in the case of artists) for fun and play. These are the years in which participation is characterized by joy and enthusiasm, and this kind of involvement mirrors (in large part) the support shown by and received from teachers or coaches. The goal here is to maintain high motivation to learn and to receive pleasure from spending energy through the chosen activity (which can be either motoric, such as performing a sport, or intellectual, such as studying or drawing). Then, in the development stage, specific techniques must be introduced by the educator/trainer to stimulate the personal involvement of the subject so that she does not just mirror learning through observation. In the case of sports, at this stage, the numbers of hours devoted to the chosen activity substantially increases, and coaches are more oriented to the technical components. In the last stage, the athletes become experts, capable of competing at the highest levels. This is the stage of perfection, in which the mind and the body are almost entirely focused on performing the chosen activity. The aim of training in this stage is to perfect—to the highest possible level—the skills and expertise the individual already possesses. This process relies on the athletes increasingly taking upon themselves the responsibility for training and competition.

Bloom's model has been refined over the years (e.g., Anderson, Krathwohl, and Bloom 2001) and a potential fourth stage has been introduced for elucidating the process of conservation of skills (Durand-Bush 2000). This fourth stage covers the years that come immediately after reaching the stage of perfection and is called the stage of maintenance. In this stage, the superior performer is asked to constantly replicate the excellent results he has achieved in the past. To do so, the performer must be part of a social environment, which motivates him to continue training with the same intensity and will.

In operational terms, these theoretical suggestions have been implemented in Canada, where practitioners developed a national program called the Long-Term Athlete Development Framework (Canadian Sport for Life 2005). This program relies on a psychosocial approach and focuses on the maturation level of an individual rather than her chronological age. Researchers and practitioners working on this developmental program have identified ten crucial factors influencing long-term athlete development (LTAD). Among these, for example, are factors such as the ten-year rule (see below), fun, specialization, trainability, and periodization.

The results of a survey of US athletes who participated in the Olympic Games during the period from 1984 to 1998 (816 athletes, 58.2 percent male and 41.7 percent female, with 283 Olympic medalists) confirmed the importance of using a long-term developmental model (such as the LTAD) for training competing athletes (Gibbons 2002). Success at the Olympic Games, the authors demonstrated, is the culmination of a complex, long-term process, which typically involves not only the athletes but also other individuals (e.g., partners, family, coaches) and organizations that are active parts of their social and cultural environments.[5] We believe that the findings presented above provide interesting ground for linking up current research in sport psychology with work on embodied cognition carried out in the cognitive sciences.

A number of theorists, as noted above, have explicitly described embodiment as a means through which extra-neural (bodily and environmental) structures come to shape cognitive processes. Among these theorists, philosopher Andy Clark (2008) is probably the one who has expended the most effort in articulating this idea. Clark argues that the body plays an important role as part of the extended mechanisms of cognition (Clark and Chalmers 1998). In his account, known as the extended mind thesis (Clark 2008; Kiverstein, Farina, and Clark 2013; Kiverstein and Farina 2011) cognition doesn't take place exclusively inside the biological boundary of the individual but, on the contrary, can arise in the dynamical (real-time) interplay between neural structures, body, and world. Clark (2013, 2008) therefore claims that the cognitive processes that make up our minds can and do sometimes reach beyond the boundaries of individual organisms to include, as proper parts, aspects of the organism's physical and sociocultural environment. In other words, structures and processes located outside the human head can become part of the machinery of cognition. This claim, in Clark's view, applies to enduring states as well as to transient processes (Clark 2008).

As Gallagher (2011) recently noted, "the physical body on Clark's account, functions as a non-neural vehicle for cognitive processes, in much the same general way that the physical processes of neurons do" (63). The body, in Clark's view, is therefore part of an extended cognitive system that begins with the brain but also requires (in most cases) the body and the environment to function properly. Interestingly, in this extended system, bodily actions (in the forms of proceduralized skills and expertise, Clark 2015) are seen as capable of shaping human cognition in important ways.

Clark's work provided the springboard for other philosophers (such as Shaun Gallagher) to explore the idea of cognition as a socially extended phenomenon. In a series of papers, Gallagher (Gallagher 2013; Gallagher and Crisafi 2009) argued that certain social practices (mental institutions) are usefully understood as extending our mind, because they help us to accomplish certain cognitive processes that we wouldn't be able to realize in their absence. Paradigmatic examples include things like legal systems, educational systems, and cultural institutions such as museums, galleries, academies, and the like. This work on socially extended cognition, we note, offers an ideal background for framing environmentalist research in sport psychology, which, as we have seen above, emphasizes the role of supportive social and cultural environments in talent development.

Clark's work also inspired interdisciplinary philosopher of mind John Sutton' research on the relations between embodied cognition and the nature of skill and expertise (Sutton 2007; Sutton et al. 2011; Christensen, Sutton, and McIlwain 2016). Sutton and colleagues formulated a synthetic and original theory of skilled actions and embodied activities (called the *Mesh* theory of cognitive control), which proposes that cognitive and automatic processes make an important contribution to skill control. In the account of Sutton and colleagues, cognitive and automatic processes work together in a closely meshed and embodied setting (in such a setting, awareness and information about body states and movements is crucial). Cognitive control typically focuses on strategic task features, whereas automatic control is responsible for its implementation. Sutton's theory is relevant to the environmentalist research discussed above for two reasons: (1) because it shows that skills are complex and necessarily multifaceted (hence not only genetically determined), and (2) because it demonstrates their inescapable embodied dimension (the fact that there is a necessity to understand them in relation with a body through which they are learned). From the analysis conducted above it is therefore clear that another crucial component (besides genetic and environmental factors) of the multidimensional model of talent we are proposing in this chapter must be embodiment.

Next, to expand the breadth and scope of this chapter, we critically assess radical environmentalist research (e.g., Ericsson, Krampe, and Tesch-Römer 1993; Ericsson 1996; Ericsson et al. 2006), that has claimed that deliberate practice (on its own) is what ultimately matters to talent and skill. In this context, the term "environmentalist" indicates a person whose stance within the classic nature-versus-nurture debate is that the environment in which a person is nurtured or reared (not his inborn nature), will largely determine his outcomes, abilities, and capacities (Sloboda 2002). We first review evidence supporting this approach and then point out a number of shortcomings that affect it.

5 How to Become Expert: Ericsson's Approach

According to Ericsson, Krampe, and Tesch-Römer (1993) deliberate practice occurs as "an effortful activity designed to optimize improvement" (363). Deliberate practice is thus a process that takes place when individuals who are highly motivated to develop and optimize their skills are engaged in a series of sequential and partly repetitive activities that are carefully designed and subsequently implemented to achieve a specific goal or acquire a certain expertise. This process often includes activities not inherently motivating and not leading to immediate social and monetary rewards, which are nevertheless recognized by the athletes as necessary for achieving their ultimate goals and/or mind-set. The deliberate practice model thus stresses the importance of training and practice and the interaction between the athlete and his or her nurturing environment over genetically prespecified endowments.

There are obviously limits for developing and producing superior performances; according to Ericsson, these are essentially related to three components. The first concerns the limits in the resources available: that is, the quality of the sessions, the coach's expertise, and the sport material. The second involves the athlete, who must overcome the limitations that could adversely affect her motivation. The third concerns the individual limits related to her commitment. Playing an activity at top level in fact requires intense mental and physical preparation, which has to be pursued over many long years. Athletes must also fully understand the ethics of hard work to avoid acquiring a mentality oriented toward doping or drug abuse. Ericsson's research (e.g., Ericsson, Krampe, and Tesch-Römer 1993; Ericsson and Charness 1994) is one of the original sources of the magic number 10,000 for the number of practice hours that everyone (including prodigies) allegedly requires to attain a superior level of performance at activities such as tennis, golf, chess, piano, and violin playing (the ten-year rule of necessary preparation recently trivialized/popularized by Gladwell 2008).

In a famous study of violinists, Ericsson, Krampe, and Tesch-Römer (1993) claimed that accumulated hours of training (both alone and with a music teacher) were the principal indicator of excellence. Practice alone, it was claimed, differentiated the best musicians from the others in term of weekly hours spent in this task. The best musicians spent, on average, twenty-five hours practicing a week, which was three times

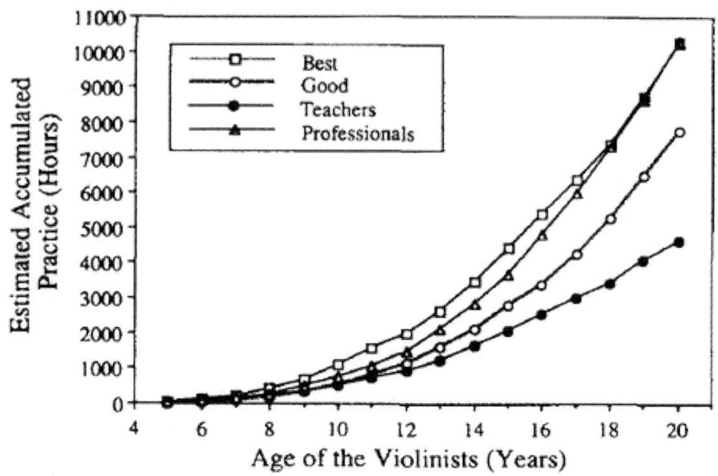

Figure 11.1

Estimated amount of time for practice alone as a function of age for the middle-aged (professional) violinists. Four categories are displayed: (1) the best expert violinists, (2) the good expert violinists, (3) the least-accomplished expert violinists, and (4) amateur violinists.
Source: Ericsson et al. (1993), 363–406.

more than the time spent by those of the same age (twenty years old) who were less expert. Ericsson found (figure 11.1) that the two best groups (top performers) had spent—overall—over 10,000 hours on practice alone (deliberate practice) compared with the 8,000 and 5,000 hours of the two less-expert groups of violinists and the 2,000 hours of the amateur violinists (Ericsson, Krampe, and Tesch-Römer 1993).

Thus, according to Ericsson and colleagues, deliberate practice is a determining factor in achieving a superior level of expertise. In other words, without a quantifiable commitment (no matter how good the genetic component is) an athlete cannot reach the level of expertise needed to compete at top level. Ericsson's results have been replicated in a number of empirical studies, and the ten-year rule has been observed in different fields of expertise, such as chess (Simon and Chase 1973), mathematics (Gustin 1985), and music (Sosniak 1985).

One set of findings on Olympic athletes further confirmed Ericsson's theory (Gibbons 2002). It has been found that, on average, it takes twelve to thirteen years of training to get on the US Olympic team. That means that athletes need a large number of years of training and education to be able to fully develop their talents. The number of months of training per year increases from the initial stages of participation to the

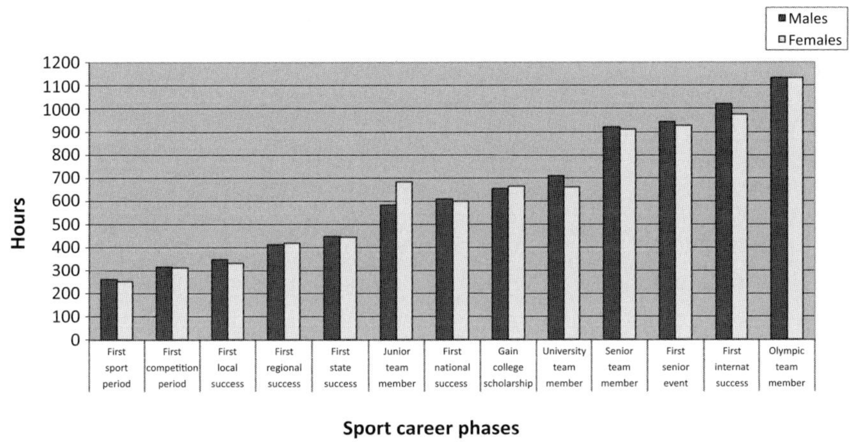

Figure 11.2
The figure shows the amount of training (in hours) of US Olympians. Subjects: 817 boys and girls. *Source*: Gibbons et al. (2003), 41.

subsequent ones. At first, the athletes train about six months a year, reaching 10.9 months when they enter the junior national team and 11.3 months per year when they are part of the Olympic team. Boys and girls train themselves for the same number of hours per year, going from 250 in the early stages to 1,130 per year in the later ones (figure 11.2).

For athletes, the coach is also extremely important when competing at national and international level: for men the influence is greatest between the ages of 18.3 and 20.8 years, while for women it is between the ages of 17.4 and 19.5 years. The two core competences wanted in a coach are teaching skill and motivation. The other two core competences are related to training knowledge and strategic planning. In addition, the study revealed that US Olympic athletes sought coaches with many years of experience and strategic knowledge regardless of their personality.

These studies certainly provide solid empirical support for Bloom's theoretical model of talent development and for many of Ericsson's claims (including the 10,000-hours-of-training rule). However, in this context, it is important not to overemphasize the reach of these results and, in turn, the overall validity of the environmentalist perspective. So, to balance out the evidence just presented, we next focus on a number of problematic issues affecting Ericsson's research. Specifically, we present three main thrusts of objections to his theory: (1) issues with the actual time and conditions for development of mastery, (2) the notion of concentration, and (3) the notion of genotypic equivalency.

First, it has been observed that Ericsson, Krampe, and Tesch-Römer's seminal study (1993) did not provide the measure of the variance of the standard deviation, and it was not clear whether his results were consistent for all the musicians tested. A follow-up study, on 104 chess players (Gobet and Campitelli 2007) of different levels of expertise ranging from master to amateur, confirmed the validity of this objection, showing (on one side) that practice was needed to become a master, but (on the other) that some players required eight times more practice to reach master level than others. To be precise, the fastest chess player in the study reported needed 3,016 hours to become master, whereas the slower needed 23,618 hours.[6]

Similar findings have been observed in dart throwing, when comparing professional and amateur performers. The results showed that only 28 percent of variance was explained by accumulated practice time—12,839 hours as opposed to 3,270 hours in fifteen years of practice, respectively, for professional and amateur players (Duffy, Baluch, and Ericsson 2004).

Analogously, studies in sport performance have revealed that elite athletes do not always complete 10,000 hours of training before reaching international levels. For example, 28 percent of elite Australian athletes reached the status of international athletes within four years of practice, while other international-level wrestlers, field hockey players, and footballers had accumulated only 6,000 hours, 4,000 hours, and 500 hours of training, respectively (Elferink Gemser et al. 2011; Phillips et al. 2010; Huijen et al. 2009).

All these studies therefore suggest that Ericsson's data are affected by a large variability and quite clearly demonstrate that there is more to talent and skill than just the sheer volume of hours practiced (Ericsson himself has noted this, see the above-mentioned three components). With regard to this point, it has been recently shown that reconsolidation is crucial to talent and skill. Wymbs, Bastian, and Celnik (2016), for instance, demonstrated that motor skills are strengthened (reconsolidated) over multiple training sessions when reactivated within an environment that increases variability and maintains the original learning context. The studies discussed above also point to the ineliminable role of innate talent (genetic inherited abilities) in developing elite performance, something advocates of the deliberate practice account (such as Ericsson) usually tend to downplay, ignore, or underestimate.

The second problematic issue affecting Ericsson's approach concerns his understanding of the notion of concentration in deliberate practice. It seems that Ericsson's theory is not falsifiable, calling into question its adherence to contemporary scientific practice. According to Ericsson (1996), "concentration is the most essential aspect" of deliberate practice (24). This suggests that sustained concentration is paramount for achieving effective training, and that it is required to keep up motivations, to monitor goals, and even to assess teacher guidance. Without sustained concentration, the inexperienced will always repeat the same mistakes (won't listen) or will practice for reasons that are imposed by others (won't train properly). Because concentration might not be easily quantifiable and there will always be dispute over whether an individual is using full concentration during deliberate practice, it is always going to be very difficult (if not impossible) to define, in scientific terms, the quality of deliberate practice. Accordingly, an advocate of Ericsson's approach could always question the quality of practice when a performer (despite intense practice) does not perform as expected, making it unfalsifiable.

The third problem with Ericsson's approach lies in his defense of the notion of genotypic equivalency. According to Ericsson and Pool (2016), everyone has the genes necessary for the acquisition of expertise provided they are able to train sufficiently; that is, on the condition that they are allowed to put in an appropriate amount of deliberate practice. This idea, however, clashes (as Baker 2007 has noted) with basic evolutionary theory (Davids and Baker 2007), which prescribes the necessity of genetic variability for ensuring natural selection over evolutionary time (in brief, the more genetically variable is a species, the higher are its chances of survival). If basic evolutionary theory is right (and it seems hard to disprove) then it follows that both random and nonrandom genetic variations in all areas of human performance and behavior (including skill and expertise) are absolutely crucial for continued species evolution. This casts serious doubts on the overall validity of Ericsson's approach (very strongly based on the idea of genetic equivalency), which—as we have seen above—does not make much sense evolutionarily.

Given these conceptual and methodological shortcomings, it is thus possible to agree with Tucker and Collins (2012) when they argue that Ericsson's model does not fully adhere to current scientific practice. In addition, we would like to note that Ericsson's theory, while grounded on the notion of embodied practices, does very little to explore the potential profitable links with the paradigm of embodied cognition in the cognitive sciences (as introduced above). We believe this is another potential shortcoming affecting Ericsson's approach and thus push (more on this below) for a more integrative perspective.

At this point, then, a question naturally arises: What does this conflicting evidence tell us about the nature of talent and skill acquisition? Is talent genetically inherited or developmentally acquired? And what role does embodiment play in talent acquisition?

In part 6, we try to answer these questions and—following Baker (Baker et al. 2003; Baker 2007) and various other researchers (e.g., Phillips, Renshaw, and Portus 2010; Vaeyens et al. 2008; Simonton 2001; Davids and Baker 2007)—we call for the development of an integrative and multidimensional model of talent and skill. This model should fuse, we claim, the best of both gene-centered and environmentalist research, while embracing a fully embodied perspective. This latter point has not been fully emphasized in the literature we reviewed in this contribution, and thus our addition constitutes an important innovation for the field.

6 Integrating Embodied Cognition and Culture for Understanding Talent and Skill

Elite performance and success, we believe, is about the coming together of dozens of different factors (see Baker and Hodges 2015; and Roth 2012, for reviews): deliberate practice, good genes, quality coaching, strategic thinking, careful planning, motivation, dedication, focus, concentration, availability of resources, time spent learning, desire to succeed, and lifestyle, along with many other physiological attributes. However, it is not presently possible to ascertain the exact relative contribution of each of these factors or attributes to elite sporting performance (Breitbach, Tug, and Simon 2014).

In our view it is also important to emphasize that, often, athletes' sensorimotor and sociocultural experiences are crucial to talent and skill acquisition. We would also like to stress the role of embodied activity in this process. Not many empirical studies to date, however, have explored the role of embodied cognition in sport psychology. Beilock (2008) has produced one excellent review that looked at the crucial role of sensorimotor experience in sport psychology, presenting cognitive science and neuroscience research (Milton et al. 2007; Calvo-Merino et al. 2006; Casile and Giese 2006; Repp and Knoblich 2004) that supports the idea that many cognitive operations are grounded in action.

Milton and colleague's 2007 paper is particularly interesting. The authors looked at youngsters who were on track to become elite performers and how they used their experiences on the field to build a mental representation of what they had to do to improve their practice. Results demonstrated that expert golfers, when mentally rehearsing the pre-shot routine, activated the superior parietal lobe, the left dorsal premotor, and occipital cortices. These areas are part of a broader action-simulation network involved in the perception, representation, and production of action. It was also shown that naïve golfers, when doing the same, activated very different areas: the posterior limbic and basal ganglion (BG) regions of the brain. BG activation was taken to be indicative that the simulation of shot-related processes and procedures were not fully automatized (Milton et al. 2007). The upshot of this research is therefore that certain routines are embodied and coded in different areas of the brain, linking practice to embodiment.

Virtually the same was observed when experts in classical ballet and Capoeira watched videos of ballet or Capoeira actions while their brains were being scanned (Calvo-Merino et al. 2005; Rizzolatti, Fogassi, and Gallese 2001). "When the brain activity of individuals who were watching their own dance style was compared to activity when individuals were watching the other dance style (e.g. ballet dancers watching ballet versus ballet dancers watching Capoeira), greater activation was seen in a network of brain regions (e.g. bilateral activation in premotor cortex and intraparietal sulcus, right superior parietal lobe, and left posterior superior temporal sulcus) thought to support both the observation and production of action" (Beilock 2008, 21). These results thus demonstrate that sensorimotor and sociocultural (embodied) experiences play a crucial role in the development of elite performance.

A subtler aspect to consider is perhaps that the sensorimotor experiences could have a different relevance in endurance sports if compared with precision sports. In the former, which are more biomechanically limited (like cycling, running, rowing) muscles, heart, and lungs (whose capacities are largely determined by genes) provide a ceiling for the ability one wants to acquire. In sports based more on accuracy and precision in the execution (like golf, billiard, shooting, or curling), on the contrary, deliberate practice might matter more and be the key to how quickly the ability can be acquired, through the continuous information linking up the sensorimotor system to the cortex.

To explain our ideas and support our call for an integrative account of talent and skill, we discuss two case studies. The first concerns the Polgar sisters, and the second, Kenyan runners. The Polgar sisters are three Hungarian sisters who were taught (from the age of four) how to play chess, first by their father, psychologist Laszlo Polgar, and then by professionals. The three girls all became outstanding chess players. Two became chess grand masters, with Judit being one of the most accomplished female chess players in history, and Susan an international master. This case is often presented in the media as a nurture-over-nature example, a case where individuals are trained to be geniuses.[7] It is therefore often said that this case study provides undisputable evidence that talent is made, not born. We disagree with this interpretation and argue instead that, even in a skill-based sport (chess), deliberate practice on its own isn't probably sufficient for elite performance. This confirms our original intuition, and the main thesis of this chapter, that genes, deliberate practice, ethical factors, sociocultural influences, and embodiment work together in the development of skill and expertise. In other words, none of them has primacy over any other and all play varying (across different sports) but crucial roles in talent development. Next we discuss problems with the standard interpretation.

First, the fact that the Polgar sisters were related does not allow us to exclude the potential contribution of genes—quite the opposite. We already exposed the reasons against gene-centrism (part 2 above); however, if talent also runs through a family (and sometimes it does: famous examples include the Bernoulli family and the Bach family), it may well be possible that the Polgar sisters had some particular genetic endowments at birth that, after being appropriately trained, favored their superior performances. But more than this, when we carefully analyze their story (and see not only what they have achieved but also at what age it was achieved) we start to understand that it is very difficult to make the case that only their many hours of training were the secret of their many successes.

When Judit Polgar was five years old, she defeated a family friend (an adult) without even looking at the chessboard. At the same age, she also defeated her father (a decent-level chess-playing adult). By age seven she had beaten a master-level player while blindfolded. At age ten she defeated an international master, and subsequently, at age eleven, she beat a grand master. If, however, one calculates the needed 10,000 hours into years, with an average of five hours a day with no breaks, the total comes to 8.3 years. Assuming that the 10,000-hour rule is correct and that Ericsson's account is accurate, this means that Judit, by age eleven, should have already put more than eight years of her life into training. This is clearly impossible. The same applies to Judit's sister, Susan, who won a Hungarian chess competition in the under-eleven category at age five and went on to a very successful career. Thus, these staggering accomplishments show that what made the sisters outstanding performers was not simply the fact that they had accumulated hours and hours of practice, but rather (most probably) that their ability to learn the skills and techniques involved in chess playing was already astonishing. Surely this ability was developed through training, but it was also somehow inherited, as this capacity is one that is not commonly observed in the majority of people.

Of course, to progress through the grand master level, and so to become the very best in the world, one has to train hard, and that certainly requires putting in an incredible amount of deliberate practice into the task.[8] However, in this case it seems clear that the trajectory of excellence was very clearly expressed in infancy, being (most likely) a symptom of an innate ability. The Polgar sisters can be therefore said to be the sporting equivalent of Michael Phelps or the musical equivalent of Mozart, incredible talents who achieve—within the first few years of age—what for others might take a lifetime to accomplish, if ever. This is not an argument for gene-centrism but a recognition that talent, at least in some cases, has to do with genes. Saying this does not negate or underestimate the value of training and practice. We believe that practice and training should be understood as the realization of genetic potential.

We also believe that this case study confirms our call for an embodied model of talent. In the case of Susan Polgar (2016), the role of embodiment has been thoroughly demonstrated through several fMRI scans (such as those conducted by Professor Joy Hirsch and shown in a National Geographic documentary aired in March 2016). In her study, Hirsch and colleagues demonstrated that in the chess player's brain, areas normally dedicated to face processing is powerfully activated when she imagines a chess game. So, in Susan Polgar's brain, the role of the fusiform area in the recognition of the chess positions represents a clear example of how embodiment models the cortex functions in relation to the experiences of the performers.

At this point a skeptical reader might object that the chess case is interesting in its own right, and that it surely forces us to acknowledge the importance of many of the components of elite performance presented earlier (including genetics), but that chess is not usually regarded as a sport (only a few national sport federations treat it as such, e.g., Cuba). Moreover, it seems that chess playing is a conceptual activity, not a physical one. In other words, a skeptical reader may point to the lack of physical prowess in chess playing and, on those grounds, question whether chess is really the best example on which to base an embodied account of talent and expertise.[9] Rather than confronting this objection head-on, which involves a lengthy excursus to show the sense in which chess playing may be considered embodied (something already hinted at above with the fMRI scans), we simply note that a number of authors before us have used chess in this fashion (Pereira et al. 2008; Dreyfus 2005).

To further strengthen our idea of an embodied and multidimensional model of talent and expertise, we discuss next another case study, which is, clearly, more robustly embodied and which shows, more directly, the relevance of environmental, sociocultural, and even ethical factors in talent acquisition and development of superior/elite performance (Voestermans and Verheggen 2013).Our second case study involves Kenyan runners.

It is widely known that Kenyan runners are dominant on endurance running competitions (twenty-five medals from long-distance running events in the Olympics of 2008 and 2012). However, this dominance is unlikely to be explained by looking at just one factor. A number of studies (e.g., Wilber and Pitsiladis 2012) have investigated the population of a small region in Western Kenya that produces most of the country's race winners. The authors of these studies have claimed that this particular geographical area has allowed Kenyans to have the "proper genes" for distance running (e.g., Larsen 2003). The studies found that individuals of this population have less mass for their height, longer legs, shorter torsos, more slender limbs, and higher cardiorespiratory fitness than Western counterparts. This set of largely inherited qualities allows them to easily outrun, after only a few months of training, most Western athletes. However, those who think that genes on their own can explain Kenyan dominance are doomed to failure (Hamilton 2000).

There are also environmental and sociocultural, hence embodied, factors (such as diet, habits, and customs; altitude, which is crucial to the capacity of the body to carry oxygen; air quality; lifestyle; etc.) that affect and determine these superior performances (Christensen and Damkjaer 2010; Wilber and Pitsiladis 2012). In addition, one may also point to ethical issues. Doping has proved problematic for Kenyan runners, with many of them testing positive for drug use recently, and even with some authorities seemingly involved. This widespread "culture of doping" shows the effects of illicit practices allowing athletes to perform beyond their "natural" talents and beyond what training affords. This point connects well to socially extended embodied practices as discussed earlier in this chapter (the situated research by Gallagher and colleagues, for example), as institutions, institutional practices, officials, and the like surely have a direct effect on how talent is expressed.

Given all the above, it seems straightforward to affirm that the successes of Kenyan athletes can only be explained by virtue of an embodied, integrative, and multidimensional model, conjugating all these different factors. Thus, the general lesson we can draw from the analysis of these two case studies is that we should not polarize the debate as if genes, embodiment, and practice approaches were mutually excluding. Instead we should recognize that there are many different paths to elite performance and that a one-size- or one-number-fits-all approach is necessarily bound to fail.

7 Conclusion

Knowing the determinants of excellent performance and predicting athletes' success have long been challenging issues in sport science. We have argued that sport performance is a complex multifactorial phenomenon, determined by many inner (e.g., genetics, health, biological and psychological profile) and outer (environmental and sociocultural and ethical factors such as coaching, sport opportunities, culture of doping, embodied practices) factors. We have thus claimed that superior sport development is likely influenced by a balanced interaction of these inner and outer variables and that embodiment plays a central role in elite performance. We would now like to wrap up this chapter by discussing future research directions.

A promising approach to talent has been one that recognizes the presence of a natural endowment. A number of studies (e.g., Pearson, Naughton, and Torode 2006) have developed effective systems for spotting young talent. Through these systems, researchers have singled out 249 genes (Bray et al. 2009) related to sport performance, as well as crucial characteristics of the body structure and psychological/environmental factors. This avenue of research is certainly very appealing. However, this research has failed to demonstrate the predominance of a single factor in talent development and has not adequately emphasized the crucial role of coaches in elite performances (Reilly et al. 2000).

Thus, from our perspective, future studies must move toward an integrated and multidimensional framework, which takes into account not only ethical considerations and genetic, psychological, embodied, and sociocultural perspectives, but also the new ecological approach, more oriented to study the interaction among individuals and between their environments (Davids et al. 2013). In other words, we agree with Ericsson and colleagues (2006) that the nature-nurture dichotomy is no longer scientifically meaningful—to us, however, this implies recognition of genetic influences, ethical and cultural factors, deliberate practice, and embodied experiences in the acquisition of expert performance.

Acknowledgments

A very special thanks must go to Massimiliano Cappuccio and to Jesús Ilundáin-Agurruza for helpful comments and keen critique on earlier drafts of this manuscript. Mirko Farina would like to express his appreciation to the British Academy for the Humanities and Social Sciences and to King's College London, for financing his research.

Notes

1. Advocates of embodied cognition (such as Anderson 2003; Sutton 2007) take as their theoretical starting point the idea that cognitive processes are deeply rooted in the body's interactions with the world (Clark 2008; Wheeler 2005). Embodied cognition thus aims to explain the full range of perceptual, cognitive, and motor capacities we possess as capacities that are dependent on aspects of an agent's body. In recent years the terms "embodied cognition" or "embodiment" have been used interchangeably to refer to a wide range of ideas and approaches that range from minimal to radical embodiment and encompass a number of positions in between. More specifically, these terms have been used to describe either standard claims about how bodily actions or

movements provide a format for neuronal representations (Goldman and Vignemont 2009; Gallese and Lakoff 2005) and help reduce computational load (Clark 2008; Wheeler 2005), or more radical proposals such as the idea that sensorimotor know-how is a constitutive part of perceptual experience (O'Regan and Noë 2001), the thought that phenomenal consciousness supervenes on the whole embodied organism in dynamic interaction with the environment (Thompson and Varela 2001), the belief that social sensorimotor interactions and social pattern of experience can be a constitutive parts of social cognition (De Jaegher, Di Paolo, and Gallagher 2010), or the thought that living systems are autopoietic (self-contained, self-organizing) systems (Maturana and Varela 1991).

2. Building on recent work in cultural and development psychology (Lerner and Overton 2010; Baltes, Reuter-Lorenz, and Rösler 2006), Farina (2016) has however attacked this understanding and defended the idea that contextualized experiences and learning, on the one hand, and brain plasticity, on the other, operate conjointly to shape the development of human cognitive functions across the entire lifespan. The multidimensional model of talent we propose in this chapter (part 4) is, at least in part, inspired by Farina's approach to human cognition (Farina 2017).

3. Latour (2004) famously asked us to focus on "what the body can do." By focusing on the body's possibilities for action we learn, according to Latour, to understand our bodies in terms of their capacities to affect and to be affected. These capacities are typically observed in embodied practices. The expression "embodied practices" thus suggests that our bodies, especially through perception, emotion, and spatiotemporal movements (Tiwari 2010) are what allows us to live and experience the world in the way we do (Wegenstein 2006).

4. Wood et al. (2014) recently demonstrated that there exists a genetic architecture for human height that is characterized by a very large but finite number (thousands) of causal variants. This built on a previous study (Weedon et al. 2007), which showed that stature is the result of the combined effects of multiple genes, enzymes, or other agents involved in different processes from bone growth to cell growth. These results demonstrated that there is no single gene for stature and suggest that there might also be embodied or cultural factors (such as diet) influencing it.

5. Cultural factors (see Baker et al. 2003) are a crucial component of the environmental equation influencing the development of expertise. Notable case studies include ice hockey in Canada (Russell 2000) and alpine skiing in Austria (Coakley 2015). Unfortunately, the contribution of these factors is often overlooked.

6. These results have also been replicated by Hambrick et al. (2014).

7. Myers 1993.

8. We would like to note, however, that we are very skeptical of any attempt to quantify this amount, for a number of reasons. First, we believe (as noted) that this amount may differ from activity to activity (or sport to sport). Second, we think it also depends, sometimes heavily, on cultural and sociological factors, which are context-dependent and unique to the individual tested.

9. Thanks to the reviewer for pressing this point.

References

Aarnio, M., T. Winter, U. M. Kujala, and J. Kaprio. 1997. "Familial Aggregation of Leisure-Time Physical Activity—A Three Generation Study." *International Journal of Sports Medicine* 18 (7): 549–556.

Abney, Mark, Mary Sara McPeek, and Carole Ober. 2001. "Broad and Narrow Heritabilities of Quantitative Traits in a Founder Population." *American Journal of Human Genetics* 68 (5): 1302–1307.

Anderson, Lorin W., David R. Krathwohl, and Benjamin Samuel Bloom. 2001. *A Taxonomy for Learning, Teaching, and Assessing: A Revision of Bloom's Taxonomy of Educational Objectives*. Boston: Allyn and Bacon.

Anderson, Michael L. 2003. "Embodied Cognition: A Field Guide." *Artificial Intelligence* 149 (1): 91–130.

Baker, Joseph. 2007. "Nature and Nurture Interact to Create Expert Performers." *High Ability Studies* 18 (1): 57–58.

Baker, Joseph, and Nicola J. Hodges, eds. 2015. "Sporting Expertise: A Festchrift in Honour of Dr. Janet Starkes Introduction." *International Journal of Sport Psychology* Part I, 46 (6).

Baker, Joseph, Sean Horton, Jennifer Robertson-Wilson, and Michael Wall. 2003. "Nurturing Sport Expertise: Factors Influencing the Development of Elite Athlete." *Journal of Sports Science and Medicine* 2 (1): 1–9.

Baltes, Paul B., Patricia A. Reuter-Lorenz, and Frank Rösler. 2006. *Lifespan Development and the Brain: The Perspective of Biocultural Co-Constructivism.* Cambridge: Cambridge University Press.

Bartmus, U., E. Neumann, and H. Demarees. 1987. "The Talent Problem in Sports," *International Journal of Sports Medicine* 1987; 8 (6): 415–416.

Beilock, Sian L. 2008. "Beyond the Playing Field: Sport Psychology Meets Embodied Cognition." *International Review of Sport and Exercise Psychology* 1 (1): 19–30.

Beunen, Gaston, and Martine Thomis. 2004. "Gene Powered? Where to Go from Heritability (h2) in Muscle Strength and Power?" *Exercise and Sport Sciences Reviews* 32 (4): 148–154.

Bloom, B., and L. Sosniak. 1985. *Developing Talent in Young People.* New York: Ballantine.

Bouchard, C., and E. P. Hoffman. 2011. "Genetic and Molecular Aspects of Sport Performance, Vol. XVIII of the IOC Encyclopeadia of Sports Medicine, an IOC Medical Commission Publication." West Sussex, UK: Wiley-Blackwell.

Bouchard, Claude, Robert M. Malina, and Louis Pérusse. 1997. *Genetics of Fitness and Physical Performance*. Champaign, IL: Human Kinetics.

Bouchard, Claude, Mark A. Sarzynski, Treva K. Rice, William E. Kraus, Timothy S. Church, Yun Ju Sung, D. C. Rao, and Tuomo Rankinen. 2011. "Genomic Predictors of the Maximal O2 Uptake

Response to Standardized Exercise Training Programs." *Journal of Applied Physiology* 110 (5): 1160–1170.

Bray, Molly S., James M. Hagberg, Louis Pérusse, Tuomo Rankinen, Stephen M. Roth, Bernd Wolfarth, and Claude Bouchard. 2009. "The Human Gene Map for Performance and Health-Related Fitness Phenotypes: The 2006–2007 Update." *Medicine and Science in Sports and Exercise* 41 (1): 35–73.

Breitbach, Sarah, Suzan Tug, and Perikles Simon. 2014. "Conventional and Genetic Talent Identification in Sports: Will Recent Developments Trace Talent?" *Sports Medicine* 44 (11): 1489–1503.

Calvo, Mar, Gil Rodas, Miguel Vallejo, Asunción Estruch, Antoni Arcas, Casimiro Javierre, Ginés Viscor, and Josep Lluís Ventura. 2002. "Heritability of Explosive Power and Anaerobic Capacity in Humans." *European Journal of Applied Physiology* 86 (3): 218–225.

Calvo-Merino, B., D. E. Glaser, J. Grèzes, R. E. Passingham, and P. Haggard. 2005. "Action Observation and Acquired Motor Skills: An FMRI Study with Expert Dancers." *Cerebral Cortex* 15 (8): 1243–1249.

Calvo-Merino, Beatriz, Julie Grèzes, Daniel E. Glaser, Richard E. Passingham, and Patrick Haggard. 2006. "Seeing or Doing? Influence of Visual and Motor Familiarity in Action Observation." *Current Biology* 16 (22): 2277.

Camporesi, Silvia. 2013. "Bend It Like Beckham! The Ethics of Genetically Testing Children for Athletic Potential." *Sport, Ethics and Philosophy* 7 (2): 175–185.

Canadian Sport for Life. 2005. "Long-Term Athlete Development. Resource Paper V2." Vancouver, BC: Canadian Sport Centres.

Casile, Antonino, and Martin A. Giese. 2006. "Nonvisual Motor Training Influences Biological Motion Perception." *Current Biology* 16 (1): 69–74.

Christensen, Dirk Lund, and Søren Damkjaer. 2010. "Traditional and Modern Running Culture among the Kalenjin of Kenya: A Historical and Anthropological Perspective." In *Anthropology of Sport and Human Movement: A Biocultural Perspective*, edited by Robert R. Sands and Linda R. Sands, 187–212. Lanham, MD: Lexington.

Christensen, Wayne, John Sutton, and Doris J. F. McIlwain. 2016. "Cognition in Skilled Action: Meshed Control and the Varieties of Skill Experience." *Mind & Language* 31 (1): 37–66.

Clark, Andy. 1998. *Being There: Putting Brain, Body, and World Together Again*. Cambridge, MA: MIT Press.

Clark, Andy. 2008. *Supersizing the Mind: Embodiment, Action, and Cognitive Extension*. New York: Oxford University Press.

Clark, Andy. 2013. *Mindware: An Introduction to the Philosophy of Cognitive Science*. 2nd ed. New York: Oxford University Press.

Clark, Andy. 2015. "What 'Extended Me' Knows." *Synthese* 192 (11): 3757–3775.

Clark, Andy, and David Chalmers. 1998. "The Extended Mind." *Analysis* 58 (1): 7–19.

Coakley, Jay. 2015. *Sport and Society: Issues and Controversies*. 7th ed. New York: McGraw-Hill.

Collins, Malcolm, and Stuart M. Raleigh. 2009. "Genetic Risk Factors for Musculoskeletal Soft Tissue Injuries." *Medicine and Sport Science* 54 (August):136–149.

Davids, Keith, Duarte Araújo, Luis Vilar, Ian Renshaw, and Ross Pinder. 2013. "An Ecological Dynamics Approach to Skill Acquisition: Implications for Development of Talent in Sport." *Talent Development and Excellence* 5 (1): 21–34.

Davids, Keith, and Joseph Baker. 2007. "Genes, Environment and Sport Performance." *Sports Medicine* 37 (11): 961–980.

De Jaegher, Hanne, Ezequiel Di Paolo, and Shaun Gallagher. 2010. "Can Social Interaction Constitute Social Cognition?" *Trends in Cognitive Sciences* 14 (10): 441–447.

Dreyfus, Hubert L. 2005. "Overcoming the Myth of the Mental: How Philosophers Can Profit from the Phenomenology of Everyday Expertise." *Proceedings and Addresses of the American Philosophical Association* 79 (2): 47–65.

Duffy, Linda J., Bahman Baluch, and K. Anders Ericsson. 2004. "Dart Performance as a Function of Facets of Practice amongst Professional and Amateur Men and Women Players." *International Journal of Sport Psychology* 35:232–245.

Durand-Bush, Natalie. 2000. *The Development and Maintenance of Expert Athletic Performance: Perceptions of Olympic and World Champions, Their Parents and Coaches*. Ontario: University of Ottawa.

Ehlert, T., D. Moser, and P. Simon. 2012. "Epigenetics in Sports: A Potent Confounder in Genetic Association Studies." *Sports Medicine* 43 (2): 93–110.

Elferink-Gemser, Marije T., Geir Jordet, Manuel J. Coelho-E-Silva, and Chris Visscher. 2011. "The Marvels of Elite Sports: How to Get There?" *British Journal of Sports Medicine* 45 (9): 683–684.

Ericsson, Anders, and Robert Pool. 2016. *Peak: Secrets from the New Science of Expertise*. Boston, MA: Houghton Mifflin Harcourt.

Ericsson, K. Anders. 1996. "The Acquisition of Expert Performance: An Introduction to Some of the Issues." In *The Road to Excellence: The Acquisition of Expert Performance in the Arts and Science, Sports and Games*, edited by K. Anders Ericsson, 1–50. Mahwah, NJ: Erlbaum.

Ericsson, K. Anders, and Neil Charness. 1994. "Expert Performance: Its Structure and Acquisition." *American Psychologist* 49 (8): 725–747.

Ericsson, K. Anders, Neil Charness, Paul J. Feltovich, and Robert R. Hoffman, eds. 2006. *The Cambridge Handbook of Expertise and Expert Performance: Its Development, Organization, and Content*. New York: Cambridge University Press.

Ericsson, K. Anders, Ralf T. Krampe, and Clemens Tesch-Römer. 1993. "The Role of Deliberate Practice in the Acquisition of Expert Performance." *Psychological Review* 100 (3): 363–406.

Farina, M. 2016. "Three Approaches to Human Cognitive Development: Neo-Nativism, Neuroconstructivism, and Dynamic Enskilment." *British Journal for the Philosophy of Science* 67 (2): 617–641. doi: 10.1093/bjps/axu026.

Farina, M. 2017. "Neural Plasticity: Don't Fall for the Hype!" *British Academy Review* 30:54–56.

Fox, P. W., S. L. Hershberger, and T. J. Bouchard Jr. 1996. "Genetic and Environmental Contributions to the Acquisition of a Motor Skill." *Nature* 384 (6607): 356–358.

Frazer, Kelly A., Sarah S. Murray, Nicholas J. Schork, and Eric J. Topol. 2009. "Human Genetic Variation and Its Contribution to Complex Traits." *Nature Reviews: Genetics* 10 (4): 241–251.

Gallagher, Shaun. 2011. "Interpretations of Embodied Cognition." In *The Implications of Embodiment: Cognition and Communication*, edited by W. Tschacher and C. Bergomi, 59–70. Exeter, UK: Imprint Academic.

Gallagher, Shaun. 2013. "The Socially Extended Mind." *Cognitive Systems Research* 25–26 (December): 4–12.

Gallagher, Shaun, and Anthony Crisafi. 2009. "Mental Institutions." *Topoi* 28 (1): 45–51.

Gallese, Vittorio, and George Lakoff. 2005. "The Brain's Concepts: The Role of the Sensory-Motor System in Conceptual Knowledge." *Cognitive Neuropsychology* 22 (3): 455–479.

Galton, Francis. 1865. "Hereditary Talent and Character." *Macmillan's Magazine* 12.157–166 :318–327.

Galton, Francis. [1869] 1992. *Hereditary Genius: An Inquiry into Its Laws and Consequences*. Cleveland: World.

Gibbons, Tim. 2002. *The Path of Excellence: A Comprehensive View of Development of U.S. Olympians Who Competed from 1984–1998*. New York: United States Olympic Committee.

Gladwell, Malcolm. 2008. *Outliers: The Story of Success*. Boston: Little, Brown.

Gobet, Fernand, and Guillermo Campitelli. 2007. "The Role of Domain-Specific Practice, Handedness, and Starting Age in Chess." *Developmental Psychology* 43 (1): 159.

Goldman, Alvin, and Frederique de Vignemont. 2009. "Is Social Cognition Embodied?" *Trends in Cognitive Sciences* 13 (4): 154–159.

Gustin, William C. 1985. "The Development of Exceptional Research Mathematicians." In *Developing Talent in Young People*, edited by Benjamin S. Bloom, 270–331. New York: Ballantine Books.

Hambrick, David Z., Frederick L. Oswald, Erik M. Altmann, Elizabeth J. Meinz, Fernand Gobet, and Guillermo Campitelli. 2014. "Deliberate Practice: Is That All It Takes to Become an Expert?" *Intelligence* 45:34–45.

Hamilton, Bruce. 2000. "East African Running Dominance: What Is behind It?" *British Journal of Sports Medicine* 34 (5): 391–394.

Hong, Y., P. M. Rautaharju, P. N. Hopkins, D. K. Arnett, L. Djousse, J. S. Pankow, P. Sholinsky, D. C. Rao, and M. A. Province. 2001. "Familial Aggregation of QT-Interval Variability in a General Population: Results from the NHLBI Family Heart Study." *Clinical Genetics* 59 (3): 171–177.

Howe, M. J., J. W. Davidson, and J. A. Sloboda. 1998. "Innate Talents: Reality or Myth?" *Behavioral and Brain Sciences* 21 (3): 399–407; discussion 407–442.

Huijgen, B. C. H., M. T. Elferink-Gemser, W. J. Post, and C. Visscher. 2009. "Soccer Skill Development in Professionals." *International Journal of Sports Medicine* 30 (8): 585–591.

Kiverstein, Julian, and Mirko Farina. 2011. "Embraining Culture: Leaky Minds and Spongy Brains." *Teorema: Revista Internacional de Filosofía* 32 (2): 35–53.

Kiverstein, Julian, Mirko Farina, and Andy Clark. 2013. *The Extended Mind* Oxford: Oxford Bibliographies Online, Oxford University Press. doi: 10.1093/OBO/9780195396577-0099.

Larsen, Henrik B. 2003. "Kenyan Dominance in Distance Running." *Comparative Biochemistry and Physiology, Part A: Molecular and Integrative Physiology* 136 (1): 161–170.

Latour, Bruno. 2004. "How to Talk about the Body? The Normative Dimension of Science Studies." *Body and Society* 10 (2/3): 205–229.

Lauderdale, D. S., R. Fabsitz, J. M. Meyer, P. Sholinsky, V. Ramakrishnan, and J. Goldberg. 1997. "Familial Determinants of Moderate and Intense Physical Activity: A Twin Study." *Medicine and Science in Sports and Exercise* 29 (8): 1062–1068.

Lerner, Richard M., and Willis F. Overton, eds. 2010. *Handbook of Life-Span Developmental Psychology*. New York: John Wiley.

Lippi, Giuseppe, Umile Giuseppe Longo, and Nicola Maffulli. 2010. "Genetics and Sports." *British Medical Bulletin* 93:27–47.

Maes, H. H., G. P. Beunen, R. F. Vlietinck, M. C. Neale, M. Thomis, B. Vanden Eynde, R. Lysens, J. Simons, C. Derom, and R. Derom. 1996. "Inheritance of Physical Fitness in 10-Yr-Old Twins and Their Parents." *Medicine and Science in Sports and Exercise* 28 (12): 1479–1491.

Maia, José A. R., Martine Thomis, and Gaston Beunen. 2002. "Genetic Factors in Physical Activity Levels." *American Journal of Preventive Medicine* 23 (2): 87–91.

Martens, Rainer. 1987. "Science, Knowledge, and Sport Psychology." *Sport Psychologist* 5 (1): 9–24.

Maturana, Humberto R., and Francisco J. Varela. 1991. *Autopoiesis and Cognition: The Realization of the Living*. Vol. 42. Berlin: Springer Science and Business Media.

McNamee, Michael John, Arno Müller, Ivo van Hilvoorde, and Søren Holm. 2009. "Genetic Testing and Sports Medicine Ethics." *Sports Medicine* 39 (5): 339–344.

Miah, Andy, and Emma Rich. 2006. "Genetic Tests for Ability? Talent Identification and the Value of an Open Future." *Sport, Education and Society* 11 (3): 259–273.

Milton, John, Ana Solodkin, Petr Hlustík, and Steven L. Small. 2007. "The Mind of Expert Motor Performance Is Cool and Focused." *NeuroImage* 35 (2): 804–813.

Missitzi, Julia, Reinhard Gentner, Angelica Misitzi, Nickos Geladas, Panagiotis Politis, Vassilis Klissouras, and Joseph Classen. 2013. "Heritability of Motor Control and Motor Learning." *Physiological Reports* 1 (7): e00188.

Montgomery, Hugh, and Latif Safari. 2007. "Genetic Basis of Physical Fitness." *Annual Review of Anthropology* 36 (1): 391–405.

Myers, Linnet. 1993. "Trained to Be a Genius, Girl, 16, Wallops Chess Champ Spassky for $110,000." *Chicago Tribune*, February 18. http://articles.chicagotribune.com/1993-02-18/news/9303181339_1_judit-polgar-boris-spassky-world-chess-champion.

Newton-Cheh, Christopher, Toby Johnson, Vesela Gateva, Martin D. Tobin, Murielle Bochud, Lachlan Coin, Samer S. Najjar, et al. 2009. "Genome-Wide Association Study Identifies Eight Loci Associated with Blood Pressure." *Nature Genetics* 41 (6): 666–676.

O'Regan, J. K., and A. Noë. 2001. "A Sensorimotor Account of Vision and Visual Consciousness." *Behavioral and Brain Sciences* 24 (5): 939–973; discussion 973–1031.

Pearson, D. T., G. A. Naughton, and M. Torode. 2006. "Predictability of Physiological Testing and the Role of Maturation in Talent Identification for Adolescent Team Sports." *Journal of Science and Medicine in Sport / Sports Medicine Australia* 9 (4): 277–287.

Peeters, M. W., M. A. I. Thomis, G. P. Beunen, and R. M. Malina. 2009. "Genetics and Sports: An Overview of the Pre-Molecular Biology Era." *Genetics and Sports* 54 (August): 28–42.

Pereira, André, Carlos Martinho, Iolanda Leite, and Ana Paiva. 2008. "iCat, the Chess Player: The Influence of Embodiment in the Enjoyment of a Game." *Proceedings of the 7th International Joint Conference on Autonomous Agents and Multiagent Systems* 3:1253–1256.

Pérusse, L., T. Rice, M. A. Province, J. Gagnon, A. S. Leon, J. S. Skinner, J. H. Wilmore, D. C. Rao, and C. Bouchard. 2000. "Familial Aggregation of Amount and Distribution of Subcutaneous Fat and Their Responses to Exercise Training in the HERITAGE Family Study." *Obesity Research* 8 (2): 140–150.

Phillips, Elissa, Keith Davids, Ian Renshaw, and Marc Portus. 2010. "Expert Performance in Sport and the Dynamics of Talent Development." *Sports Medicine* 40 (4): 271–283.

Plomin, Robert, Nicholas G. Shakeshaft, Andrew McMillan, and Maciej Trzaskowski. 2014. "Nature, Nurture, and Expertise." *Intelligence* 45 (July): 46–59.

Polgar, Susan. 2016. "National Geographic Chess Documentary 'My Brilliant Brain.'" *Chess Daily-News*, May 15. https://chessdailynews.com/national-geographic-chess-documentary-my-brilliant-brain/.

Régnier, Guy. 1987. "Un modèle conceptuel pour la détection du talent sportif." Unpublished PhD diss., University of Montreal, Canada.

Reilly, T., A. M. Williams, A. Nevill, and A. Franks. 2000. "A Multidisciplinary Approach to Talent Identification in Soccer." *Journal of Sports Sciences* 18 (9): 695–702.

Repp, Bruno H., and Günther Knoblich. 2004. "Perceiving Action Identity: How Pianists Recognize Their Own Performances." *Psychological Science* 15 (9): 604–609.

Rizzolatti, G., L. Fogassi, and V. Gallese. 2001. "Neurophysiological Mechanisms Underlying the Understanding and Imitation of Action." *Nature Reviews: Neuroscience* 2 (9): 661–670.

Roth, Stephen M. 2012. "Critical Overview of Applications of Genetic Testing in Sport Talent Identification." *Recent Patents on DNA and Gene Sequences* 6 (3): 247–255.

Rowland, T. W. 1998. "The Biological Basis of Physical Activity." *Medicine and Science in Sports and Exercise* 30 (3): 392–399.

Russell, Scott. 2000. *Ice time: A Canadian Hockey Journey*. New York: Viking.

Salmela, John H., Bernard Petiot, and T. Blaine Hoshizaki, eds. 1987. *Psychological Nurturing and Guidance of Gymnastic Talent*. Montréal: Sport Psyche Éditions.

Silventoinen, Karri. 2003. "Determinants of Variation in Adult Body Height." *Journal of Biosocial Science* 35 (2): 263–285.

Simon, Herbert A., and William G. Chase. 1973. "Skill in Chess." *American Science* 61:394–403.

Simonton, Dean Keith. 1999. "Talent and Its Development: An Emergenic and Epigenetic Model." *Psychological Review* 106 (3): 435–457.

Simonton, Dean Keith. 2001. "Talent Development as a Multidimensional, Multiplicative, and Dynamic Process." *Current Directions in Psychological Science* 10 (2): 39–43.

Sloboda, John. 2002. "Michael Howe (1940–2002)." *The Psychologist* 15 (3): 146.

Sosniak, Lauren A. 1985. "Learning to Be a Concert Pianist." In *Developing Talent in Young People*, edited by Benjamin Bloom, 19–67. New York: Ballantine Books.

Sutton, John. 2007. "Batting, Habit and Memory: The Embodied Mind and the Nature of Skill." *Sport in Society* 10 (5): 763–786.

Sutton, John, Doris McIlwain, Wayne Christensen, and Andrew Geeves. 2011. "Applying Intelligence to the Reflexes: Embodied Skills and Habits between Dreyfus and Descartes." *Journal of the British Society for Phenomenology* 42 (1): 78–103.

Thompson, Evan, and Francisco J. Varela. 2001. "Radical Embodiment: Neural Dynamics and Consciousness." *Trends in Cognitive Sciences* 5 (10): 418–425.

Thorburn, A. W., and J. Proietto. 2000. "Biological Determinants of Spontaneous Physical Activity." *Obesity Reviews* 1 (2): 87–94.

Tiainen, Kristina, Sarianna Sipilä, Markku Alén, Eino Heikkinen, Jaakko Kaprio, Markku Koskenvuo, Asko Tolvanen, Satu Pajala, and Taina Rantanen. 2005. "Shared Genetic and Environmental Effects on Strength and Power in Older Female Twins." *Medicine and Science in Sports and Exercise* 37 (1): 72–78.

Tiwari, Reena. 2010. "*Space Body Ritual: Performativity in the City*." Lanham, MD: Lexington Books.

Tucker, Ross, and Malcolm Collins. 2012. "What Makes Champions? A Review of the Relative Contribution of Genes and Training to Sporting Success." *British Journal of Sports Medicine* 46 (8): 555–561.

Vaeyens, Roel, Matthieu Lenoir, A. Mark Williams, and Renaat M. Philippaerts. 2008. "Talent Identification and Development Programmes in Sport: Current Models and Future Directions." *Sports Medicine* 38 (9): 703–714.

Voestermans, Paul, and Theo Verheggen. 2013. *Culture as Embodiment: The Social Tuning of Behavior*. Hoboken, NJ: John Wiley and Sons.

Weedon, Michael N., Guillaume Lettre, Rachel M. Freathy, Cecilia M. Lindgren, Benjamin F. Voight, John R. B. Perry, Katherine S. Elliott, et al. 2007. "A Common Variant of HMGA2 Is Associated with Adult and Childhood Height in the General Population." *Nature Genetics* 39 (10): 1245–1250.

Wegenstein, Bernadette. 2006. *Getting Under the Skin: The Body and Media Theory*. Cambridge, MA: MIT Press.

Wheeler, Michael. 2005. *Reconstructing the Cognitive World: The Next Step*. Cambridge, MA: MIT Press.

Wilber, Randall L., and Yannis P. Pitsiladis. 2012. "Kenyan and Ethiopian Distance Runners: What Makes Them So Good?" *International Journal of Sports Physiology and Performance* 7 (2): 92–102.

Williams, Alun G., and Jonathan P. Folland. 2008. "Similarity of Polygenic Profiles Limits the Potential for Elite Human Physical Performance." *Journal of Physiology* 586 (1): 113–121.

Wood, Andrew R., Tonu Esko, Jian Yang, Sailaja Vedantam, Tune H. Pers, Stefan Gustafsson, Audrey Y. Chu, et al. 2014. "Defining the Role of Common Variation in the Genomic and Biological Architecture of Adult Human Height." *Nature Genetics* 46 (11): 1173–1186.

Wymbs, Nicholas F., Amy J. Bastian, and Pablo A. Celnik. 2016. "Motor Skills Are Strengthened through Reconsolidation." *Current Biology* 26 (3): 338–343.

12 Emerging Technologies for Sport Performance Enhancement: Embodied Cognition and Manipulation of Brain Rhythms

Miriam Reiner

1 Introduction

Physical performance and cognitive abilities are intertwined. Executive skills such as problem solving, decision making, and inhibition correlate with expert performance in sport (Jacobson and Matthaeus 2014). One of the more interesting examples of intellectual emergence intertwined with embodied mechanisms is a cognitive mechanisms known as a "thought experiment."

Thought experiments happen in imagination. Their power is in the thinker's capacity to convincingly "see," with the mind's eye, the "results" of an action performed in thought. For instance, we can easily predict the course of motion of a ball thrown at us, and catch or move away, so not to be hit. Thought experiments have a strong epistemological power in constructing knowledge (Reiner and Gilbert 2000; Reiner 2000; Reiner and Burko 2003). To better see into their embodied-intellectual mentation process, it is beneficial to look at their role in a drastically different discipline, physics reasoning. Thought experiments were a central mechanism in physics innovation (Reiner 2008), and although performed in thought only, their results and conclusions were convincing, shared by all, and became cornerstones of new theories such as the special relativity theory.

For instance, Einstein's thought experiment on simultaneity shares many embodied faculties with sport imagery. It requires the reader to imagine motion, and what she would see if she were located in two different positions: in a fast-moving train and on an embankment. The story is that two strokes of lightning are emitted from two symmetrical points at her left and right, while she is either inside a very fast train moving toward the right lightning or at rest on the embankment. Will she witness identical events while in the train and on the embankment? Will she see the two strokes simultaneously while in the train? While on the embankment? Or, stated differently, the reader is asked to judge whether reality is different when one is in the reference frame of the train compared with on the embankment.

The answer is that, while being in the train moving toward the lightning, she would see the right lightning first and the left lightning, which is "chasing her," would be seen later. However, if she were on the embankment, she would see both left and right lightning—that is, both events—simultaneously. Thus simultaneity is defined by the frame of reference. Two simultaneous events in one frame of reference might be non-simultaneous in another, and each body-reference has its own time; unless we are told what the body-reference is, there is no meaning in a statement of the time of an event. This "result," obtained in thought only, was powerful enough to lead to a paradigm shift in the physics community, that is, the sequence of events and results were uniformly viewed by all readers. Maintaining in imagination the physical constitution of our body, in the perceptual situated context of the environment, contributed a significant portion of the information-processing traditionally attributed to higher cognitive processing alone.

Perceptual patterns of bodily engagement in the environment provide specific tools for remembering, thinking, and perceiving in imagination and for constructing mental "results" that are valid in the physical world. The internal imaginary stimuli and resulting affordances of the body-in-the-environment are replicated in the imaginary world to generate both optimally efficient movements, as in sport, and intellectual physics constructs, as described in the cognitive-ecological affordance approach by Gibson (1979).

Imagery is often triggered by physical sensory cues. For instance, sensation of forces determines bodily motion (Reiner 1999; Reiner and Gilbert 2000), as in throwing a spear, manipulating a hammer in a throw, or manipulating the body in a jump. But how do we know what to be attentive to? After all, the environment is a series of constantly, ongoing, active stimuli—how do we select what to attend to? More specifically, what are the neural processes that underlie the selection of relevant internal stimuli that make this uniform human perceptual mentation possible? It is probably more than just a single function, beyond a specific brain region, engaging a variety of well-orchestrated functionalities, of multiple regions. For instance, Sauseng et al. (2009) suggested that retention of relevant information depends on a coupling between theta and gamma rhythms, and suppression of irrelevant information depends on the alpha rhythm. They further show that increased alpha band was correlated with increased suppression of irrelevant information resulting in enhanced performance.

Similar processes of selection occur in any interaction with the environment, allowing mental prediction of results of action (Bartlett, Wheat, and Robins 2007). It is therefore not surprising that imagery has been mentioned as a central procedure in research of sport psychology. Training assumes that a memory is mentally created and is accessible: repetitive physical and imagery training on a movement pattern requires accessing an existing mental movement pattern. Thus a crucial precondition to performing a motion pattern, either in thought or physically, is the existence of a relevant memory of the movement. How are patterns of movement memory generated? What are the processes of memory consolidation? Why would repetition in imagination alone further improve the physical performance?

Beyond memory patterns, other mental processes are involved in embodied manipulation in sport, such as mental rotation, mental load, motor control, and erring. In the parts that follow I discuss processes and technologies for enhanced performance by controlling brain rhythms. Four aspects are presented: (1) memory consolidation with theta neurofeedback training (NFT); (2) enhanced mental rotation with NFT; (3) enhanced movement performance by reducing mental load in real time; and (4) the role of erring in estimation of optimal performance. The conclusion integrates all four angles taken above into the framework of the recently emerging technologies of embodiment of virtual and augmented reality.

2 Neurofeedback and Memory Consolidation of Movement

Imagine for instance that you just completed a long training on a newly learned Chopin prelude. You move your fingers, play on your imaginary piano, and simultaneously hear the music in your imagination. By doing that, you activate a *motor plan*, a process by which you activate brain mechanisms and muscular components, resulting in a sequential motion of your fingers. Your fingers move in a pattern that was generated during training, while you physically played the piano. If you were tested immediately afterward, and then in the evening and again in the morning, your performance would be best in the morning (Wilson and McNaughton 1994). The reason is that the motor plan is registered during training, stabilized during the following few hours, then consolidated during sleep (Dudai 2004).

A large body of research has consistently shown that sleep enhances memory consolidation—mostly night sleep, but even day naps improve consolidation (e.g., Stickgold and Walker 2005; Dudai 2004; Rauchs et al. 2005). Sleep was found to explain 70 percent of variance in memory consolidation as measured by quality of performance (Stickgold and Walker 2005). In addition, a high correlation, in the range of 0.56–0.95, between performance and sleep, across varying tasks, supports the crucial role of sleep in motor memory consolidation (Stickgold and Walker 2005). These processes are uniquely correlated with sleep and were not found in awake daytime hours. Memory formation, such as memory of sequential movement, evolves in two steps (Dudai 2004; Albouy et al. 2008). A first initial registration of the training motion occurs in the hippocampus, within minutes to hours after starting the training process. This registration is stabilized within two to eight hours after training. The second phase occurs off-line, hours to days after training, without additional training beyond the test.

Performance resulting from the first phase is rapidly improved, and the delta compared to a pretraining stage is large. This first hippocampal registration phase is known as neural memory formation (although both stages are correlated with induced changes in neural activity) and mainly takes place in the hippocampal and neorcortical systems. Sh(0) and Sc(0) represent the strength of the initial hippocampal and neocortical traces, respectively. The hippocampal representation later becomes active during sleep, but interestingly, also during recall, as during imagination: that is, in the process of "running" the movement in a thought experiment (Dudai 2004).

This first registration creates a neocortical trace, which, in the second phase, the system-consolidation phase, is reorganized in long-lasting memories (Albouy et al. 2008; Maquet 2001) and consolidated through a process of theta resonance between the hippocampus and remote areas. The hippocampus and the striatum become engaged in a process of mutual resonance, at the frequency of 4–8 Hz, which eventually results in consolidation of the movement pattern. Two processes occur now in parallel: the memory trace, Sh(1), is increasingly strengthened in the striatum, and, in parallel, the memory trace in the hippocampus, Sc(0), decays much faster (Dudai 2004).

The second stage above, of memory consolidation, is dependent on night sleep (Albouy et al. 2008; Dudai 2004; Stickgold and Walker 2005; Fischer et al. 2002; Maquet 2001). For instance, the movement pattern of an ordered sequence of finger tapping (somewhat similar to playing piano), known as the finger-tapping task (FTT, e.g., Korman et al. 2003), was improved significantly when comparing performance after night sleep with performance immediately after training (Boyce et al. 2016; Heib et al. 2015; Diekelmann and Born 2010; Censor, Karni, and Sagi 2006; for a review see Cohen et al. 2015). Korman et al. (2007) showed that even a short day nap contributes to memory consolidation. The memory trace of the movement is continuously consolidated with each reactivation of the neuronal circuits that were involved in the first registration (encoding) (Albouy et al. 2008), which may explain why reactivation during imagery contributes to performance.

Memory of motion patterns and muscle activations are at the heart of sport training. Only a limited number of well-validated studies on sport enhancement are available, and even fewer studies on self-manipulation of brain oscillation bands, such as in neurofeedback studies, have been published. Cannon et al. (2014) argue that the neural mechanisms that generate specific frequency bands help communicate signals within and among brain regions, thereby making possible specific cognitive functions, depending on the brain regions and frequency bands involved. If so, can we train people to enhance particular wave bands to activate neural mechanisms? This is the idea behind neurofeedback—users are trained to modulate the frequency of specific brain oscillations. Neurofeedback mechanisms and their function are still not well understood, in spite of recent advances. A review by Vernon (2005) states that, "due to a range of methodological limitations and a general failure to elicit unambiguous changes in baseline EEG activity, a clear association between neurofeedback training and enhanced performance has yet to be established" (1).

Since then, both methodological advances and a better understanding of the neural mechanisms and oscillations have provided new results. A pioneering study that brought evidence for the correlations of theta power and performance was provided by Egner and Gruzelier (2003). They studied neurofeedback theta/alpha effects for enhancing normal function in music performance under stressful conditions of conservatory students and brought evidence that expert subjective ratings in musical performance in a student group that underwent neurofeedback were highly correlated with a progressive rise in theta/alpha amplitudes. Encouraged by studies on the role of theta in sleep memory consolidation and by the Egner and Gruzelier (2003) pioneering results, it seemed feasible to test whether elevated theta oscillations during awake hours would correlate with similar consolidation effects.

This assumption was tested by Reiner, Rozengurt, and Barnea (2014). They asked whether the first memory registration of a still unstable, just-learned sequence of movements can be consolidated beyond the first registration, during awake time, if, in some way, theta resonance across the hippocampus and striatum is enhanced. So the hypothesis tested was whether higher intensity of the theta amplitude during awake hours enhances memory consolidation. In the experiment, a conditioning protocol was applied, in which the participants received a visual feedback on their intensity of theta/beta level and were trained to increase the ratio. The task was a sequence of finger movements. They were instructed to touch the thumb of their left hand, with their fingers, in the sequence 4-1-3-2-4.

The experimental design included three groups (one experimental group and two control groups) and four phases: training on the movement until plateau; test; neurofeedback training (NFT); and tests immediately after NFT, 24 hours after NFT, 48 hours after NFT, and a week after NFT.

Results showed a clear and significant enhanced performance of the motion pattern in the theta group, when compared with performance prior to the neurofeedback process, but not in the two control groups. Performance in the beta group showed a minor deterioration and a minor nonsignificant improved performance in the control group. Changes in performance are shown in figure 12.1 below.

Each point represents the average number of sequences completed in thirty seconds. Four connected points represent the four blocks of one test. The vertical lines represent the error. The study reports a significant improvement in performance in the theta group, relative to the beta and control groups, immediately after NFT. Performance was further improved after night sleep in all groups, with a significant advantage favoring the theta group. Indeed, theta power during training was correlated with the level of improvement, indicating a clear relationship between memory consolidation and theta NFT.

Will the same experimental protocol apply to larger patterns of movement sequences, as in sport? For instance, think of learning golf: it requires mastering the precise pattern of grip, tilting the body, bending the knees, and swinging the ball, all in a smooth continuous motion. Can the ordered sequence of movements and overall smoothness of motion be enhanced? Will neurofeedback of theta/beta change the neural activation to generate a memory trace that is superior, beyond a standard physical-imagery training? Indeed, these results suggest a theoretical framework of memory consolidation of movement during awake hours with neurofeedback.

An interesting approach, suggesting the individualization of EEG neurofeedback protocol, comes from Arns et al. (2008). They assumed that each individual has an EEG

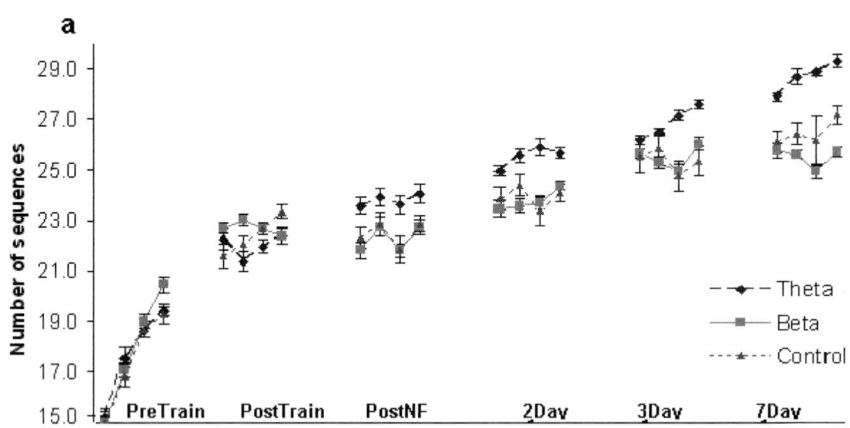

Figure 12.1
Average performance of four blocks in each group: before training on the sequence of movement, after training, after NFT, and 24 hours, 48 hours, and a week after NFT.

fingerprint that correlates with the person's successes and another that correlates with the person's failures. Accepting this approach dictates first identifying the specific oscillation patterns that characterize each individual in successful versus failure states, then using neurofeedback to enhance the individual signature specific to success.

Arns et al. (2008) applied such an individualized protocol to study enhancement of golf, with personal signature of EGG correlated with successful putts. They then trained each player to raise their individual success markers using neurofeedback during golf putting, according to the individual EEG markers. The overall percentage of successful putts was significantly larger in the neurofeedback series of training compared with the control series, and most participants improved their performance by an average of 25 percent. It would be interesting to look at the individual EEG frequency component to extract the overlap across users and conclude whether a common mechanism underlies the individual patterns.

A special kind of sequence of movement is dancing. Dancing with music is different from learning a sequence of movements such as in golf because of the music cues that correlate with the sequence of movements. Neurofeedback to elevate the ratio of alpha/theta rhythms was correlated with gains of dancers from novice to expert, and the control-SMR group showed an effect mainly on novices, with a higher effect on lower abilities (Fitts and Posner 1967). Movement might be enhanced by lowering anxiety, when anxiety is a factor in performance. Singer (2004) showed that dancers' anxiety was reduced following thirty sessions of a broadband 11–16 Hz (T3/4) training with inhibits of 2–7 Hz and 23–38 Hz activity. Gruzelier et al. (2014) studied anxiety and creativity in a dancing task: they found enhanced performance in dancing correlated with a reduction in anxiety following heart rate variability (HRV) training, and showed that alpha/theta training was correlated with expressive creativity elaboration.

The core difference between the effects of alpha (relative to theta) and theta neurofeedback on performance are rooted in the underlying mechanism. The first, alpha relative to theta intensity, is correlated with creativity, and the effects of performance are on parameters of creativity rather than on duration and accuracy. The effects of elevated alpha on enhanced creativity might result in slight changes to movements, while the effect of theta is on fast and accurate performance. Thus neurofeedback to enhance theta amplitude, leading to faster performance and enhanced accuracy, would fit some sports, whereas elevated alpha would better fit creative sport performance such as dance.

Additional protocols related to motor memory consolidation used transcranial magnetic stimulation (TMS)—a noninvasive method for stimulating the brain. When applied at 10 Hz, results show an entrainment of alpha rhythms (Robertson 2009), which increased participants' capacity to suppress irrelevant stimuli and enhanced working memory capacity (Sauseng et al. 2009).

An exciting potential angle on enhancement during sleep comes from Ngo et al. (2013), who tested whether sound stimuli modify slow oscillations during sleep. Their results show that sound stimuli that are in phase with slow oscillations induce enhanced slow oscillatory activity in the brain, which in turn enhances spindle activity coupled with slow oscillations, resulting in enhanced sleep-dependent memory consolidation. Are appropriate sound stimuli tools to induce rhythms that correlate with memory consolidation? The underlying mechanism that correlates auditory frequencies with induced oscillation bands is not well understood. This is a potentially exciting option, not yet well understood, that requires additional research.

3 Enhancing Mental Rotation with Brain Rhythms

One of the essential cognitive abilities for everyday spatial activities, and in sport, relates to predicting the position of a rotated object: that is, imagining the act of rotation of an object, without the actual rotation. This operation is known as mental rotation, and it has been studied extensively over the years. Mental rotation is involved in acts such as orientation in unfamiliar places or finding a route on a map, and has an important role in cognitive processes associated with learning and training, as in academic and analytic tasks. For instance, success in mathematics and physics is positively correlated with mental rotation skills (Delgado and Prieto 2004).

This skill is fundamental to sport performance, enabling efficient manipulation and interaction with objects in the surrounding space. The interplay between manipulation of an object in imagination, relative to the position and posture of the body, are also at the heart of embodiment. In many sport activities, embodiment is related to the ability to "see" the bodily motion required for the desired result—such as the motion required to set the ball bouncing into a golf hole, or to throw a boomerang, or the coordination between the jumping body and a flying swing in athletics. The time needed for imaginary rotation is crucial: the faster and more accurate mental rotation is, the faster and more accurate is the response. Time needed for mental rotation increases with the angle of rotation (Shepard and Metzler 1971) and with the changes in perceived shape created by motion compared with the original (Cooper and Shepard 1973; Shepard and Cooper 1982).

People differ in their mental rotation abilities—that is, in their accuracy and the time needed to predict the course of rotation or recognize rotated objects (Thomas and Kail 1991; Lizarraga and Ganuza 2003). Motor imagery and motor execution share similar motor-related neural networks (Neuper et al. 2005; Gerardin et al 2000; Guillot et al. 2008). Does this imply that "execution" in imagination will result in enhanced motion execution? When the effects of imagery on motor execution in the context of relearning after stroke have been tested, some results have shown improved performance and some have failed to show significant improvement compared with control conditions (Ietswaart et al. 2011). In studying imagery in sport, results show consistent benefits (Lebon, Collet, and Guillot 2010; Higuchi, Shimada, and Rekimoto 2011; for a review see Schuster et al. 2011). Mental rotation is a central function in imagery.

Moreau et al. (2011) tested the relationship between motor performance in sport and mental rotation in problem solving. Highly performing athletes completed a series of tests that measured mental rotation and sport-specific training measures and found a significant relationship between sport performance, sport-specific training, and mental rotation, with a gendered effect favoring males. High-achieving athletes also used flexible strategies to improve their mental rotation problem-solving tasks, which pointed to their mental rotation strategies in sport. Similarly, Pietsch (2012) compared mental rotation skills in three groups of students from a variety of backgrounds: music, sport, and education. The results showed a better mental rotation performance for music and sport students compared with the education students. As above, the gender difference effect favoring males was found here, too, with the exception of the music students. Skill at mental rotation enhances sport performance, but the other way around works too: spatial ability, especially mental rotation, is enhanced through practice in sport (Moreau 2012), and coordination in manipulating the self-body in space is correlated with mental rotation (Jansen et al. 2010). Motor neural structures are activated during nonphysical tasks such as during imagery, mental rotation (Ganis et al. 2000) relating imagery, with mental rotation and with enhanced performance.

Given the crucial fundamentality of mental rotation, can it be enhanced? Indeed some studies suggest that training might enhance mental rotation ability (Ericsson, Nandagopal, and Roring 2005), and motor training that includes cognitive functions of rotation in imagery has an effect on scores achieved in a mental rotation test (Moreau 2012). Similar results were reported on the effect of games on improved mental rotation (De Lisi and Wolford 2002; Cherney 2008).

Recent studies suggest a method that affects the underlying mechanism of mental rotation and is independent of training: manipulation of specific brain rhythms. Based on previous results suggesting a role of the upper alpha frequencies in mental rotation ability (Hanslmayr et al. 2005; see Vernon 2005 for an overview), Zoefel, Huster, and Herrmann (2011) used neurofeedback training (NFT) as an operant conditioning protocol to train participants to control their own brain oscillations. Their assumption was that the amplitude of the upper alpha frequency band is correlated with mental rotation. They trained participants to raise their individually determined upper alpha band during five consecutive days, one session per day. Participants completed a mental rotation test before the first and after the last session. The neurofeedback group increased the amplitude of the individual upper alpha band and showed a correlated enhanced mental rotation performance, confirming their initial assumptions on the role of enhanced alpha in mental rotation.

The alpha band was also examined in a dance study by Gruzelier et al. (2014). Using an alpha/theta neurofeedback protocol, they found that alpha/theta training increased cognitive creativity with the test of unusual uses (Gruzelier et al. 2014), which might be associated with enhanced mental rotation ability correlated with elevated alpha activity. Another interesting study focused on the effects of mindfulness meditation. Mindfulness meditation has been recently shown to correlate with enhanced alpha frequencies, similar to the effects of alpha-neurofeedback (Chow et al. 2017). Mindfulness meditation is the ability to maintain attention toward a process or object and ignore distractions. As attentional control is improved by mindfulness meditation (Lutz et al. 2008), mental rotation capacity might be affected. No studies have yet tested this effect, but because mindfulness meditation is such a simple, noninvasive technique, its possible effects on mental rotation and sport performance raise an extremely interesting research question and potential enhancement method.

4 Coping with the Negative Effect of Excessive Mental Load in Movement Performance

Mental load is correlated with decreased attentional control, and increases with the number of items in working memory. It is affected by anxiety, mental fatigue, environmental distractors such as background noise, sensory ambiguity such as blurriness, cognitive ambiguity, and level of task difficulty, and results in deterioration of performance when mental load exceeds a specific level or is lower than a particular threshold. Thus, it seems that enhanced performance happens within a window between levels of mental load. If so, identifying the conditions of enhanced performance would involve identifying the mechanism underlying increased or decreased mental load. Linden et al. (2003) overloaded participants' memory in an fMRI experiment and looked for the correlated activations, hoping to identify an underlying mechanism for overload that is correlated with excess items in the working memory. Increases in response to memory load were observed. Their results showed correlated increases in activations of the dorsolateral prefrontal cortex (DLPFC) and the pre-supplementary motor area (pre-SMA).

The more interesting result was that the activity in the frontal eye fields (FEFs) and in areas along the intraparietal sulcus peaked when mental load was lower—that is, when the number of objects in the working memory was two or three, and decreased when the number of items in memory increased. This result suggests that performing cognitive tasks under high load fails to support visual working memory. Are there any implications at all for enhancement of sport performance? The above results suggest that overload in sensory environmental stimuli, within the range levels of excessive visual cues in the Linden et al. experiment (2003), is detrimental to performance.

Yet, once performance becomes automatic, the distracting environmental stimuli would need to be powerful to penetrate and disrupt automatic performance. The prefrontal cortex, and intraparietal sulcus and FEF, are correlated with attention, and hence it would be feasible to assume that the attention networks are affected. Overload impedes attention, and less mental effort is dedicated to the task compared with conditions of lower load on working memory. Following Linden et al. (2003), several additional studies have confirmed the relation between excess mental load and performance. Depending on the task, excess mental load has a major effect on sport decision making and performance (Duncan et al. 2015; Marcora, Staiano, and Manning 2009). The effect on performance is not linear, and the assumption that the higher the mental load the lower the level of performance is incorrect (Peifer et al. 2014). Very high and very low mental load have a similar effect on performance (Arent and Landers 2003; Sandi 2013; Mekari et al. 2015). Arent and Landers (2003) brought empirical findings suggesting that the inverted-U hypothesis predicts optimal performance at the level of 60 to 70 percent of maximum arousal; enhancing performance, according to this result, would suggest keeping the arousal at this level.

What type of methodology would allow control of the mental load level to keep the level of arousal optimal? Real-time neural measures of mental load might provide an appropriate technology. Real-time measures of mental load are tricky, especially if the measure is nonsubjective and uses tools other than questionnaires. A method for real-time measures of mental load is briefly described below.

One major issue in mental load was the objectivity of measures. Mental load has been traditionally measured with post-performance questionnaires (Homer, Plass, and Blake 2008), which limited both the validity and the ability to extract event-related changes in mental load. Recent studies suggest a high temporal resolution measurement of mental load, using EEG techniques (Dan and Reiner 2016). Using an EEG index of mental load, Dan and Reiner (2016) showed that performance of complex tasks that require processing of excessive high-density sensory cues requires higher mental efforts, resulting in reduced performance. Stress adds to mental load, and hence reduces performance too (Hatfield, Haufler, and Contreras-Vidal 2009). Environmental "noise" such as light flashes, sounds and voices, inner stress, and blurred views or limited visibility increase mental load and reduce performance. In a study in the context of surgery in a virtual environment, in which high accuracy of a movement was crucial to performance, we tested transferability of training and learning from a low-immersive environment to a high-immersive environment and found that whereas learning of movements in a low-immersive/high mental load environment is limited in transferability to practice, and vice versa, learning from high-immersive/low mental load to low immersive environments is well transferred (Lev and Reiner 2012).

Berka et al. (2008) looked at the neurophysiological measure of anxiety, as measured by the power spectral density of heart rate variability (HRV), in experts and novices, in an attempt to discover whether anxiety is a factor in performance in rifle marksmanship. They found that novices had higher mean heart rates compared with experts, with a more pronounced level of HRV at 0.15 Hz in novices, and concluded that average anxiety of novices tends to be higher compared with experts. They suggested employing procedures to reduce anxiety to improve novice performance. This might work if novices had the experience that allowed developing the memory trace of the motor movement of the pattern needed for execution; otherwise, lower anxiety will just allow optimal execution of the limited and preliminary existing relevant movement sequence (Reiner, Rozengurt, and Barnea 2014; Reiner 2004). Berka et al. (2008) further report preliminary results on an increase in alpha and theta correlated with expert shooting, with a slight increase in mental load for experts. However this preliminary data is obtained from an extremely small sample, with no statistical significance (three participants in each group), and hence is of low validity. The lower mental load in novices compared with experts is inconsistent with both theory and previous results.

Can we train to reduce mental load, and if so, what would be an optimal training system? The stronger the memory trace, the less it is subject to interference caused by attentional distractions as associated with excess demands on working memory. There are few studies on controlled working load and performance. Current studies on mastering physical performance in interaction with objects in virtual environments (similar to hammer throwing) are reported by Reiner and Gelfeld (2014). They measured mental load by recording the changes in pupil dynamics with a high-resolution eye tracker (SMI 500) and found that mental load was increased and performance was reduced in the condition of unpredictable variables in the task—for example, if there was no clear indication of the mass of the virtual object that was to be thrown, or if the visual cues of the virtual object to be thrown were not clear enough to indicate the object properties.

However, in predictable, low-ambiguity conditions, mental load dropped and, after performance of a critical number of repetitions, participants achieved an "automatic" performance condition, similar to the conditions of "flow" performance. This further suggests that both performance and training conditions must be highly predictable to achieve automation, and that training should be conducted up to the automation point, and not beyond, since at this point mental load tends to drop to the U-shaped low levels of performance, because of lower attentional focus.

5 Virtual Reality, Enhanced Sport Performance, and Embodiment

Virtual reality brings an exciting, ecologically valid setup for training in sport. Virtual worlds, being fully controllable and flexible, allow inclusion of conditions that are not easily replicated in reality, such as foggy vision, multiple players, sensory stimuli, and subliminal cues that generate—when designed appropriately—affordances with lasting effects. In the following we review studies and report the findings of sport training in virtual worlds. Not many studies are reported on virtual reality, embodiment, and sport, hence we bring here examples of movement training in other domains that require fine and complex movements with high precision, then apply the conclusions to sport. To conclude, we link the findings to the new emerging virtual and augmented technologies for superior training in sport.

Mental load and the efficacy of training for enhanced movement in VR: Is VR better than flat-screens for motion training? The first example shows the results of a recently completed first controlled study on training for fine movements of surgical skills in a virtual world, which we carried out at the VR.NeuroCog lab (http://vrneurocog.wixsite.com/vrneurocog). The description and results are discussed in the context of similar training scenarios in sport movements. We designed a surgical environment in virtual reality (see the setup in figure 12.2). The purpose of the study was to test the effects of 2-D compared with 3-D virtual reality on performance and mental load. The study was especially designed to test whether there is any superior advantage in using 3-D virtual worlds for training compared with 2-D flat-screens: Is training in a 2-D video interactive environment less or more efficient compared with training in a 3-D virtual interactive environment? Is 3-D virtual immersive technology indeed needed for high-level training, or is it just another technological unfulfilled premise? Ten subjects (age 27.2, s.d. 3.7, gender-balanced) participated in the experiment for payment. The virtual world presented a 3-D (with depth) virtual realistic abdominal cavity. The flat interactive training environment was identical, but the image was presented on a flat-screen with no depth, similar to the conditions in laparoscopic OR surgery. The VR here was highly immersive and ecologically valid, in the sense that it highly resembles realistic setups. The user experienced visual, auditory, and force-feedback sensations. Force feedback created the feel of force exerted on the arm when touching or dissecting a tissue/blood vessel with a virtual surgical tool. The force feedback was enabled by a robotic arm—the Phantom Force Feedback device (by SensAble). The robotic arm was placed under the space where the virtual abdomen was seen and was invisible to the eye during the experiment (see figure 12.2). Both the haptic (touch) and visual display were rendered using the lab's proprietary application programming interface, based on OpenGL.

Participants had the shutter glasses on, which enabled 3-D vision, and were asked to perform a sophisticated motion pattern as quickly and accurately as possible. The motion patterns included linear motion, accurate touch, and rotation and required avoidance of touching the abdominal wall. The purpose was to dissect several virtual lumps located in increasingly hard-to-reach positions on the digestive tract. They repeated the task, with random repositioning of the lumps, in two blocks of thirty-one trials each.

Environmental cues and display (2-D flat-screen versus 3-D virtual world) were manipulated by adding or reducing depth. Half the participants performed the task in an immersive 3-D virtual world and half performed the task in a 2-D video interactive world. Electroencephalogram (EEG) was recorded with the Mitsar-EEG-202 system from nineteen electrodes placed on the skull according the standard 10–20 system. After artifact removal, we calculated mental load indices from the EEG measures and timed the duration of task completion and accuracy.

Results show that the duration of time needed in a highly ambiguous environment (interactive 2-D training) was correlated with longer time duration and lower accuracy

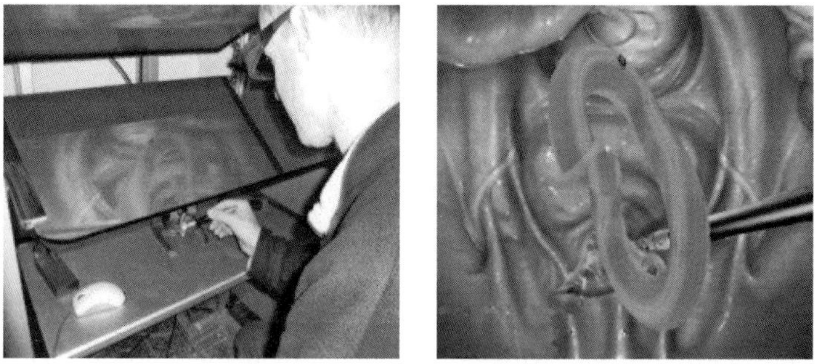

Figure 12.2
Left, the setup of the VR; right, the visuals.

Table 12.1
Comparison of mental load indices among training in VR, with a flat-screen, and rest conditions.

	Mean	Std. Deviation	N
Dislocation Theta/Alpha	1.6150	.35415	10
Collocation Theta/Alpha	1.1261	.42167	10
REST_Theta/Alpha	.7224	.44445	10

compared with the 3-D virtual environment. The mental load EEG indices were calculated from the ratio of frontal theta and parietal alpha. The mental load index for 2-D presentation was significantly higher compared with training in 3-D virtual reality ($F=58.5$; $p<0.001$), and the mental load index of training in virtual reality was higher ($F=53.4$; $p<0.001$) compared with rest conditions (see table 12.1).

Implications for sport are that training in 2-D is associated with increased mental load compared with a 3-D immersive virtual reality training environment. The mental load increases because of the lack of depth, which increases ambiguity. Similar results regarding the higher mental load and lower accuracy in 2-D versus 3-D were obtained in other studies with varying tasks and conditions (Dan and Reiner 2016; Reiner and Gelfeld 2014; Lev and Reiner 2012). There is a large overlap between learning fine movement patterns in contexts such as learning in surgery and fine movement patterns of the hand in throwing a spear, and it suggests that training in 2-D is not only more demanding and less efficient, but also not transferable to 3-D (Lev and Reiner 2012). It further suggests that low ambiguity (and predictability) is crucial for lower mental load, and that the central most important point in training—transferability—is low in ambiguous, ecologically nonvalid environments. The reason is probably that the embodiment functions that humans recruit for efficient interaction with the environment are not valid, or hardly helpful, in non-ecologically-valid environments. Ecological validity—the level of similarity between the training environment and the performance environment—is crucial.

6 Enhanced Performance in VR: Can We Predict Errors?

The ability to predict who makes more errors, and the type of errors typical to an individual (the "erring profile" in sport), provides an interesting and powerful tool for identifying optimal trainees, and targeting the types of errors made, for enhanced performance. A recent technology based on EEG allows identification of such errors in the course of performance of a sport action, such as playing tennis. The unique power of virtual reality is in the ability to measure, in real time, event-related EEG signals, known as event related potentials (ERP) that correlate with the different categories of errors. Yazmir and Reiner (2016) designed a virtual world in which participants played a tennis game. The virtual environment was highly immersive, ecologically valid, and included visual, auditory, and touch cues. While playing, participants performed a series of natural errors. After artifact removal and noise reduction, we identified the ERPs correlated with each type of error, in an attempt to find out whether each type of error has a unique ERP marker, or whether error ERPs are independent of the type of error. Results showed a strong correlation between the types of error and the ERP signals—in terms of peaks, latency, amplitude, and correlated rhythms (Yazmir and Reiner 2016; Yazmir et al. 2016). Results further suggested categories of "performers," such as slow responders, when compared to the average. Their response time seem to be correlated to brain network responses, since we found a relatively late ERP (compared to the average of the populations), correlated with their manual response time. Is this tendency trainable? It might be a natural tendency suggesting a ceiling effect, meaning that trainees differ by their highest ceiling ability.

7 Conclusion

Virtual reality now provides tools for a realistic, virtual, human-size coach, demonstrating a motion. For instance, current technology provides the tools to create a three-dimensional model of a coach, send it over the web to a remote location, and then reconstruct it in the remote location, so that the locals will see the remote person as if face-to-face, in front of them (for a description, please see Dan and Reiner 2016). For instance, see figure 12.3. The two women are not standing there in reality. Their 3-D model was built, sent over the web, and reconstructed in the location of the viewer, "coming out" of the screen as if face-to-face.

The above representation is in real time, meaning that each motion of the two models will be seen in real time. Can we use this for a remote coach to interact in real time with multiple golf trainees in VR? Or might a coach follow and monitor very accurately the 3-D motion in real time of each trainee? And what if this is enhanced with EEG systems that provide in real time the level of difficulty in addition to the brain signature of the upcoming or performed errors? And, further, suppose that we measure in real time the level of mental load, and adapt the virtual training world to perform at the level of 60–70 percent of the U-shaped mental load curve, for optimal training? This is a whole new paradigm for training for excellence.

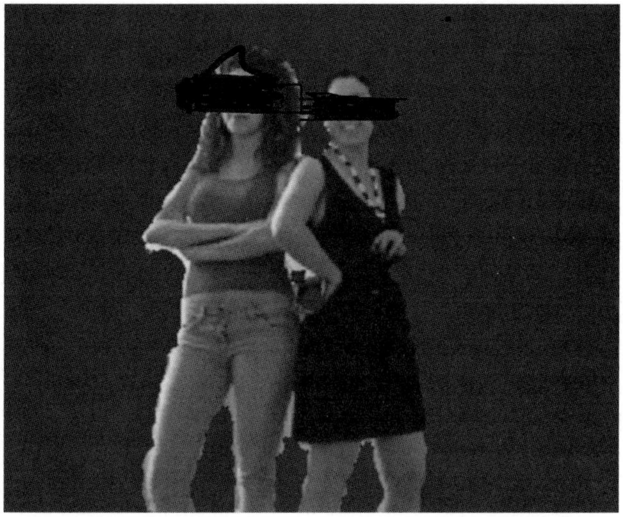

Figure 12.3
Real-time virtual representation of the two remote women propriety software of the VR and neurocognition lab.

Another exciting option is to use the programmable capacity of the VR to adapt to the user. Imagine, for instance, that the VR provides feedback for theta neurofeedback to target enhanced motor memory. It will require real-time connection to an EEG system, appropriate algorithms, and integration of the data from the VR and EEG, yet this is doable (as in brain-computer interface systems).

How is this related to embodiment? Especially in sport? According to Gibson (1979), affordances are built in real time through adaptation to the environmental cues, affecting both physical and cognitive performance. These patterns are activated in imagination, too, for reconsolidation of the desired pattern. VR is not different from a perceptual point of view; however, it is powerful, in that the environmental cues are controllable, through programming, and hence provide a new tool to provide the appropriate environmental, Gibsonian cues to activate the relevant brain functions for enhanced performance. Virtual reality can be programmed to provide an image and analysis of the individual act performance, for real-time correction. In this way VR becomes a tool to support and improve performance in imagination and extend the power of experimenting in thought for enhanced memory consolidation. Once motion patterns are registered in memory, they become tools for training and retraining—in imagination and physically. Thus the integration of the recent new findings from brain research with the emerging technologies of virtual reality and brain-computer interfaces are exciting tools that might change the training efficacy paradigm for excellence in performance in sport.

References

Albouy, Geneviève, Virginie Sterpenich, Evelyne Balteau, Gilles Vandewalle, Martin Desseilles, Thanh Dang-Vu, Annabelle Darsaud, et al. 2008. "Both the Hippocampus and Striatum Are Involved in Consolidation of Motor Sequence Memory." *Neuron* 58 (2): 261–272.

Arent, Shawn M., and Daniel M. Landers. 2003. "Arousal, Anxiety, and Performance: A Reexamination of the Inverted-U Hypothesis." *Research Quarterly for Exercise and Sport* 74 (4): 436–444.

Arns, Martijn, Michiel Kleinnijenhuis, Kamran Fallahpour, and Rien Breteler. 2008. "Golf Performance Enhancement and Real-Life Neurofeedback Training Using Personalized Event-Locked EEG Profiles." *Journal of Neurotherapy* 11 (4): 11–18.

Bartlett, Roger, Jon Wheat, and Matthew Robins. 2007. "Is Movement Variability Important for Sports Biomechanists?" *Sports Biomechanics / International Society of Biomechanics in Sports* 6 (2): 224–243.

Berka, Chris, Gkwk Chung, Sam O. Nagashima, Adrienne Musacchia, Gene Davis, Robin Johnson, and Djordje Popovic. 2008. "Using Interactive Neuro-Educational Technology to Increase the Pace and Efficiency of Rifle Marksmanship Training." In *Annual Meeting of the American Educational Research Association*. New York: Advanced Brain Monitoring. https://pdfs.semanticscholar.org/4f62/a5378bf52017c92d235d466683733e5c0477.pdf.

Boyce, Richard, Stephen D. Glasgow, Sylvain Williams, and Antoine Adamantidis. 2016. "Causal Evidence for the Role of REM Sleep Theta Rhythm in Contextual Memory Consolidation." *Science* 352 (6287): 812–816.

Cannon, Jonathan, Michelle M. McCarthy, Shane Lee, Jung Lee, Christoph Börgers, Miles A. Whittington, and Nancy Kopell. 2014. "Neurosystems: Brain Rhythms and Cognitive Processing." *European Journal of Neuroscience* 39 (5): 705–719.

Censor, Nitzan, Avi Karni, and Dov Sagi. 2006. "A Link between Perceptual Learning, Adaptation and Sleep." *Vision Research* 46 (23): 4071–4074.

Cherney, Isabelle D. 2008. "Mom, Let Me Play More Computer Games: They Improve My Mental Rotation Skills." *Sex Roles* 59 (11/12): 776–786.

Chow, Theodore, Tanaz Javan, Tomas Ros, and Paul Frewen. 2017. "EEG Dynamics of Mindfulness Meditation versus Alpha Neurofeedback: A Sham-Controlled Study." *Mindfulness* 8 (3): 572–584. doi:10.1007/s12671-016-0631-8.

Cohen, Noga, Liat Pell, Micah G. Edelson, Aya Ben-Yakov, Alex Pine, and Yadin Dudai. 2015. "Peri-Encoding Predictors of Memory Encoding and Consolidation." *Neuroscience and Biobehavioral Reviews* 50 (March): 128–142.

Cooper, Lynn A., and Roger N. Shepard. 1973. "Chronometric Studies of the Rotation of Mental Images." In *Visual Information Processing*, edited by William G. Chase, 75–176. Cambridge, MA: Academic Press.

Dan, Alex, and Miriam Reiner. 2016. "EEG-Based Cognitive Load of Processing Events in 3D Virtual Worlds Is Lower than Processing Events in 2D Displays." *International Journal of Psychophysiology* (August). doi:10.1016/j.ijpsycho.2016.08.013.

Delgado, Ana R., and Gerardo Prieto. 2004. "Cognitive Mediators and Sex-Related Differences in Mathematics." *Intelligence* 32 (1): 25–32.

De Lisi, Richard, and Jennifer L. Wolford. 2002. "Improving Children's Mental Rotation Accuracy with Computer Game Playing." *Journal of Genetic Psychology* 163 (3): 272–282.

Diekelmann, Susanne, and Jan Born. 2010. "The Memory Function of Sleep." *Nature Reviews: Neuroscience* 11 (2): 114–126.

Dudai, Yadin. 2004. "The Neurobiology of Consolidations, or, How Stable Is the Engram?" *Annual Review of Psychology* 55:51–86.

Duncan, Michael J., Nicholas Fowler, Oliver George, Samuel Joyce, and Joanne Hankey. 2015. "Mental Fatigue Negatively Influences Manual Dexterity and Anticipation Timing but Not Repeated High-Intensity Exercise Performance in Trained Adults." *Research in Sports Medicine* 23 (1): 1–13.

Egner, Tobias, and John H. Gruzelier. 2003. "Ecological Validity of Neurofeedback: Modulation of Slow Wave EEG Enhances Musical Performance." *NeuroReport* 14 (9): 1221–1224

Ericsson, K. Anders, Kiruthiga Nandagopal, and Roy W. Roring. 2005. "Giftedness Viewed from the Expert-Performance Perspective." *Journal for the Education of the Gifted* 28 (3/4): 287–311.

Fischer, Stefan, Manfred Hallschmid, Anna Lisa Elsner, and Jan Born. 2002. "Sleep Forms Memory for Finger Skills." *Proceedings of the National Academy of Sciences of the United States of America* 99 (18): 11987–11991.

Fitts, Paul Morris, and Michael I. Posner. 1967. *Human Performance*. Pacific Grove, CA: Brooks/Cole. http://psycnet.apa.org/psycinfo/1967-35040-000.

Ganis, Giorgio, Julian P. Keenan, Stephen M. Kosslyn, and Alvaro Pascual-Leone. 2000. "Transcranial Magnetic Stimulation of Primary Motor Cortex Affects Mental Rotation." *Cerebral Cortex* 10 (2): 175–180.

Gerardin, E., A. Sirigu, S. Lehéricy, J. B. Poline, B. Gaymard, C. Marsault, Y. Agid, and D. Le Bihan. 2000. "Partially Overlapping Neural Networks for Real and Imagined Hand Movements." *Cerebral Cortex* 10 (11): 1093–1104.

Gibson, James J. 1979. "The Theory of Affordances." In *The Ecological Approach to Visual Perception*, 127–143. Boston: Houghton Mifflin.

Gruzelier, J. H., T. Thompson, E. Redding, R. Brandt, and T. Steffert. 2014. "Application of Alpha/Theta Neurofeedback and Heart Rate Variability Training to Young Contemporary Dancers: State Anxiety and Creativity." *International Journal of Psychophysiology* 93 (1): 105–111.

Guillot, Aymeric, Christian Collet, Vo An Nguyen, Francine Malouin, Carol Richards, and Julien Doyon. 2008. "Functional Neuroanatomical Networks Associated with Expertise in Motor Imagery." *NeuroImage* 41 (4): 1471–1483.

Hanslmayr, Simon, Paul Sauseng, Michael Doppelmayr, Manuel Schabus, and Wolfgang Klimesch. 2005. "Increasing Individual Upper Alpha Power by Neurofeedback Improves Cognitive Performance in Human Subjects." *Applied Psychophysiology and Biofeedback* 30 (1): 1–10.

Hatfield, B., A. Haufler, and J. Contreras-Vidal. 2009. "Brain Processes and Neurofeedback for Performance Enhancement of Precision Motor Behavior." In *Foundations of Augmented Cognition: Neuroergonomics and Operational Neuroscience*, edited by Dylan D. Schmorrow, Ivy V. Estabrooke, and Marc Grootjen, 810–817. Lecture Notes in Computer Science. Berlin: Springer Berlin Heidelberg.

Heib, Dominik P. J., Kerstin Hoedlmoser, Peter Anderer, Georg Gruber, Josef Zeitlhofer, and Manuel Schabus. 2015. "Oscillatory Theta Activity during Memory Formation and Its Impact on Overnight Consolidation: A Missing Link?" *Journal of Cognitive Neuroscience* 27 (8): 1648–1658.

Higuchi, Keita, Tetsuro Shimada, and Jun Rekimoto. 2011. "Flying Sports Assistant: External Visual Imagery Representation for Sports Training." *Proceedings of the 2nd Augmented Human International Conference* 7:1–4. doi:10.1145/1959826.1959833.

Homer, Bruce D., Jan L. Plass, and Linda Blake. 2008. "The Effects of Video on Cognitive Load and Social Presence in Multimedia-Learning." *Computers in Human Behavior* 24 (3): 786–797.

Ietswaart, Magdalena, Marie Johnston, H. Chris Dijkerman, Sara Joice, Clare L. Scott, Ronald S. MacWalter, and Steven J. C. Hamilton. 2011. "Mental Practice with Motor Imagery in Stroke Recovery: Randomized Controlled Trial of Efficacy." *Brain: A Journal of Neurology* 134 (Pt 5): 1373–1386.

Jacobson, Jed, and Leland Matthaeus. 2014. "Athletics and Executive Functioning: How Athletic Participation and Sport Type Correlate with Cognitive Performance." *Psychology of Sport and Exercise* 15 (5): 521–527.

Jansen, Petra, Stefanie Pietsch, and Others. 2010. "Physical Activity Improves Mental Rotation Performance." *Creative Education: Cost Effectiveness and Resource Allocation* 1 (1): 58–61.

Klimesch, Wolfgang, Paul Sauseng, and Christian Gerloff. 2003. "Enhancing Cognitive Performance with Repetitive Transcranial Magnetic Stimulation at Human Individual Alpha Frequency." *European Journal of Neuroscience* 17 (5): 1129–1133.

Korman, Maria, Julien Doyon, Julia Doljansky, Julie Carrier, Yaron Dagan, and Avi Karni. 2007. "Daytime Sleep Condenses the Time Course of Motor Memory Consolidation." *Nature Neuroscience* 10 (9): 1206–1213.

Korman, Maria, Naftali Raz, Tamar Flash, and Avi Karni. 2003. "Multiple Shifts in the Representation of a Motor Sequence during the Acquisition of Skilled Performance." *Proceedings of the National Academy of Sciences of the United States of America* 100 (21): 12492–12497.

Lebon, Florent, Christian Collet, and Aymeric Guillot. 2010. "Benefits of Motor Imagery Training on Muscle Strength." *Journal of Strength and Conditioning Research / National Strength and Conditioning Association* 24 (6): 1680–1687.

Lev, Dror David, and Miriam Reiner. 2012. "Is Learning in Low Immersive Environments Carried Over to High Immersive Environments?" *Advances in Human-Computer Interaction* (September): 16. doi:10.1155/2012/521521.

Linden, David E. J., Robert A. Bittner, Lars Muckli, James A. Waltz, Nikolaus Kriegeskorte, Rainer Goebel, Wolf Singer, and Matthias H. J. Munk. 2003. "Cortical Capacity Constraints for Visual Working Memory: Dissociation of fMRI Load Effects in a Fronto-Parietal Network." *NeuroImage* 20 (3): 1518–1530.

Lizarraga, M. L. Sanz de Acedo, and J. M. García Ganuza. 2003. "Improvement of Mental Rotation in Girls and Boys." *Sex Roles* 49 (5/6): 277–286. doi:10.1023/A:1024656408294.

Lutz, Antoine, Heleen A. Slagter, John D. Dunne, and Richard J. Davidson. 2008. "Attention Regulation and Monitoring in Meditation." *Trends in Cognitive Sciences* 12 (4): 163–169.

Maquet, P. 2001. "The Role of Sleep in Learning and Memory." *Science* 294 (5544): 1048–1052.

Marcora, Samuele M., Walter Staiano, and Victoria Manning. 2009. "Mental Fatigue Impairs Physical Performance in Humans." *Journal of Applied Physiology* 106 (3): 857–864.

Mekari, Saïd, Sarah Fraser, Laurent Bosquet, Clément Bonnéry, Véronique Labelle, Philippe Pouliot, Frédéric Lesage, and Louis Bherer. 2015. "The Relationship between Exercise Intensity, Cerebral Oxygenation and Cognitive Performance in Young Adults." *European Journal of Applied Physiology* 115 (10): 2189–2197.

Moreau, David. 2012. "The Role of Motor Processes in Three-Dimensional Mental Rotation: Shaping Cognitive Processing via Sensorimotor Experience." *Learning and Individual Differences* 22 (3): 354–359.

Moreau, David, Annie Mansy-Dannay, Jérôme Clerc, and Alain Guerrien. 2011. "Spatial Ability and Motor Performance: Assessing Mental Rotation Processes in Elite and Novice Athletes." *International Journal of Sport Psychology* 42 (6): 525–547.

Neuper, Christa, Reinhold Scherer, Miriam Reiner, and Gert Pfurtscheller. 2005. "Imagery of Motor Actions: Differential Effects of Kinesthetic and Visual-Motor Mode of Imagery in Single-Trial EEG." *Brain Research: Cognitive Brain Research* 25 (3): 668–677.

Ngo, Hong-Viet V., Thomas Martinetz, Jan Born, and Matthias Mölle. 2013. "Auditory Closed-Loop Stimulation of the Sleep Slow Oscillation Enhances Memory." *Neuron* 78 (3): 545–553.

Peifer, Corinna, André Schulz, Hartmut Schächinger, Nicola Baumann, and Conny H. Antoni. 2014. "The Relation of Flow-Experience and Physiological Arousal under Stress—Can U Shape It?" *Journal of Experimental Social Psychology* 53:62–69.

Pietsch, Stefanie, and Petra Jansen. 2012. "Different Mental Rotation Performance in Students of Music, Sport and Education." *Learning and Individual Differences* 22 (1): 159–163.

Rauchs, Géraldine, Béatrice Desgranges, Jean Foret, and Francis Eustache. 2005. "The Relationships between Memory Systems and Sleep Stages." *Journal of Sleep Research* 14 (2): 123–140.

Reiner, M. 2004. "The Role of Haptics in Immersive Telecommunication Environments." *IEEE Transactions on Circuits and Systems for Video Technology* 14 (3): 392–401.

Reiner, M., and J. Gilbert. 2000. "Epistemological Resources for Thought Experimentation in Science Learning." *International Journal of Science Education* 22 (5), 489–506.

Reiner, Miriam. 1999. "Conceptual Construction of Fields through Tactile Interface." *Interactive Learning Environments* 7 (1): 31–55.

Reiner, Miriam. 2000. "Thought Experiments and Embodied Cognition." In *Developing Models in Science Education*, edited by John K. Gilbert and Carolyn J. Boulter, 157–176. Amsterdam: Springer Netherlands.

Reiner, Miriam. 2008. "Seeing through Touch: The Role of Haptic Information in Visualization." In *Visualization: Theory and Practice in Science Education*, edited by John K. Gilbert, Miriam Reiner, and Mary Nakhleh, 73–84. Models and Modeling in Science Education 3. Amsterdam: Springer Netherlands.

Reiner, Miriam, and Lior M. Burko. 2003. "On the Limitations of Thought Experiments in Physics and the Consequences for Physics Education." *Science and Education* 12 (4): 365–385.

Reiner, Miriam, and Tatiana M. Gelfeld. 2014. "Estimating Mental Workload through Event-Related Fluctuations of Pupil Area during a Task in a Virtual World." *International Journal of Psychophysiology* 93 (1): 38–44.

Reiner, Miriam, and John K. Gilbert. 2004. "The Symbiotic Roles of Empirical Experimentation and Thought Experimentation in the Learning of Physics." *International Journal of Science Education* 26 (15): 1819–1834.

Reiner, Miriam, Roman Rozengurt, and Anat Barnea. 2014. "Better than Sleep: Theta Neurofeedback Training Accelerates Memory Consolidation." *Biological Psychology* 95 (January): 45–53.

Robertson, Edwin M. 2009. "Brain Rhythms: Enhancing Memories." *Current Biology* 19 (21): R992–994.

Sandi, Carmen. 2013. "Stress and Cognition." *Wiley Interdisciplinary Reviews: Cognitive Science* 4 (3): 245–261.

Sauseng, P., W. Klimesch, K. Heise, W. R. Gruber, E. Holz, A. A. Karim, M. Glennon, C. Gerloff, N. Birbaumer, and F. C. Hummel. 2009. "Human Brain Oscillations Dissociate Memory Storage from Information Selection Processes and Predict Short-Term Memory Capacity." *Current Biology* 19:1846–1852.

Schuster, Corina, Roger Hilfiker, Oliver Amft, Anne Scheidhauer, Brian Andrews, Jenny Butler, Udo Kischka, and Thierry Ettlin. 2011. "Best Practice for Motor Imagery: A Systematic Literature Review on Motor Imagery Training Elements in Five Different Disciplines." *BMC Medicine* 9 (June): 75.

Sharma, Nikhil, Valerie M. Pomeroy, and Jean-Claude Baron. 2006. "Motor Imagery: A Backdoor to the Motor System after Stroke?" *Stroke: A Journal of Cerebral Circulation* 37 (7): 1941–1952.

Shepard, R. N., and J. Metzler. 1971. "Mental Rotation of Three-Dimensional Objects." *Science* 171 (3972): 701–703.

Shepard, Roger N., and Lynn A. Cooper. 1982. *Mental Images and Their Transformations*. Cambridge, MA: MIT Press.

Singer, Kenedy. 2004. "The Effect of Neurofeedback on Performance Anxiety in Dancers." *Journal of Dance Medicine and Science* 8 (3): 78–81.

Smith, Mitchell R., Samuele M. Marcora, and Aaron J. Coutts. 2015. "Mental Fatigue Impairs Intermittent Running Performance." *Medicine and Science in Sports and Exercise* 47 (8): 1682–1690.

Stickgold, Robert, and Matthew P. Walker. 2005. "Memory Consolidation and Reconsolidation: What Is the Role of Sleep?" *Trends in Neurosciences* 28 (8): 408–415.

Thomas, Hoben, and Robert Kail. 1991. "Sex Differences in Speed of Mental Rotation and the X-Linked Genetic Hypothesis." *Intelligence* 15 (1): 17–32.

Vernon, David J. 2005. "Can Neurofeedback Training Enhance Performance? An Evaluation of the Evidence with Implications for Future Research." *Applied Psychophysiology and Biofeedback* 30 (4): 347–364.

Wilson, M. A., and B. L. McNaughton. 1994. "Reactivation of Hippocampal Ensemble Memories during Sleep." *Science* 265 (5172): 676–679.

Yazmir, Boris, and Miriam Reiner. 2016. "Neural Correlates of User-Initiated Motor Success and Failure—A Brain-Computer Interface Perspective." *Neuroscience: Neurofeedback*. http://www.sciencedirect.com/science/article/pii/S0306452216306005.

Yazmir, Boris, Miriam Reiner, Hillel Pratt, and Miriam Zacksenhouse. 2016. "Brain Responses to Errors during 3D Motion in a Hapto-Visual VR." *Lecture Notes in Computer Science* 9775:120–130. https://doi.org/10.1007/978-3-319-42324-1_12.

Zoefel, Benedikt, René J. Huster, and Christoph S. Herrmann. 2011. "Neurofeedback Training of the Upper Alpha Frequency Band in EEG Improves Cognitive Performance." *NeuroImage* 54 (2): 1427–1431.

IV The Intersubjective Dimension of Skill: Mutual Understanding, Coordination, and Empathy in Team Sports

13 Action Understanding, Motor Resonance, and Embodied Simulation in Sports: Bridging Ecological and Neuroscientific Approaches

Ana Maria Abreu, Pedro Tiago Esteves, and Salvatore Maria Aglioti

1 Introduction

The study of performance has long been at the center of research interests for sport scientists. Professional athletes have been used as models in neuroscientific studies of expertise. Performance in cognitive neuroscience, however, is not confined to the action of a player, but involves decision-making skills related to anticipating the consequences of the actions of others or reacting to an opponent or teammate. Accordingly, observing "social" actions is of paramount importance in both sport science and neuroscience settings. In keeping with the embodied cognition theory, the ability to represent the meaning of gestures of another is based on the possibility that one is able to reactivate, in one's own motor system, the programs associated with the observed action.

The grounded cognition theory maintains that the motor system of a passive observer automatically tends to internally simulate the observed action (for review, see Barsalou 2008). The ecological approach to cognition, on the other hand, builds on dynamical systems tools to understand human cognitive processes by considering multiple internal and external influences. The embodied perspective of a situated agent as a dynamical system posits that people, by virtue of their central nervous system and other physical body properties, interact with the environment at different levels, such as when contracting muscle fibers to generate locomotion or picking up visual information to intercept a flying ball. As these interactions recur over time, structural congruence is achieved between an individual and its immediate environment. In other words, a stronger individual-environment coupling leads to meaningful changes in the individual and magnifies the potential of interaction. In this vein, cognition is considered to extend beyond the agents' brain and body limits, across the level of interaction with the objects and agents of the world. Such an ecological approach to embodiment would benefit from expanding research on the exploration of action possibilities during human intentional behaviors and social interactions. Here we incorporate these two theoretical approaches to draw new perspectives, in order to advance the understanding of how meaning emerges from individual-environment interactions at different scales of analysis.

The concept of embodiment has become a useful tool for sport scientists who use it to try to understand proficient performance and motor expertise. However, there seems to be a divide between ecological and neuroscientific approaches to embodiment that should be accounted for in the field of sport science. An ecological approach to human behavior adopts dynamical systems tools for understanding the unfolding nature of the human cognitive processes at the level of individual-environment interactions. This approach seeks to analyze how coordinated patterns of behavior evolve over time under multiple internal and external influences. It therefore takes mind, body, and environment to be conceived as highly interactive systems. A neuroscientific approach, on the other hand, seeks to explain human behavior in view of the boundaries and possibilities of neural functioning.

However, neural functioning does not operate in isolation. It is embedded in a specific environment, where internal and external influences interact. Thus, it is a mistake to think that these approaches represent different interpretations of embodiment (one in which cognition occurs beyond the brain and one in which cognition occurs within the brain). In fact, the extant gap between approaches stems from the different levels of analysis as well as from the distinct sources of knowledge employed by each contender. When scrutinizing each approach, we find that each is not only consistent with, but also significantly contributes to, strengthening the argument of the other. This suggests that we might benefit from integrating knowledge and information from both points of view. In the discussion that follows, we guide you through the neuroscientific and ecological stands on embodiment and suggest that although cognition may extend beyond the brain, into the body, this does not imply the need to disregard brain function or the environment with which the brain is interacting. In fact, even Pavlovian reactions are mediated by the brain. As such, there is great potential in considering a complementary perspective of these two conceptual beliefs. The marriage of these two approaches is of paramount importance, as it allows sport scientists to focus on the process of embodiment instead of focusing on the definition of embodiment according to each approach. Understanding how these two approaches might merge into one single comprehensive theory might endow sport scientists with the knowledge to fully investigate embodiment from brain to affordances, from the inside out.

2 A Neuroscientific Approach to Embodied Cognition: From Theory of Mind to Embodied Practice

As we marvel in the face of extraordinary sporting feats and seemingly effortless motor accomplishments, we might wonder how elite athletes adapt to opponents or the environment. In previous work, we have discussed how this adaptation is based on a simple action-reaction system, wherein one must correctly identify and adapt to constraints (Abreu and Duarte 2015). But how can one correctly identify these constraints? How can an expert player recognize the important cues given by a teammate or an opponent in order to modulate his or her own behavior in anticipation of the consequences that will ensue? We have previously argued that action anticipation in sport may be regulated by early, finely tuned pattern-recognition processes that are based on quick saliency-driven responses and result from motor resonance mechanisms, associated with expertise (Abreu 2014). However, there is much to be said about these motor resonance mechanisms that do not merely allow athletes to read the minds of others, but also put athletes in the state of vicariously feeling the body of another and thus affording the correct prediction concerning the outcome of another's motion. Could there be a more eloquent mechanism to allow for a true understanding of the other or the world around us?

When it comes to understanding the minds of others, it has been mostly considered that we need to make attributions concerning our own mental states and the mental states of others. The ability that allows us to understand, interpret, and predict the behavior of others has been termed theory of mind (ToM) (Premack and Woodruff 1978). Nonetheless, there has been great discussion concerning ToM and whether it might alone possess the role of understanding the mental states of others. Take empathy, for example. ToM and empathy seem to be closely related. While ToM endows us with the ability to attribute and reason about the mental states of others (Premack and Woodruff 1978), empathy entails an affective reaction component. This allows us to feel what one "takes" the other to be feeling as a form of automatic contagion or resulting from imagination processes (Prinz 2011). However, there are many definitions of empathy (De Vignemont and Singer 2006), and this is but one of the many that abound. As such, it might be difficult to establish a clear-cut distinction between empathy and ToM.

Singer (2009) sheds some light on this issue by suggesting that although our abilities to mentalize and empathize are mostly used in tandem (when we need to understand other people's desires, intentions, beliefs, and feelings), these two abilities actually rely on different neural circuitries (ToM—medial prefrontal cortex, temporal poles, superior temporal sulcus, and temporoparietal junction; empathy—anterior cingulate cortex, anterior insula, and secondary somatosensory cortex). Despite these findings, others have shown that the same neural substrate—the right temporoparietal junction—subtends both ToM and cognitive empathy (e.g., Mai et al. 2016, 380), suggesting that inferring intentions and emotions shares a conceptual as well as neural overlap. Such heterogeneity in results might imply that either the concept definition or the methods used to investigate these concepts are still unclear. It is thus not unexpected that philosophers have questioned what sources should be considered for understanding others. Some suggest that empathy and ToM are two different (albeit cooperative) mechanisms at work and that it is crucial to consider different levels of empathy (e.g., Songhorian 2013). Others reflect on the different accounts of ToM (e.g., Zahavi 2010), probing theory ToM (led by inferences) and simulation ToM (considered to use one's own mind as a model to understand the minds of others). One account of simulation ToM suggests that it is implicit and sub-personal (e.g., Gallese 2007). Gallagher (2005) states that neither account (theory ToM versus simulation ToM) suffices in isolation and proposes an alternative "interaction theory" that is neither singularly theoretical nor dependent on internal simulation, but is rather a form of embodied practice.

3 Simulation and Embodied Cognition

These phenomenological issues nicely translate to the theory of grounded cognition, by which simulation mechanisms constitute the bases for different cognitive processes (Barsalou 2008). Though many have conceptually muddled grounded cognition and embodied cognition, Wilson and Golonka (2013) submit that embodied cognition is a fairly radical affair, and Wilson (2013) makes a point to distinguish these terms, stating that although shaped by the body, grounded cognition still considers the existence of mental representations, whereas embodied cognition substitutes representations for the role of the body in constructing cognition. Hence, we enter the domain of body-dependent motor action and motor experience.

Based on the aforementioned ideas, we arrive at the theory of embodied cognition, according to which the observation of a human motor action can lead to the reactivation of the action systems associated with the observed action. Thus, the ability to represent the meaning of gestures of another is based on the possibility that one is able to reactivate, in one's own motor system, the programs associated with the observed action (Gallese and Lakoff 2005). Many studies (behavioral, EEG, neuroimaging, and neurophysiology) have shown that the motor system of a passive observer automatically tends to internally simulate the observed action (Rizzolatti and Craighero 2004).

This theory has enormous implications in sport, as we might envision that if one excels at a certain motor action, one will be able to better recognize, understand, and predict the outcome of that same action produced by another. Nonetheless, there is probably more to motor cognition, since action recognition does not always depend on the ability to produce that action (Mahon and Caramazza 2005).

4 The Neural Correlates of Embodied Cognition: What (Don't) We Know?

With the discovery of the mirror neuron system (MNS), a neural system that is activated both during motor action and during action observation (e.g., Di Pellegrino et al. 1992; Gallese et al. 1996), Gallese's simulation ToM gained new strength. The borders between ToM and empathy become less obvious, and it is suggested that empathy is based on mirror-matching mechanisms (Gallese 2003). Recent imaging studies have shown that, indeed, the MNS plays a role in understanding more than only human action and intention, but also emotions, feelings, imitation, and speech (see, for example, Fabbri-Destro and Rizzolatti 2008). The MNS (involving the inferior parietal lobule, the ventral premotor cortex, and the inferior frontal gyrus), as well as the behavioral implications of shared activation between observed and performed actions, have largely been investigated (see for example, Abreu 2014). Specifically, the so-called action observation network (AON), mainly subtending the inferior frontal gyrus and the premotor ventral cortex, activates both in-action and action-observation situations (Neal and Kilner 2010). The effect of passive mirroring (during action observation) as indexed by corticospinal excitability modulations (enhanced muscle-motor-evoked potentials) (Fadiga et al. 1995) was later replicated by Urgesi and others (2006b) using still images with implied motion. In another transcranial magnetic stimulation (TMS) study, Urgesi and collaborators (2006a) show a functional correspondence between action execution and observation given by the similar influence of the observer's hand posture (postural congruency) in both action execution and action observation.

Crucially, it seems that the AON has implications that go beyond a simple coupling between action execution and action observation. Specifically, the simple observation of movies with human motor action content brings about some of the same benefits given by actual motor practice, such as improvement in attention-related cognitive skills and disengagement from mental effort (Oliveira, Araújo, and Abreu 2014). Importantly, when speaking of neural simulation of action, one should note that not only observed but also imagined actions (covert), as well as actual actions, share some cortical areas implicating the subliminal activation of the motor system (Jeannerod 2001). Previous findings from motor imagery studies suggested just that, since imagined and executed actions share the same central structures (e.g., Decety 1996).

In their lesion-symptom mapping studies meta-analysis, Urgesi, Candidi, and Avenanti (2014) find that damage to three main nodes of the AON (inferior frontal cortex, inferior parietal cortex, and middle/superior temporal cortex) consistently leads to difficulties in action perception and understanding. Again, these findings lend support to the implication of the AON in action processing through embodiment. However, Hickok (2009) suggests otherwise. According to Hickok, there is no convincing evidence that actions are understood through motor representation, either because mirror neurons code not actions, but goals (and goals can be achieved by means of several different actions), or because motor representations are not the foundation of action understanding. In line with this, Mahon and Caramazza (2008) suggest that mirror neuron activity might simply reflect pure Pavlovian sensory-motor pairings or abstract representations that can be influenced by sensorimotor knowledge but do not singly depend on the motor system. Despite much evidence that action and action observation are coupled (e.g., Calvo-Merino et al. 2006), these heterogeneous findings suggest that more research is needed to pinpoint the neural correlates of embodied cognition. Nonetheless, independent of whether the mirror properties of the AON subtend all motor understanding, such a system certainly seems to play a role in embodiment. In support of this, Candidi and coworkers (2010) show, in a TMS study, that the semantic derivation of motor skills leads to limb-specific reduction of motor evoked potential (MEP) amplitude. Crucially, these findings confirm that even abstract action knowledge is embodied in the motor system.

Although a shared neural network would nicely explain action-understanding mechanisms, the putative absence of such a network does not challenge the existence of a tuned reactivation system supported by the motor resonance theory. This theory suggests that motor and sensory expertise go hand in hand with a greater capacity to anticipate the motor behavior of another (Aglioti et al. 2008). Indeed, Abreu and collaborators (2012) show that expertise in anticipating the consequences of actions of another goes beyond the MNS and implies a functional reorganization subtending a close relationship among expertise, error detection, body awareness, and action anticipation. Notably, action anticipation and understanding is of paramount importance in sport (particularly in dyadic or team interactions) where athletes constantly need to predict the outcome or consequences of the action of others (Abreu 2014; Abreu and Esteves 2014). In this sense, Daprati and others (2010) propose that motor simulation can afford the development of motor inferences that are of critical importance in the decision-making process.

5 Embodied Cognition in Sport

Despite the promise that the theory of embodiment might shed new light on the body-grounded mechanisms involved in sporting and exercise activities and come to explain motor development and expertise, this promise seems largely underrealized (Allen-Collinson 2009). Specifically, and although there is much research recruiting athletes and expert sport people, most findings have led to, or dwelled on, the phenomena of motor expertise and embodiment, and not on the implications of the sport in question in relation to the concept of embodiment. An exception to this is a study by Agans and collaborators (2013), in which the authors discuss the importance of embodiment in positive movement experiences (i.e., movement experiences that are mutually beneficial when considering individual/context relations) that might serve as a new paradigm for exercise, sport adherence, and a healthier lifestyle.

The suggestion of such a theoretical framework based on the concept of embodiment is of paramount importance because it suggests that it is possible to have positive movement experiences when the characteristics of the individual and those of the context are aligned. Despite this example, knowledge concerning the concept and functioning of embodiment is seldom applied, and most studies simply recruit athletes or musicians as selected groups of motor experts. In line with this, Ong and others (2014) have shown, in their study with ice-hockey players (action experts) and fans (visual experts), that embodiment effects were not only based on sensorimotor expertise but could also result from knowledge derived from visual experience. This tells us that the contextual experience (interaction with the context) can be modulated by several means to feed the embodiment processes.

Independent of whether we are already at a point where we might be able to apply our knowledge concerning the embodied nature of action, many have discussed and suggested how this knowledge might serve to enhance performance (Toner and Moran 2014). Ready or not, we should start testing our suggestions in order to benefit those that we have long been studying.

6 An Ecological Approach to Embodied Cognition

Over the last few decades there has been an increase in criticism of what might be called the "egocentric" approach to human behavior that somewhat neglects body and environmental influence (Richardson, Marsh, and Schmidt 2010). This position reflects a biased approach to human behavior such that cognitive abilities are deemed as *disembodied* (Richardson et al. 2008). Cognitive science has been urged to place greater attention on how cognitive activity proceeds as a situated activity by means of a meaningful interaction among the human body, its action system, and the changing environment (e.g., Clark 1999; Chrisley and Ziemke 2006). The considerable amount of research in embodiment and situated cognition strongly motivates the move to considering cognition in its broader environment (e.g., Clark 2008; Varela, Thompson, and Rosch 1991). As Mace (1977) has provokingly put it: "Ask not what's inside your head, but what your head is inside of" (43). Dynamical approaches (e.g., Thelen and Smith 1996; van Gelder 1998) have done exactly this and made profound contributions to human cognition by considering the close interdependence between brain, individual, and environment.

From a theoretical perspective, this approach is grounded on the ecological scale between the individual and the environment, originally proposed by James Gibson in the late sixties (Gibson 1966). Gibson's seminal work has stimulated a comprehensive body of research aligned with the ecological psychology rationale. This perspective stands for a holistic account of human behavior in the sense that it favors the "whole" and the links between its components rather than its components per se (Sanders 1996). In practical terms, both individual and environment change and are changed by each other over time such that they are so strongly coupled that they can be considered as a single system (Chemero 2001). The individual-environment system evolves upon the creation of meaningful links between perception and action processes on a reciprocal and mutual basis. This functional organization between the individual and environment is named synergy (Turvey, Shaw, and Mace 1978; Turvey 1981, 2007).

Consider the following illustrative example of a synergy in sport. Typically, in futsal,[1] players of the same team interact among themselves and with the players of the opponent team to achieve a given objective such as scoring a shot at the goal. An interesting study aimed at understanding how movement trajectories of players of two opposing teams were coordinated over time during a futsal practice match (Travassos et al. 2011). With this scope in mind, movement trajectories of players from the same team and between opposing teams were considered. Results showed that defenders of the same team revealed a consistent level of synchrony in their movements (i.e., simultaneous actions) especially in the lateral direction (i.e., toward the lateral line of the pitch). In this case, the performers mutually influenced each other by synchronizing their movements in space and time, probably as a result of picking up the same kind of information to guide their behaviors (Travassos et al. 2011).

This mutual influence obtained by synchronization is defined as a synergy. This same phenomenon has been reported in different domains such as rocking chairs (Richardson et al. 2007), or clapping (Fitzpatrick, Schmidt, and Carello 1996). For instance, in one early synchrony study (Richardson et al. 2007), participants were asked to sit side by side and to rock their chairs in two conditions: intentional and unintentional coordination. Findings indicate that even in the absence of a shared intention to coordinate, in the second experimental condition, rocking movements were synchronized upon the availability of visual information about the movements of the participant seated nearby. Importantly, a synergetic relation between individuals was noticeable irrespective of an implicit intention to coordinate. Certainly, we have all noticed how, if we clap long enough, we end up clapping together. The synergetic relation between individuals can thus explain this surprising effect: that is, independent of intent or conscious awareness, we affect and are affected by others.

Consider a series of metronomes placed on a thin board supported by two horizontally positioned soda cans. Although the metronomes might start out at different paces, because they are placed over the same media (thin board over cans), the metronomes influence the sway of the soda cans that, in turn, influence the metronomes' movements, eventually leading to metronome synchrony (Abreu and Duarte 2015). Thus, we might consider the mutual influence (cans over metronomes and metronomes over cans), leading to synchronization, to be a synergy.

A central premise of dynamic approaches to human cognition and behavior is the ability of the individual to directly access *meaningful* properties of the environment through the information conveyed by structured energy patterns (e.g., acoustic, visual) (Gibson 1979). These energy arrays remain unchanged despite modification of the evolving conditions, which create an invariant structure to be used for action purposes. By these means, individuals can be *aware* of their surroundings through perception-action couplings, despite the variation of environmental conditions (Michaels and Carello 1981). As the individual and the environment engage in continuous interactions over time, this flow of information permits a functional coupling that allows the stabilization of behavior patterns (Warren 2006).

7 Contribution of Dynamical Systems Theory to a Dynamic Approach to Cognition

A dynamical perspective on a situated, embodied individual considers the close interplay between the nervous system, body, and environment as interactive *systems* that evolve over time (Van Gelder 1998; Beer 2000). Within this scope, proponents of the dynamics approach to cognition have applied tools of dynamical systems theory (DST) (e.g., Haken 1983; Kelso 1995; Haken, Kelso, and Bunz 1985), originally conceived in the domain of physics of complex systems. This theory may be of great value to clarify embodied cognitive functions. The object of study of a dynamical approach to cognition is related to how behavior proceeds over time at different interactive system levels (neural, cognitive, or social). In other words, how the different states of organization of the individual-environment system emerge, dissolve, and persist (Kugler and Turvey 1987). Within this approach, mathematical modeling is used to acknowledge how the intertwined couplings between brain, body, and environment support the dynamics of behavior patterns (Haselager, Bongers, and van Rooij 2003; Warren 2006).

Worthy of note is that these states of organization are considered to arise directly from the dynamics of the system itself, reflecting intrinsic tendencies for self-organization, which are not rooted on a specific cognitive structure (Van Orden, Holden, and Turvey 2003). Here lies also one of the distinctive aspects of this approach: the study of how cognitive function unfolds over time as a result of a shared influence of context, body, and brain (Port 2002).

8 Closing the Gaps between Mind, Body, and Environment: Embodiment and Embeddedness

Embodiment and embeddedness are key concepts within the dynamic approach to cognition. Interaction between an individual and its environment is expressed by means of its body and action system (Richardson et al. 2007). In this sense, the act of embodying is viewed as an extension of the couplings between perception and action processes, wherein information from the environment is picked up by *body components* (e.g., visual and motor systems) to regulate upcoming actions. An immediate consequence is that the occurring actions change circumstances of the mind and body, and perception thereafter (van Orden, Holden, and Turvey 2003). In turn, this co-implication between the individual and the environment, expressed at different levels such as mind, perceptions, and actions, is illustrative of the embeddedness of the individual in the environment (Richardson, Marsh, and Schmidt 2010).

There is a promising stream of research dedicated to the study of embodied cognition aligned with a DST approach. The majority of these studies involve everyday tasks like standing, walking, and reaching to study how coordinated rhythmic movements assemble both at individual and interpersonal levels. One such experiment required participants to make judgments about reachability of an object placed on a table while handling rods of different lengths (van Rooij, Bongers, and Haselager 2002). Results showed that judgements were importantly affected by different constraints such as the order of presentation of the rods with varying lengths, reaching distance, and distance of the participants from the object. From these experimental findings it is possible to elaborate on how cognition (i.e., judgement based on the imagined action) might arise beyond particular elements (e.g., mental representation) as a result of an information linkage between the individual and the environment (Richardson, Marsh, and Schmidt 2010).

Instead of focusing on the internal processes occurring inside the brain, the focus of this approach is directed to how *brain and body* use meaningful information to regulate cognition processes and, in turn, purposive behavior (Varela, Thompson, and Rosch 1993). This approach challenges either neuronal or environmental explanations of cognition to consider the emergence of meaning at the scale of individual-environment interactions (Marsh et al. 2009). Nonetheless, how does meaning come about? This approach recognizes the fundamental role of the body in providing support for mind and meaning but, at the same time, stresses the embeddedness of the body in relation to the environment, which provides an additional context of meaningfulness (Marsh et al. 2009). In line with this view, cognition is considered to decisively expand the limits of the agent's brain and body across the level of interaction with the environment (Beer 2000). As such, cognitive phenomena, like perceiving and acting, can transcend the biological and anatomical boundaries, implicating behavior as a property that emerges from the individual-environment system (Richardson, Marsh, and Schmidt 2010). These principles hold relevant implications for considering embodied cognition within a dynamic rationale. One such implication relates to the concept of affordances (Hirose 2002).

9 How Might the Concept of Affordances Enlighten Cognitive Functioning?

A central tenet of a dynamic approach to human behavior must include the notion that the interaction between an individual and the environment evolves upon the exploration of opportunities of action (i.e., affordances) (Fajen, Riley, and Turvey 2009). In this sense, cognition moves away from planning and problem solving to the detection and exploration of affordances (Haselager, Bongers, and van Rooij 2003). Affordances are properties of the environment taken with reference to the individual. Thus, to perceive an affordance is to access what a given environmental property means to the individual (Gibson 1979). Affordances are perceived by means of the structured information (i.e., visual, auditory, and so on) that remains invariant despite absolute variations of the perceiver and environment. For instance, the rate of change of the (optical) angle between an individual and an object of interest (e.g., scoring target in teams sport) remains *invariant* across different distances to the target, permitting regulation of locomotion across different conditions. This premise opens up the possibility that the individual might acknowledge which action modes are possible or not, without the mediational role of internal structures of knowledge, by detecting invariant information (Turvey 1992).

In view of the previous example, the rate of turning is informative on the sufficiency of actual movement to approach the desired target. Worthy of note is that the detection of and action on affordances depends on the *fit* between the perceiver and the action-related properties of the environment itself. For instance, for an individual to successfully jump over an obstacle while running, the locomotor system must be able to comply with the demands of the obstacle, both in body dimensions (e.g., leg length) and body abilities (e.g., strength, agility). Such capabilities of an individual, in relation with the environment, are named *effectivities* (Shaw and Turvey 1981). Hence, by perceiving the evolving affordances, an individual is able to update his state of relation with the environment in such a way that he directly perceives what he can or cannot do. For example, in athletic sport, a *jumpable* obstacle is readily informative (i.e., meaningful), for a given athlete, concerning the possibility to perform a jump upon its physical features (e.g., shape, size, and consistency).

The study of affordances has been proposed as a viable approach to better understand cognitive function in various domains in sport science (Marsh et al. 2009). An extensive stream of research has been devoted to the study of affordances in different tasks, such as walking through apertures (e.g., Warren and Whang 1987), reaching (Pepping and Li 2000), or dyadic interaction in sport (e.g., Esteves, de Oliveira, and Araújo 2011). In a paradigmatic experiment, participants were asked to attach 10 cm blocks to their shoes and judge whether the heights of various surfaces afforded sitting or climbing (Mark 1987). Results showed that judgment of these action boundaries (to sit or to climb) was influenced by information relative to the bodily features of the participants, whose sitting abilities were changed by the use of blocks attached to their shoes. Interestingly, the perceived maximum seat height underestimated the actual maximum sitting height, as a result of wearing blocks. Interestingly, in a later study using a similar experimental setting, Mark and others (1990) reported that, as trials proceeded, individuals were able to retune their judgments of maximum sitting height in a way that it corresponded to their actual conditions (i.e., while with blocks attached to their shoes). These results show that even without specific training practice, blocks appeared to be progressively *embodied* by the individuals, a condition that may have permitted better exploration of the evolving possibilities for action. The evidence in favour of perception of affordances being based on the participant's body features reinforces an embodiment viewpoint on cognition wherein meaningful properties of the environment are used to regulate behavior with reference to the individual.

Research has also focused on how action capabilities of performers influence the exploration of affordances. A recent study has considered how individuals may estimate walkable distances according to their bioenergetics resources (Zadra, Weltman, and Proffitt 2016). The use of carbohydrate supplementation was associated with a decrease on distance estimates, when compared with a placebo condition. Importantly, physiological measures that express physical fitness of participants proved to robustly predict distance estimates, irrespective of experimental manipulations. Additional support for the influence of action capabilities on the detection of affordances has also been reported in sport environments (e.g., Dicks, Davids, and Button 2010). In this experiment, football goalkeepers attempted to intercept a penalty kick (i.e., a shot to score a goal) with deceptive and nondeceptive movements of the penalty taker. Interestingly, the timing and accuracy of movement response behaviors of the goalkeepers appeared to be influenced by their individual action capabilities, especially in terms of speed. While slower goalkeepers tended to initiate their movement earlier to intercept the ball, faster goalkeepers initiated their movements closer to the moment the penalty taker touched the ball. The exploration of the affordance to intercept the penalty kick appeared to be mainly dependent on the use of information concerning the capabilities of the perceiver with respect to a specific set of environmental conditions.

Of particular interest is the use of tools as a means to amplify the effectivities of the individual. This may occur because changes in the body allow exploring a greater range of possibilities of action (i.e., affordances) (Hirose 2002). From a conceptual point of view, the use of tools may greatly extend cognition beyond the individual's body limits (Marsh et al. 2009). For example, the use of customized tools, like a cane, may facilitate visually impaired people to explore different possibilities for locomotion in terms of route selection and collision avoidance. Another interesting example may refer to a hockey player moving a ball with a stick, in the direction of the target to score a shot while avoiding upcoming opponents.

Considering the above, the stick may be conceived to integrate the perception-action system as it expands the process of information pickup of the environment (i.e., ball, ground) to contribute to the regulation of player displacements. As this process of perceiving and using information to guide behavior is progressively refined, the stick may, at a certain level, be considered as an extension of the arm and hand of the player. Hove, Riley, and Shockley (2006) investigated this domain by asking participants with different levels of expertise to produce accurate judgements of the suitability of different weighted hockey sticks for performing power and precision actions. Participants were asked to hold the hockey stick with two hands and verbally rate its suitability to perform the power and precision tasks in different conditions: (1) while wielding the stick; (2) before and after striking a street hockey puck. Results showed that, irrespective of expertise, participants were sensitive to the influence of the stick's mass distribution on its suitability for performing the different actions. This evidence is in line with the use of tools as a means to extend cognition (i.e., detecting and exploring affordances) possibly by engaging the haptic system in the process of accessing relevant information to support action.

The concept of affordances and interaction with one's surroundings discussed here does not, in any way, negate the neuroscientific findings discussed above. Actually, dynamic approaches have also devoted attention to the role of neural substrates on behavior and cognition processes (e.g., Kelso and Tognoli 2009). When considering cognition/behavior in light of the dynamics approach, the relevance of the neural processes is determinant (as in cases of strategic behavior or symbolic recognition). In such cases, cognition may derive less from information available from the context (of the world) and more from information about the world (allocated in the brain—in the form of memories). Indeed, it is unquestionable that past experiences and symbols act as relevant constraints on the regulation of cognitive processes and, in turn, purposive behaviors.

This proposition may be explicitly validated as sport performers, for instance, participate in competitive environments regulated by on-field referees who use visual or auditory cues to validate (or not) a given behavior. One such example may be a basketball referee who uses hand signals to represent a specific meaning to the players (e.g., illegal use of physical contact toward an opponent). Another illustrative example consists of the strategic instructions (i.e., verbal or graphical) given by the coaches to the athletes, in the dressing room before the competition, as a means to be better prepared in view of the opponents' strengths. In this sense, insights from neuroscientific approaches might be of interest in the move toward a more comprehensive perspective of embodied cognition.

10 Conclusion

It seems clear that both ecological and neuroscientific approaches largely contribute to the understanding of embodied cognition and that these views are both not only extremely informative, but also complementary. Embodied cognition is viewed by the dynamic approach as an evolving process expanded over different interactive levels of the system: mind, body, and environment. Within this perspective, cognitive functioning is deemed to emerge from the scale of interaction between the environment and the individual, and not from a particular structural locus. Although dynamic explanations of embodied cognition tend to emphasize the interdependence between body and environment in the acquisition of meaning through the exploration of affordances, these explanations do not disregard the implication of the brain in processing meaningfulness.

Interestingly, similar insights have been collected from neuroscientific views of embodiment. Indeed, the aforementioned motor resonance mechanisms, supported by the mirror properties of the AON, imply that expertise in a particular motor domain should lead to expertise in the anticipation of the consequences of the action of another by using visual rather than motor cues. In other words, experts learn to detect opportunities (e.g., specific visual features concerning both bodies and contexts) in order to better interact with the environment. The mechanism supporting such phenomenon is the reactivation of the action systems implicated in the observed action, which nicely fits the interactional concept of the dynamic model.

Thus, there seems to be a promising pathway to be explored to advance the current state of knowledge. One possibility would imply further investigating the link between affordances and cognition by means of customized tools within informationally rich environments. This goal could also be achieved by manipulating action capabilities and considering collaborative work along the exploration of affordances. It is time to acknowledge that findings from dynamic as well as neuroscientific approaches contribute to a cohesive body of evidence for embodied cognition.

Acknowledgments

We would like to acknowledge funding from the Ministry of University and Research (PRIN: Progetti di Ricerca di Rilevanza Nazionale NAZIONALE—Bando 2015 Prot. 20159CZFJK) to SMA.

Note

1. Futsal is a variation of association football in which two teams, composed of five players each, aim to score a shot on the opponents' goal.

References

Abreu, Ana Maria. 2014. "Action Anticipation in Sports: A Particular Case of Expert Decision-Making." *Trends in Sport Sciences* 21 (1): 5–11.

Abreu, Ana Maria, and Ricardo Duarte. 2015. "Expertise in Sports: Reconciling Sports Sciences with Findings from Experimental and Social Psychology and Neuroscience." *Annals of Sports Medicine and Research* 2 (3): 1020.

Abreu, Ana Maria, and Pedro Esteves. 2014. "Bases neurocientíficas de la toma de decisiones en el deporte." In *El entrenamiento táctico y decisional en el deporte*, edited by F. Del Villar Álvarez and L. García-González, 59–79. Madrid: Editorial Síntesis.

Abreu, Ana Maria, Emiliano Macaluso, Rúben T. Azevedo, Paola Cesari, Cosimo Urgesi, and Salvatore Matia Aglioti. 2012. "Action Anticipation beyond the Action Observation Network:

A Functional Magnetic Resonance Imaging Study in expert Basketball Players." *European Journal of Neuroscience* 35 (10): 1646–1654. doi:10.1111/j.1460-9568.2012.08104.x.

Agans, Jennifer P., Reidar Säfvenbom, Jacqueline L. Davis, Edmond P. Bowers, and Richard M. Lerner. 2013. "Chapter Ten: Positive Movement Experiences: Approaching the Study of Athletic Participation, Exercise, and Leisure Activity through Relational Developmental Systems Theory and the Concept of Embodiment." *Advances in Child Development and Behavior* 45:261–286. doi:10.1016/B978-0-12-397946-9.00010-5.

Aglioti, Salvatore M., Paola Cesari, Michela Romani, and Cosimo Urgesi. 2008. "Action Anticipation and Motor Resonance in Elite Basketball Players." *Nature Neuroscience* 11 (9): 1109–1116. doi:10.1038/nn.2182.

Allen-Collinson, Jacquelyn. 2009. "Sporting Embodiment: Sports Studies and the (Continuing) Promise of Phenomenology." *Qualitative Research in Sport and Exercise* 1 (3): 279–296. doi:10.1080/19398440903192340.

Barsalou, Lawrence W. 2008. "Grounded Cognition." *Annual Review of Psychology* 59:617–645. doi:10.1146/annurev.psych.59.103006.093639.

Beer, Randall D. 2000. "Dynamical Approaches to Cognitive Science." *Trends in Cognitive Sciences* 4 (3): 91–99. doi:10.1016/S1364-6613(99)01440-0.

Calvo-Merino, Beatriz, Julie Grèzes, Daniel E. Glaser, Richard E. Passingham, and Patrick Haggard. 2006. "Seeing or Doing? Influence of Visual and Motor Familiarity in Action Observation." *Current Biology* 16 (19): 1905–1910. doi:10.1016/j.cub.2006.07.065.

Candidi, Matteo, Carmelo Mario Vicario, Ana Maria Abreu, and Salvatore Maria Aglioti. 2010. "Competing Mechanisms for Mapping Action-Related Categorical Knowledge and Observed Actions." *Cerebral Cortex* 20 (12): 2832–2841. doi:10.1093/cercor/bhq033.

Chemero, Anthony. 2001. "Dynamical Explanation and Mental Representations." *Trends in Cognitive Sciences* 5 (4): 141–142.

Chrisley, Ronald, and Tom Ziemke. 2006. "Embodiment." *Encyclopedia of Cognitive Science*. Hoboken, NJ: John Wiley and Sons. doi:10.1002/0470018860.s00172.

Clark, Andy. 1999. "An Embodied Cognitive Science?" *Trends in Cognitive Sciences* 3 (9): 345–351. doi:http://dx.doi.org/10.1016/S1364-6613(99)01361-3.

Clark, Andy. 2008. *Supersizing the Mind: Embodiment, Action, and Cognitive Extension*. Oxford: Oxford University Press.

Daprati, Elena, Daniele Nico, Sylvie Duval, and Francesco Lacquaniti. 2010. "Different Motor Imagery Modes Following Brain Damage." *Cortex: A Journal Devoted to the Study of the Nervous System and Behavior* 46 (8): 1016–1030. doi:10.1016/j.cortex.2009.08.002.

Decety, Jean. 1996. "Do Imagined and Executed Actions Share the Same Neural Substrate?" *Brain Research: Cognitive Brain Research* 3 (2): 87–93. doi:10.1016/0926-6410(95)00033-X.

De Vignemont, Frederique, and Tania Singer. 2006. "The Empathic Brain: How, When and Why?" *Trends in Cognitive Sciences* 10 (10): 435–441. doi:10.1016/j.tics.2006.08.008.

Dicks, Matt, Keith Davids, and Chris Button. 2010. "Individual Differences in the Visual Control of Intercepting a Penalty Kick in Association Football." *Human Movement Science* 29 (3): 401–411. doi:10.1016/j.humov.2010.02.008.

Di Pellegrino, Giuseppe, Luciano Fadiga, Leonardo Fogassi, Vittorio Gallese, and Giacomo Rizzolatti. 1992. "Understanding Motor Events: A Neurophysiological Study." *Experimental Brain Research* 91 (1): 176–180. doi:10.1007/BF00230027.

Esteves, Pedro Tiago, Rita F. de Oliveira, and Duarte Araújo. 2011. "Posture-Related Affordances Guide Attacks in Basketball." *Psychology of Sport and Exercise* 12 (6): 639–644. doi:10.1016/j.psychsport.2011.06.007.

Fabbri-Destro, Maddalena, and Giacomo Rizzolatti. 2008. "Mirror Neurons and Mirror Systems in Monkeys and Humans." *Physiology* 23 (3): 171–179. doi:10.1152/physiol.00004.2008.

Fadiga, Luciano, Leonardo Fogassi, Giovanni Pavesi, and Giacomo Rizzolatti. 1995. "Motor Facilitation during Action Observation: A Magnetic Stimulation Study." *Journal of Neurophysiology* 73 (6): 2608–2611.

Fajen, Brett R., Michael A. Riley, and Michael T. Turvey. 2009. "Information, Affordances, and the Control of Action in Sport." *International Journal of Sport Psychology* 40 (1): 79–107.

Fitzpatrick, Paula, R. C. Schmidt, and Claudia Carello. 1996. "Dynamical Patterns in Clapping Behavior." *Journal of Experimental Psychology: Human Perception and Performance* 22 (3): 707–724. doi:http://dx.doi.org/10.1037/0096-1523.22.3.707.

Gallagher, Shaun. 2005. *How the Body Shapes the Mind*. Oxford: Oxford University Press.

Gallese, Vittorio. 2003. "The Roots of Empathy: The Shared Manifold Hypothesis and the Neural Basis of Intersubjectivity." *Psychopathology* 36 (4): 171–180. doi:10.1159/000072786.

Gallese, Vittorio. 2007. "Before and Below 'Theory of Mind': Embodied Simulation and the Neural Correlates of Social Cognition." *Philosophical Transactions of the Royal Society of London B: Biological Sciences* 362 (1480): 659–669. doi:10.1098/rstb.2006.2002.

Gallese, Vittorio, Luciano Fadiga, Leonardo Fogassi, and Giacomo Rizzolatti. 1996. "Action Recognition in the Premotor Cortex." *Brain* 119 (2): 593–609. doi:10.1093/brain/119.2.593.

Gallese, Vittorio, and George Lakoff. 2005. "The Brain's Concepts: The Role of the Sensory-Motor System in Conceptual Knowledge." *Cognitive Neuropsychology* 22 (3): 455–479. doi:10.1080/02643290442000310.

Gibson, James Jerome. 1966. *The Senses Considered as Perceptual Systems*. Oxford: Houghton Mifflin.

Gibson, James Jerome. 1979. *The Ecological Approach to Visual Perception*. Boston, MA: Houghton Mifflin.

Haken, Hermann. 1983. *Synergetics*. Berlin: Springer Verlag.

Haken, Hermann, J. A. Scott Kelso, and Heinz Bunz. 1985. "A Theoretical Model of Phase Transitions in Human Hand Movements." *Biological Cybernetics* 51 (5): 347–356. doi:10.1007/BF00336922.

Haselager, Pim, Raoul M. Bongers, and Iris van Rooij. 2003. "Cognitive Science, Representations, and Dynamical Systems Theory." In *The Dynamical Systems Approach to Cognition: Concepts and Empirical Paradigms Based on Self-Organization, Embodiment, and Coordination Dynamics*. Studies of Nonlinear Phenomena in Life Science, edited by W. Tschacher and J-P. Dauwalder, vol. 10, 229–242. Singapore: World Scientific.

Hickok, Gregory. 2009. "Eight Problems for the Mirror Neuron Theory of Action Understanding in Monkeys and Humans." *Journal of Cognitive Neuroscience* 21 (7): 1229–1243. doi:10.1162/jocn.2009.21189.

Hirose, Naoya. 2002. "An Ecological Approach to Embodiment and Cognition." *Cognitive Systems Research* 3 (3): 289–299. doi:10.1016/S1389-0417(02)00044-X.

Hove, Philip, Michael A. Riley, and Kevin Shockley. 2006. "Perceiving Affordances of Hockey Sticks by Dynamics Touch." *Ecological Psychology* 18 (3): 163–189.

Jeannerod, Marc. 2001. "Neural Simulation of Action: A Unifying Mechanism for Motor Cognition." *NeuroImage* 14 (1pt2): S103–S109. doi:10.1006/nimg.2001.0832.

Kelso, J. A. Scott. 1995. *Dynamic Patterns: The Self-Organization of Brain and Behavior*. Cambridge, MA: MIT Press.

Kelso, J. A. Scott, and Emmanuelle Tognoli. 2009. "Toward a Complementary Neuroscience: Metastable Coordination Dynamics of the Brain." In *Downward Causation and the Neurobiology of Free Will*, edited by N. Murphy, G. Ellis, and T. O'Connor, 103–124. Berlin: Springer. doi:10.1007/978-3-642-03205-9_6.

Kugler, Peter Noble, and Michael T. Turvey. 1987. *Information, Natural Law, and the Self-Assembly of Rhythmic Movement*. Hillsdale, NJ: Lawrence Erlbaum.

Mace, William M. 1977. "James J. Gibson's Strategy for Perceiving: Ask Not What's Inside Your Head, but What Your Head's Inside Of." In *Perceiving, Acting, and Knowing*, edited by Robert Shaw and John Bransford, 43–65. Hillsdale, NJ: Erlbaum.

Mahon, Bradford Z., and Alfonso Caramazza. 2005. "The Orchestration of the Sensory-Motor Systems: Clues from Neuropsychology." *Cognitive Neuropsychology* 22 (3): 480–494. doi:10.1080/02643290442000446.

Mahon, Bradford Z., and Alfonso Caramazza. 2008. "A Critical Look at the Embodied Cognition Hypothesis and a New Proposal for Grounding Conceptual Content." *Journal of Physiology-Paris* 102 (1): 59–70. doi:10.1016/j.jphysparis.2008.03.004.

Mai, Xiaoqin, Wenli Zhang, Xinmu Hu, Zhen Zhen, Zhenhua Xu, Jing Zhang, and Chao Liu. 2016. "Using tDCS to Explore the Role of the Right Temporo-Parietal Junction in Theory of Mind and Cognitive Empathy." *Frontiers in Psychology* 7 (March): 380. doi:10.3389/fpsyg.2016.0038.

Mark, Leonard S. 1987. "Eyeheight-Scaled Information about Affordances: A Study of Sitting and Stair Climbing." *Journal of Experimental Psychology: Human Perception and Performance* 13 (3): 361–370. doi:http://dx.doi.org/10.1037/0096-1523.13.3.361.

Mark, Leonard S., James A. Balliett, Kent D. Craver, Stephen D. Douglas, and Teresa Fox. 1990. "What an Actor Must Do in Order to Perceive the Affordance for Sitting." *Ecological Psychology* 2 (4): 325–366. doi:10.1207/s15326969eco0204_2.

Marsh, Kerry L., Lucy Johnston, Michael J. Richardson, and R. C. Schmidt. 2009. "Toward a Radically Embodied, Embedded Social Psychology." *European Journal of Social Psychology* 39 (7): 1217–1225. doi:10.1002/ejsp.666.

Michaels, Claire F., and Claudia Carello. 1981. *Direct Perception*. Englewood Cliffs, NJ: Prentice-Hall.

Neal, Alice, and James M. Kilner. 2010. "What Is Simulated in the Action Observation Network When We Observe Actions?" *European Journal of Neuroscience* 32 (10): 1765–1770.

Oliveira, Patricia A., Duarte Araújo, and Ana Maria Abreu. 2014. "Proneness for Exercise, Cognitive and Psychophysiological Consequences of Action Observation." *Psychology of Sport and Exercise* 15 (1): 39–47. doi:10.1016/j.psychsport.2013.09.008.

Ong, Nicole T., Keith R. Lohse, Romeo Chua, Scott Sinnett, and Nicola J. Hodges. 2014. "A Test of Motor Skill-Specific Action Embodiment in Ice-Hockey Players." *Acta Psychologica* 150 (July): 61–68. doi:10.1016/j.actpsy.2014.04.005.

Pepping, Gert-Jan, and Franqois-Xavier Li. 2000. "Sex Differences and Action Scaling in Overhead Reaching." *Perceptual and Motor Skills* 90 (3 pt 2): 1123–1129.

Port, Robert F. 2002. "Dynamical Systems Hypothesis in Cognitive Science." In *Encyclopedia of Cognitive Science,* edited by L. Nadel, 1027–1032. London: MacMillan.

Premack, David, and Guy Woodruff. 1978. "Does the Chimpanzee Have a Theory of Mind?" *Behavioral and Brain Sciences* 1 (4): 515–526. doi:http://dx.doi.org/10.1017/S0140525X00076512.

Prinz, Jesse. 2011. "Is Empathy Necessary for Morality?" In *Empathy: Philosophical and Psychological Perspectives*, edited by A. Coplan and P. Goldie, 211–229. Oxford: Oxford University Press.

Richardson, Michael J., Kerry L. Marsh, Robert W. Isenhower, Justin R. L. Goodman, and Richard C. Schmidt. 2007. "Rocking Together: Dynamics of Intentional and Unintentional Interpersonal Coordination." *Human Movement Science* 26 (6): 867–891. doi:10.1016/j.humov.2007.07.002.

Richardson, Michael J., Kerry L. Marsh, and R. C. Schmidt. 2010. "Challenging the Egocentric View of Coordinated Perceiving, Acting, and Knowing." In *The Mind in Context*, edited by Batja Mesquita, Lisa Feldman Barrett, and Eliot R. Smith, 307–333. New York: Guilford.

Richardson, Michael J., Kevin Shockley, Bret R. Fajen, Michael A. Riley, and Michael T. Turvey. 2008. "Ecological Psychology: Six Principles for an Embodied-Embedded Approach to Behavior." In *Elsevier Handbook of Cognitive Science: An Embodied Approach*, edited by Paco Calvo and Toni Gomila, 161–187. New York: Elsevier.

Rizzolatti, Giacomo, and Laila Craighero. 2004. "The Mirror-Neuron System." *Annual Review of Neuroscience* 27:169–192. doi:10.1146/annurev.neuro.27.070203.144230.

Sanders, John T. 1996. "An Ecological Approach to Cognitive Science." *Electronic Journal of Analytic Philosophy* 4 (Spring): 1–11.

Shaw, Robert E., and Michael T. Turvey. 1981. "Coalitions as Models for Ecosystems: A Realist Perspective on Perceptual Organization." In *Perceptual Organization*, edited by Michael Kubovy and James Pomeranz, 343–415. Hillsdale, NJ: Erlbaum.

Singer, Tania. 2009. "Understanding Others: Brain Mechanisms of Theory of Mind and Empathy." In *Neuroeconomics: Decision Making and the Brain*, edited by P. W. Glimcher, C. F. Camerer, E. Fehr, and R. A. Poldrack, 251–268. San Diego, CA: Academic Press.

Songhorian, Sarah. 2013. "How Do We Understand Others? Empathy and Theory of Mind as Two Different, but Cooperative, Mechanisms for Sensibility." *Phenomenology and Mind* 4:104–112.

Thelen, Esther, and Linda B. Smith. 1996. *A Dynamic Systems Approach to the Development of Cognition and Action*. Cambridge, MA: MIT Press.

Toner, John, and Aidan Moran. 2014. "In Praise of Conscious Awareness: A New Framework for the Investigation of 'Continuous Improvement' in Expert Athletes." *Frontiers in Psychology* 5 (July): 769. doi:10.3389/fpsyg.2014.00769.

Travassos, Bruno, Duarte Araújo, Luís Vilar, and T. McGarry. 2011. "Interpersonal Coordination and Ball Dynamics in Futsal (Indoor Football)." *Human Movement Science* 30 (6): 1245–1259. doi:10.1016/j.humov.2011.04.003.

Turvey, Michael T. 1992. "Affordances and Prospective Control: An Outline of the Ontology." *Ecological Psychology: A Publication of the International Society for Ecological Psychology* 4 (3): 173–187. doi:10.1207/s15326969eco0403_3.

Turvey, Michael T. 2007. "Action and Perception at the Level of Synergies." *Human Movement Science* 26 (4): 657–697. doi:10.1016/j.humov.2007.04.002.

Turvey, Michael T., Robert E. Shaw, and William Mace. 1978. "Issues in the Theory of Action: Degrees of Freedom, Coordinative Structures and Coalitions." In *Attention and Performance VII*, edited by Jean Requin, 557–595. Hillsdale, NJ: Lawrence Erlbaum.

Urgesi, Cosimo, Matteo Candidi, and Alessio Avenanti. 2014. "Neuroanatomical Substrates of Action Perception and Understanding: An Anatomic Likelihood Estimation Meta-Analysis of Lesion-Symptom Mapping Studies in Brain Injured Patients." *Frontiers in Human Neuroscience* 8 (May): 344. doi:10.3389/fnhum.2014.00344.

Urgesi, Cosimo, Matteo Candidi, Franco Fabbro, Michela Romani, and Salvatore M. Aglioti. 2006a. "Motor Facilitation during Action Observation: Topographic Mapping of the Target Muscle and Influence of the Onlooker's Posture." *European Journal of Neuroscience* 23 (9): 2522–2530. doi:10.1111/j.1460-9568.2006.04772.x.

Urgesi, Cosimo, Valentina Moro, Matteo Candidi, and Salvatore M. Aglioti. 2006b. "Mapping Implied Body Actions in the Human Motor System." *Journal of Neuroscience* 26 (30): 7942–7949. doi:http://dx.doi.org/10.1523/JNEUROSCI.1289-06.2006.

Van Gelder, Tim. 1998. "The Dynamical Hypothesis in Cognitive Science." *Behavioral and Brain Sciences* 21 (5): 615–665.

Van Orden, Guy C., John G. Holden, and Michael T. Turvey. 2003. "Self-Organization of Cognitive Performance." *Journal of Experimental Psychology: General* 132 (3): 331–350. doi:http://dx.doi.org/10.1037/0096-3445.132.3.331.

Van Rooij, Iris J. E. I., Raoul M. Bongers, and Willem F. G. Haselager. 2002. "A Non-Representational Approach to Imagined Action." *Cognitive Science* 26 (3): 345–375.

Varela, Francisco, Evan Thompson, and Eleanor Rosch. 1991. *The Embodied Mind: Cognitive Science and Human Experience*. Cambridge, MA: MIT Press.

Varela, Francisco, Evan Thompson, and Eleanor Rosch. 1993. *The Embodied Mind*. Cambridge, MA: MIT Press.

Warren, William H. 2006. "The Dynamics of Perception and Action." *Psychological Review* 113 (2): 358–389. doi:http://dx.doi.org/10.1037/003-295X.113.2.358.

Warren, William H., and Suzanne Whang. 1987. "Visual Guidance of Walking through Apertures: Body-Scaled Information for Affordances." *Journal of Experimental Psychology: Human Perception and Performance* 13 (3): 371–383. doi:http://dx.doi.org/10.1037/0096-1523.13.3.371.

Wilson, Andrew. 2013. *Grounded vs. Embodied Cognition: A (Hopefully Uncontentious) Note on Terminology*. Notes from Two Scientific Psychologists. http://psychsciencenotes.blogspot.pt/2013/07/grounded-vs-embodied-cognition.html.

Wilson, Andrew D., and Sabrina Golonka. 2013. "Embodied Cognition Is Not What You Think It Is." *Frontiers in Psychology* 4 (February): 58. doi:10.3389/fpsyg.2013.00058.

Zadra, Jonathan R., Arthur L. Weltman, and Dennis R. Proffitt. 2016. "Walkable Distances Are Bioenergetically Scaled." *Journal of Experimental Psychology: Human Perception and Performance* 42 (1): 39–51. doi:http://dx.doi.org/10.1037/xhp0000107.

Zahavi, Dan. 2010. "Empathy, Embodiment and Interpersonal Understanding: From Lipps to Schutz." *Inquiry: A Journal of Medical Care Organization, Provision and Financing* 53 (3): 285–306. doi:10.1080/00201741003784663.

14 Action Imitative and Prediction Error–Induced Contagions in Human Actions

Tsuyoshi Ikegami, Hiroki Nakamoto, and Gowrishankar Ganesh

1 Introduction

The next time you see a corner kick in a soccer match, make note of a strange and funny behavior; when the ball flies into the goal area, you will notice that it is not just the strikers and defenders (around the strikers) who jump to try to head the ball, but in fact most of the players on the field, even those who are nowhere near the ball, execute a jump in synchrony. The jumps by the other players are smaller, unconscious (players asked later report not being aware they had done it), and obviously serve no purpose, as they are far from the ball, sometimes even outside the penalty area. The behavior shows that our own actions are affected by environmental cues and behaviors observed in others, probably due to an overlap of action production and action perception processes in the brain (Rizzolatti and Craighero 2004; Blakemore and Frith 2005). This overlap leads to a blurring of differences in the sensorimotor system, between one's actions and perceptions of other's actions, and is a core feature of embodied cognition (Shapiro 2010).

Right from birth, action observation and subsequent imitation (Meltzoff and Moore 1977; Cook et al. 2014; Stahl and Feigenson 2015; Piaget 1954) play a key role in the development of our motor behaviors. *Imitation learning* is an explicit process wherein an individual consciously copies actions he or she observes in others, and it is believed to be crucial for optimizing behaviors in high dimensional systems, like our body (Schaal 1999; Schaal, Ijspeert, and Billard 2003). However, there exists a second category of observation-induced action modifications, like the soccer example, that are unconscious, affect behavior without an individual willing it, sometimes serve no discernible purpose, and often occur even without an individual realizing it. These so-called *motor contagions* include a wide range of effects on an individual's action intention, goal, or kinematics and are arguably still not completely understood. In this chapter we review the different motor contagions reported in the literature. We show that, while most contagions are driven by features like the kinematics, intentions, or goals of observed actions, and lead to an increase in similarity between one's actions and those observed in others, other contagions do not manifest as an increase in similarity to observed actions. We discuss the possible mechanisms underlying this second category of motor contagions and propose an extended conceptual model to explain the complete contagion spectrum. Based on these discussions, we then analyze how athletes may control, prevent, and compensate for these contagions during performance.

2 Previous Characterization of Motor Contagion

Over the past two decades, studies have identified a variety of motor contagions in adult human behavior (Kilner, Paulignan, and Blakemore 2003; Blakemore and Frith 2005; Chartrand and Bargh 1999; Heyes 2011). These have been characterized and given different names depending on the action feature that they affect and the context in which they are activated. We start by reviewing these characterizations.

2.1 Automatic Imitation

Automatic imitation is a covert form of imitation in which the observation of task-irrelevant body movements involuntarily facilitates one's own performance of similar movements in terms of kinematics (Heyes 2011, 2013). Stürmer, Aschersleben, and Prinz (2000) examined hand opening and closing by participants while they viewed one of two hand actions on a computer screen. The color of the viewed hand changed abruptly from flesh color to either blue or red. Participants were asked to respond to the blue stimulus by opening their hand, and respond to the red stimulus by closing their hand. Although the observed action (open or close) was task-irrelevant, responses were faster when the action of the stimulus hand was compatible with the correct response than when the stimulus action was response-incompatible. Observation of a compatible action clearly facilitated action execution. Brass et al. (2000) asked participants to rest their fingers on a table and observe a movie that showed the left hand of a human model on the screen and facing the participant. The participants were instructed to lift their right index finger when they observed the numeral "1" on a screen, and lift their right middle finger when they observed a "2." The experiment included three observation conditions: in the congruent condition, the model lifted a finger corresponding to the presented number (i.e., index finger for 1 and middle finger for 2); in the incongruent condition, the model lifted a finger that did not correspond to the presented number (i.e., the middle finger for 1 and index finger for 2); and finally, in the baseline condition, the model did not lift any finger. The participants showed a shorter reaction time to initiate their finger movements in the congruent condition compared with the baseline condition, whereas they showed a longer reaction time in the incongruent condition compared with the baseline condition.

Automatic imitation is believed to be modulated by a similarity in topographical properties of body movements (Heyes 2011, 2013) such that observation of index finger movements by the model affects the participant's index but not middle finger movements. However, the same result may also be explained by the phenomenon of spatial stimulus-response compatibility (Craighero et al. 1996; Fitts and Seeger 1953; Simon 1969), wherein a sensory stimulus facilitates the accuracy or speed of a response with similar spatial characteristics. To exclude this possibility, Brass, Bekkering, and Prinz (2001) repeated their previous experiment (Brass et al. 2000) with a different set of movies of the human model that were flipped upside down (figure 14.1). Even though the flipping made the observed movement incongruent in external space, the authors observed that the participants again showed a shorter reaction time when lifting or tapping a finger congruent with what they observed in the movie. This experiment indicates that automatic imitation cannot be explained only by spatial stimulus-response compatibility, and is rather a consequence of topographical movement features of observed body stimuli.

The above automatic imitation phenomena were caused by task-irrelevant stimuli that were presented over the task-relevant stimuli. On the other hand, Leighton and Heyes (2010) confirmed that automatic imitation takes place even when the task-irrelevant stimulus is presented on the left and right sides of the monitor, that is, in the peripheral visual field, while the participant attended to a small task-relevant stimulus on the center of a computer monitor. This result shows that automatic imitation can occur when observers do not intend to pay direct spatial attention to the action stimuli and hence has the potential to affect team sports like soccer, basketball, and hockey, without players realizing it.

Automatic imitation leads not only to temporal interference (i.e., a change in reaction time), but also spatial interference. Kilner et al. (2003) reported an interference effect of observed biological movements on one's own movements. In their experiments, participants made rhythmic arm movements in a vertical or horizontal direction while observing an experimenter who made either similar (congruent) or orthogonal (incongruent) arm movements in front of them (facing the participants). The variability of the participant's own movements was observed to be larger in the incongruent condition, compared with the congruent condition and no observation (baseline) condition. Interestingly, this interference effect was not observed when participants observed incongruent but biologically implausible movements performed by a robot.

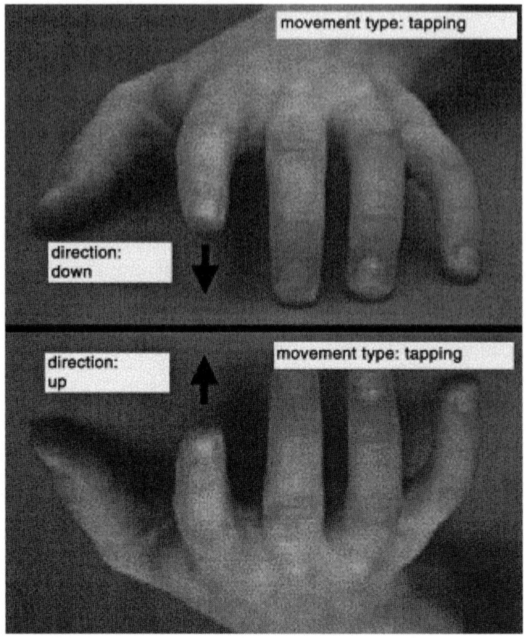

Figure 14.1
Presented stimulus of normal (upper) and flipped (lower) hand orientation in the experiment by Brass, Bekkering, and Prinz (2001). During presentation of the normal hand orientation, both the topographical movement features (the finger movements shown in the stimulus) and movement direction (lift or drop of finger) in the stimulus were congruent with the tapping movement by participants. In the flipped presentation, while the topographical movement features were still congruent, the movement direction was not, and the finger-drop movement in the stimulus was now visually incongruent with a finger drop (during tapping) by the participants. The reaction time of participants was, however, reportedly decreased during observation of the finger-drop stimulus while viewing the flipped hand orientation, even though it was visually incongruent to their tap. This result suggests that automatic imitation is modulated by the topographical movement features of observed body stimuli.

To examine whether automatic imitation is really automatic, Cook and colleagues (2012) developed a unique experimental paradigm using the rock-paper-scissors game. Their paradigm involved only two of the three rock, paper, and scissors conditions. Participants were exposed to a strategic context in which imitating the opponent's gesture (i.e., a draw) led to a suboptimal monetary reward. One or both players were blindfolded in their experiment. The frequency of a draw was at chance level (50 percent) when both players were blindfolded, but the researchers observed a significantly higher (than chance) level of draws when only one player was blindfolded. This result suggests that the observation of the blindfolded opponent made the player with vision unconsciously imitate the opponent's gesture even though it resulted in a loss in his or her monetary reward. Similar evidence for the automatic nature of automatic imitation is also presented by the work of Belot, Crawford, and Heyes (2013).

Automatic imitation can be theoretically explained by interactions between the two routes of the *dual route model* of sensorimotor processing (figure 14.2) (Heyes 2011, 2013). This theoretical account originates from studies on stimulus-response compatibility (Zorzi and Umiltà 1995). The model proposes two sensorimotor processing routes. One process is via a conscious or conditional route (dashed line in figure 14.2). This conscious route is based on short-term associations between sensory representations and motor representations that can be formed immediately and flexibly through task instructions. This route accounts for task relevant actions. The other process is via an unconscious or unconditional route, which is developed by long-term associations between sensory representations and motor representations developed through experience (Heyes et al. 2005; Catmur, Walsh, and Heyes 2007). This unconscious route cannot be altered directly by intentional processes and is thus automatically driven, even by a task-irrelevant stimulus. During action observation, the unconscious route processes the observed action kinematics (such as movement trajectory, velocity, or posture of body parts). The sensory (visual) representations of the actions then automatically activate corresponding motor representations, consequently resulting in an action with the same kinematics as the one observed. Therefore, when both task-irrelevant and task-relevant stimuli activate the same motor representation (i.e., in congruent conditions), the task performance is facilitated. However, when the task-irrelevant and task-relevant stimuli result in the activation of different motor representations (i.e., in incongruent conditions), the task performance is hampered because of a competition between the two representations.

It is important to note here that the dual route model is not the only model proposed in the literature to explain contagions (Heyes 2011, 2013). We will, however, limit our discussions to the dual route model in this chapter because of its simple structure and because the issues relevant to the dual route model are valid for multiple possible mechanisms.

2.2 Emulation (Intention/Goal Imitation)

Emulation (Byrne and Russon 1998; Whiten et al. 2009) leads to imitation of the intention or goal of an observed action. Emulation thus requires not just action observation, but also action understanding (Blakemore and Decety 2001; Rizzolatti and Craighero 2004; Brass et al. 2007) and has been suggested to play a role in various social functions.

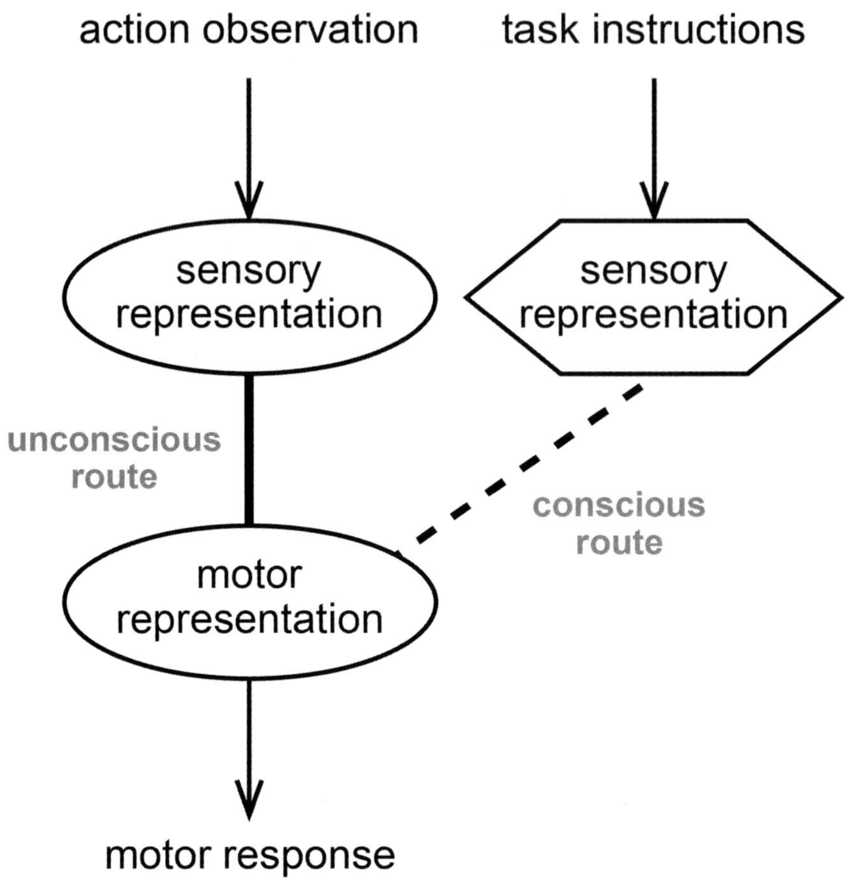

Figure 14.2
The dual route model suggests that motor contagions are caused by an interference between the conscious and unconscious routes of sensorimotor processing. The conscious route is driven by short-term sensorimotor associations (dashed line), which can be formed immediately based on task instructions. The unconscious route is driven by action observation and is caused by the long-term sensorimotor associations (solid line) that develop through experience or learning.

In the experiments by Bekkering and his colleagues (Bekkering, Wohlschläger, and Gattis 2000; Gleissner, Meltzoff, and Bekkering 2000), preschool children were instructed by an experimenter: "Try to imitate me as if you were my mirror. You do what I do." The experimenter then touched either his left or right ear with either his ipsilateral or contralateral hand. The children consistently touched the correct ear but predominantly used their ipsilateral hand to do so, even when the experimenter used his contralateral hand. In other words, the subjects successfully imitated the goal of the observed action but did not imitate the action kinematics.

To confirm that the error in contralateral touch imitation was not caused by difficulty in touching the ears across one's body, the authors manipulated the saliency of the observed goal in their stimulus. They performed a control experiment in which experimenters reached, not for their ears but, for a space in air near the ear with their contralateral hands. In this case, the same children successfully imitated the action kinematics, making significantly more contralateral touches than before. These results suggest that even preschool children can hierarchically decompose observed actions into subcomponents—at least the goal and kinematics—and when they are asked to imitate a goal-directed observed action, they tend to imitate the goal rather than the kinematics. On the other hand, they tend to imitate the kinematics for actions that are not perceived to have a goal.

Goal-imitation has also been observed in adults. Bird et al. (2007) examined imitation errors in adult participants using the pen-and-cup task that was originally developed by Wohlschlager, Gattis, and Bekkering (2003). The participants were asked to observe actions performed by a model in the video and imitate it in an anatomically compatible but egocentrically incompatible way. The observed actions were experimentally manipulated into three hierarchical action subcomponents: object (hierarchically high), effector (middle), movement path (low). In the video, the model moved a centrally located pen into one of two colored cups (objects) using either their right or left hand (effector). The action was performed with one of two different grasps (the thumb pointing up or pointing down) leading to different arm movement trajectories. The participants showed fewer object errors than effector errors and fewer effector errors than grip errors, which is consistent with the idea that imitation of a hierarchically higher action component takes priority over the imitation of a lower one.

While the above studies explicitly instructed participants to imitate actions performed by others, a series of studies by Castiello and his colleague have shown that emulation can be implicit. Edwards, Humphreys, and Castiello (2003) asked participants to observe an experimenter performing a goal-oriented action to reach and grasp either a large or small object, and then the participants performed the same grasping action for an object of similar size (congruent condition) or an object of different size (incongruent condition). The participants took a shorter time to reach peak velocity in grasps in the congruent compared with the incongruent condition, implying that the observed congruent actions implicitly facilitated the participant's action performance. This observation effect appears to be similar to automatic imitation, but a clear distinction was observed in a second experiment in which the participants did not observe the reaching action but observed only the reached object. Interestingly, even in the absence of an action, the time taken to reach peak velocity by participants was reduced during the congruent (object observation) condition compared with the incongruent condition. This result is therefore referred to as "automatic emulation" (Heyes 2011). Assuming that, similar to proposals for automatic imitation, a representation coding an object as an action goal may automatically activate a corresponding motor representation leading to an action required for the same goal achievement, automatic emulation may also be explained by the presence of the unconscious sensorimotor processing route, as in figure 14.2.

How does the understanding of intentions (hierarchically higher than the goal) behind observed actions affect one's own actions? To address this issue, Castiello (2003) developed an experiment paradigm involving motor interference due to a *distractor*. In the previous work (Castiello 1999), they had showed that a goal-directed action to a task-relevant target is implicitly affected by objects acting as distractors; when a target to be grasped by participants is presented alongside a distractor of a different size, the amplitude of peak grip aperture increased with increase in the size of the distractor. Based on this result, Castiello (2003) examined whether the interference effect was transferred between individuals through action observation or not. Participants were first asked to observe a human model who reached and grasped an object presented either in isolation or flanked by a smaller object (the distractor). They were subsequently asked to make the same action for the same target object presented in isolation. The results showed a significant transfer of interference effects from the model to the observer; the amplitude of the participant's peak grip aperture was modulated by the size of the distractor for observed actions performed by the model. Importantly, the interference effects were found even after the participants observed catch trials where the target and distractor were presented to the model, but he or she did not move (though the model was allowed to look at the objects).

Additional experiments confirmed that the interference effects occurred only when the observer could monitor the gaze direction of the model. The effects were suppressed when the upper part of the model's body was visible but with the face invisible or when the model's gaze was constrained by asking the model to fixate on the target while performing the action. These results suggested that the motor intention of the model could be inferred by monitoring the model's gaze and, importantly, that the understanding of the model's intention could affect the observer's own actions.

Similar to goal emulation, intention emulation probably also results from the activation of motor representations corresponding to the representations coding the intention of the observed action. Therefore, this contagion may also be characterized as automatic emulation. To summarize, the observations reviewed here indicate that emulation is a motor contagion that results in individuals imitating the intention or goal of observed actions.

2.3 Outcome Mimicry

Another type of motor contagion has been reported to affect one's action outcomes (De Maeght and Prinz 2004). In a virtual reality experiment setup with baseball batters (Gray 2002), Gray and Beilock (2011) asked batters of varied experience to hit a baseball toward center field following observation of one of three stimuli: (1) *action,* in which a simulated ball was shown traveling from the home plate to the left, right, or center field, (2) *outcome,* in which a ball was shown resting in either the left, right, or center field, and (3) *verbal,* in which the word "left," "right," or "center" was shown on the screen. Note that the stimuli did not include any human action and consisted only of a ball traveling to a particular location, a stationary ball at a particular location in the baseball field, or a textual message merely indicating the location that the ball had landed. The researchers observed that the hits of the "experienced" batters were affected by the action and outcome stimuli, whereas those of the "less experienced" batters were affected only by the action stimuli. Specifically, if a batter observed a ball traveling to the left field, her subsequent hit was more to the left even though she was instructed to hit toward the center field, and if the batter observed a ball traveling right, then her subsequent hit was more to the right. These results can be interpreted as mimicry of the observed outcome, which we will refer to as outcome mimicry, and may partly explain the belief in baseball that "hitting is contagious" (Bock, Maewal, and Gough 2012).

Outcome mimicry has been shown of not just observed outcomes, but also anticipated outcomes. Previous studies in sport psychology have demonstrated that expert athletes can anticipate domain-specific action outcomes rapidly and accurately by visually detecting and extracting kinematic cues inherent to an opponents' action (Abernethy and Zawi 2007; Jackson and Mogan 2007; Huys et al. 2009). Takeuchi and colleagues (2014) investigated the effect on outcome mimicry of the degree of difficulty in anticipating the outcome of a hammer throw. In their experiment, varsity hammer throwers watched videos of model hammer throwers who made throws to the left, right, or center of the field. The actual flight of the hammer was occluded in the videos such that the participants could observe only the throwing action but not the hammer trajectory. Some of the throws in the video were purposely made with exaggerated actions to facilitate the anticipation. Following the video, the participants were asked to make throws to the center of the field. There was no evidence of imitation of the model's kinematics by the participants. Outcome mimicry however, was observed. Participant throws were biased toward the direction they anticipated for the model's throw. Crucially, this bias was observed only after the videos in which the throws were easy to anticipate.

Again, like automatic imitation, goal imitation, and intention imitation, the reported outcome mimicry is also implicit and unintentional. Although both the aforementioned studies explicitly instructed participants to hit or throw a ball toward a specific direction, participants ended up being biased by the observed outcome even though it did not directly assist their own task.

Gray and Beilock (2011) reported that highly experienced batters are more affected by the outcome of others' actions because experienced athletes are expected to have a stronger link between an observed outcome and the motor action required to achieve that outcome. These results can again be explained by the unconscious sensorimotor processing route: a representation that codes for an observed outcome may automatically activate a corresponding motor representation, consequently resulting in an action corresponding to the same outcome (figure 14.2).

2.4 Motor Mimicry

It has been known for a long time that humans are prone to mimic an observed individual's body postures and mannerisms without intention (Charny 1966; Condon and Ogston 1967; Kendon 1970; LaFrance and Broadbent 1976) during social interactions. Such automatic imitation or mimicry in social situations is referred to as *motor mimicry* and also known as the *chameleon effect* (Chartrand and Bargh 1999). In contrast to automatic imitation, emulation, and outcome imitation, which manifest as changes in reaction time and/or accuracy of movements, motor mimicry manifests as changes in behaviors and behavioral choices. These changes are usually quantified by the frequency of occurrence of certain actions or behaviors (Heyes 2011).

Chartrand and Bargh (1999) provided the first valid demonstration of motor mimicry by showing a cause-and-effect relationship between observed behaviors and one's own behaviors in a social context. Their experiments manipulated the *cause*: the mannerisms and behaviors of partners (confederates of the experiment), and examined the *effect* on the occurrence (frequency) of the same mannerisms in interacting participants. Participants in their experiment took turns with a confederate to describe a series of photographs in two sessions. In one session, the confederate rubbed his face but did not shake his foot, whereas in the other session, the confederate shook his foot but did not rub his face. The experiment observed that participants rubbed their face more often in the session with the face-rubbing confederate than in the session with the foot-shaking confederate, whereas they shook their foot more often in the session with the foot-shaking confederate than in the session with the face-rubbing confederate. This result provided the first causal evidence to show that individuals unintentionally mimic behaviors or mannerisms of another individual with whom they interact.

Motor mimicry has been linked to increased liking, rapport, or prosocial attitude (van Baaren et al. 2004; Chartrand and Bargh 1999) during social interactions and has been proposed as an important unconscious communication tool used by humans. Chartrand and Bargh (1999, experiment 2) conducted another experiment in which a confederate mimicked mannerisms of participants during the same social interaction as the above-mentioned main experiment. After the interaction with the confederate, the participants who were mimicked reported the confederate to be more likable and the interactions to be smoother, even though they had not been aware of being mimicked.

Van Baaren et al. (2004) performed experiments similar to the second experiment by Chartland and Bargh (1999) to examine whether mimicry makes an individual more prosocial. In their experiment, confederates mimicked mannerisms or body postures of a participant during a social interaction, following which that confederate, or a new confederate, "accidentally" dropped six pens in front of the participant. The participants who had been mimicked were observed to pick up more pens, in comparison to those who had not been mimicked. These results suggest that mimicry makes an individual show more favorable rapport, or prosocial attitude, toward not only the individual who performed the mimicry, but also toward other people. The finding that motor mimicry enhances prosocial behavior suggests that it serves to strengthen social bonds and may play an important role in the building of any close-knit community, such as a sport team.

Finally, although there is still no direct evidence that motor mimicry is based on the same mechanism as automatic imitation, emulation, or outcome imitation, motor mimicry has been explained by a perception-behavior link assuming the existence of an automatic connection between representations coding observed behaviors and motor representations enabling the same behaviors (Chartrand and Bargh 1999).

3 A New Type of Contagion

The four types of motor contagion that have been studied predominantly in the past, and which we reviewed above, are induced simply by the observation of actions and have a signature characteristic—they cause certain features of one's action to become similar to that of the observed action in terms of kinematics, outcome, goal or intention, or overall behavior. For this reason, we characterize them here as *action-imitative contagions* (or AICs). We now introduce a new type of contagion that is induced not simply by action observation, but when the observation is accompanied by *prediction errors*—differences between actions one observes and those one predicts or expects. In other words, with these contagions, a given action can cause vastly different motor effects in an observer depending on what the observer has predicted about the action. These contagions, which we call *prediction error–induced contagions* (or PECs), are thus fundamentally different from AICs.

In a study with darts experts, Ikegami and Ganesh (2014) asked darts experts to watch videos of a novice thrower. Part of the video was masked such that while a novice thrower was visible to the experts, his dart flight trajectory and dartboard were not. The experts were asked to predict the outcome of the novices' throws (in terms of the location on the dartboard) by viewing the novices' throw kinematics. In their first experiment, the authors showed that the experts' own throws progressively deteriorated after repeated video observation-prediction sessions. Interestingly, they observed that the deterioration was correlated with the improvement in the action prediction by the experts.

To test these observations further, the authors modulated the improvement in the experts' prediction of the observed novices' throws in a second experiment, and examined its effect on their darts performance. They manipulated two prediction errors that helped the experts improve their outcome prediction. The first is the *outcome prediction error*—the difference between the outcome predicted by the expert from the observed novice's action and the actual outcome provided to the expert orally by the experimenter. The second is the *kinematics prediction error*—the difference between the novice kinematics the expert actually observed and the kinematics expected by the expert based on the goal she believed the novice was aiming for. The outcome prediction error was suppressed by not providing the experts with the actual outcome of the novices' throws. The kinematics prediction error was suppressed by altering the experts' beliefs about the novice's goals—the authors misinformed the expert at the start of the experiment that "the novice does not always aim for the board center but aims for unknown targets provided by us," and that "only the trials in which the novice was successful are presented." This misinformation was expected to remove any prior goal belief that the experts may have had.

In the absence of these two prediction errors, the experts' prediction ability did not change over the course of the experiment. Interestingly, the darts performance of the experts was also observed to remain unchanged in this experiment, even though the experts watched the same darts videos as in the first experiment. These results indicated that the experts' darts performance was affected not by the observation of the novices' dart throws but rather by the prediction errors during the observation, which suggests the presence of PEC.

PEC-like behaviors have also been reported in several observational motor-learning results. Gribble and his colleagues (Mattar and Gribble 2005; Brown, Wilson, and Gribble 2009; Brown et al. 2010; McGregor, Cashaback, and Gribble 2016) have reported that observation can help individuals learn the dynamics of a novel task—the so-called *internal model* of the task environment (Kawato 1999; Wolpert, Ghahramani, and Jordan 1995; Shadmehr and Wise 2005)—faster. In their studies, they observed that participants who observed another individual performing the same adaptation task showed faster adaptation to the so called viscous-curl force field (Shadmehr and Mussa-Ivaldi 1994), in comparison to control participants who did not observe anybody, or participants who observed an individual adapting to a different force field. Wanda, Li, and Thoroughman (2013) performed a similar experiment in which participants were asked to watch individuals learning to make straight reaching movements toward a single target in the viscous-curl force field. A straight movement in this field requires one to learn a pattern of lateral hand forces corresponding to their reach velocity. Then the observing participants are subsequently asked to make reaching movements toward the same target. Utilizing the error clamp technique (Scheidt et al. 2000) that allows for the measurement of lateral hand forces during reaching movements, Wanda and colleagues showed that the participants can reproduce the temporal pattern of force characterizing the movement that they observed without any physical experience of the force field. That is, they developed an internal model corresponding to an observed movement simply though action observation. Numerous studies on human motor learning have shown that learning of internal models is driven by prediction errors: differences between actions actually performed and those predicted by a participant. Similar prediction errors—but in this case differences between observed actions performed by another individual and actions the observer participant predicts that individual to produce—may contribute to the participant learning the internal model by observation (Brown et al. 2010).

To examine possible changes in internal models (though at a more trial-by-trial level) during their darts study, Ikegami and Ganesh analyzed the interactions between the expert's ability to predict the outcome of observed actions and their ability to *self-estimate* the outcome of their own actions (Ikegami and Ganesh 2017). The self-estimation was measured as the distance between where experts' darts landed and where the experts self-estimated them to have landed (in a no-visual feedback condition). First, the authors observed that the improvement in the experts' outcome-prediction ability caused a deterioration in self-estimation accuracy. The experts tended to always self-estimate their throws to be near the center of the dartboard, even when their throws landed far from the center. Interestingly, however, this self-estimation was not random and, though wrong, showed a significant correlation with where their darts landed. Next, the authors showed that the trial-by-trial qualitative changes in the darts performance, self-estimation, and the corresponding correlation by each expert can be explained by a state-space model that assumes that the self-estimation is used by the experts as feedback (in the absence of vision) to regulate their dart throws. Critically, the quantification of their model revealed that the deterioration was caused by a specific change in the expert's *outcome forward model*, a mapping between throw action kinematics and consequence (dart landing position on the dartboard). On the other hand, the changes observed in the experts' ability to make action corrections corresponding to the (erroneous) self-estimation, usually attributed to the controller or darts *inverse model* (a mapping from a dart landing position to the throw action kinematics), were minimal.

While further studies are required to check if and how observations affect the forward and inverse models differently, the above results support the claim that PECs are caused by modifications of sensorimotor mappings or internal models. Crucially, note that these modifications are aimed at reducing prediction errors and depend not only on the observed action, but also on what the observer predicts. Thus PECs may not lead to imitation of the observed action features. For example, in the study of Wanda, Li, and Thoroughman (2013), the force output profiles indicated that the observer's reaching movements were biased after observation, not toward the same direction as the observed movements, but in the opposite direction to the observed movement (see figure 14.3). Although, in their simple two-dimensional movement experiment, the prediction-driven contagion leads, in a sense, to an *anti-imitation,* or mirroring of an observed action feature (specifically, hand forces), the effects can be difficult to predict in high-dimensional tasks involving multiple joints. Thus, PECs may not manifest as similarities between observed and performed action kinematics or outcomes. Next, we consider these results to analyze how the changes in motor representations may be reconciled with the dual route model (Heyes 2011, 2013).

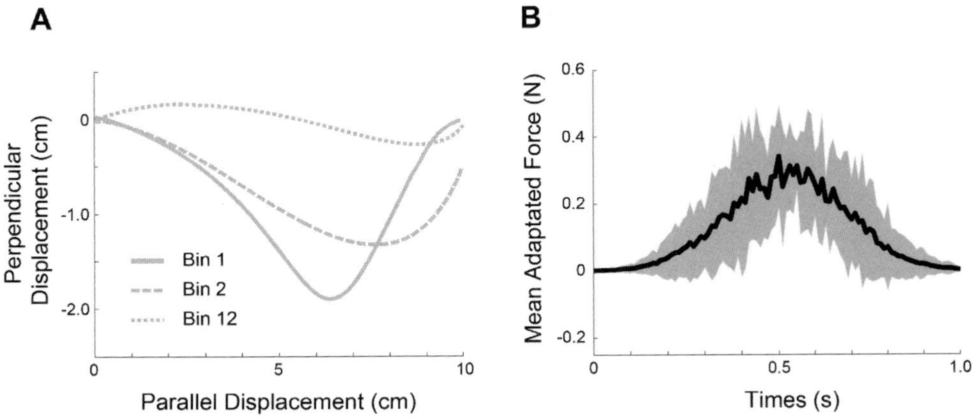

Figure 14.3
Representative reproductions of figures 3 and 4 from Wanda, Li, and Thoroughman (2013). (A) Participants from an observation learning group watched hand movements of a model actor adapting to a viscous-curl force field before performing the task themselves. In the first learning bin (Bin 1: trials 1–8), the hand trajectory of the model (orange solid line) was largely distorted by the force field, toward the right (downward direction in the figure). The trajectory slowly converges to a straight line as the model learns the new force environment (Bin 2: trials 9–16; Bin 12: trials 89–96). (B) The mean force (black line) generated by the participants who observed the model and later worked under the "error clamp condition" that allows measurement of the lateral hand forces during reaching movements. Although they had not experienced the force field themselves, they generated substantial lateral forces when they subsequently made reaching movements in the force field. These forces can be considered to be a motor contagion. Importantly, the direction of their generated forces indicates that the participants' reaches tended to move toward the direction opposite (left) to the movements they observed in the model (compare with movement direction in [A]).

4 Comparing Prediction Error–Induced Contagion and Action-Imitative Contagion

The core cause of AIC is believed to be associations between representations that encode features of an observed action, such as kinematics, outcome, goals, or intentions, and motor representations of actions with those same features. These associations are assumed to develop through long-term experience or learning, and possibly to be genetically predisposed (Cook et al. 2014), enabling an automatic transformation of an observed action feature to the corresponding motor response (Heyes 2011). Observation of an action first activates a representation that encodes a feature of the action; this in turn automatically activates the corresponding motor representation that leads to a movement with the same feature. Which feature leads to contagion probably depends on the saliency of the task and attentional characteristics of the observer (see part 2.2). From the behavioral view point, AICs lead to an increase in the similarity between one or more features of one's actions and of actions observed in others.

On the other hand, evidence suggests that PECs are caused by prediction errors (differences between what one expects and what one sees). PECs may not lead to direct imitation of any movement feature, and may in fact lead to effects mirroring the observed movement features (Wanda, Li, and Thoroughman 2013). Furthermore, they have been reported to persist for several action trials after action observations (Wanda, Li, and Thoroughman 2013; Ikegami and Ganesh 2014). These characteristics, combined with the fact that prediction errors are known to critically influence sensorimotor mappings or internal models (Wolpert and Kawato 1998; Tseng et al. 2007), suggest that, in contrast to AICs, PECs lead to a change in the motor representations in the brain (Ikegami and Ganesh 2014, 2017). To explain these two types of motor contagions, we therefore propose an extension of the dual route model of figure 14.2.

We propose to extend the dual route model by highlighting the role of predictions, by the brain, about observed actions (figure 14.4).

According to the original dual route model (Heyes 2011, 2013), the interaction between the unconscious route, triggered by the "action observation," and the conscious route, triggered by the "task instructions," induce AICs in the observer. The extended model hypothesizes that, in parallel, the prediction system utilizes the same "action observation" and "task instructions" to predict or estimate subsequent action features in the observed agent. Discrepancies between the predicted features and actual features seen in the observed agent generate *prediction errors* that lead to a modification of the prediction system. It has been suggested that the motor system is at least partially involved in prediction of observed actions (represented by dashed enclosing line) (Wolpert, Doya, and Kawato 2003; Aglioti et al. 2008; Ikegami and Ganesh 2014, 2017; Ganesh and Ikegami 2016), which suggests that the changes in the prediction system (double line with arrow in figure 14.4) are equivalent to changes in the motor representations in the brain. Our extended model thus suggests that PECs are caused by the prediction-error-driven modifications of the motor representations in the brain. An interesting implication of this conceptual model is that, in the presence of prediction errors, both AICs and PECs can occur in parallel. However, this possibility remains to be tested in practice.

The dal route model proposes that observed actions automatically activate corresponding motor representations in the brain. This suggestion is supported by the *common coding theory* introduced by Prinz (1997) and by recent neural recordings in studies

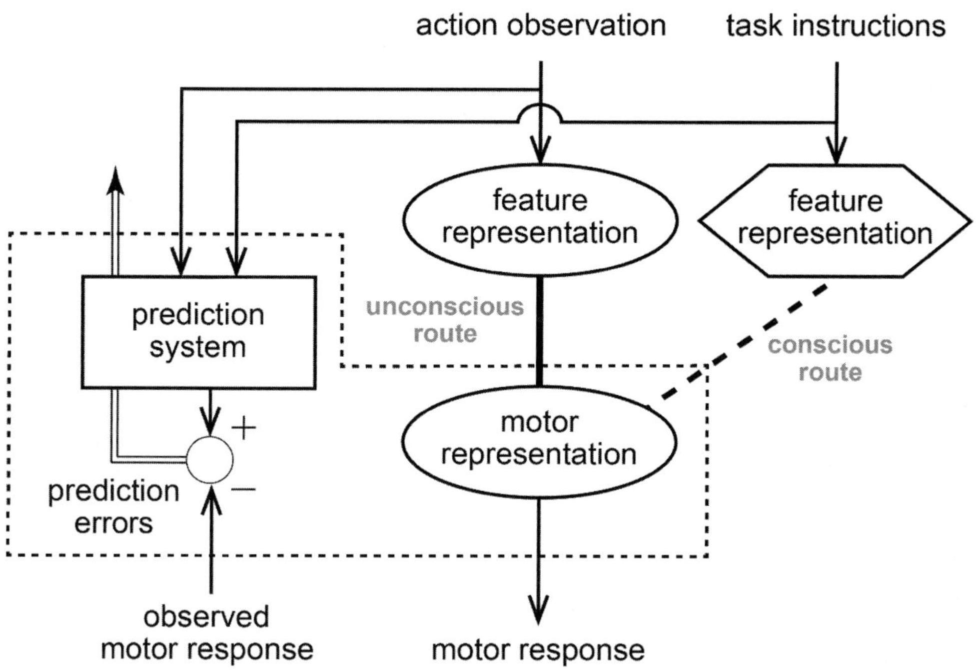

Figure 14.4
Extended dual route model. The prediction system is added to the original dual route model. Both the action observation and task instructions are used to predict features of an observed individual's motor response. Prediction errors—differences between the predicted and actual feature/s of a motor response—change the prediction system. The model proposes that the motor system is at least partially involved in action prediction (shown by the dashed enclosure). That is why the prediction error–induced changes in the prediction system can modify motor representations and, in turn, cause PECs. Note that here we choose to use the term "feature representation" instead of "sensory representation" as in the original dual route model (figure 14.2), to clarify the fact that the representations may include different features of an observed action (such as its kinematics, goal, or intention). The model represents only the observer, who is assumed to observe the actions of another agent and receive the same task instructions as the observed agent.

investigating the so-called mirror neurons (Rizzolatti and Craighero 2004; Rizzolatti and Sinigaglia 2010). Our proposed extended model (figure 14.4) goes a step further and suggests that action observations can in fact change motor representations in the brain. Ikegami and Ganesh (2017) showed that this change occurs in the so-called outcome forward model in the brain. Overall, these ideas agree well with the proposed theme of *conceptualization* in embodied cognition (Shapiro 2010, 2013). Details about this theme are available in other chapters in this book.

5 Application to Sports

Athletes and coaches have often claimed to have experienced contagion during training and games. Some anecdotal experiences have been reported by researchers. In one of his interviews, Ichiro Suzuki, one of the most consistent batters in major league baseball in recent times, disclosed that he refrains from closely watching poor batters on his team before playing because it affects his own batting performance (June 19, 2007, *Yukan Fuji*, reported in Ikegami and Ganesh 2014). Gray and Beilock (2011) reported similar comments from coaches in US major league baseball: "One guy starts hitting well, the other guys are gonna catch on" (Tommy Lasorda, Los Angeles Dodgers); "Absolutely, hitting is contagious. You get a bunch of these guys hitting, hopefully the guys that aren't hitting right now will catch on fire" (Charlie Puleo, New York Mets).

In addition to factors like mood contagion (Totterdell 2000) and social contagion (Boss and Kleinert 2015), motor contagions, both AICs and PECs, are arguably the key causes of these empirical observations in sports. Therefore, an understanding of why motor contagion occurs not only contributes to our theoretical understanding of sensorimotor representations and plasticity in the brain, but also sheds light on whether and how individuals can control motor contagions in order to improve their sport performance and alleviate unwanted performance decrements. Here, we discuss issues regarding the controllability of motor contagions and the applicability and relevance of motor contagion research to sport performance and motor learning.

5.1 Controlling Motor Contagion

Athletes in professional sports need to obtain maximum performance and to resist any adverse effects from motor contagions, while capitalizing on any favorable ones. As discussed above, numerous studies have shown that motor contagions can affect one's actions, goals, and intentions very implicitly and unconsciously. It would seem as if motor contagions are uncontrollable. However, it is common knowledge that although we imitate some actions, we don't imitate others. Several studies have thus proposed the presence of an inhibitory mechanism and/or an action-control mechanism that prevents us from imitating all the time (Brass and Heyes 2005; Schütz-Bosbach et al. 2009; Spengler et al. 2010; Cross et al. 2013).

Though the exact mechanism driving motor contagions is still unclear, as we have discussed, contagions arguably result when an observed action activates a corresponding motor representation. Brass, Ruby, and Spengler (2009) investigated the existence of functional mechanisms in the brain that control the activations of motor representations caused by action observation. They reported that a reduced imitative response in an imitation-inhibition task (i.e., reduced contagion) was accompanied by increased activation (Brass et al. 2000) (see details in part 2.1 in this chapter) in the medial prefrontal cortex (mPFC) (see also, Brass and Heyes 2005; Spengler, von Cramon, and Brass 2009). Furthermore, they reported an overlap between the brain activations during reduced contagions and the brain activations related to self-related processing and/or complex social-cognitive tasks. These overlaps were observed in the anterior frontomedian cortex (aFMC) and the temporoparietal junction (TPJ). From these results they hypothesized that information processing about one's self may increase the ability to achieve one's own motor intentions and resist motor contagions. That is, self-related processing may play a fundamental role in the control of motor contagions (see also, Schütz-Bosbach et al. 2009).

Based on this hypothesis, Spengler and colleagues (2010) investigated whether self-focus enhances control of one's own actions and/or inhibits motor contagion during an imitation-inhibition task. In their study, self-focus was elicited by engaging participants in a self-referential task, namely judging evaluative statements (e.g., "Leipzig is a pleasant town"). On the other hand, the non-self-focus tasks involved judgments of neutral statements that required retrieval of semantic memory ("Leipzig is the capital of Germany"). Participants performed alternating trials of the self-referential (or non-self-referential) task and an imitation-inhibition task. Researchers observed that contagion (visible as interference in the inhibition-imitation task) was reduced after the self-focus tasks. Furthermore, Schütz-Bosbach and colleagues (2009) reported a decrease in motor evoked potential induced by transcranial magnetic stimulation (TMS) of primary motor areas when observed actions are attributed to oneself, compared with when the same actions are attributed to another agent. These findings suggest that self-related processing can enhance the resistance of actions to motor contagions.

As described in part 2.1, automatic imitation describes a special case of the stimulus-response compatibility effect. Traditional stimulus-response compatibility studies have suggested that automatic response activation can be suppressed in preparation for trials in which the automatic response to an observed action is likely to interfere with task-relevant behavior (e.g., Vu and Proctor 2004). To investigate whether such suppression in preparation also occurs for automatic imitation, Cross and Iacoboni (2014) measured muscle-specific cortico-spinal excitability during action observation, by using TMS when participants prepared to execute imitative or counter-imitative responses to action stimuli. They found that cortico-spinal excitability was suppressed during the preparation of counter-imitation actions, compared with the preparation of imitative actions. Automatic imitation, therefore, can be suppressed when the automatic response is likely to interfere with a task goal.

Similar to the above AIC studies, there is evidence that PECs can be controlled and suppressed as well. PEC in darts experts (see part 3; Ikegami and Ganesh 2014) was observed when an expert's prediction about the kinematics and outcome of an observed action differed from the kinematics and outcome the expert actually observed. In contrast, when specific goal beliefs or feedback about outcomes were removed during observation, PEC was attenuated. In their study, the authors removed the outcome feedback by withholding information about the outcome of the actions the darts experts observed, while they altered experts' beliefs about the model's goal by misinforming the darts experts about the intention of the observed model. Their results suggest that PECs can be suppressed by not predicting observed actions. This suppression has important implications for sports that frequently include action predictions (more on this point later).

Motor contagions are not always detrimental, but can also facilitate performance. Eaves, Turgeon, and Vogt (2012) showed that passive observation of a rhythmical action can bias the frequency of the observer's subsequently performed rhythmical actions. In their subsequent study, the authors investigated how action frequency was further modulated by simultaneous motor imagery of one's own action during observation of an action performed by others. In the study, participants were required to execute an instructed rhythmical action (e.g., slow actions), following observation of a rhythmical distractor movie (e.g., of fast actions). They report that motor imagery, during action observation, of an action synchronized to the observed rhythmic action, induces a more pronounced imitation bias compared with passive observation and also in comparison to static unsynchronized imaging. On the neural side, this observation is supported by a recent neurophysiological study (Nedelko et al. 2012) that demonstrated that simultaneous imagery of action execution during action observation activates a larger cortical motor region compared with mere observation without imagery.

A study by van Leeuwen and colleagues (2009) provides an alternate possibility for controlling motor contagions, by controlling available working memory. Working memory refers to the cognitive system that retains (a small amount of) information in an active state for use in ongoing tasks (for a review, see Baddeley 2007). Working memory is also believed to influence attentional control: the capacity to focus, to divide, and to switch attention (Baddeley 1996). The dorsolateral prefrontal cortex in humans has been known to be involved in inhibitory control (Aron, Robbins, and Poldrack 2004) and working memory (Courtney et al. 1998; Owen et al. 2005). In the study by Brass et al. (2003), considering the fact that patients with damage to the lateral frontal region are more prone to spontaneous imitation, the authors hypothesized that a large load on working memory could increase susceptibility to motor contagion, specifically automatic imitation. To test their hypothesis, they examined how participant behavior in an imitation-inhibition task was affected by a secondary task that loaded working memory (Brass et al. 2000). As expected, a higher working memory load facilitated reaction times for congruent stimuli (i.e., facilitated automatic imitation).

5.2 Preventing Motor Contagion in Sports

Often in sports, coaches and teammates ask players to "avoid making the same mistakes [made by others]," or "repeat the same action [as others]." Is it possible to capitalize on motor contagion in order to facilitate these desired behaviors? Next, we summarize what the discussion in part 5.1 tells us about how one can prevent motor contagion before it occurs and how one can compensate for a motor contagion that has or will occur in sports.

5.2.1 Focusing on self Although there are few studies that have directly investigated the attenuation of motor contagion in sports, laboratory experiments that have simulated a sport-like scenario (or part of one) can give us important ideas for successful performance in sports. For example, according to Spengler et al. (2010), enhanced focus on one's own goals and intentions might help attenuate unwanted motor contagion. This result is supported by a study (Obhi et al. 2014) that reported that individuals with high narcissistic tendencies, who tend to display an excessive self-focus and reduced concern for others, demonstrate reduced automatic imitation in an imitation-inhibition task. There is some experimental evidence to show that this procedure can also work in sports. In their study with hammer throwers (discussed in part 2.3), Takeuchi et al. (2014) demonstrated that varsity hammer throwers mimic the predicted outcome of models they watch in a video. In the second part of their study, the authors investigated the effects of self-focus on the observed motor contagion. Hammer throwers were asked to say out loud either, "I'll do my best!" (in the self-focus condition), or "Make a mistake!" (in the non-self-focus condition), when they viewed the video of the model hammer thrower. The authors reported that the outcome mimicry observed in their first experiment was reduced only in the self-focus condition, similar to that reported in the Spengler et al. (2010) study. While this result has not been tested for other sports, it does suggest that athletes can attenuate motor contagion by focusing on self-centered ideas and on their own performance.

5.2.2 Manipulation of prior information and planning A recent study (Andrieux and Proteau 2016) shows that information about an observed individual's performance ability—that is, whether he or she is a "skilled" or "unskilled" performer—facilitates the effect of observational learning. The authors suggest that informing the observers of what they are about to see may enable them to select whether the goal of an observation is to imitate or to detect errors or weaknesses in the model's performance, and hence facilitate action-adaptation processes. In combination with the results from a previous study (Cross and Iacoboni 2014) that suggested that automatic imitation can be suppressed when the automatic response is likely to interfere with a task goal (see part 5.1), this result suggests that prior information (or maybe misinformation) about an observed individual's ability may be used to control motor contagions. Such a method may be most useful to reduce motor contagions in sports like baseball, darts, curling, and archery in which individuals perform immediately after observing the performance of other players (Gray and Beilock 2011).

The study with darts professionals (Ikegami and Ganesh 2014) shows the critical importance of instructions on PECs. PECs are caused by a difference between the predicted and observed action features of an observed individual. Predictions about actions of an observed individual are made with the knowledge of the observed individual's goal and intention (which may be inferred from a specific situation). The study shows that a lack of information about the goal (or misinformation about it) can help attenuate PECs. For sports like curling, darts, and golf, where the goal of an action is critically dependent on the results, athletes can avoid a goal belief (and hence PECs) by avoiding watching the game too intently.

5.2.3 Working memory manipulation It has been suggested that motor contagions are increased when working memory is occupied (van Leeuwen et al. 2009). Thus, training to increase the capacity of working memory may help attenuate motor contagion. An early model of motor learning hypothesizes that motor learning occurs in three distinct stages that differ in their cognitive demand (so-called cognitive, associative, and autonomous stages) (Fitts and Posner 1967). It has been hypothesized that working memory involvement diminishes with progression in motor learning (Fitts and Posner 1967), with the autonomous stage utilizing hardly any working memory at all. Therefore, it seems reasonable to assume that simply concentrating on improving one's skills in one's sport can increase resistance to motor contagion. On the other hand, in sports, some skills rely on the use of working memory. Furley and Memmert (2010) distinguish between sport skills that rely on working memory, such as tactical decision making in football and basketball, and skills that do not rely heavily on working memory (i.e., automated sensorimotor skills, such as controlling the ball or a basketball free shot). While an increase in working memory can benefit both these types of skills, obviously, developing skill can help prevent motor contagion only in the latter type.

5.3 Compensating for Motor Contagion in Sports

5.3.1 Planning for contagion Preventing motor contagion would obviously be the preferred choice for most athletes, but this may not always be feasible. Another option is to anticipate contagions and compensate for them during action planning. This, however, requires a good understanding of the various forms of contagions affecting the actions, intentions, and outcomes in any particular sport. Motor actions are generally agreed to involve distinct planning and execution phases (Ganesh and Burdet 2013). Roughly, planning refers to the process of selection of a particular action, while execution refers to the process of generating the planned action. Because of extensive training, whereas action selection can still be flexibly and promptly changed by the athletes, execution changes proceed slowly and are affected by so called motor-memory effects (Ganesh et al. 2010; Kodl, Ganesh, and Burdet 2011) or use-dependent motor processes (Diedrichsen et al. 2010; Classen et al. 1998). Therefore, when contagion is expected, or the presence of contagion is detected, it is important for the athlete to explicitly change her plan to compensate for the error in order to attenuate it. Plan changes may be particularly effective for single or team player sports that involve alternating or one-at-a-time performance by individuals, such as baseball, archery, darts, shooting, and field athletics.

5.3.2 Post-action correction Finally, in many sport settings, athletes do not know whether a positive or negative contagion would affect their actions during a competition. More importantly, the contagion may not be a simple effect on particular action features, but may present itself as multiple simultaneous and non-trivial changes in one's action features. This is particularly true for team sports involving multiple players performing at the same time, like soccer, basketball and hockey. Compensating for the contagion by means of plan changes may not be intuitive in such cases. Furthermore, athletes often suffer from pressure during competitions, which affects their effective working-memory functions. Performance pressure in particular is widely known to put a heavy load on the working memory of athletes (Beilock and Gray 2007), and as described previously, working-memory loads can modulate motor contagion (van Leeuwen et al. 2009). One suggestion for the attenuation of detected contagions was presented in a study (Gray and Beilock 2011) that showed that the effect of motor contagion is short-lived. In this study of baseball hitting, motor contagions affecting hit direction were eliminated after four pitches in the case of more-experienced hitters and after two pitches in the case of less-experienced hitters. These results suggest that if a negative contagion is detected, it would be advantageous for an athlete to take a break, such as a time-out, if possible.

6 Conclusion

In conclusion, obviously the optimal strategy for avoiding contagion in sports is to avoid watching the actions of other individuals before one's own performance. However, this is not an option in many scenarios. The next best option is to understand the various motor contagions and their causes and, with this knowledge, develop procedures to prevent, attenuate, and/or compensate for the contagions. In this regard, studies in sport science and psychology over the past decades have isolated and explained many types of motor contagions that lead to implicit imitation of the kinematics, goals, intentions, and outcomes of observed human actions. In this chapter we categorized these previous findings as action-imitative contagions or AICs, as they are caused by various features of an observed action. We then introduced a new type of motor contagion, which we call prediction error–induced contagions or PECs, that are also induced by observations of other's behaviors but differ fundamentally from AICs in terms of their cause and effect.

Based on the available data on PECs, we proposed a possible extension (figure 14.4) to the dual route model to incorporate and explain the AICs and PECs. However, being a relatively new discovery, many features of PEC are still not well understood. Further studies are required to investigate the full range of PECs affecting human behaviors, and how these are modulated by an observer's (athlete's) skill, visual perspective, and level of attention, and the observed agent's anatomy, skill, and style (as well as the observer's prior knowledge about these characteristics of the agent).

An interesting aspect of our extended model (figure 14.4) is that it shows how the discovery of PECs links motor contagion studies that, until now, have viewed contagion as automatic activation in already present sensorimotor associations, with motor neuroscience studies that have concentrated on understanding the development and adaptations of sensorimotor associations. The PEC link highlights that a collaborative approach by sport psychologists, motor neuroscientists, and social neuroscientists is required for a better understanding of the complete spectrum of motor contagions, and of how they develop and shape our behaviors in society and during sports.

Acknowledgments

This work was partially supported by JSPS KAKENHI Grant 16H05916 and 26120003 (to T. I.), 16K12999 and 26702025 (to H. N.), and 25282248 and 15K12623 (to G. G.). The authors declare no competing financial interests.

References

Abernethy, Bruce, and Khairi Zawi. 2007. "Pickup of Essential Kinematics Underpins Expert Perception of Movement Patterns." *Journal of Motor Behavior* 39 (5): 353–367. doi:10.3200/jmbr.39.5.353-368.

Aglioti, Salvatore M., Paola Cesari, Michela Romani, and Cosimo Urgesi. 2008. "Action Anticipation and Motor Resonance in Elite Basketball Players." *Nature Neuroscience* 11 (9): 1109–1116.

Andrieux, Mathieu, and Luc Proteau. 2016. "Observational Learning: Tell Beginners What They Are about to Watch and They Will Learn Better." *Frontiers in Psychology* 7 (January): 51. doi:10.3389/fpsyg.2016.00051.

Aron, Adam R., Trevor W. Robbins, and Russell A. Poldrack. 2004. "Inhibition and the Right Inferior Frontal Cortex." *Trends in Cognitive Science* 8 (4): 170–177. doi:10.1016/j.tics.2004.02.010.

Baddeley, Alan. 1996. "Exploring the Central Executive." *Quarterly Journal of Experimental Psychology A* 49 (1): 5–28.

Baddeley, Alan. 2007. *Working Memory, Thought, and Action*. Vol. 45. Oxford: Oxford University Press.

Beilock, Sian L., and Rob Gray. 2007. "Why Do Athletes Choke Under Pressure?" In *Handbook of Sport Psychology*, edited by Gershon Tenenbaum and Robert C. Eklund, 425–444. Hoboken, NJ: John Wiley and Sons.

Bekkering, Harold, Andreas Wohlschlager, and Merideth Gattis. 2000. "Imitation of Gestures in Children is Goal-Directed." *Quarterly Journal of Experimental Psychology A* 53 (1): 153–164.

Belot, Michèle, Vincent P. Crawford, and Cecilia Heyes. 2013. "Players of Matching Pennies Automatically Imitate Opponents' Gestures against Strong Incentives." *Proceedings of the National Academy of Sciences of the United States of America* 110 (8): 2763–2768. doi:10.1073/pnas.1209981110.

Bird, Geoffrey, Rachel Brindley, Jane Leighton, and Cecilia Heyes. 2007. "General Processes, Rather than 'Goals,' Explain Imitation Errors." *Journal of Experimental Psychology: Human Perception and Performance* 33 (5):1158–1169.

Blakemore, Sarah-Jayne, and Jean Decety. 2001. "From the Perception of Action to the Understanding of Intention." *Nature Reviews: Neuroscience* 2 (8): 561–567. doi:10.1038/35086023.

Blakemore, Sarah-Jayne, and Chris Frith. 2005. "The Role of Motor Contagion in the Prediction of Action." *Neuropsychologia* 43 (2): 260–267. doi:10.1016/j.neuropsychologia.2004.11.012.

Bock, Joel R., Akhilesh Maewal, and David A. Gough. 2012. "Hitting Is Contagious in Baseball: Evidence from Long Hitting Streaks." *PLoS ONE* 7 (12):e51367. doi:10.1371/journal.pone.0051367.

Boss, Martin, and Jens Kleinert. 2015. "Explaining Social Contagion in Sport Applying Heider's Balance Theory: First Experimental Results." *Psychology of Sport and Exercise* 16 (3): 160–169. http://dx.doi.org/10.1016/j.psychsport.2014.10.006.

Brass, Marcel, Harold Bekkering, and Wolfgang Prinz. 2001. "Movement Observation Affects Movement Execution in a Simple Response Task." *Acta Psychologica* 106 (1/2): 3–22.

Brass, Marcel, Harold Bekkering, Andreas Wohlschlager, and Wolfgang Prinz. 2000. "Compatibility between Observed and Executed Finger Movements: Comparing Symbolic, Spatial, and Imitative Cues." *Brain and Cognition* 44 (2): 124–143. doi:10.1006/brcg.2000.1225.

Brass, Marcel, Jan Derrfuss, Gabriele Matthes-von Cramon, and D. Yves von Cramon. 2003. "Imitative Response Tendencies in Patients with Frontal Brain Lesions." *Neuropsychology* 17 (2): 265–271.

Brass, Marcel, and Cecilia Heyes. 2005. "Imitation: Is Cognitive Neuroscience Solving the Correspondence Problem?" *Trends in Cognitive Sciences* 9 (10): 489–495. http://dx.doi.org/10.1016/j.tics.2005.08.007.

Brass, Marcel, Perrine Ruby, and Stephanie Spengler. 2009. "Inhibition of Imitative Behaviour and Social Cognition." *Philosophical Transactions of the Royal Society of London B: Biological Sciences* 364 (1528): 2359–2367. doi:10.1098/rstb.2009.0066.

Brass, Marcel, Ruth M. Schmitt, Stephanie Spengler, and György Gergely. 2007. "Investigating Action Understanding: Inferential Processes Versus Action Simulation." *Current Biology* 17 (24): 2117–2121. doi:S0960-9822(07)02343-3 [pii] 10.1016/j.cub.2007.11.057.

Brown, Liana E., Elizabeth T. Wilson, and Paul L. Gribble. 2009. "Repetitive Transcranial Magnetic Stimulation to the Primary Motor Cortex Interferes with Motor Learning by Observing." *Journal of Cognitive Neuroscience* 21 (5): 1013–1022. doi:10.1162/jocn.2009.21079.

Brown, Liana E., Elizabeth T. Wilson, Sukhvinder S. Obhi, and Paul L. Gribble. 2010. "Effect of Trial Order and Error Magnitude on Motor Learning by Observing." *Journal of Neurophysiology* 104 (3): 1409–1416. doi:10.1152/jn.01047.2009.

Byrne, Richard W., and Anne E. Russon. 1998. "Learning by Imitation: A Hierarchical Approach." *Behavioral and Brain Sciences* 21 (5): 667–684; discussion 684–721.

Castiello, Umberto. 1999. "Mechanisms of Selection for the Control of Hand Action." *Trends in Cognitive Sciences* 3 (7): 264–271.

Castiello, Umberto. 2003. "Understanding Other People's Actions: Intention and Attention." *Journal of Experimental Psychology: Human Perception and Performance* 29 (2): 416–430.

Catmur, Caroline, Vincent Walsh, and Cecilia Heyes. 2007. "Sensorimotor Learning Configures the Human Mirror System." *Current Biology* 17 (17): 1527–1531. doi:S0960-9822(07)01782-4 [pii] 10.1016/j.cub.2007.08.006.

Charny, E. Joseph. 1966. "Psychosomatic Manifestations of Rapport in Psychotherapy." *Psychosomatic Medicine* 28 (4): 305–315.

Chartrand, Tanya L., and John A. Bargh. 1999. "The Chameleon Effect: The Perception-Behavior Link and Social Interaction." *Journal of Personality and Social Psychology* 76 (6): 893–910.

Classen, Joseph, Joachim Liepert, Steven P. Wise, Mark Hallett, and Leonardo G. Cohen. 1998. "Rapid Plasticity of Human Cortical Movement Representation Induced by Practice." *Journal of Neurophysiology* 79 (2): 1117–1123.

Condon, William S., and William D. Ogston. 1967. "A Segmentation of Behavior." *Journal of Psychiatric Research* 5 (3): 221–235.

Cook, Richard, Geoffrey Bird, Caroline Catmur, Clare Press, and Cecilia Heyes. 2014. "Mirror Neurons: From Origin to Function." *Behavioral and Brain Sciences* 37 (2): 177–192. doi:10.1017/S0140525X13000903.

Cook, Richard, Geoffrey Bird, Gabriele Lunser, Steffen Huck, and Cecilia Heyes. 2012. "Automatic Imitation in a Strategic Context: Players of Rock-Paper-Scissors Imitate Opponents' Gestures." *Proceedings of the Royal Society B: Biological Sciences* 279 (1729): 780–786. doi:10.1098/rspb.2011.1024.

Courtney, Susan M., Laurent Petit, James V. Haxby, and Leslie G. Ungerleider. 1998. "The Role of Prefrontal Cortex in Working Memory: Examining the Contents of Consciousness." *Philosophical Transactions of the Royal Society of London B: Biological Sciences* 353 (1377): 1819–1828.

Craighero, Laila, Luciano Fadiga, Carlo A. Umiltà, and Giacomo Rizzolatti. 1996. "Evidence for Visuomotor Priming Effect." *NeuroReport* 8 (1): 347–349.

Cross, Katy A., and Marco Iacoboni. 2014. "To Imitate or Not: Avoiding Imitation Involves Preparatory Inhibition of Motor Resonance." *NeuroImage* 91 (May): 228–236. doi:10.1016/j.neuroimage.2014.01.027.

Cross, Katy A., Salvatore Torrisi, Elizabeth A. Reynolds Losin, and Marco Iacoboni. 2013. "Controlling Automatic Imitative Tendencies: Interactions between Mirror Neuron and Cognitive Control Systems." *NeuroImage* 83:493–504. doi:http://dx.doi.org/10.1016/j.neuroimage.2013.06.060.

De Maeght, Sara, and Wolfgang Prinz. 2004. "Action Induction through Action Observation." *Psychological Research* 68 (2/3): 97–114. doi:10.1007/s00426-003-0148-3.

Diedrichsen, Jörn, Olivier White, Darren Newman, and Niall Lally. 2010. "Use-Dependent and Error-Based Learning of Motor Behaviors." *Journal of Neuroscience* 30 (15): 5159–5166. doi:30/15/5159[pii]10.1523/JNEUROSCI.5406-09.2010.

Eaves, Daniel L., Martine Turgeon, and Stefan Vogt. 2012. "Automatic Imitation in Rhythmical Actions: Kinematic Fidelity and the Effects of Compatibility, Delay, and Visual Monitoring." *PLoS ONE* 7 (10):e46728. doi:10.1371/journal.pone.0046728.

Edwards, Martin G., Glyn W. Humphreys, and Umberto Castiello. 2003. "Motor Facilitation Following Action Observation: A Behavioural Study in Prehensile Action." *Brain and Cognition* 53 (3): 495–502.

Fitts, Paul M., and Michael I. Posner. 1967. *Human Performance*. Pacific Grove, CA: Brooks/Cole.

Fitts, Paul M., and Charles M. Seeger. 1953. "S-R Compatibility: Spatial Characteristics of Stimulus and Response Codes." *Journal of Experimental Psychology* 46 (3): 199–210.

Furley, Philip Alexander, and Daniel Memmert. 2010. "The Role of Working Memory in Sport." *International Review of Sport and Exercise Psychology* 3 (2): 171–194. doi:10.1080/1750984X.2010.526238.

Ganesh, Gowrishankar, and Etienne Burdet. 2013. "Motor Planning Explains Human Behaviour in Tasks with Multiple Solutions." *Robotics and Autonomous Systems* 61 (4): 362–368.

Ganesh, Gowrishankar, Masahiko Haruno, Mitsuo Kawato, and Etienne Burdet. 2010. "Motor Memory and Local Minimization of Error and Effort, Not Global Optimization, Determine Motor Behavior." *Journal of Neurophysiology* 104 (1): 382–390. doi:jn.01058.2009[pii]10.1152/jn.01058.2009.

Ganesh, Gowrishankar, and Tsuyoshi Ikegami. 2016. "Beyond Watching: Action Understanding by Humans and Implications for Motion Planning by Interacting Robots." In *Dance Notations and Robot Motion*, edited by Jean-Paul Laumond and Naoko Abe, 139–167. Springer Tracts in Advanced Robotics 111. New York: Springer.

Gleissner, Brigitte, Andrew N. Meltzoff, and Harold Bekkering. 2000. "Children's Coding of Human Action: Cognitive Factors Influencing Imitation in 3-Year-Olds." *Developmental Science* 3 (4): 405–414. doi:10.1111/1467-7687.00135.

Gray, Rob. 2002. "Behavior of College Baseball Players in a Virtual Batting Task." *Journal of Experimental Psychology: Human Perception and Performance* 28 (5): 1131–1148.

Gray, Rob, and Sian L. Beilock. 2011. "Hitting Is Contagious: Experience and Action Induction." *Journal of Experimental Psychology: Applied* 17 (1): 49–59. doi:10.1037/a0022846.

Heyes, Cecilia. 2011. "Automatic Imitation." *Psychological Bulletin* 137 (3): 463–483. doi:10.1037/a0022288.

Heyes, Cecilia. 2013. "Imitation: Associative and Context Dependent." In *Action Science: Foundations of an Emerging Discipline*, edited by Wolfgang Prinz, Miriam Beisert, and Arvid Herwig, 309. Cambridge, MA: MIT Press.

Heyes, Cecilia, Geoffery Bird, Helen Johnson, and Patrick Haggard. 2005. "Experience Modulates Automatic Imitation." *Brain Research: Cognitive Brain Research* 22 (2): 233–240. doi:10.1016/j.cogbrainres.2004.09.009.

Huys, Raoul, Rouwen Canal-Bruland, Norbert Hagemann, Peter J. Beek, Nicholas J. Smeeton, and A. Mark Williams. 2009. "Global Information Pickup Underpins Anticipation of Tennis Shot Direction." *Journal of Motor Behavior* 41 (2): 158–171. doi:10.3200/jmbr.41.2.158-171.

Ikegami, Tsuyoshi, and Gowrishankar Ganesh. 2014. "Watching Novice Action Degrades Expert Motor Performance: Causation between Action Production and Outcome Prediction of Observed Actions by Humans." *Scientific Reports* 4 (November): 6989. doi:10.1038/srep06989.

Ikegami, Tsuyoshi, and Gowrishankar Ganesh. 2017. "Shared Mechanisms in the Estimation of Self-generated Actions and the Prediction of Other's Actions by Humans." *eNeuro* 4 (6). doi:10.1523/ENEURO.0341-17.2017.

Jackson, Robin C., and Peter Mogan. 2007. "Advance Visual Information, Awareness, and Anticipation Skill." *Journal of Motor Behavior* 39 (5): 341–351. doi:10.3200/jmbr.39.5.341-352.

Kawato, Mitsuo 1999. "Internal Models for Motor Control and Trajectory Planning." *Current Opinion in Neurobiology* 9 (6): 718–727. doi:S0959-4388(99)00028-8 [pii].

Kendon, Adam. 1970. "Movement Coordination in Social Interaction: Some Examples Described." *Acta Psychologica* 32 (2): 100–125.

Kilner, James M., Yves Paulignan, and Sarah-Jayne Blakemore. 2003. "An Interference Effect of Observed Biological Movement on Action." *Current Biology* 13 (6): 522–525.

Kodl, Jindrich, Gowrishankar Ganesh, and Etienne Burdet. 2011. "The CNS Stochastically Selects Motor Plan Utilizing Extrinsic and Intrinsic Representations." *PLoS ONE* 6 (9):e24229. doi:10.1371/journal.pone.0024229 PONE-D-11-03462 [pii].

Lafrance, Marianne, and Maida Broadbent. 1976. "Group Rapport: Posture Sharing as a Nonverbal Indicator." *Group and Organization Studies* 1 (3): 328–333.

Leighton, Jane, and Cecilia Heyes. 2010. "Hand to Mouth: Automatic Imitation across Effector Systems." *Journal of Experimental Psychology: Human Perception and Performance* 36 (5): 1174–1183. doi:10.1037/a0019953.

Mattar, Andrew A., and Paul L. Gribble. 2005. "Motor Learning by Observing." *Neuron* 46 (1): 153–160. doi:10.1016/j.neuron.2005.02.009.

McGregor, Heather R., Joshua G. Cashaback, and Paul L. Gribble. 2016. "Functional Plasticity in Somatosensory Cortex Supports Motor Learning by Observing." *Current Biology* 26 (7): 921–927. doi:10.1016/j.cub.2016.01.064.

Meltzoff, Andrew N., and M. Keith Moore. 1977. "Imitation of Facial and Manual Gestures by Human Neonates." *Science* 198 (4312): 75–78. doi:10.1126/science.198.4312.75.

Nedelko, Violetta, Thomas Hassa, Farsin Hamzei, Mircea Ariel Schoenfeld, and Christian Dettmers. 2012. "Action Imagery Combined with Action Observation Activates More Corticomotor Regions than Action Observation Alone." *Journal of Neurological Physical Therapy* 36 (4): 182–188. doi:10.1097/NPT.0b013e318272cad1.

Obhi, Sukhvinder S., Jeremy Hogeveen, Miranda Giacomin, and Christian H. Jordan. 2014. "Automatic Imitation Is Reduced in Narcissists." *Journal of Experimental Psychology: Human Perception and Performance* 40 (3): 920–928. doi:10.1037/a0034056.

Owen, Adrian M., Kathryn M. McMillan, Angela R. Laird, and Ed Bullmore. 2005. "N-Back Working Memory Paradigm: A Meta-analysis of Normative Functional Neuroimaging Studies." *Human Brain Mapping* 25 (1): 46–59. doi:10.1002/hbm.20131.

Piaget, Jean. 1954. *The Construction of Reality in the Child.* Translated by Margaret Cook. New York: Basic Books. doi:10.1037/11168-000.

Prinz, W. 1997. "Perception and Action Planning." *European Journal of Cognitive Psychology* 9:129–154.

Rizzolatti, Giacomo, and Laila Craighero. 2004. "The Mirror-Neuron System." *Annual Review of Neuroscience* 27:169–192. doi:10.1146/annurev.neuro.27.070203.144230.

Rizzolatti, Giacomo, and Corrado Sinigaglia. 2010. "The Functional Role of the Parieto-frontal Mirror Circuit: Interpretations and Misinterpretations." *Nature Reviews: Neuroscience* 11 (4): 264–274. doi:nrn2805[pii]10.1038/nrn2805.

Schaal, Stefan. 1999. "Is Imitation Learning the Route to Humanoid Robots?" *Trends in Cognitive Sciences* 3 (6): 233–242.

Schaal, Stefan, Auke Ijspeert, and Aude Billard. 2003. "Computational Approaches to Motor Learning by Imitation." *Philosophical Transactions of the Royal Society of London B: Biological Sciences* 358 (1431): 537–547. doi:10.1098/rstb.2002.1258.

Scheidt, Robert A., David J. Reinkensmeyer, Michael A. Conditt, W. Zev Rymer, and Ferdinando A. Mussa-Ivaldi. 2000. "Persistence of Motor Adaptation during Constrained, Multi-Joint, Arm Movements." *Journal of Neurophysiology* 84 (2): 853–862.

Schütz-Bosbach, Simone, Alessio Avenanti, Salvatore Maria Aglioti, and Patrick Haggard. 2009. "Don't Do It! Cortical Inhibition and Self-Attribution during Action Observation." *Journal of Cognitive Neuroscience* 21 (6): 1215–1227. doi:10.1162/jocn.2009.21068.

Shadmehr, Reza, and Ferdinando A. Mussa-Ivaldi. 1994. "Adaptive Representation of Dynamics during Learning of a Motor Task." *Journal of Neuroscience* 14 (5 Pt 2): 3208–3224.

Shadmehr, Reza, and Steven P. Wise. 2005. *The Computational Neurobiology of Reaching and Pointing.* Cambridge, MA: MIT Press.

Shapiro, Lawrence. 2010. *Embodied Cognition.* London: Routledge/Taylor and Francis.

Shapiro, Lawrence A. 2013. "Dynamics and Cognition." *Minds and Machines* 23 (3): 353–375. doi:10.1007/s11023-012-9290-2.

Simon, J. Richard. 1969. "Reactions toward the Source of Stimulation." *Journal of Experimental Psychology* 81 (1): 174–176.

Spengler, Stephanie, Marcel Brass, Simone Kuhn, and Simone Schütz-Bosbach. 2010. "Minimizing Motor Mimicry by Myself: Self-Focus Enhances Online Action-Control Mechanisms during Motor Contagion." *Conscious and Cognition* 19 (1): 98–106. doi:10.1016/j.concog.2009.12.014.

Spengler, Stephanie, D. Yves von Cramon, and Marcel Brass. 2009. "Control of Shared Representations Relies on Key Processes Involved in Mental State Attribution." *Human Brain Mapping* 30 (11): 3704–3718. doi:10.1002/hbm.20800.

Stahl, Aimee E., and Lisa Feigenson. 2015. "Cognitive Development: Observing the Unexpected Enhances Infants' Learning and Exploration." *Science* 348 (6230): 91–94. doi:10.1126/science.aaa3799.

Stürmer, Birgit, Gisa Aschersleben, and Wolfgang Prinz. 2000. "Correspondence Effects with Manual Gestures and Postures: A Study of Imitation." *Journal of Experimental Psychology: Human Perception and Performance* 26 (6): 1746–1759.

Takeuchi, Tatsuya, Hiroki Nakamoto, Sachi Ikudome, and Shiro Mori. 2014. "Cause and Solution of Motor Contagion in Hammer Throwing." Paper presented at The 65th Conference of the Japanese Society of Physical Education, Health and Sports Sciences, Iwate University, Japan, August 27.

Totterdell, Peter. 2000. "Catching Moods and Hitting Runs: Mood Linkage and Subjective Performance in Professional Sport Teams." *Journal of Applied Psychology* 85 (6): 848–859.

Tseng, Ya-weng, Jörn Diedrichsen, John W. Krakauer, Reza Shadmehr, and Amy J. Bastian. 2007. "Sensory Prediction Errors Drive Cerebellum-Dependent Adaptation of Reaching." *Journal of Neurophysiology* 98 (1): 54–62. doi:00266.2007 [pii] 10.1152/jn.00266.2007.

van Baaren, Rick B., Rob W. Holland, Kerry Kawakami, and Ad van Knippenberg. 2004. "Mimicry and Prosocial Behavior." *Psychological Science* 15 (1): 71–74.

van Leeuwen, Matthijs L., Rick B. van Baaren, Douglas Martin, Ap Dijksterhuis, and Harold Bekkering. 2009. "Executive Functioning and Imitation: Increasing Working Memory Load Facilitates Behavioural Imitation." *Neuropsychologia* 47 (14): 3265–3270. http://dx.doi.org/10.1016/j.neuropsychologia.2009.06.005.

Vu, Kim-Phoung, and Robert W. Proctor. 2004. "Mixing Compatible and Incompatible Mappings: Elimination, Reduction, and Enhancement of Spatial Compatibility Effects." *Quarterly Journal of Experimental Psychology A: Human Experimental Psychology* 57 (3): 539–556. doi:10.1080/02724980343000387.

Wanda, Paul A., Gang Li, and Kurt A. Thoroughman. 2013. "State Dependence of Adaptation of Force Output Following Movement Observation." *Journal of Neurophysiology* 110 (5): 1246–1256. doi:10.1152/jn.00353.2012.

Whiten, Andrew, Nicola McGuigan, Sarah Marshall-Pescini, and Lydia M. Hopper. 2009. "Emulation, Imitation, Over-Imitation and the Scope of Culture for Child and Chimpanzee." *Philosophical Transactions of the Royal Society of London B: Biological Sciences* 364 (1528): 2417–2428. doi:10.1098/rstb.2009.0069.

Wohlschlager, Andreas, Meredith Gattis, and Harold Bekkering. 2003. "Action Generation and Action Perception in Imitation: An Instance of the Ideomotor Principle." *Philosophical Transactions of the Royal Society of London B: Biological Sciences* 358 (1431): 501–515. doi:10.1098/rstb.2002.1257.

Wolpert, Daniel M., Kenji Doya, and Mitsuo Kawato. 2003. "A Unifying Computational Framework for Motor Control and Social Interaction." *Philosophical Transactions of the Royal Society of London B: Biological Sciences* 358 (1431): 593–602. doi:10.1098/rstb.2002.1238.

Wolpert, Daniel M., Zoubin Ghahramani, and Michael I. Jordan. 1995. "An Internal Model for Sensorimotor Integration." *Science* 269 (5232): 1880–1882.

Wolpert, Daniel M., and Mitsuo Kawato. 1998. "Multiple Paired Forward and Inverse Models for Motor Control." *Neural Networks* 11 (7/8): 1317–1329. doi:S0893-6080(98)00066-5 [pii].

Zorzi, Marco, and Carlo Umiltà. 1995. "A Computational Model of the Simon Effect." *Psychological Research* 58 (3): 193–205.

15 Planning Together and Playing Together

Lincoln J. Colling

1 Introduction

Sonny Bill Williams, one of the most captivating players in world rugby, has become known as a proponent of the offload, a quick pass executed after being tackled by an opponent but before being brought to ground. Performing an offload is often made more impressive when the player receiving the ball is outside of the passer's direct field of view. Furthermore, successfully performing this maneuver on the rugby field requires that it be done at high speed and while trying to retain possession of the ball. This feat of coordination requires the passer to know, or at least anticipate, exactly where his teammate will be, and when they will be there. Only if he and his teammates coordinate their actions precisely will they be successful, and any failure might result in an interception by the opposition and his team conceding points.

The skillful coordination exhibited by Sonny Bill Williams and his teammates is an example of what philosophers and psychologists have referred to as *joint action*. One definition of joint action, provided by Sebanz, Bekkering, and Knoblich (2006), suggests that joint action is "any form of social interaction whereby two or more individuals coordinate their actions in space and time to bring about some change in the environment." Butterfill (2016) offers a simpler and somewhat broader definition: "A joint action is an event grounded by two or more agents' actions." It is the mechanisms that underlie joint action, particularly of the kind found on the sport field, that are the target of this chapter.

Philosophical interest in joint action has tended to focus rather narrowly on notions of *collective intentionality* and on using these notions to differentiate joint actions from seemingly similar acts that are not joint actions. For example, Searle (1990) uses the example of a group of people converging on a single point in a park. This behavior could either be a joint action or a collection of individual behaviors. What differentiates the two are the intentions that cause the behavior. If the people each have the intention,

"It is raining and I am running to shelter," then it would be a collection of individual behaviors. However, it might be possible that each person has a different intention, a collective intention, of the form, "We intend to get ready to perform a ballet by means of *me* running to the gazebo" (Searle 1990). Similarly, in understanding team coordination, the sport psychology literature has focused on issues such as communication in teams and social factors that might influence team cohesion (e.g., see Eccles and Tenenbaum 2004). Or they have taken an information-processing approach rather than examining details of joint action planning (e.g., Reimer, Park, and Hinsz 2006).

2 An Embodied Account of Joint Action

Work by philosophers examining collective intentionality and joint action has traditionally been done by analyzing the propositional content of the intentions thought to ground joint action (e.g., Bratman 1993; Searle 1990). The approach that we adopt is different, however. Rather than analyzing propositions, we attempt to explain skillful joint action with an approach that is firmly grounded in the tradition of *embodied cognition*. Embodied cognition is a term that has come to mean many things (e.g., Wilson 2002), and, therefore, it is reasonable to ask, In what sense is ours an embodied approach?

Our approach fits within an approach to embodiment that emphasizes the close links between perception and action. It draws inspiration from theoretical concepts found in the common coding approach to perception and action (Prinz 1997; Hommel 2009), mirror systems theory (Rizzolatti and Craighero 2004), computational accounts of motor control based on internal models (Wolpert 1997), and the emulation theory of representation (Grush 1997, 2004).

It is an embodied approach in at least three senses, according to Wilson's (2002) criteria. First, unlike accounts based on collective intentionality, our account is aimed at explaining joint action by examining the mechanisms that *guide action*. Second, rather than propositional, symbolic, or amodal representations found in classical cognitive science approaches—those in the intellectual tradition of, for example, Newell and Simon (1997), Fodor and Pylyshyn (1988), and Block (2009)—our approach favors body-based or sensorimotor representations, particularly as outlined by Grush (1997, 2004). Third, our approach stresses that *cognition is time-pressured*, and, therefore, we aim to explain how joint action can happen rapidly and without conscious deliberation.

Coordination on the sport field thus provides the ideal context for answering our question. As our opening example illustrates, to be successful on the sport field, a player needs to anticipate how their teammate will move in response to opposition players and the changing environment, and they must be able to adjust their actions appropriately. To do this, she will have to consider not only her own goals and actions, but also the goals and actions of her teammates and how these might change in response to changes on the field. This cannot be done through conscious deliberation or involve negotiation of each player's role through sharing of knowledge and beliefs or through verbal communication. These adjustments need to be made too rapidly. Therefore, to understand how people adjust their plans in response to the goals, plans, and actions of others, we need to identify mechanisms that do not rely on conscious deliberation, mechanisms that allow people to achieve rapid and effortless skillful coordination.

What are these mechanisms, and what is the evidence for their existence? We argue that, to achieve the kind of coordination evident on the sport field, people sometimes include others in their planning by representing others' goals and actions in much the same way as they represent their own goals and actions. These shared representations, which we call *co-representations*, are actually plans for the other's part of a joint action. We will show, with evidence from the joint task literature, that in simple joint tasks we represent the tasks of others in the same way that we represent our own tasks and plan the actions of others in much the same way as we plan our own actions.

In more complex tasks, however, it may be the case that we actually engage in collective planning, which involves representing tasks and planning actions as collective actions that are to be performed by two agents, just as we might plan bimanual actions as actions to be performed by two hands. Finally, we argue that planning others' actions allows us to co-opt the mechanisms that we use for controlling and predicting our own actions to generate predictions about the unfolding action dynamics of others in real time, permitting us, in ideal circumstances, to align our actions with minimal delays.

Talk of planning may initially seem misplaced if we conceive of planning as the conscious deliberative processes that shape our actions. While this notion of planning is common in the philosophical literature (e.g., Bratman 1987), there is a broader notion of planning found in the psychological and neuroscience literature, particularly the literature on motor control. Here the term planning is used to include all processes involved in performance and monitoring of action that compute means from ends (e.g., Pacherie 2008; Grafton and Hamilton 2007), and these processes do not all involve conscious deliberation (Prinz 1997; Pacherie 2006; Jeannerod 1994). This is the notion of planning on which we rely.

3 Planning a Teammate's Task

Planning is sometimes guided by representations that link events to actions. Suppose, for example, that I intend to take a mark in Australian Rules football. The role of this intention is to predispose me to act in a certain way when particular conditions arise—in this example, it would be to jump up with outstretched arms when the ball approaches. We call this link between events—the ball approaching and the action of jumping—a *task representation.*

Task representations are links between events and actions that serve to trigger preparation for an action in response to the occurrence of an event.[1] When taking a mark in an area of open field, the actions of my teammates might be of no concern to me, and what they plan to do might have no bearing on my actions. However, in other situations, my teammate and I might each have a different role to play. One example might be when my teammate and I are standing side by side and we intend to take possession of a ball that has been kicked by another player. I, being the taller player, would ordinarily jump up to take a mark when the ball is sailing high through the air. My shorter teammate, however, might be given the responsibility of retrieving the ball if it approaches by rolling along the grass. Here, I might have a task representation that links a high ball to a jump, such that when a high ball approaches it triggers preparation for my jump without deliberation. Similarly, my teammate might have a task representation that links a low ball to crouching, such that when a low ball approaches it triggers preparation for crouching.

These task representations may be sufficient when my teammate and I are standing some distance from each other, so that any event could be acted on by only one of us and not the other; however, when standing side by side, it might be useful for me to plan my actions around my teammate's and for my teammate to plan his action around mine, thus decreasing the likelihood of delays or interference. In order for us to plan our actions *around* each other, it would be useful for each of us to have a task co-representation of each other's task. A task co-representation is just a task representation that each agent shares.

Thus, if I have a task representation that links a high ball to jumping and my teammate similarly has a task representation that links a high ball to jumping, then *we* can be said to have a task co-representation linking a high ball to jumping. If we further have a task co-representation that links a low ball to crouching, then *we* can be said to have a task co-representation of each other's task. But what evidence is there for the existence of task co-representation?

4 Evidence for Task Co-representation

One line of evidence that supports the existence of task co-representation comes from the joint task literature. The basic logic of the paradigms used in the joint task literature is to compare how people respond to events that are linked to only their own action with how people respond to events that may be linked to their and their partner's actions. This comparison can be revealing, because if you represent only your own task, then, all other things being equal, what your partner's task is should have no influence on how you respond to events. For example, the nature of your partner's task should not have an influence on the speed and accuracy of your responses.

However, if your partner's task does have an influence, this would suggest that you are in some sense representing your partner's task. One example of a paradigm that employs this logic is the joint flanker task developed by Atmaca, Sebanz, and Knoblich (2011). The traditional flanker task involves a participant responding to target stimuli presented centrally (with different target types requiring different responses) while ignoring distractor stimuli flanking the central stimulus. The key finding is that when the central stimulus and the flanking stimuli are from categories that require different responses—for example, the central stimulus might come from a category that requires a left button press and the flanking stimuli might come from a category that requires a right button press—responses are slower relative to the case where the flankers and target come from categories that require the same response. This is because when the target and distractors signal different responses, each stimulus activates an action. One of these actions—the action triggered by the distractor stimuli—must then be suppressed, and this results in response conflict (see Eriksen 1995).

In the *joint flanker task*, two participants respond to letters flanked by distractors. Each participant responds to a specific letter with a key press, and the two participants are assigned different letters. Sometimes, a participant encounters an event in which their assigned letter is surrounded by distractors that are irrelevant to their partner's task: this is an event that is linked to only that participant's action. But sometimes the participant will encounter an event in which their letter is surrounded by distractors made up from their partner's target letter: this is an event that is linked to not only that participant's action but also to their partner's action.

Atmaca, Sebanz, and Knoblich (2011) found that when this occurred, participant responses were slower relative to the case where the event was linked to their action only. This suggests that the participant's responses were influenced by what their partner's task was, and this is taken as evidence that they represent their partner's task—that is, that the participant and partner have a task co-representation of the joint task. Sebanz, Knoblich, and Prinz (2005) provide further evidence using the same logic but with a different paradigm, the *joint Simon task*.

There might, however, be an alternative explanation for the effect found in the joint flanker task. For example, it might be that the presence of an additional person somehow changes the task in a way that gives rise to the effect but without the participant representing their coactor's task. To examine this possibility, Atmaca, Sebanz, and Knoblich (2011) ran a further condition in which participants were led to believe that, although their coactor appeared to respond to specific targets on the screen, their coactor's movements were not under intentional control and were instead controlled by electromagnets placed under their fingers.

If it is really the case that the effect is driven by the participant representing their coactor's task, then this condition should abolish the effect, because the coactor would no longer have a task representation that the participant could share. That is, task co-representation would, by definition, be absent when the other's movements are externally controlled. Importantly, everything else was kept identical, with the only difference being that participants believed that their coactor's actions were unintentional. The results showed that this belief was able to extinguish the effect, suggesting that the effect is driven by task representations rather than other differences between conditions.

Another paradigm that provides evidence that people sometimes have task representations about other's tasks is the *joint Navon task* (Böckler, Knoblich, and Sebanz 2012). In the joint Navon task, two participants are asked to respond to a stimulus that is composed of a local and a global dimension. For example, the stimulus might be several small "S"s (local dimension) arranged in the shape of a single large "F" (global dimension). Participants are asked to press a response key when they see a specified letter in a given dimension. In the standard Navon task, the finding is that when participants are asked to respond to one dimension (e.g., the global dimension) by, for example, pressing the left button in response to one letter and pressing the right button in response to another letter, their responses are slower when the ignored dimension (in this example, the local dimension) signals a response that is incongruent with the response signaled by the relevant dimension. In the joint Navon task, each participant is assigned different letters (to rule out response conflict), but sometimes both participants attend, and respond, to the same feature (e.g., the global feature) while at other times they attend to different features (i.e., one to the local feature and the other to the global feature). If each participant represents only their own task, then whether the other's task concerns the same or different dimension should not matter.

However, the findings of Böckler, Knoblich, and Sebanz (2012) show that this does matter. Participants were slower to respond to their targets when they and their coactor were attending to different dimensions. Böckler, Knoblich, and Sebanz (2012) suggest that this is a result of attentional conflict. In effect, representing the other's task—responding to events by attending to the other dimension—causes a conflict between the participant's required focus of attention and his or her partner's focus.

But might it be the case that the difference in response times between the same focus and different focus conditions is merely the result of the task instructions increasing the salience of the other dimension? To rule out this possibility, Böckler, Knoblich, and Sebanz (2012) had participants perform the task alone. However, in this individual version, participants saw the same instructions as the joint version, but they were told that they would be performing the task alone and that the instructions were just a carry-over from a previous experiment in which participants acted in pairs. In this follow-up experiment, the nature of instructions—to adopt the same or different attentional focus—had no influence on task performance, suggesting that it was the presence of a coacting partner that made the difference, and not just the instructions.

One final source of evidence supporting the existence of task co-representation comes from measuring the brain activity of participants when they encounter an event to which they do not themselves have to respond, but to which their coactor may or may not have to respond. If participants did not represent the other's task, then they would be unlikely to know how the other would act, and it would certainly not be possible to plan the other's actions. But there is evidence that participants do plan the other's action. In an fMRI study, Ramnani and Miall (2003) found that regions related to planning one's own actions were also active in response to events that required a response from a hidden partner, but, consistent with Atmaca, Sebanz, and Knoblich (2011), only when the hidden partner was an intentional agent. Since it would be a mistake to actually perform the planned action, it might also be possible to observe markers of response inhibition when encountering an event to which another must respond.

Research examining electrophysiological markers of response inhibition do show greater response inhibition when encountering events requiring responses from another person relative to events to which no one should respond (Tsai et al. 2008; Sebanz et al. 2006).

5 Alternative Explanations in the Joint Task Literature

While the joint task literature has usually been used to support the existence of task co-representation, at least two criticisms of this interpretation have been raised. They are, first, that at least some of the effects from the joint task literature can be explained by *turn confusion*—that is, participant's being unsure whose turn it is to act (e.g., Wenke et al. 2011). And, second, that the effects are not social in nature, but are instead driven by nonsocial factors such as the mere presence of another individual—or any other salient object—changing the way the participant represents her own responses (e.g.,

Dolk et al. 2013; Dolk et al. 2014). We will deal with each of these briefly in turn and show that these criticisms are valid for only some paradigms and some situations, and they don't undermine our claim about the existence of task co-representation.

Since both criticisms have focused primarily on the joint Simon task, we begin by first outlining this paradigm. In the Simon task (see Simon 1969), a participant is asked to make a response to one feature of a stimulus (e.g., the color of an arrow) while ignoring an irrelevant spatial dimension of the stimulus (e.g., the direction in which the arrow is pointing). The typical finding is that when participants are asked to respond to the target feature while ignoring the irrelevant spatial feature, the spatial feature facilitates the response when it is spatially compatible with the response. For instance, a response with a right button press would be facilitated by a right pointing arrow. Importantly, this facilitation effect is not found if the responses do not have a spatial dimension. For instance, if participants perform a go/no-go task, in which they respond to one target stimulus with a single button while withholding their responses to other stimuli, the irrelevant spatial dimension of the stimulus has no effect (Kornblum, Hasbroucq, and Osman 1990).

In the joint version of the Simon task, the standard two-choice task is distributed across two individuals, and each responds to one color while ignoring their partner's target color. As each participant responds to only one color, while withholding their response to the other color, each participant performs a go/no-go task. However, Sebanz, Knoblich, and Prinz (2003) found that, when individuals performed this go/no-go task as part of a pair, the results mirrored the individual two-choice task, with a participant's response being facilitated when the spatial dimension of the stimulus overlapped with the spatial location of the response button. The explanation that was first suggested by Sebanz, Knoblich, and Prinz (2003) is that participants represent not only their own task but also the task of their coactor. By representing the task as a task requiring both a left and a right response (although now split between two people), each participants' nonspatial response took on a spatial dimension. Thus, the finding could be taken as evidence for co-representation.

Contrary to this explanation, Wenke et al. (2011) have argued that, during the joint Simon task, the spatial dimension of the stimulus can also be used as a cue to indicate whose turn it is to respond. During compatible trials, the arrow, or other spatial stimulus, is overlapping with the spatial location of the actor whose turn it is to respond. Liepelt et al. (2010) found that the size of the joint Simon effect was modulated by the nature of the previous trial, so that when the previous trial was compatible and the current trial was also compatible, then the magnitude of the effect increased. This suggests the participants were learning to use the spatial cue as a turn cue even though in the long run the spatial cue was not informative.

While turn confusion may be able to account for at least some of the findings in the joint task literature—and Wenke et al. (2011) also claim that turn confusion rather than task co-representation may be the cause of several null findings in other joint task paradigms—turn confusion cannot explain all the joint task findings. In particular, the findings from the joint Navon task (Böckler, Knoblich, and Sebanz 2012) are difficult to reconcile with an account based on turn confusion. In the joint Navon task, participants are required to have either a global or a local focus of attention, and joint task effects are seen when the coactor holds a different focus of attention. Here the effect results from the presence of the coactor's target letter in the other stimulus dimension—for example, the global dimension when the participant was responding to the local dimension. Therefore, before any turn confusion could occur, participants would first need to shift their focus of attention to this other dimension. That is, any turn confusion would be able to arise only after the participant had already implemented the confederate's task rule, and thus task co-representation, rather than turn confusion, provides a more satisfactory account of these results.

While Wenke et al. (2011) has argued for an alternative, but still social, explanation for some joint task effects, others have suggested that the effect could be nonsocial in nature. For instance, Guagnano, Rusconi, and Umiltà (2010) have suggested that spatial proximity to another person is the primary driver of some of the effects seen in the joint task literature. Guagnano, Rusconi, and Umiltà (2010) found that similar effects could be observed when participants merely sat next to a confederate who was performing a different task, and that these effects disappeared as the confederate moved out of peripersonal space. They argued that the presence of another individual changed the way in which participants represented their own actions and that this, rather than task co-representation, was responsible for the effects.

Similarly, Dolk et al. (2013) have argued that joint task effects are not social at all—that is, they do not require the presence of another person—and that similar effects can be produced by placing any salient stimulus in close proximity to the participant. For example, Dolk et al. (2013, experiment 1) had participants perform a go/no-go version of the joint Simon task in the presence of a salient object (a small ornamental cat with a waving hand) located to one side of the participant. The participant performed a go/no-go task in response to two acoustic signals that were played over left and right loudspeakers (with location serving as the irrelevant spatial dimension). The results showed that responses were facilitated when the go stimulus was played from the speaker congruent with the participant's location relative to when the stimulus was played from the same side of space as the cat. On the basis of this, Dolk et al. (2013) argued that the results in the joint Simon task could be explained by participants spatially coding their own response with reference to the salient object. While it is true that effects similar to joint task effects can be produced by placing participants in close proximity to other people or other salient stimuli, other evidence suggests that joint task effects can be produced even in the absence of another individual, as long as participants *believe* that they are performing the task with another person.[2]

One line of evidence that has been used to support this claim has been the hidden coactor versions of joint task paradigms. For instance, Tsai et al. (2008) employed a version of the joint Simon task in which participants believed that they were coacting with either a hidden human coactor or a computer. In both cases, the part of the coactor was played by a computer, so the only thing that differed was whether the participant conceived of themselves as coacting with an intentional agent or a nonintentional machine. The results showed that only when participants believed that they were coacting with a human did the joint Simon effect emerge (similar effects have also been reported by Vlainic et al. 2010; however, see Welsh et al. 2007 for an example of where the belief manipulation may not have been strong enough). In the discussion of joint intention, we discuss further examples that can be used to argue against nonsocial interpretations of joint task effects.

6 Planning Tasks with Joint Outcomes

The task representations that we have discussed up until this point have been fairly simple. They have just linked events to actions—for instance, the occurrence of a high ball with the action of jumping. But a more complex form of task representation might be possible. In particular, it might be possible for task representations to link events to joint outcomes. Joint outcomes can be thought of as two (or more) distinct outcomes with some relation between them, or as a single outcome with specified sub-outcomes. It is the addition of this *relation* between the outcomes or the grouping of the outcomes together in a unified whole that is the feature that distinguishes joint outcomes from the outcomes specified by ordinary task representations.

Why might joint task co-representations be necessary, and how might they be useful? Let us take an example from beach volleyball, where two players work together as a team. You and Lily are teammates, and one of your opponents has just struck the ball and it is sailing over the net toward your side of the court. You might have a task representation linking this event to an action, such as moving toward the back of the court and preparing to set the ball. This would be a task co-representation if Lily also had a task representation linking this event to an equivalent action. As we have seen, Lily having such a task representation would result in Lily planning this action upon the occurrence of the event. However, for you and Lily to be successful in a game of volleyball, Lily will need to perform an action that is different from yours, and, as we have shown above, task co-representation can lead to interference in selecting and executing the appropriate action.

Might it instead be possible for you and Lily to coordinate your plans so that the occurrence of the event is linked to an outcome that is jointly specified? What might such a representation look like? We suggest that one possibility is that there is a task representation that links the event of the ball sailing over the net on your side of the court to a set of related actions, such as you moving into position to bump the ball and, simultaneously, Lily getting into position to spike the ball. Here the outcome is jointly specified because it specifies an action for you and an action for Lily, along with a relation between the two actions—for example, that they are to occur at the same time. We can say that two agents have a joint task co-representation just in case there is a joint task representation that each of them share. What distinguishes joint task co-representation from task co-representation is that, rather than an event triggering an outcome and then, at the same time, the same event triggering a different outcome—as with task co-representation—joint task co-representation specifies the outcome as a single unified entity.

7 Evidence of Joint Plans

What would count as evidence for the existence of joint task co-representation? Direct evidence for joint task co-representation is difficult to find; however, the critical feature of joint task co-representation, that outcomes must be jointly specified, may be more amenable to experimental investigation. To understand what is meant by this—that the *goal* or *plan* must be jointly specified—let us consider the case of a bimanual task that involves performing two actions, one with each hand.

First, we can ask whether the outcome is represented jointly or as two actions. That is, whether there is one plan or two plans. Paradigms using *automatic imitation* tasks have been used to probe the structure of plans, and it might be possible to use these to probe the structure of putative joint plans. Second, we might ask whether a task that is learned with a joint outcome can still be performed when only a single outcome is possible. In our bimanual example, this would be equivalent to learning a task bimanually and then testing performance on half the task when it is performed unimanually.

Would performance with, for example, the left hand be equivalent regardless of whether the right hand is still engaged in its part? Paradigms employing joint skill learning could be used to answer this question in the context of joint tasks. Experiments by Tsai, Sebanz, and Knoblich (2011) have adopted automatic imitation approach to examine the structure of joint task co-representations. Before we can consider how Tsai, Sebanz, and Knoblich (2011) modified the automatic imitation paradigm to examine the structure of joint goal representations, it is first necessary to understand how the automatic imitation paradigm can be used to examine the structure of goal representations.

One example of a study that employs the automatic imitation paradigm to probe the structure of plans comes from Liepelt, Von Cramen, and Brass (2008a). In this study, the authors examined the consequences of participants ascribing particular goals to other people. In the standard version of the automatic imitation paradigm, participants respond to a target stimulus by producing an action while simultaneously observing a task-irrelevant action—for example, participants might be asked to respond to the appearance of a "2" by raising their index finger, with the target numeral displayed over a hand shown with a raised index finger or raised middle finger (see Brass et al. 2000). The general finding in these paradigms is that people respond more quickly to the target stimulus when the irrelevant action matches the response action—for example, people are quicker to respond to the target stimulus by raising their index finger when the irrelevant action stimulus also depicts a raised index finger (congruent condition) than when it depicts a raised middle finger (incongruent condition).

The question that Liepelt, Von Cramon, and Brass (2008) examined was whether it was the observation of the action itself that facilitated the response or whether it was the goal attributed to the observed action that was driving the effect. To do this, they examined automatic imitation under different conditions that were designed so that participants would ascribe different goals to the observed agents. Crucially, the observed actions themselves were held constant.

The critical comparison was between two conditions that depicted a finger being *partially* raised in a task where the participant was required to fully raise their finger. The first condition was the *attempted-movement condition*, in which the finger was shown with restraints that prevented more than partial raising. And the second condition was the *micro-movement condition*, in which these restraints were absent. Thus, participants would be able to infer that in the micro-movement condition the intended goal was to partially raise the finger whereas in the attempted-movement condition it was to fully raise the finger. That is, only in the attempted-movement condition would the observed agent have the same set of goals or tasks as the observing participant.

If the effect relied on the participant and observed agent having congruent *goals*, rather than merely performing congruent *movements*, then response facilitation should only occur in the attempted-movement condition and not the micro-movement condition. This is indeed what was observed. This finding is important because it demonstrates that when an observer is engaged in a task, responses produced by particular action plans can be facilitated by observing actions that are produced by congruent action plans. Therefore, by examining when actions are facilitated and when they are not, it is possible to probe how actions and goals are represented.

By extending the logic of Liepelt, Von Cramon, and Brass (2008), it might be possible to examine if and when participants, and a coactor, are capable of having a joint goal by examining how participant's responses are facilitated when observing actions performed by dyads and individuals. The crucial comparisons needed to examine this question are found in Tsai, Sebanz, and Knoblich (2011). The authors ran a series of experiments wherein participants, acting with a confederate, viewed two hands, one on each side of a display, belonging to two other agents. The participant's task was simply to imitate the key pressing action performed by the hand on their side of the display and to withhold their responses when that hand did not move.

The findings of Liepelt, Von Cramon, and Brass (2008) suggest that responses should be facilitated only when the goal of the participant matches the goals of the observed agent. It might be possible to manipulate whether the participant has a joint goal or an individual goal by manipulating whether the participant acts with the confederate (joint goal) or alone (individual goal). Similarly, it might be possible to manipulate whether a joint goal or an individual goal can be inferred from the observed actions by manipulating whether the observed agents act together or alone. To manipulate whether the participant acted alone or together, the confederate's task was modified so that they either moved with the participant (acting together) or moved when the participant withheld their response (acting alone).

Importantly, the participant's task never changed, and they always responded to the movements of the hands on their side of the display. To manipulate whether the observed agents acted alone or together, Tsai, Sebanz, and Knoblich (2011) varied whether the two hands moved in isolation (acting alone) or simultaneously (acting together). By manipulating these factors, it was possible to vary the task context so that there was either a match between the observers' and the observed agents' tasks (both acting alone or both acting together) or a mismatch (for example, the observers acting alone and the observed agents acting together).

The critical comparison was whether the responses of the participant would be modulated by the match between their own task context and the observed task context.

The results confirmed this prediction. When observing the agents acting together, participants responded faster when the confederate was also required to make a response. Conversely, when observing agents acting alone—that is, when the observed hands moved one at a time—participants were quicker to make a response when only they were required to act. Importantly, it was not just the observation of two hands moving simultaneously that facilitated responses when the participant and the confederate acted together. Rather, when the observed actions were altered so that they appeared to belong to a single individual—and of course a single individual can only act alone—the confederate's task had no effect.

Taken together, these results show that participants can plan their actions as part of a pair, with a joint goal, because observing actions that are similarly controlled by a joint goal facilitates the production of these actions. While these findings don't show unequivocally that there is something like joint task representation, or joint task co-representation, they do show that there is something like a jointly specified outcome.

Further evidence of people representing something like joint action outcomes comes from a study that used a transfer of learning paradigm (Loehr and Vesper 2016). The aim of this paradigm was to examine whether a skill learned in the context of a joint action, where actions produce joint outcomes, would transfer to a context where the same action was performed alone. To do this, novice piano players learned to play a piano melody as part of a duet, which they were subsequently tested on in either a joint or individual context. Ordinarily, when learning an action, the actions are represented in terms of their outcomes (Prinz 1997; Hommel 2009). For individual actions, these outcomes are individual outcomes. However, it is possible that in the joint learning context, any actions produced by the participant would realize joint outcomes—a series of temporally coordinated complementary tones—and the actions would be learned and represented in terms of these joint outcomes. When the participant subsequently performed the same actions in an individual context, the previously learned actions would no longer produce the joint effects, or realize the joint outcomes, to which they are linked, and this might result in decreased performance accuracy. Alternatively, if joint outcome representations do not exist, and actions learned in joint contexts are just represented in terms of their individual effects and outcomes, then there should be no difference in performance between the individual and the joint test conditions.

The results from Loehr and Vesper (2016) showed that joint learning did not transfer to individual performance, suggesting that joint actions can be represented in terms of their joint outcomes. Taken together, the findings on joint imitation and joint piano performance suggest that people can indeed represent tasks in terms of jointly specified actions. More evidence is needed to confirm the existence of joint task co-representation, but if joint task co-representation can be confirmed, then there will be important implications for how we think about planning in joint tasks. Rather than simply planning one's own action, or planning one's own action with knowledge of how a co-actor might behave, joint task representation suggests that, in joint tasks, people might represent their own task and the tasks of their partners in a single unified fashion. It is this ability to have a plan of another's action that might be vitally important for how we predict the actions of others. It is this question of action prediction that we turn our attention to next.

8 Anticipating a Teammate's Actions

What is the purpose of representing others' goals? As we have already hinted, representing the goals of others might help us predict their actions. Action prediction is particularly important on the sport field, where timing can be critical and any delay in responding can result in conceding points or, worse, losing the game. Therefore, being able to plan an action early by anticipating what a teammate will do is vitally important for success. But how exactly is action prediction achieved? One possibility is that action prediction is achieved through motor emulation. While many different formulations of the motor emulation approach to action prediction exist, each differing slightly in its details, the approach outlined here draws most of its details from the approach formulated by Colling and Williamson (2014), Colling, Knoblich, and Sebanz (2013), and Wilson and Knoblich (2005).

The motor emulation approach to action prediction relies heavily on notions developed in the motor control literature—in particular, inverse and forward models—and notions borrowed from the common coding literature (Prinz 1997; also see Hommel 2009 and Hommel et al. 2001 for a slightly different formulation). Inverse and forward models are concepts that made their way into the motor control literature by way of control theory. Control theory is the general engineering approach to controlling and predicting the behavior of *control systems* (see Golnaraghi and Kuo 2010 for an introduction to control theory). In a basic control system, known as open-loop control, inverse models act as *controllers* by performing an *inverse* mapping from a goal state to the control commands required to bring about that goal state. The controlled system itself performs a *forward* mapping by transforming these control commands into the desired output or goal state.

In more complex control systems, known as closed-loop control, the output from the target system can be fed back into the controller so that any discrepancy between the actual output and the desired output can be corrected by updating the control commands. Feedback control is useful for bringing about goal states in the target system without having to specify the exact control commands at the outset. For example, when trying to heat an oven to a desired temperature without feedback, precise knowledge about how much energy to apply, and for how long to apply it, would be needed. By using feedback from a thermostat, which can monitor the difference between the actual state and the goal state, this process can be simplified. Feedback control is useful in many situations, but for it to work correctly, some conditions must be met. Critically, it must be possible to gain access to accurate information about the current state of the system. Information about the current state of the system can be inaccurate for at least two reasons. First, sensors that detect the current state of the system might not be of sufficiently high fidelity—for example, the thermometer may be subject to noise and thus be unable to distinguish between 100°C and 150°C. Second, the information about the state of the system might be outdated—for example, the thermometer might be slow to react and instead display the temperature as it was at some time in the past. In order to accurately control a system that exhibits these types of problems, an approach known as pseudo-closed-loop control can be used.

Pseudo-closed-loop control differs from closed-looped control by the addition of a *forward model*. A forward model, like the target system, performs a forward mapping from the control commands to the goal state—that is, it replicates how the controlled system would behave if it had received those control commands. Because forward models respond to control commands in the same way the controlled system would, forward models can be used to *simulate* the behavior of a system. Or, to use the terminology of Grush (1997), forward models can serve as an emulator. With a forward model, or emulator, in place, the control system need not only rely on sensor readings for feedback. Rather, by sending a second copy of any control commands to the forward model, the predictions generated by the forward model can be used as feedback.

If feedback from the forward model is more readily available than actual feedback, then it can be used as a substitute, thereby bypassing sensory delays. Simulated feedback can also be combined with sensory feedback—with each source weighted according to its expected accuracy—to provide a more accurate estimate of the true current state than either source could provide alone. In the context of motor control, inverse models act as planners. Inverse models take a goal as their input and generate the motor commands required to bring about that goal.[3] Forward models serve as predictors that capture the relationship between motor commands and motor outputs. Forward models serve many functions in action control. For instance, predictions generated by forward models can be used to predict and then cancel out the sensory effects of a movement, thereby making it possible to distinguish between the sensory effects of self-movements and external events. Forward models can also generate predictions about the movements themselves, with these predictions able to serve as feedback, thereby overcoming the large delays that result when waiting for feedback from the periphery (Wolpert 1997).

9 Emulator Account of Action Prediction

According to the emulator account of action prediction, the computational mechanisms that underlie action control serve a role in the prediction of others' actions. If the story that we have laid out about co-representation is correct, then co-representation might link events to actions through something like an inverse model, and this in turn might drive forward models that facilitate coordination.

9.1 Inverse Models in Action Prediction

Csibra (2008) has suggested that this mapping from (others') goal states to motor commands relies crucially on the mirror neuron system. To support this claim, Csibra (2008) draws on evidence that shows that activity in the mirror system is modulated by the goals that have been ascribed to an observed agent.[4] For example, Umiltà et al. (2001) had macaque monkeys view a reach-to-grasp movement either in the presence or absence of a food object. The data showed that activity in the mirror neuron system was modulated by the presence of the food. Importantly, however, it was not merely the observation of the food that modulated the activity. To demonstrate this, the reach-to-grasp actions were repeated with the final target of the action—the location where the food would be—hidden from view. Critically, the monkey was given information about the presence of food behind the occluder before the action took place. This manipulation showed that activity in the mirror neuron system was modulated by the action goal with activity being dependent on whether the monkey knew that the action was directed toward grasping food or not. Similar results have also been found in the human neuroimaging literature. For example, Iacoboni et al. (2005) conducted an fMRI study where observers viewed actions performed in two different context conditions (the presence of additional objects in the visual scene was used to indicate context). In both contexts, observers viewed the same reaching action; however, the action context was used to indicate that different intentions, or different ultimate goals, might be present. For example, in the "drinking tea" context, observers could infer that the action was directed at the cup with the intention of picking up the cup and drinking tea from it. This was in contrast to the "washing up" context, which led observers to infer that the goal was to pick up the cup to take it away and clean it. The results showed that regions in the mirror neuron system were sensitive to the inferred intention. Taken together, finding such as these, Csibra (2008) argues, show that the mirror neuron system is involved in determining the motor commands that would be used to realize the goal of an observed agent—that is, the mirror neuron system implements an inverse model for the actions of others.

9.2 Forward Models in Action Prediction

Once the goal has been represented, and some motor commands have been generated, the task of actually generating a prediction about the co-actor's action—or the consequences of their action—is performed by something like a forward model. As outlined above, forward models replicate the input-output relations of the motor system, and they can be used to predict the unfolding dynamics of an action or the sensory consequences of an action. Wilson and Knoblich (2005) and Colling and colleagues (Colling, Knoblich, and Sebanz 2013; Colling and Williamson 2014) have suggested these forward models might also be used to generate predictions about the actions of others.

What is the evidence that the motor system is involved in action prediction? Several lines of evidence have been used to support the claim that the motor system is involved in action prediction. One line of study has examined differences in action-prediction abilities between novices and movement experts—for example, expert basketball or tennis players. The general finding has been that experts are more accurate at predicting the outcomes of actions (Aglioti et al. 2008; Isaacs and Finch 1983; Sebanz and Shiffrar 2009; Abernethy 1990).

Another approach has relied on interference paradigms. The logic of these paradigms is that if motor control and action prediction rely on common mechanisms, then the two tasks should cause interference with each other (e.g., Springer et al. 2011). While these studies do provide evidence for the involvement of the motor system in action prediction, the motor emulation approach argues something more specific than that the motor system is merely *involved* in action prediction. Rather, the claim is that action prediction works by internally simulating the to-be-predicted action using the same mechanisms that ordinarily support action prediction during motor control. That is, the emulator framework suggests that the mechanisms that are used to anticipate the observed action are the same mechanisms specific to the production of that action.

As a consequence, this framework makes very clear predictions about the nature of the predictions that people will generate. Specifically, features or idiosyncrasies of the observer's motor system should "leak out" into the predictions that they generate. For instance, the kinematic match between the observer and the observed agent should have an influence on anticipation accuracy. Or, similarly, movements that are easier for an observer to produce should be easier for them to predict. One paradigm that has been used to test the predictions of the emulator theory is the *real-time prediction* paradigm.

Originally developed by Flach, Knoblich, and Prinz (2003), the real-time prediction paradigm requires participants to generate ongoing predictions of coactors actions. Prediction accuracy is measured by examining how accurately participants are able to align an action response with the to-be-predicted action. The use of action responses is important, because evidence suggests that response modality—whether, for example, participants respond verbally or with an action—matters (see Mann, Abernethy, and Farrow 2010). Consequently, the use of an action response ensures that the paradigm taps into the same mechanisms that underlie prediction for coordination rather than prediction more generally (cf, Aglioti et al. 2008).

The first prediction of the emulator account, that anticipation accuracy should be influenced by the kinematic match between the observer and the observed agent, was tested by Colling, Thompson, and Sutton (2014). This experiment was split into two phases. In the first phase, participants were asked to perform a series of arm movements as if they were drawing zigzags on a blackboard. While performing this action, their movements were recorded with motion capture, and these motion-capture recordings were later rendered as stick figures to be used as stimuli in the second phase. In the second phase, participants viewed these recorded movements while attempting to align a button press with a particular critical point in the stimulus. These critical points corresponded to the apex of each upward movement in the zigzag pattern. Importantly, each participant viewed recordings of their own movements as well as recordings of the movement of another person. If participants use a forward model of their own kinematics, as suggested by the emulator hypothesis, then responses should be more accurately aligned with the stimulus when participants view recordings of their own actions, because the same forward model that was used to produce the observed action would also be used to predict the observed action. This is indeed what was found.

Colling, Knoblich, and Sebanz (2013; see also Colling, Thompson, and Sutton 2016) have suggested that action prediction relies on something like a reperformance of past actions. To support this claim, Colling, Thompson, and Sutton (2016) demonstrated how experience might influence action anticipation using the real-time prediction paradigm. Participants were split into two groups. An experienced group first received practice performing the action they would later be asked to generate predictions about, while the naïve group went straight to the alignment task.

In the alignment task, participants viewed moving displays that either depicted a stick figure performing an action or a single moving point that replicated the dynamics of the stick figure's hand. If action anticipation relies on general-purpose mechanisms, rather than action-specific mechanisms, then alignment accuracy should be roughly equal for both types of displays, because the additional information in the stick figure displays does not provide any additional cues about the dynamics of the hand. However, if action prediction relies on action-specific mechanisms, then one might expect that the addition of extra information about how the action is performed—for example, the configuration of the limbs and joints used to produce the dynamics of the hand—should assist prediction, because it allows the observer to more accurately internally reenact the observed action. The results of the study showed that whether this additional limb and joint information was useful was dependent on whether the participant had experience producing the movement. Furthermore, experienced participants were also better at predicting the fine-grained temporal dynamics of the observed action—the dynamics that would be replicated with an action-specific mechanism.

The final line of evidence that has been used to support the emulator theory of action prediction relies on the logic that if action-specific mechanisms support action anticipation, then movements that are easier to produce should also be easier to anticipate. When producing actions, the motor system is subject to certain constraints, resulting in certain idiosyncratic features being present in all movements. One such example comes from the two-thirds power law. The two-thirds power law describes the relationship between the angular velocity of a curved movement and the curvature of the movement trajectory (Viviani and Terzuolo 1982).

Interestingly, this law not only constrains action production, but has also been shown to influence perceptual judgements (Viviani and Stucchi 1992). In particular, when participants are asked to judge whether a moving point, tracing out an elliptical trajectory, was moving at a constant velocity, they were systematically biased toward trajectories conforming to the two-thirds power law. That is, participants judged trajectories to be constant velocity if they conformed to the velocity profile that would be found if somebody was asked to *produce* a constant-velocity trajectory. Importantly, for our purposes, the two-thirds power law also influences action prediction, with observers being able to more accurately predict stimuli adhering to this constraint (Knoblich et al. 2002; Colling, Thompson, and Sutton 2014).

Another example of biomechanical constraint in action production is found in reaching movements. Several studies have observed hemispatial differences in reaching movements. Specifically, it has been demonstrated that reaching movements performed to the same side of the body as the reaching hand are quicker, have a higher peak velocity, and, importantly, are more accurate than cross-body reaching movements (Prablanc et al. 1979; Carson, Goodman, and Elliott 1992; Carey, Hargreaves, and Goodale 1996). Initial theories suggested a role for hemispheric processing differences in these effects (see Malfara and Jones 1981); however, recent work has suggested that these findings are more readily explained by the biomechanical constraints inherent in cross-body reaching (Gordon et al. 1994; Carey and Otto-de Haart 2001).

Specifically, Gordon et al. (1994) argue that these performance asymmetries are a result of differences in the inertial forces experienced by the limb, a model that has been supported by Carey and Otto-de Haart (2001). An increase in inertial forces results in more noise in the system and a greater degree of variability in the underlying representations (Franklin and Wolpert 2011). If these past motor representations are reactivated during action prediction, as claimed by the emulator hypothesis, then we can expect the hemispatial asymmetries found in action production to also be found in action prediction. Colling and Dall'Acqua (2016) tested this hypothesis, using the real-time prediction paradigm, by asking participants to align button-press responses with the critical points in a zigzag movement that was directed to either the contralateral or ipsilateral side of space. Importantly, the actual kinematics of the reaching movements was held constant either by time-reversing ipsilateral movements to create contralateral movements (experiment 1) or by time-reversing contralateral movements to create ipsilateral movements (experiment 4).

The results replicated the findings found in reaching studies, and alignment was more accurate when generating predictions about ipsilateral movements. Taken together, the results from the real-time prediction paradigm provide support for the role of motor emulation in action prediction. Importantly, the results show that action anticipation mechanisms operate fast enough to plausibly support joint action coordination on the sport field.

One line of evidence that has been used to address these questions comes from a paradigm that has used a robot coactor. Stenzel et al. (2012) had participants perform a version of the joint Simon task with robot coactor while manipulating the beliefs that the participant had about how the robot's actions were controlled. In the humanlike condition, participants were told that the robot had been designed to function in a biologically inspired manner, whereas in the machinelike condition, participants were told that the robot operated in a purely deterministic manner. That is, in the humanlike condition, participants were encouraged to attribute humanlike intentions and decision processes to the robot. A debriefing questionnaire, in which participants were required to indicate their agreement with phrases such as "The robot acted intentionally" and "The robot decided actively when to respond to a stimulus," confirmed that this manipulation did indeed have the desired effect. The results showed that only under the humanlike instructions did the joint task effects emerge. This is to be expected if co-representation only occurs when the coactor is capable of acting according to intentions. That is, co-representation might be dependent on an actor having a belief that he or she is doing something *with another intentional agent*, and, therefore, might be dependent on a preexisting joint intention.

10 Conclusion

The framework we have outlined suggests that during joint action coordination on the sport field, we plan our teammates' actions, and represent our teammates' goals and tasks, using much the same mechanisms that we use to plan and represent our own. Furthermore, we have suggested that actually predicting the timing and unfolding dynamics of our teammates' actions rely on the same mechanisms that we use to predict our own actions during action control.

What implications does our account have for understanding success and failure on the sport field? There is a well-known distinction between an expert team and a team of experts (see Eccles and Tenenbaum 2004). For instance, the Spanish national football team was regularly filled with star players; however, between their fourth-place finish in the 1950 football World Cup and raising the cup in the 2010 football World Cup Final, they regularly failed to achieve success in major tournaments.

Salas, Cannon-Bowers, and Johnston (1997) offer a number of suggestions as to how a team of experts might be turned into an expert team. These include team training to foster shared and compatible mental models, training of situational awareness and communication, and training team leaders to maintain shared situational awareness. However, a final suggestion offered by Salas, Cannon-Bowers, and Johnston (1997), which is most compatible with the view we have outlined here, is to train team members in each other's roles. Our account argues that coordination on the sport field involves representing the goals of others so that we can plan our actions with them and anticipate their actions.

Only when a player knows what task their teammates will perform is it possible to co-represent that task. If the account we have presented here is correct, it might also provide insight into understanding team failure. Team cohesion, defined by Carron, Brawley, and Widmeyer (1998, 213) as the "tendency for a group to stick together," has been recognized as an important part of team success (e.g., Carron, Bray, and Eys 2010). The view we have presented here might be able to provide an account of mechanisms behind team failure when cohesion breaks down.

It may be the case that disharmony in a team actually has the effect of making it less likely that players include others in their planning. For instance, Costantini and Ferri (2013; see also Aquino et al. 2015) found that social exclusion could modulate the effects found in the joint Simon task, suggesting that when people felt excluded they were less likely to include their coactor in their planning. Furthermore, our claims about the mechanisms that underlie action prediction might also have implications for coaching or team selection in sports that rely heavily on action anticipation or interpersonal alignment such as, for example, rowing.

Our account of action prediction suggests that these mechanisms are grounded in the motor control system and carry traces of an actor's motor experience and biomechanics. If this is true, then it may be the case that, if certain people are better matched in terms of biomechanics or other anthropometric factors, then this might have an influence on how accurately they can predict or align with each other. If future research is able to accurately determine these factors, then it might be possible to incorporate these into crew or team selection so as to benefit from any prediction or alignment advantage.

Acknowledgments

The work presented here has been greatly influenced by collaborative projects with Stephen Butterfill, Natalie Sebanz, John Sutton, and William F. Thompson. I am greatly indebted to their input; however, any mistakes I have made are my responsibility alone. Thank you also to Zhivan Alach for his comments on the manuscript.

Notes

1. Note that some authors, such as, for example, Pacherie (2006) distinguish between different types of intentions in an intention hierarchy. In this view, the intention to take a mark, the intention to jump up when the ball approaches, and the intention to perform a particular set of movements that result in jumping would all be different kinds of intention, with different roles, and different kinds of content. These three levels map roughly onto what we will call intentions, tasks, and motor plans.

2. We revisit the influence of beliefs later in the context of joint intentions.

3. Although approaches such as optimal feedback control (see Franklin and Wolpert 2011) do not explicitly rely on inverse models, they can be thought of as implicitly invoking inverse models (see Wolpert and Kawato 1998).

4. The mirror neuron system is also the putative neural substrate of automatic imitation effects discussed earlier (e.g., see Liepelt, Von Cramon, and Brass 2008).

References

Abernethy, Bruce. 1990. "Anticipation in Squash: Differences in Advance Cue Utilization between Expert and Novice Players." *Journal of Sports Sciences* 8 (1): 17–34. doi:10.1080/02640419008732128.

Aglioti, Salvatore M., Paola Cesari, Michela Romani, and Cosimo Urgesi. 2008. "Action Anticipation and Motor Resonance in Elite Basketball Players." *Nature Neuroscience* 11 (9): 1109–16. doi:10.1038/nn.2182.

Aquino, Antonio, Daniele Paolini, Stefano Pagliaro, Daniele Migliorati, Annemarie Wolff, Francesca Romana Alparone, and Marcello Costantini. 2015. "Group Membership and Social Status Modulate Joint Actions." *Experimental Brain Research* 233 (8). doi:10.1007/s00221-015-4316-7.

Atmaca, Silke, Natalie Sebanz, and Günther Knoblich. 2011. "The Joint Flanker Effect: Sharing Tasks with Real and Imagined Co-Actors." *Experimental Brain Research* 211 (3–4). doi:10.1007/s00221-011-2709-9.

Block, Ned. 2009. "The Mind as the Software of the Brain." In *Science Fiction and Philosophy: From Time Travel to Superintelligence*, ed. Susan Schneider, 126–169. UK: John Wiley & Sons.

Böckler, Anne, Günther Knoblich, and Natalie Sebanz. 2012. "Effects of a Coactor's Focus of Attention on Task Performance." *Journal of Experimental Psychology: Human Perception and Performance* 38 (6): 1404–1415. doi:10.1037/a0027523.

Brass, Marcel, Harold Bekkering, Andreas Wohlschläger, and Wolfgang Prinz. 2000. "Compatibility between Observed and Executed Finger Movements: Comparing Symbolic, Spatial, and Imitative Cues." *Brain and Cognition* 44 (2): 124–143. doi:10.1006/brcg.2000.1225.

Bratman, Michael E. 1987. *Intention, Plans, and Practical Reason*. Cambridge, MA: Harvard University Press.

Bratman, Michael E. 1993. "Shared Intention." *Ethics* 104 (1): 97–113.

Butterfill, Stephen A. 2016. "Coordinating Joint Action." In *Routledge Handbook on Collective Intentionality*, edited by Ludwig Kirk and Jankovic Marija. London: Routledge.

Carey, David P., Eric L. Hargreaves, and Melvyn A. Goodale. 1996. "Reaching to Ipsilateral or Contralateral Targets: Within-Hemisphere Visuomotor Processing Cannot Explain Hemispatial Differences in Motor Control." *Experimental Brain Research* 112 (3): 496–504.

Carey, David P., and E. Grace Otto-de Haart. 2001. Hemispatial Differences in Visually Guided Aiming Are Neither Hemispatial nor Visual. *Neuropsychologia* 39 (9): 885–894. doi:10.1016/S0028-3932(01)00036-7.

Carron, Albert V., Lawrence R. Brawley, and William N. Widmeyer. 1998. "The Measurement of Cohesiveness in Sport Groups." In *Advances Sport and Exercise Psychology Measurement*, edited by Joan L Duda, 213–226. Morgantown, WV: Fitness Information Technology.

Carron, Albert V., Steven R. Bray, and Mark A. Eys. 2010. "Team Cohesion and Team Success in Sport." *Journal of Sports Sciences* 20 (2): 119–126.

Carson, Richard G., David Goodman, and Digby Elliott. 1992. "Asymmetries in the Discrete and Pseudocontinuous Regulation of Visually Guided Reaching." *Brain and Cognition* 18 (2): 169–191. doi:10.1016/0278-2626(92)90077-Y.

Colling, Lincoln, and Tommaso Dall'acqua. 2016. "Biomechanical Constraints of Action Production also Influence Predictions of Observed Actions." Presentation from the 2014 Australasian Experimental Psychology Conference (Brisbane). *Figshare*. doi:10.6084/m9.figshare.3207241.v1.

Colling, Lincoln J., Günther Knoblich, and Natalie Sebanz. 2013. "How Does 'Mirroring' Support Joint Action?" *Cortex: A Journal Devoted to the Study of the Nervous System and Behavior* 49 (10): 2964–2965. doi:10.1016/j.cortex.2013.06.006.

Colling, Lincoln J., William F. Thompson, and John Sutton. 2014. "The Effect of Movement Kinematics on Predicting the Timing of Observed Actions." *Experimental Brain Research* 232 (4): 1193–1206. doi:10.1007/s00221-014-3836-x.

Colling, Lincoln J., and Kellie Williamson. 2014. "Entrainment and Motor Emulation Approaches to Joint Action: Alternatives or Complementary Approaches?" *Frontiers in Human Neuroscience* 8 (September): 754. doi:10.3389/fnhum.2014.00754.

Colling, Lincoln John, William F. Thompson, and John Sutton. 2016. "Mechanisms for Action Prediction Operate Differently in Observers with Motor Experience." *BioRxiv*. doi:10.1101/044438.

Costantini, Marcello, and Francesca Ferri. 2013. "Action Co-Representation and Social Exclusion." *Experimental Brain Research* 227 (1): 85–92. doi:10.1007/s00221-013-3487-3.

Csibra, Gergely. 2008. "Action Mirroring and Action Understanding: An Alternative Account." In *Sensorimotor Foundations of Higher Cognition*, edited by Patrick Haggard, Yves Rossetti, and Mitsuo Kawato, 435–459. New York: Oxford University Press.

Dolk, Thomas, Bernhard Hommel, Wolfgang Prinz, and Roman Liepelt. 2013. "The (Not so) Social Simon Effect: A Referential Coding Account." *Journal of Experimental Psychology: Human Perception and Performance* 39 (5): 1248–1260. doi:10.1037/a0031031.

Dolk, Thomas, Bernhard Hommel, Wolfgang Prinz, and Roman Liepelt. 2014. "The Joint Flanker Effect: Less Social Than Previously Thought." *Psychonomic Bulletin and Review* 21 (5): 1224–1230. doi:10.3758/s13423-014-0583-8.

Eccles, David W., and Gershon Tenenbaum. 2004. "Why an Expert Team Is More Than a Team of Experts: A Social-Cognitive Conceptualization of Team Coordination and Communication in Sport." *Journal of Sport and Exercise Psychology* 26 (4): 542–560.

Eriksen, Charles W. 1995. "The Flankers Task and Response Competition: A Useful Tool for Investigating a Variety of Cognitive Problems." *Visual Cognition* 2 (2/3): 101–118. doi:10.1080/13506289508401726.

Flach, Rüdiger, Günther Knoblich, and Wolfgang Prinz. 2003. "Off-Line Authorship Effects in Action Perception." *Brain and Cognition* 53 (3): 503–513. doi:10.1016/S0278-2626(03)00211-2.

Fodor, Jerry A., and Zenon W. Pylyshyn. 1988. "Connectionism and Cognitive Architecture: A Critical Analysis." *Cognition* 28 (12): 3–71. doi:10.1016/0010-0277(88)90031-5.

Franklin, David W., and Daniel M. Wolpert. 2011. "Computational Mechanisms of Sensorimotor Control." *Neuron* 72 (3): 425–442. doi:10.1016/j.neuron.2011.10.006.

Golnaraghi, M. F., and Benjamin C. Kuo. 2010. *Automatic Control Systems*. 9th ed. Hoboken, NJ: Wiley.

Gordon, James, Maria Felice Ghilardi, Scott E. Cooper, and Claude Ghez. 1994. "Accuracy of Planar Reaching Movements." *Experimental Brain Research* 99 (1): 112–130. doi:10.1007/BF00241416.

Grafton, Scott T., and Antonia F. de C. Hamilton. 2007. "Evidence for a Distributed Hierarchy of Action Representation in the Brain." *Human Movement Science* 26 (4): 590–616. doi:10.1016/j.humov.2007.05.009.

Grush, Rick. 1997. "The Architecture of Representation." *Philosophical Psychology* 10 (1): 5–23. doi:10.1080/09515089708573201.

Grush, Rick. 2004. "The Emulation Theory of Representation: Motor Control, Imagery, and Perception." *Behavioral and Brain Sciences* 27 (3): 377–396; discussion, 396–442. doi:10.1017/S0140525X04000093.

Guagnano, Delia, Elena Rusconi, and Carlo Arrigo Umiltà. 2010. "Sharing a Task or Sharing Space? On the Effect of the Confederate in Action Coding in a Detection Task." *Cognition* 114 (3): 348–355. doi:10.1016/j.cognition.2009.10.008.

Hommel, Bernhard. 2009. "Action Control According to TEC (Theory of Event Coding)." *Psychological Research* 73 (4): 512–526. doi:10.1007/s00426-009-0234-2.

Hommel, Bernhard, Jochen Müsseler, Gisa Aschersleben, and Wolfgang Prinz. 2001. "The Theory of Event Coding: A Framework for Perception and Action Planning." *Behavioral and Brain Sciences* 24 (5): 849–878; discussion, 878–937. doi:10.1017/S0140525X01000103.

Iacoboni, Marco, Istvan Molnar-Szakacs, Vittorio Gallese, Giovanni Buccino, John C. Mazziotta, and Giacomo Rizzolatti. 2005. "Grasping the Intentions of Others with One's Own Mirror Neuron System." *PLoS Biology* 3 (3): e79. doi:10.1371/journal.pbio.0030079.

Isaacs, Larry D., and Alfred E. Finch. 1983. "Anticipatory Timing of Beginning and Intermediate Tennis Players." *Perceptual and Motor Skills* 57 (2): 451–454. doi:10.2466/pms.1983.57.2.451.

Jeannerod, Marc. 1994. "The Representing Brain: Neural Correlates of Motor Intention and Imagery." *Behavioral and Brain Sciences* 17 (2): 187–202. doi:10.1017/S0140525X00034026.

Knoblich, Günther, Eva Seigerschmidt, Rüdiger Flach, and Wolfgang Prinz. 2002. "Authorship Effects in the Prediction of Handwriting Strokes: Evidence for Action Simulation during Action Perception." *Quarterly Journal of Experimental Psychology A: Human Experimental Psychology* 55 (3): 1027–1046. doi:10.1080/02724980143000631.

Kornblum, Sylvan, Thierry Hasbroucq, and Allen Osman. 1990. "Dimensional Overlap: Cognitive Basis for Stimulus-Response Compatibility: A Model and Taxonomy." *Psychological Review* 97 (2): 253–270. doi:10.1037/0033-295X.97.2.253.

Liepelt, Roman, D. Yves Von Cramon, and Marcel Brass. 2008. "What Is Matched in Direct Matching? Intention Attribution Modulates Motor Priming." *Journal of Experimental Psychology: Human Perception and Performance* 34 (3): 578–591. doi:10.1037/0096-1523.34.3.578.

Liepelt, Roman, Dorit Wenke, Rico Fischer, and Wolfgang Prinz. 2010. "Trial-to-Trial Sequential Dependencies in a Social and Non-Social Simon Task." *Psychological Research* 75 (5): 366–375. doi:10.1007/s00426-010-0314-3.

Loehr, Janeen D., and Cordula Vesper. 2016. "The Sound of You and Me: Novices Represent Shared Goals in Joint Action." *Quarterly Journal of Experimental Psychology* 69 (3): 535–547. doi:10.1080/17470218.2015.1061029.

Malfara, Anthony, and Bill Jones. 1981. "Hemispheric Asymmetries in Motor Control of Guided Reaching with and without Optic Displacement." *Neuropsychologia* 19 (3): 483–486. doi:10.1016/0028-3932(81)90081-6.

Mann, David L., Bruce Abernethy, and Damian Farrow. 2010. "Action Specificity Increases Anticipatory Performance and the Expert Advantage in Natural Interceptive Tasks." *Acta Psychologica* 135 (1): 17–23. doi:10.1016/j.actpsy.2010.04.006.

Newell, Allen, and Herbert A Simon. 1997. "Computer Science as Empirical Inquiry: Symbols Are Search." In *Mind Design II: Philosophy, Psychology, Artificial Intelligence*, edited by John Haugeland, 81–110. Cambridge, MA: MIT Press.

Pacherie, Elisabeth. 2006. "Towards a Dynamic Theory of Intentions." In *Does Consciousness Cause Behavior*, edited by Susan Pockett, William P. Banks, and Shaun Gallagher, 145–167. Cambridge, MA: MIT Press.

Pacherie, Elisabeth. 2008. "The Phenomenology of Action: A Conceptual Framework." *Cognition* 107 (1): 179–217. doi:10.1016/j.cognition.2007.09.003.

Prablanc, Claude, J. F. Echallier, Egli Komilis, and Marc Jeannerod. 1979. "Optimal Response of Eye and Hand Motor Systems in Pointing at a Visual Target." *Biological Cybernetics* 35 (2): 113–124. doi:10.1007/BF00337436.

Prinz, Wolfgang. 1997. "Perception and Action Planning." *European Journal of Cognitive Psychology* 9 (2): 129–154. doi:10.1080/713752551.

Ramnani, Narender, and R. Christopher Miall. 2003. "A System in the Human Brain for Predicting the Actions of Others." *Nature Neuroscience* 7 (1): 85–90. doi:10.1038/nn1168.

Reimer, Torsten, Ernest S. Park, and Verlin B. Hinsz. 2006. "Shared and Coordinated Cognition in Competitive and Dynamic Task Environments: An Information-Processing Perspective for Team Sports." *International Journal of Sport and Exercise Psychology* 4 (4): 376–400.

Rizzolatti, Giacomo, and Laila Craighero. 2004. "The Mirror-Neuron System." *Annual Review of Neuroscience* 27 (1): 169–192. doi:10.1146/annurev.neuro.27.070203.144230.

Salas, Eduardo, Janis A. Cannon-Bowers, and Joan Hall Johnston. 1997. "How Can You Turn a Team of Experts into an Expert Team? Emerging Training Strategies." In *Naturalistic Decision Making*, edited by Caroline E. Zsambok and Gary Klein, 359–370. Hillsdale, NJ: Erlbaum.

Searle, John. 1990. "Collective Intentions and Actions." In *Intentions in Communication*, edited by Philip R. Cohen, Jerry Morgan, and Martha E. Pollack, 401–415. Cambridge MA: MIT Press.

Sebanz, Natalie, Harold Bekkering, and Günther Knoblich. 2006. "Joint Action: Bodies and Minds Moving Together." *Trends in Cognitive Sciences* 10 (2): 70–76. doi:10.1016/j.tics.2005.12.009.

Sebanz, Natalie, Günther Knoblich, and Wolfgang Prinz. 2003. "Representing Others' Actions: Just Like One's Own?" *Cognition* 88 (3): B11–21.

Sebanz, Natalie, Günther Knoblich, and Wolfgang Prinz. 2005. "How Two Share a Task: Corepresenting Stimulus-Response Mappings." *Journal of Experimental Psychology: Human Perception and Performance* 31 (6): 1234–1246. doi:10.1037/0096-1523.31.6.1234.

Sebanz, Natalie, Günther Knoblich, Wolfgang Prinz, and Edmund Wascher. 2006. "Twin Peaks: An ERP Study of Action Planning and Control in Coaching Individuals." *Journal of Cognitive Neuroscience* 18 (5): 859–870. doi:10.1162/jocn.2006.18.5.859.

Sebanz, Natalie, and Maggie Shiffrar. 2009. "Detecting Deception in a Bluffing Body: The Role of Expertise." *Psychonomic Bulletin and Review* 16 (1): 170–175. doi:10.3758/PBR.16.1.170.

Simon, J. Richard. 1969. "Reactions toward the Source of Stimulation." *Journal of Experimental Psychology* 81 (1): 174–176. doi:10.1037/h0027448.

Springer, Anne, Simone Brandstädter, Roman Liepelt, Teresa Birngruber, Martin A. Giese, Franz Mechsner, and Wolfgang Prinz. 2011. "Motor Execution Affects Action Prediction." *Brain and Cognition* 76 (1): 26–36. doi:10.1016/j.bandc.2011.03.007.

Stenzel, Anna, Eris Chinellato, Maria A. Tirado, Ángel P. del Pobil, Markus Lappe, and Roman Liepelt. 2012. "When Humanoid Robots Become Human-Like Interaction Partners: Corepresentation of Robotic Actions." *Journal of Experimental Psychology: Human Perception and Performance* 38 (5): 1073–1077. doi:10.1037/a0029493.

Tsai, Chia-Chin, Wen-Jui Kuo, Daisy L. Hung, and Ovid J. L. Tzeng. 2008. "Action Co-Representation Is Tuned to Other Humans." *Journal of Cognitive Neuroscience* 20 (11): 2015–2024.

Tsai, Jessica Chia-Chin, Natalie Sebanz, and Günther Knoblich. 2011. "The GROOP Effect: Groups Mimic Group Actions." *Cognition* 118 (1): 135–140. doi:10.1016/j.cognition.2010.10.007.

Umiltà, Maria A, Evelyne Kohler, Vittorio Gallese, Leonardo Fogassi, Luciano Fadiga, Christian Keysers, and Giacomo Rizzolatti. 2001. "I Know What You Are Doing: A Neurophysiological Study." *Neuron* 31 (1): 155–165. doi:10.1016/S0896-6273(01)00337-3.

Viviani, Paolo, and Natalie Stucchi. 1992. "Biological Movements Look Uniform: Evidence of Motor-Perceptual Interactions." *Journal of Experimental Psychology: Human Perception and Performance* 18 (3): 603–623. doi:10.1037/0096-1523.18.3.603.

Viviani, Paolo, and Carlo Terzuolo. 1982. "Trajectory Determines Movement Dynamics." *Neuroscience* 7 (2): 431–437. doi:10.1016/0306-4522(82)90277-9.

Vlainic, Elize, Roman Liepelt, Lorenza S Colzato, Wolfgang Prinz, and Bernhard Hommel. 2010. "The Virtual Co-Actor: The Social Simon Effect Does Not Rely on Online Feedback from the Other." *Cognition* 1:208. doi:10.3389/fpsyg.2010.00208.

Welsh, Timothy N., Laura Higgins, Matthew Ray, and Daniel J. Weeks. 2007. "Seeing vs. Believing: Is Believing Sufficient to Activate the Processes of Response Co-Representation?" *Human Movement Science* 26 (6): 853–866. doi:10.1016/j.humov.2007.06.003.

Wenke, Dorit, Silke Atmaca, Antje Holländer, Roman Liepelt, Pamela Baess, and Wolfgang Prinz. 2011. "What Is Shared in Joint Action? Issues of Co-Representation, Response Conflict, and Agent Identification." *Review of Philosophy and Psychology* 2 (2): 147–172. doi:10.1007/s13164-011-0057-0.

Wilson, Margaret. 2002. "Six Views of Embodied Cognition." *Psychonomic Bulletin and Review* 9 (4): 625–636.

Wilson, Margaret, and Günther Knoblich. 2005. "The Case for Motor Involvement in Perceiving Conspecifics." *Psychological Bulletin* 131 (3): 460–473. doi:10.1037/0033-2909.131.3.460.

Wolpert, Daniel M. 1997. "Computational Approaches to Motor Control." *Trends in Cognitive Sciences* 1 (6): 209–216. doi:10.1016/S1364-6613(97)01070-X.

Wolpert, Daniel M., and Mitsuo Kawato. 1998. "Multiple Paired Forward and Inverse Models for Motor Control." *Neural Networks* 11 (7/8): 1317–1329. doi:10.1016/S0893-6080(98)00066-5.

V Enculturated, Gendered, and Disciplined Bodies: Approaches to Performance and Motivation in the Social Sciences

16 Excellence without Mental Representation: High Performance in Risk Sports and Japanese Swordsmanship

Jesús Ilundáin-Agurruza, Kevin Krein, and Karl Erickson

1 Introduction

The most common explanations of cognition in sport rely on the idea that mental representation plays a central role in explaining athletic skill (Ericsson 2006; Sutton 2007; Beilock 2008). Next ensues a strawman account: sportspersons internally represent in their brain the situations they face. As they perceive changes in their environment, they process pertinent information and determine how to respond. Then, the brain organizes the motor response. We may ask, regarding the skills of a white-water kayaker going over a hundred-foot waterfall, how is this possible? What many philosophers, and cognitive or sport scientists, mean is, what mechanisms underlie the activity and are causally responsible for the behavior? It is often thought that an adequate explanation must involve the kayaker having an internal representation of his or her kayak, paddle, waterfall, and landing. His or her senses indicate where the waterfall lip is, and the brain, processing this information, directs his body to get in a position to safely hit the water below. Training has imprinted routines that allow for efficient moves in a fluid sequence. Embodied cognition and enactivism proponents argue that cognition does not fundamentally involve representation in this way. Rather, mental representation comes later, as part of an enculturated and scaffolded framework.

The above representational account, extremely simplified, even simplistic, could be filled in and strengthened with far more detail. Presently we limit ourselves to a contextualizing overview and circumvent enhancements to such accounts (Fodor 1987; Fodor and Pylyshyn 2014). Likewise, we sidestep an in-depth review of critiques of representational theories, as others have engaged in such dispute (Chemero 2009; Hutto and Myin 2013). Our goal is to explore new terrain. The problem to be solved concerns the cognitive engagements of expert performers in risky endeavors. Characterized by intense focus and the ability to react subtly and suitably to unexpected threats, these engagements present challenges because they involve high-level functioning, intentionality, and creative spontaneity. Relying on an enactive stance, and following phenomenological accounts of martial arts masters and sportspersons, as well as current empirical research in sport psychology, we argue that mental content or representation—in a traditional sense—is not involved, specifically during intense "full on" moments.

To examine this, we develop two ideas. One, we evaluate the extent to which activities that require high levels of performance in dangerous contexts—presently outdoor risk sports and Japanese swordsmanship (*kenjutsu*)—may require a different sort of explanation, arguing that such cases do not result from processing internal representations. An enactive account mostly in agreement with Hutto and Myin's (2013) radically enactive cognition (REC), a view that considers that basic minds operate without recourse to mental content, is especially suited to this task. Two, we explore how this enactive understanding of cognition in highly skilled performance relates to cultural context in certain cognitive and performing states called flow and *mushin* (mindful fluid awareness) in the sport and martial arts worlds, respectively.

Part 2 below specifies the kinds of sports and martial arts under consideration and discusses the underlying holistic framework. Part 3 delves into mental representation and introduces enactivism in order to set up the version we endorse, REC. Part 4 centers on REC, delineating the relationship between cognition and high performance. Part 5 argues that flow and *mushin* states, emblematic of expert-level performers in risk sports and martial arts, embody an enactive nonrepresentational cognition in action. Then, it delves into the specific challenges that risk sports and swordsmanship face, relating these to cognition. Part 6 explores the role of culture, paying particular attention to how the representational and nonrepresentational interact, centering on the Buddhist framework in Japanese martial arts.

2 Preliminary Explanations

A basic premise is that risk sports and traditional Japanese martial arts meaningfully overlap in terms of performance requirements and phenomenology, particularly in high performance. Risk sports and adventure activities are understood presently as those in which danger of serious injury or death is a *constitutive* element (Ilundáin-Agurruza 2007; Russell 2005). The extreme specificity and diversity of sports requires prudence when making general claims about them. Of particular interest here are "nature sports" (Krein 2007, 2014), for which the awesome size and power of natural features provides clear examples of life-threatening situations that require fast adaptation to quickly changing situations and call on decisive fluidity in action: for example, wingsuit flying, BASE jumping, outdoor luge, or big wave surfing. This brings the analysis closer to the dynamics of swordsmanship. Other risk sports rely on different skill sets. For instance, mountaineering calls for careful planning in protracted sorties that can last days or even weeks and, once at altitude, a slow pace because of low oxygen levels. Nonetheless, much of our discussion regarding mental representation extends to these risk activities and other safer outdoor activities and sports, but making this overt is beyond the scope of this chapter.

Concerning martial arts, and to be detailed for those unfamiliar, the focus lies on *koryū* (古流), *traditional* martial arts in the spirit of *bujutsu* (武術), or combat techniques, expressly on *kenjutsu* (剣術), swordsmanship techniques, before the Meiji Restoration of 1868. These practices radically differ, functionally and philosophically, from modern counterparts under the aegis of *budō* (武道)—for example, judo—and even more so from "sportified" martial arts or *kakutogi* (格闘技), such as karate. Contemporary martial arts have taken clear steps to minimize harm, whereas in *koryū*, injury was but part of practice: serious damage was common, and death remained a possibility in *kenjutsu* even when using *bokken* (木剣), wooden swords. When engaged as intended, in duels or fights, *kenjutsu* would often result in the death of one or both opponents.

These activities are chosen for several reasons. If sports are unique by virtue of their superfluous limitation of permissible means to achieve their ends (they make things harder than they need to be), risk sports gratuitously add danger to the formula. Whereas killing lions or bears with a spear or bow and arrow has been done throughout history out of necessity, the sportsperson does so even when she has access to better technology such as guns. This structural superfluity turns the utilitarian hunt into a sport. Both are risky; only the latter is done "for fun." This unnecessary courting of risk has interesting consequences for performance and cognition, as part 5 shows.

As for *kenjutsu*, as a martial art, it traditionally sought lethal efficacy and efficiency: no gratuitous movements no matter how beautiful. But, this effectiveness was bound by a strict code of behavior (*bushidō* 武士道) that required honorability and also codified battlefield and duel encounters.[1] Moreover, as *kenjutsu* evolved into *kendō* (剣道 way of the sword) from the sixteenth to the eighteenth centuries—a period that for many marks the apex of Japanese swordsmanship, and on which we focus—it moved from warfare techniques to the way of the sword as a perennial path toward self-flourishing, achievement, and self-perfection intensely focused on the present.[2] Aikido founder Ueshiba Morihei's words speak to this: "Those who are enlightened never stop forging themselves" (Ueshiba 1992, 52). This aligns the art of the sword with the view of sport as a striving toward excellence under the aegis of Ancient Greek *areté* (ἀρετή).

Importantly for our purposes, most phenomenologically incisive treatises belonging to *kenjutsu* are from the sixteenth to the eighteenth centuries. This literature provides insight into the mental states of fighters and how these states were understood in their own historical and cultural context. It also proves revealing for contemporary athletes in fast-paced high-risk sports.

A holistic framework underlies this inquiry (Ilundáin-Agurruza 2016, 2017). We eschew intellectualist and dualist stances that separate body and mind as distinct substances, bring inner/outer splits, and make cognition mind (brain) bound. The mind/body dualism often generates "representational theories of mind and cognition" wherein representations are internal and about or directed to other representations and states of affairs in the world (Johnson 2007, 113–114). Instead, this holism advances a pragmatic (Dewey 1988) and phenomenologically (Gallagher 2005; Sheets-Johnstone 2011) informed understanding. It upholds continuities of phenomena between extremes rather than drawing up a division of "kind" between mutually exclusive poles. The continuity extends from simple organisms to persons, between cognitive processes and mechanisms, and between nonrepresentational and enculturated cognition. This bypasses dualist accounts in terms of mind and/or body or brain/body (the last of which also implies a dualism of its own, with the brain acting as the mind, the seat of cognition; see Bennett and Hacker 2003 for this charge). Additionally, instead of reductive accounts that limit explanations to neuronal processes, mechanisms, and constituents, this holism incorporates these as part of a broader view attuned to the fluid dynamics of our interacting ways in the world.

To capture this, the holistic stance posits a comparative analysis that views us as integrative *bodyminds* (Ilundáin-Agurruza 2016). Dewey congruently wrote of the "body-mind," such that body and mind are not separate things but "abstractions from our ongoing, continuous, interactive experience" (Johnson 2007, 140). "Bodymind" here excises Dewey's hyphen to better accentuate the underlying unity. It is best viewed as a verb form that functionally describes the varying degree of psychophysical integration of performers according to level of skillful expertise. "Bodyminding," and "bodyminded," if more gauche, better render the idea that this is about ongoing *living* and *lived* processes. Crucially, bodymind is not a claim about the ontology of persons; rather it is a phenomenological designatum that avoids metaphysical polemics to focus on describing how performances and experiences thereof are structured, felt, and expressed.

In short, an integrated bodymind indicates a performative achievement that in turn is evidence of superior psychosomatic unity. Being able to elicit flow and *mushin* states is a trademark of expertly integrated bodyminded experience and performance. As such, the state is amenable to and dependent on practice and skill development. This is rooted on East Asian holistic notions of persons (Yuasa 1987). Accordingly, we are better or worse integrated psychosomatically and with the environments with which we engage in relation to present abilities: in sport, for example, being in shape or not has marked consequences. Superb performers evince high degrees of integration. Novices, athletes who choke on game day, and those suffering from injuries or pathological conditions such as schizophrenia incarnate the flip side, a "dis-integrated" bodymind.

Successful big wave surfing, where swells top 60 feet (20 meters), calls on superior integration. Big wave surfers must handle the exacting kinematics and coordination needed to stay on a board sliding at 40 mph (65 km/h), and also need to steel themselves emotionally to handle the anxiety of facing five-story-high masses of fast-moving water. Their integration also assimilates the board, which is inclusive of but not limited to their body schema (see Gallagher 2005). Garrett McNamara's accomplishment in Nazaré (Portugal) in 2013—when he surfed the tallest wave on record, a 99-foot (30-meter) behemoth—embodied such highly fluid bodyminding.

3 Mental Representation and Enactivist Views

The role that representation plays in human action has dominated philosophical inquiries of mind for much of the last century. Whichever the theory of mind endorsed, it has seemed that mental activities must happen in minds, and minds, whatever they are, are where thoughts, beliefs, and attitudes take place. These may be about the external world, but should not be confused with it. A memory of a tree in front of a house should not be mistaken for the actual tree. Shapiro presents the philosophical view at its most fundamental: "Most basically, a representation is a 'stand-in' for something else" (2011, 142). That is, a representation is whatever it is in the mind that stands for the "thing" represented. Thus, much of the debate in philosophy of mind has concerned what properties could make something be a representation of something else. This is usually cast in terms of truth conditions, veridicality, and related notions, the gist of which is that representation must mirror, or be liable to being mapped onto, what is represented. Many contemporary philosophers, partisans of naturalistic views, see this in terms of *what* could make a particular neural structure represent or stand for something else. Generally, most philosophical theories of mind, until recently, have assumed that cognition necessarily involves content or representations (Drestke 1995; Fodor 1987), and even embodied cognition partisans (Shapiro 2011) favor some form of mental representation. Two reasons for this are fairly straightforward.

The first is a kind of inference to the best explanation. If we ask how wingsuit fliers coordinate with other fliers to make formations, where they should position themselves in three-dimensional space as they free-fall, it seems that they must have internal representations of their and the other fliers' locations in airspace. Misjudgment of distance to ground, cliffs, or each other, or mistakes because of expectations of flight paths that differ from what other fliers actually do, can be attributed to flaws in the internal representation of the situation.

This argument has lost some of its pull as better explanations have been developed. Many advances in computation and artificial intelligence have brought very different approaches. In 1991, roboticist Rodney Brooks commented, on the systems he was the working on, "When we examine very simple level intelligence we find that explicit representations and models of the world simply get in the way. It turns out to be better to use the world as its own model" (1991, 140). Building a model of the external world into a system, which must be updated and then somehow internally evaluated by the system, is an extra step when the world with which the system interacts already exists. Hence, such an internal representation does not seem necessary for all systems.

This may be true of simple systems, but the second reason to think that internal representations must be necessary applies to more complex systems and concerns knowledge and self-awareness. Even if we can imagine nonrepresentational systems that interact with their environments in complex and interesting ways, it is hard to see how such systems could ever have knowledge of what they are doing. Slackliners walk on suspended lines, sometimes between cliff walls hundreds of feet off the ground (and not always tethered). If they have knowledge that they are on a line off the ground at all, that knowledge must be within them. If it is, it seems that they must have an internal representation of the world. Without such a representation, it is difficult to see how they could understand what they are doing.

In many theories, the content of internal representations is determined, at least partially, by factors external to the system within which the representations occur. For some, internal representations have the content they have because they covary or are caused by rapport with certain types of things in the world: boulder representations are such because they occur in the proximity of boulders, or because boulders cause them. What is needed for internal representation is not that the content of internal states be fully determined internally, only that there be such an internal content. Much of what humans do, especially concerning explicit conscious thought, seems to depend on having internal representations of the environment and the things in it. Perhaps as a result of this, it has been held as standard that cognition, including perception, is only possible for systems that form internal representations. Put otherwise, the class of beings who think and experience the world includes only those that form and act on internal representations. According to this view, noncognitive systems may act in complex but not intelligent ways. Brooks's robotic AI systems may be able to perform complex tasks but are not able to know that they are performing those tasks or have thoughts about them. That is, there is no cognition involved. In short, higher-level thought and action-involving cognition require representations.

Hubert Dreyfus (1992, 1999) has pioneered a critique of cognitivist computational AI views of the mind and representational accounts. For him, much of human (and animal) cognition and successful action is guided not by rules but rather by pragmatic engagements with the world. He has set the alternative agenda, but his views also need revision. Dreyfus describes highly skilled action without conscious direction as "absorbed coping." For example, driving to the grocery store or tying shoelaces, unaware of either the steps involved or remembering doing so. It would be a mistake, however, to think that expert athletes fit Dreyfus's examples.

Gunnar Breivik (2013) argues that expert athletes are anything but absorbed in Dreyfus's way. Instead, and in addition to automatic or off-line processes, they also constantly monitor their bodies, kinesthetic sensations, and environmental cues (see also Christensen, Sutton, and McIlwain 2016). Unlike everyday engagements, which fit the Dreyfusian model of competency and may be performed in an absorbed state, sport generally, and adventure sports particularly, are not mundane. Jørgen Eriksen (2010) extols the many virtues of Dreyfus's stance, from how it rightly makes room for the role of deliberation in sport at the initial stages of skill learning, or when time allows for it, to how experts dispose of representations and rules. But, criticizing his failure to account for skill specificity and its effect on the role of deliberation in sports, he argues how risky sports in fact expose the weakness in his account: these prevent deliberation *while* relying on focused attention. As Eriksen explains, "It appears than the only circumstances when these exemptions [that allow for deliberate behavior] do not offer a sufficient explanation are situations containing risk and danger, or if much is at stake" (2010, 77). Psychological research found that in these cases performers opt for extensive conscious control over automated routines "even if they have practiced the actions thousands of times" (77) Ericsson (2006) actually theorizes that experts do this through complex mental representation. Having to integrate different cognitive behaviors, in Eriksen's view, brings Dreyfus closer to more traditional cognitive views.

If these critiques are largely sympathetic to Dreyfus's overall aim, there has been also a cognitivist pushback. One such response is that Dreyfus's paradigmatic activities are, in fact, *literally* mindless, a black box of automatized responses (a process sometimes referred to as "reinvestment" in motor skill acquisition research; see Masters and Maxwell 2008),[3] The systems go on autopilot—subroutines kick in and take over while "the mind" is elsewhere. Sympathetic refinements and interpretations of Dreyfus, such as Mark Wrathall's (2014), have brought some light into the black box and refined the analysis of expertise. Regardless of such polemics, the fact is that any account that relies too heavily on automatized processes for expert skill does not fit Japanese swordsmanship and risk sports: these require complete *focus,* attendant awareness, and a capacity for improvisation attuned to high-stakes, rapidly changing situations. There can be no checking out.

When Kilian Jornet *runs* up and down Mont Blanc in less than five hours, he constantly scans the terrain ahead, monitors the rock, snow, and ice under his feet, and assesses his kinesthetic dynamics, collecting and paying attention to relevant phenomena. As his foot makes impact, he relies on his automatized leg stroke pattern. But, if he encounters something "unpredictable," his response can become deliberate and customized. Should an ice patch compromise the landing of his foot, to correct the situation his attention focuses on the slippage at the most basic level possible, combining automatized responses and explicit kinetic judgments. Noticing a precarious-looking cornice on his chosen line, he gauges and adapts his response—circumvent, jump over, tread carefully, plow through—in relation to his *present* ability, fatigue, and assessment of the cornice's potential peril. Consider autopilot on airplanes. It works very well in standard conditions and specific environments, but for difficult and unpredictable situations, the pilot must take control. The situations under discussion are some of the most demanding and unpredictable situations humans encounter, and are far from commonplace. They are the last place one wants a subroutine to take over.

To be sure, experts take time to deliberate in many sports and on many occasions, and also make use of mental representations—for example, an offshore solo sailor plotting a particular course based on weather conditions or reports. But, when the "heat is on" in sport generally, and with the added urgency of danger in risk sports, this precludes deliberation and declarative content, and vacates mental representation sub-personally too. This holds true even in a sport where there is more opportunity for deliberation, such as climbing. When Alex Honnold free-soloes a mountain face—no rope or safety equipment—he does stop to ponder potential moves when facing crux moments, but once he acts we simply find fully committed movement unfolding, as his account of his "very private hell" climbing Half Dome in Yosemite shows (Honnold and Roberts 2015). Of course, even if deliberation is excluded, it does not rule out sub-personal representation. To explain this process requires rethinking cognition radically. Enactivism, and within it, REC, we argue, is the best option.

Enactivism falls under the theoretical umbrella of embodied cognition, typically traced to Varela, Rosch, and Thompson (1991). Essentially, it is the view that action is a constitutive aspect of cognition and perception. Or, as Evan Thompson puts it, enactivism entails "the performance or carrying out of an action" (2007, 13). This emphasis on action is readily amenable to a view of high performance within the holistic framework, which, following Dewey's continuity hypothesis, advances continuities rather than divisions of actual processes while still permitting to draw meaningful demarcations (see Johnson 2007).

Among the various enactive stances, we favor Hutto and Myin's radical enactivism. Noë argues, without recourse to representations, that perception is something we do, a way of acting. Noë reduces phenomenal experience to sensorimotor contingencies and embodied skills, but there is clearly more to the body than this, as Gallagher (2012) argues. And Noë brings representations back into the theory after repudiating them, as Hutto and Myin (2013) point out. Thompson's autopoietic enactivism (2007) posits that organisms and life share organizational properties wherein the former self-organize themselves in relation to their environment normatively and cognitively, and that the human mind parallels. But Thompson's position remains taxonomically and conceptually anchored in a dualistic framework. Additionally, Sheets-Johnstone (2011) charges that Thompson ignores the connection with emotions or affects and, further, that he adopts a view of movement where kinesthetic dynamics are labeled as mere acts that hide the rich qualitative dynamics essential to a proper description and understanding of movement.

If Hutto and Myin's account is preferable, it is not without problems. For one, as John Sutton (2014) advances, REC, no matter the merit of its criticisms of content-bearing views, lacks a positive research program. And, it is also liable to Laurence Kirmayer's assessment that the enactive approach "is well-equipped to consider the ways in which mindfulness involves embodied and socially situated practice but has not sufficiently taken on board the cultural framing of experience" (2015, 459). But, in a case of mutually beneficial symbiosis, our present application of REC, while benefitting from its cognitive model, addresses both concerns, developing positively its agenda and incorporating culture.

It might be argued that both theories of mental representation and enactivism are not about phenomenal consciousness but about how our brains or embodied cognition, respectively, allow us to function in the world. Further, it may be adduced that lack of *experience* of propositional content does not entail lack of representational states. We agree that there is much that is correct in this view. This is clearly the case for enculturated states, precisely those we engage when planning a mountaineering sortie or doing philosophy, such as reading a chapter on risk sports and representation. But, in the case of flow and *mushin* states characteristic of adventure sports and *kenjutsu* experts, this deserves a closer look that assesses whether, or the extent to which, representational states are present or absent. The challenge is to explain intelligent, creative, and aware performance in dire situations that cut no slack. Next, we make the enactive case for non-contentful cognition in the context of expertise.

4 Radical Enactivism and High Performance

REC eliminates representations or mental content from basic minds. For REC, representation is not necessary for cognition or intelligent behavior, and to think that it is deeply misunderstands cognition. Representation can be involved in enculturated intelligent behavior, but it is not what makes behavior intelligent or sophisticated across most pragmatic contexts. "To think otherwise, as many do, is to ascribe features and characteristics to basic minds that belong only to enculturated, scaffolded minds that are built atop them" (Hutto and Myin 2013, ix). Supporters of enactivism argue that in fact what such systems do *is* cognition, and that higher order thought is built on the basic cognition that forms the foundation of intelligent behavior. Differently said, if we want to understand cognition, we should not start with representation. This is significant because we argue that enactive accounts best explain some of the most intelligent and creative activities humans perform, those that require most acute and informed perception. In other words yet, the sportspersons and martial artists we are considering should be described as effecting intentional action without content. What these highly skilled performers do, premised on intense and prolonged training, is very sophisticated and involves focus, awareness, improvisation, responsiveness, and intention. The question becomes, Is this a special type of enactive cognition?

REC conceptualizes basic minds "in terms of capacities," as Hutto and Myin (2013, 151) aver, that "do not represent conditions that the world might be in" (ix). These capacities are but skills refined over time in changing situations that require agents to suitably adapt. There is no skill development without confronting conditions that go beyond present capacities. This is a constitutive element that takes on added relevance in dire scenarios typical of risk sports and swordsmanship. Competitive swimmers, who practice in very controlled conditions, resort to interval workouts of varying combinations and diverse technique drills in order to improve. Because their environment is much more complex, it includes perilous currents, powerful waves, challenging temperatures, and even dangerous creatures, open-water swimmers must develop additional and very different skills that include varying stroke speeds and kinematics as well as emotional temperance to handle risk-elicited anxieties. Such skill development starts early—and simply.

Developmentally, we begin as basic minds, with our history of skillful worldly engagements allowing us to build more refined skills on top of this. Instead of a difference in kind, there is a continuity from basic organisms (even lowly bacteria and paramecia) to us, as Dewey argued. If we are endowed with much more sophisticated cognitive powers than even our closest primate "cousins," in our pragmatic worldly engagements we interact enactively. As Hutto and Myin explain, what gives organisms' perceptual experiences intentionality and phenomenality is not any kind of knowledge (either propositional or even embodied know-how), but "the concrete ways in which organisms actively engage with their environments. But in so engaging with their environments there is not a set of facts that organisms know, or need to know, at any level" (2013, 30). Interactions with the environment are intentional, both as being intended and being about something, but need not be *intensional* in terms of being semantically meaningful or having content premised on truth conditions obtaining. Thus there can be cognitive processes that skirt representational content. Even if we act before we think (to paraphrase Hutto and Myin), this does not make such action noncognitive. Precisely, cognition becomes enacted.

Clearly, sports and martial arts, as complex cultural activities, involve facts of many kinds that are content-based, from specific strategies and plays in, say, rugby to the history and tactics of varied schools of swordsmanship. Yet, at the level of *actual* performance, there are many situations when facts and content are irrelevant and best left behind, as when having to improvise and meet an unexpected move by the opposing team that throws the best-laid-out plans into disarray, dropping on a surprisingly steep skiing line, or trying to parry an oncoming blade from a unusual line of cut. In advance of examining sub-personal mental representation, it is expeditious to draw some theoretical connections with sport psychology now.

Recent theories offer similar and amenable analyses. The concept of implicit motor learning, in contrast to rule-based explicit models of learning, suggests a nonconscious sensitizing to features of an experienced situation paired with action over time, and that such implicitly learned skills are robust to challenges of variability, adaptability, and stress (Masters, van der Kamp, and Capio 2013). Taken further, by combining aspects of dynamic systems with ecological psychology, the ecological dynamics perspective in sport psychology argues that motor skills generally, and skilled performance in sport more specifically, must be understood as a coordinated system of performer and context through time, neither irreducible to either element in isolation nor divorced from action (Araújo, Davids, and Hristovski 2006; Davids et al. 2015). Humans, at least, also develop complex linguistic and conceptual capacities that allow articulating and understanding (and misinterpreting sometimes) matters in very rich and sophisticated ways. Some of these types of capacities require representations, of course. But as argued above, this is neither foundational nor fundamental but rather derivative and delayed developmentally.

Yet, where do we specifically find contentless—representationally empty—cognition in all of this? It is clear that experientially there are times when mental representations are not operative during performance. As Sutton and McIlwain explain (2015) not all sportspeople's expert knowledge is declarative nor do their representations involve language necessarily. As pointed out earlier, lack of phenomenological *experience* of representational content does not mean that it may not be a sub-personal affair. True enough. Relegating representation to the catacombs of cognition is a very appealing strategy. Closer scrutiny reveals that the devil hides in the details and the depths.

Because phenomenological accounts cannot account for processes below the threshold of awareness, we need to consider alternative sources. Minding this, Mark Johnson (2007) relies on neuroscientific, psychological, and linguistic research but also endorses a nonrepresentational and enactive account (based on James and Dewey). He develops what he calls "image schemas" to account for sub-personal phenomena. But, even these, which are patternings realized in topological neural maps, and hence incorporate brain/neural processes, are still nonrepresentational in the sense that they do not mirror, re-present, or map onto truth conditions of the world. As he explains, "What we (as scientists) theoretically recognize and describe as an organism's maps are not—for that organism internal representations that can correspond to external realities. Rather, what we call sensorimotor and somatosensory maps (whether in multicellular organisms, monkeys, or humans) are for that organism precisely its structures of experience and reality" (2007, 130).

Taking the physiological road of brain/neural processes and structures, or the modeling path of cognitive mechanisms, to bypass, supplement, or alleviate the limitations of phenomenological accounts does not necessarily lead to or equate with representational content in the standard philosophical sense.

If we reduce the scope of representations to action, we could argue that content or representation is superfluous in the context of action-oriented representations. Anthony Chemero's discussion of a cricket game posits that outfielder, ball, and light reflected from the ball are but one coupled system to which representation adds nothing (2009). As an alternative then, covariance is often invoked to bring representation in a rigorous-enough sense. But, as Hutto and Myin point out, "Anything that deserves to be called content has special properties—e.g., truth, reference, implication—that make it logically distinct from and not reducible to, mere covariance relations holding between states of affairs" (2013, 67). The issue is not with covariance itself, vital for scientific explanation, but rather with the fact that "it isn't able to do the required work of explaining content" (67). In short, covariance does not have truth-bearing properties, something content minimally requires.

An alternative response to keep representation at any level, sub-personal or not, by those who would naturalize cognition, is to develop a biological account. Thus, teleofunctionalism and teleosemantics purport to bring representations, respectively, as internal states that have semantic content by virtue of their indicating how things stand with the world, and as actually indicating truth conditions (see Millikan 1984, for example). But as Hutto and Myin (2013) argue, these biological accounts "lack the right resources for naturalizing mental states with properly semantic properties, such as truth and reference" (81). The hang-up involves truth conditions, which need to obtain. Sporting and martial action often operate without such conditions obtaining. This is problematic for those aspiring to make mental representation and content necessary for cognition (a discussion of *mushin* in part 5 adds more detail). Even if we ignore this issue with truth, there are further problems.

Habit raises another challenge. For REC, habit is a primary way that sophisticated mentality and performance arises. Not only are habits imprints of the organism's history of environmental interactions, but also these are how skilled prowess develops. Hutto and Myin consider it is much more plausible that "we become handy through a prolonged history of interactive encounters—through practice and habit. An individual's manual know-how and skills are best explained entirely by appealing to a history of previous engagements and not by the acquisition of some set of internally stored mental rules and representations" (2013, 47).

This aligns with Dewey's (1988) retooled view of habit, which, far from being a repetitive and unreflective affair, is actually an explicit, dynamic, responsive capacity to meet environmental challenges by efficiently restricting possibilities. Sportspeople in particular work within the boundaries of superfluous restrictions willingly embraced for the sake of the activity these make possible (Suits 2005). These also elicit the creative engagements that characterize expert action, for in willingly working with(in) these restrictions, performers invent novel ways of overcoming such rule-imposed limitations: consider, for example, the first person who came up with the bicycle kick, or eleven-time world surfing champion Kelly Slater improvising the first ever 720 (denotes degrees of rotation) during a freesurf session in Portugal.[4] If the rules of the sport are codified and understood representationally, the movements themselves dispose of such content. These kinetic creations arise from that history of previous engagements in the soccer or surfing environments; they do not arise from the application of internal representations or rules, since by their very nature and genesis—they are inventions—such accomplishments lie outside the scope of *re*-presentation, iteration, or rule application.

Sporting and martial contests also bring a high degree of unpredictability that, predictably, increase risk. Examining this further makes the case for a nonrepresentational account as well. Unpredictable conditions require immediate, spontaneous, and effective responses. Appealing to internally stored rules and representations does not help. Consider the unpredictability of a duel, wherein the goal is to surprise the opponent, or the shifting conditions typical of ice climbing and kayaking rapids. Conceptually, from a Wittgensteinian perspective, rules neither determine their own application nor establish the criterion for interpretive correctness. As such, correct response to environmental challenges cannot be obtained from rules alone. From a procedural and practical perspective, experts need to improvise *outside* of rules.

Spontaneous response and improvisational adaptation to changing conditions that often allow no time for pondering means leaving rules behind. This is not simply a matter of lacking the time to deliberate but also an issue of nonrepresentational action. Neither animals nor humans use mental representations when involved in such scenarios: strictly and nonfiguratively, there are no truth or veridicality conditions to be satisfied when hunting, fighting, or simul-climbing (part 5 delves further into this via *kenjutsu*). Sheets-Johnstone eloquently describes the kinetic dynamics of one such scenario, a lion hunting, from an enactive stance:

> Hunting lionesses notice and understand movement—kinetic comportments—as lines of force and correlatively, as potential increases or decreases in vulnerability … *straightaway*. A hunting lioness does not wonder: "What did that mean?" when its prey changes direction.… There is an *immediacy of meaning* that bespeaks a ready and sharp kinetic intelligence not to be confounded either with stimulus-response models of behavior or with an intelligence devoid of thought, that is, a mere sensorimotor intelligence. (2010, 176; emphases added)

The immediacy, instability, and potential lethality of lion hunts are no different from what is encountered in a duel or many sport scenarios. We find direct agent-environment interactions and no representations. Moreover, such behavior, as Sheets-Johnstone goes on to explain,

> is not run off by a motor program.… A hunt is not and cannot be a specific and repeatable sequence of actions, both because the world is not the same from one day to the next or possibly even from moment to moment with respect to terrain or weather, for example, and

> because the movement of living creatures is not the same from one day to the next or even from moment to moment. In essential ways, it is unpredictable. (2010, 176)

Predictably coming full circle, it may be considered a platitude to say that no two situations are exactly the same, and that we face unpredictability all the time. But, in the do-or-die situations under consideration, this is no banal platitude but sobering realization: a minuscule change can have fateful consequences. Fanning the flames, recognizing this possibility can recursively affect the performance as anxiety mounts and focus is lost.

To handle these situations, experts develop unique personal kinetic repertoires (PKRs). These endow them with "patternings"—sequential movements dynamically developed and performed in response to environmental stimuli. Patternings include but are not reducible to brain/neural processes, as their scope also contains the enactive and kinetic histories of the performer. As they encounter changing conditions, experts skillfully switch and combine among pertinent skills proper of both basic and enculturated minds. But, the primary level of engagement is enactive and "empty" at the interface between skills and needs. REC is in line with the ecological dynamics approach in sport psychology (Araújo, Davids, and Hristovski 2006; Davids et al. 2015), whereby skilled performance in complex, dangerous environments is the product of fundamentally and dynamically intertwined relations among cognition, perception, and action. Once acknowledged, the underlying holistic continuity does not exclude experiential distinctions and boundaries, as these make sense within the encompassing context of streaming phenomena. Alongside representations of the world and deliberation, expert movement *emerges* moment to moment from the immediate and dynamic interplay between performer and environment.

The path toward expertise, in this view, results from gradually increasing perceptual attunement to environmental affordances—a more thorough, context-sensitive, and dynamic bodyminded integration. Empirical research in sport psychology (Wulf 2007) shows that external focus on movement rather than internal (e.g., attending to turning the cranks at faster rpm rather than trying to move more forcefully) results in better performance from novice to experts. But skilled performers' rich PKRs allow them to freely and spontaneously toggle throughout the full attentional range, much as gifted organ players move through the different levels of keyboards, switching attentional foci and lifting appropriate feedback from the internal (kinesthetic and proprioceptive dynamics) to the external (target- or movement-effect focused). Differently said, performers are not enslaved by attentional focus per se, letting it roam while spontaneously adjusting it as need be. This is a *relational* process between performer and environment.

None of the above means that representations are eradicated forever and completely from the realm of high performance, of course. Indeed, a truly holistic account must include them as part of the continuous patternings. The very dynamic engagements of these sport and martial practices make ample room for them, before, after, and even during performance. But not at those crux moments where, we could say, brilliant intelligence-on-the-move puts life on the line.

One virtue of this account is that it bypasses the controversial issue of whether cognitivist accounts and their computational models can process information fast enough during expert sport performance (Moe 2007). Or rather, it makes it a nonissue by cleanly avoiding any concerns regarding processing speed: without representational content there is no-thing to process.

Disposing of representations as declarative and propositional content is the easy trick. Making these disappear sub-personally is harder. But, when it comes to making things vanish, the really difficult and interesting trick is to make mental content dissolve while keeping the hands in the open under the full light of focused awareness. Flow states and *mushin* spirit away content in this way. Whether these states are empty of content in the way that enactivism propounds needs to be carefully considered.

5 Risk Sports and Japanese Swordsmanship—*Kenjutsu*

Here we develop the argument for states of flow and *mushin* as experiential windows into nonrepresentational action when life is on the line. Crucially, the connection between REC's contentless cognition and the "emptiness" characteristic of these states, especially *mushin*, is spelled out. Japanese swordsmanship and its seminal treatises play a vital role as windows into the phenomenology of expertise under duress. This is related to concrete adventure-sport examples, specifically in the context of death, injury, and the predictable anxiety.

In the West, flow reflects subjective optimal experience. Flow experiences are usually analyzed into nine characteristics (Csíkszentmihályi 1990; Jackson 1996), not jointly necessary but paradigmatic. Those most pertinent phenomenologically include the merging of action and awareness, utmost concentration in the present task, confident sense of being in control, a distorted sense of time, and an intrinsic enjoyment of the activity. Ceteris paribus, the more that these characteristics are present, the stronger the experience. Csíkszentmihályi (1990) construes flow as a balance between skills and challenge: the closer the task brings performers close to their limits the better the engagement. Going below the optimum level of challenge results in boredom, and going above leads to anxiety. There is a range or continuum to flow in which skill refinement correlates with more difficult challenges. What is interesting is how some performers manage to purposely and purposefully get in such states in dreadfully risky and scary situations.

Questions easily arise concerning the experience of fear in such scenarios. A typical response is that as soon as one drops into a ski line, the fear disappears; all that is experienced then is the slope. When things go well, actions from that point happen smoothly, often as if by themselves. At that point, there is simply skiing. Other sports give similar accounts. Describing his performances, climber, BASE jumper, and wingsuit flier (among other daring activities) Dean Potter said, "I get to a place where I disappear completely, where I merge with the rock, when time slows down, my senses are unbelievably heightened, and I feel that oneness, that full-body psychic connection to the universe. It took risking my life to get there, but mission accomplished, it was worth it. That's why I climb" (quoted in Kotler 2014, 47). This disappearance of the self and holistic feelings of oneness with the environment are not unusual in nature sports (but are central in martial arts). Flow (and *mushin*) states agree with findings in sport psychology and studies of expertise (Sutton and McIlwain 2015) that highlight the inherent flexibility, adaptability, and dedication characteristic of such mastery. Of course, this does not mean that representations are not present in flow states. *Mushin* and its literature make the case for contentless cognition in action transparent.

Going then to the Japanese archipelago, samurai readiness to die at any moment required more than mere psychological advice, tactical smarts, and swordsmanship techniques: it needed a reconceptualization of how the self, life, and death were conceived. Zen Buddhism addressed this. Additionally, it afforded keen analyses of consciousness and associated phenomena like attentional focus. Two seventeenth-century contemporaries carry out the sharpest examination of mind-set and underlying psychophysical states: the legendary Yagyū Munenori (Yagy 2003) and the accomplished Rinzai Zen priest Takuan Sōhō (1986). Takuan's analyses were as pointed as Munenori's *katana*. Both treatises stress the point that, to be successful, action must be fluid and swift: any gaps lead to failure, which most likely means death.

If the Buddhist strategy was, in accordance with its soteriological aim (concerned with salvation), to facilitate enlightenment (*satori* 悟り) and instill disregard for the self and death, the hands-on method involved training to facilitate a state referred to in the martial arts as *mushin* 無心, literally "no-mind" but better rendered as a fluid yet attentive awareness unhindered by unnecessary and distracting thoughts. Munenori and Takuan are very clear that this is not a state of inattentiveness. Rather, performers are hyperaware and able to react immediately and with their *whole* being. Takuan says, "It is called No-Mind when the [heart-mind] has neither discrimination nor thought but wanders about the entire body and extends throughout the entire self" (Takuan 1986, 33).[5] Heart-mind here refers to the Japanese *shin* 心, which is analogous to bodyminded integration: emotion, will, and intellect blend psychosomatically, and superior achievement expresses this. As *shin* extends throughout the entire body, neither brain nor mind are singled out as sources of discrimination. Such readiness for action is fulsome in terms of the continuities involved. Munenori helps clarify: "When you have exclusively learned the various practices and techniques and made great efforts in disciplined training, there will be actions in your arms, legs, and body but none in your [heart-mind]. You will be unaware of where your [heart-mind] is.... Training is done for the purpose of reaching this state. With successful training, training falls away. This is the secret principle toward which all Ways progress" (Yagyu 2003, 75).[6]

This is not about not experiencing mental representations phenomenologically; rather these are found nowhere. When there is no discrimination, and our attention is not caught up with any one "thing," in contemporary terms this means that truth conditions are not applicable. Essential to content is that it be true or false, but, engaged in the thick of action—parrying a cut—truth and falsity are unimportant for the fighter. Drawing up such distinctions means getting caught up, or rather, cut up. This is not a matter of what is but rather of what *can* the swordsperson be aware of in terms of epistemic and normative content. Lacking correspondence to a state of affairs, representation of action and applicable mental content are eliminated. In such moments, there is neither sub-personal nor explicit content: the requisite conceptual and normative conditions for mental representation are not satisfied. Even at the physiological level, the brain is quite active but its processes do not carry content (and mapping meaning onto them is problematic, as discussed). What applies for truth conditions not being applicable and not obtaining applies to veridicality and related notions.

A swordswoman may have a number of internal models about the external environment, and if asked, she may visualize and explain tactics and techniques. In the middle of a duel, however, in a state of *mushin*, these are completely irrelevant and inoperative. Her state of readiness has nothing to do with appeals to truth or having her internal models correspond to the external world. Discriminating between true and false representations, the point for representational content becomes irrelevant. From an enactive standpoint, these have disappeared as if into nothing: there is only the urgency and immediacy of response to the situation. As such, this nondiscriminating state is analogous to a REC contentless mind. Suitably, the treatises cast it in terms of "emptiness."

Takuan writes that, in *kenjutsu*, "For the striking sword, there is no [heart-mind]. For myself, who is about to attack, there is not [heart-mind]. The attacker is Emptiness. His Sword is Emptiness. I, who am about to be struck, am Emptiness" (1986, 37).[7] Turning opponent, sword, and even oneself into emptiness involves complete nondiscrimination. To achieve this, concern with, and the relevance and role of, truth and falsity must go. Paradoxically appropriate, such extreme divestment, wherein even caring for one's life dissolves, is what makes room for anxiety-free action. Simply put, emptiness forecloses situational categorization and vacates representations.

This brings up an important point of connection among REC, *mushin,* and a triad of concepts that relate to emptiness and, by extension, lack of content. All have epistemic and metaphysical ramifications with many rich and varied translations and connotations. Given the exegetical complexity, the following merely highlights key pertinent ideas (see appendix in Ilundáin-Agurruza 2016). The first is the Chinese *wu* 無, rendered as nothing, nil, hollowness, or emptiness. Its Daoist lineage connects it with *wuwei* 無為, effortless action, which is closely related to *mushin* and peerless performance. The second is *kōng* 空, which refers to the emptiness that underlies worldly phenomena in the Buddhist sense of *sunyata.* Thus it ascribes emptiness to the very fabric of reality and subtracts it from epistemic contexts. The third is a Daoist concept, *xū* 虛. It can be translated as emptiness, void, unoccupied, and even false. Interestingly, for Daoist sage Zhuangzi (1968), whose views influenced Zen Buddhism, *xū* is a vital constituent of the *zhēnrén* 真人, a superior person. As sagely role model, she acts perfectly attuned to her environment with the fluidity and efficacy of *mushin* states in all kinds of contexts, from social to artistic or martial.

These concepts divest content not just phenomenologically, but epistemically and normatively. When emptiness, nothingness, and void concern the state of mind of the performers, the latter are supposed to adapt seamlessly to their situation much like water adopts a container's shape. The sage, privy to the ultimate emptiness of reality, does not attempt to mirror reality cognitively, as there is nothing to correspond to. Instead, and here *wu* and *xū* become pertinent, the sage adapts her responses, much as for swordsmen the idea of a correspondence between internal model/truth conditions/external world becomes superfluous. To cite samurai and author Issai Chozansi, "Following the perceptions of the [heart-mind], the speed of practical application is like opening a door and the moonlight immediately shining in.... Victory and defeat are the traces of practical application. But if you don't have *conceptualization,* form will not have aspect" (2006, 118; emphasis added).[8] Indeed, this lack of conceptualization bespeaks of lack of content all the way down: if victory and defeat / truth and falsity fall by the wayside, dueling swordsmen (or risk sportspersons) act best without representations, as REC endorses.

As mentioned, grave injury and death are constitutive in these sporting and martial practices, not merely contingent. In other sports and martial arts (e.g., tae kwon do), failure may be equated metaphorically with death, but in risk sports and *kenjutsu*, it could mean *actual* death or very serious injury. This is pertinent because such perils are a primary source of tension and distraction. Additionally, it discloses further the connection between a REC-ish (but not reckless) contentless cognition and activities that court danger. Next follow descriptions of wingsuit flying, snowboarding, and luge. These illustrate varying degrees of confrontation with the grim reaper in risk sports. Since *kenjutsu*'s raison d'être was to kill an opponent, who likely had trained for years to kill before being killed, it is patently clear that mortality was always looking over the shoulder of the swordsmen, ergo a description is obviated.

How we face our mortality, as Martin Heidegger (1962) makes clear, has deep existential consequences. This in turn directly affects performance, which has phenomenological import for the readiness and capacity to focus of the performer. Sportspersons and martial artists have the same objective in this regard—emotional temperance and equanimity—but seek this usually through different methods and for dissimilar reasons. More germane to our interests, this spills over to cognition. If mental representation is not only ill-advised at the explicit level of declarative or propositional content, or ultimately not found at the sub-personal level in intense action, then adding deadly risk accentuates this.

To begin with wingsuit flying, skydivers need to acquire extensive experience, hundreds of jumps, before progressing to wingsuit flying. Wingsuit flying is basically controlled falling, with horizontal speeds that can top 200 mph (300 kp/h), with minimal movements of head, neck, torso, and limbs controlling direction and speed. It is also one of the deadliest sports, with about two hundred deaths between 1981 and 2012 (www.wingsuitfly.com). As the website Wingsuitfly (under)states, "It is generally accepted that wingsuiting adds a degree of complexity to skydiving, with risks such as flat-spins (uncontrollable spinning), burble (a vortex in the parachute deployment area), tail-strikes (hitting an aircraft's tail on exit), twists (a spinning parachute), extra material to manage during a malfunction, and difficulty in depressurising wings prior to parachute deployment. Failure to handle these issues has been known to cause fatal injury" (2017).

The year 2016 has been the deadliest on record so far for wingsuit fliers: by midsummer, there had been thirty-one deaths (Bisharat 2016). Small wonder the title of a *New York Times* article: "It's More Like a Suicide Than a Sport" (Caesar 2013). With statistics like these, its potential lethality is so unquestionable that one better be at peace before deciding to jump.

Professional snowboarders and free-skiers make their living by riding steep and dangerous lines while being filmed. Death, if less common, is no stranger to these sportspersons either: Swedish free-skier Matilda Rapaport, filming in Chile, died a few days after the July 14, 2016, avalanche caught her (Pursell 2016). The slopes are typically of such a sustained steep pitch that snow slides with the riders in the form of sluff avalanches, large amounts of snow that travel alongside riders at high rates of speed. If they fall, they may slide as far as 500–1000 feet (200 to 350 meters). Of course, in addition to the steepness and fast-moving snow, there are large cliffs, crevasses or deep fissures, cornices where an overhanging mass of hardened snow sits at the edge of a precipice, and slab avalanches, in which a section of the slope breaks loose at the same time, and often can result in the skier's burial and demise.

The sport of luge, if considerably less deadly, makes the relevance of intensity and fast reaction times under duress more explicit. As lugers sled supine and feet-first, they negotiate tight turns at speeds ranging from 70 to 90 mph (110–150 km/h). Besides the familiar Olympic luge in artificial tracks, there is a natural track version that uses mountain roads and paths with ice walls carved and built on the sides. In either one, the lugers must make use of continuous bodily micro-adjustments (e.g., shifting their weight) and the steering system to sled in the ideal line while maintaining focus as the track's roughness and the turns' high g-forces beat them. Common across these high-speed sliding sports, such as free-skiing, snowboarding, luge, or big-wave surfing, is the reality that the tiniest of these micro-adjustments can mean the split-second difference between an exceptional clean ride and a sudden crash likely to have fatal or maiming consequences. Research with luge athletes (Erickson et al. 2015) and extreme sport athletes (Brymer and Schweitzer 2013) highlights the constantly negotiated interplay between fear and optimal performance in such risk sports.

Given the dangers involved, anxiety about their demise or severe harm is at the forefront of such sportspersons and duelists' concerns. Analyzing anxiety or fear, Cappuccio and Wheeler (2012) examine Heideggerian existential angst, regarding which, "When the human agent forgets about the network of endless open questions in which it is trapped in Angst, it buries the fundamental sense of uncanniness under its habitual commerce with worldly things, and becomes 'tranquillized': it can then go back to its skilled coping with the world" (2012, 31).[9] In simpler words, when we are anxious, in this case about our end (timely or not), our inauthentic response is to ignore this as best we can through everyday distractions. For sportspersons it may involve busying themselves with the equipment not so much to check it but to divert thoughts from an upcoming competition or challenge. Or, it may involve belittling the issue. Spencer Seabrooke broke the world record for crossing a slackline untethered, walking across a chasm 210 feet (64 meters) wide and 950 feet (300 meters) high. When asked if he was afraid of death, his blasé response sounds more inauthentic than anything: "No, are you? … We are all gonna die someday. I am not reckless. I feel more in control free soloing on a slackline [walking it without a tether] than driving down the highway" (Yan 2017). Contrariwise, Potter admitted that his demise was no light matter: "That's always been the scariest part of climbing, falling … or right when you are gonna fall.… That would be it, it would be my death" (2011). (Potter died in a wingsuit accident in 2016.) He compensated for this with his moments in flow and holistic experiences.

Comparatively, Shi Dejian, a contemporary kung fu master who courts death as samurai would, regularly performs his moves standing on cliff faces hundreds of feet high. Peter Gwin narrates seeing Dejian standing on the ledge of a cliff: "He smiles at me. 'You are afraid?' he asks, seeing the look on my face. 'Kung Fu is not only training the body; it is also about controlling fear.' He hops lightly from one foot to the other, lunging, punching, spinning, each step inches from a horrifying fall. His eyes widen as he concentrates.… 'You cannot defeat death,' he says.… 'But you can defeat your fear of death'" (2011, 112). Such practice nurtures Dejian's ability to educe *mushin* (*wushin* for him, being Chinese) when "death anxiety" would normally interfere, and truly confront it.

Indeed, risk sports and *kenjutsu* have a way of directly slicing through everydayness. While the urge to distract oneself is even stronger, they also make our attempts at self-deception all the more obvious. In a more positive light, they open up the possibility of confronting the reaper and making peace with him. That is, they afford the possibility of responding to the two ways death confronts us, abstractly and concretely. As to the former, it means encountering *our* death at the most fundamental level of our existence, an exeunt from this world—which for Heidegger is ontological angst. Concerning the latter, we face death at the concrete level of the specific way in which we may die, peacefully in bed, falling from a great height—which brings anxiety in what Heidegger calls the ontic level. While risk sportspeople often focus on anxiety and a specific death, angst is an existentially vital human condition we all face.

The effect of anxiety is clearest and starkest in cases of sport choking (choking occurs in other contexts also). When choking, skills already mastered are compromised. Regardless of whether the causes may be excessive self-monitoring, distraction, a combination thereof, or an ecologically broader palette, the emotionally decisive factor, phenomenologically, is fear (Ilundáin-Agurruza 2015). This is relevant because if performers go back to a novice-like reliance on consciously controlled rule implementation instead of expert focus, spontaneity, and automatism, they will choke and fail. If some consummate athletes choke and spectacularly fail when facing a penalty kick or a difficult shot on the golf course or tennis court, what to say of those who face *truly* hazardous situations?

Handling these requires strategies for performance as well as a personal philosophy of life. The latter is very clear in the Japanese case (part 6). Some advise visualization as a way to desensitization. Samurai were encouraged to picture daily their death in all kinds of exquisite and gory detail, as famed *Hagakure* author Tsunetomo Yamamoto advised (1979). This has been appropriated nowadays by sport psychology. Schack et al. (2014), for example, rely on mental action representations to advance motor imagery training (albeit this is a potential representational imbroglio we stay out of for reasons of scope).

A way to handle matters that opens the door to authenticity is by confronting our mortality explicitly before and after the performance while finding a way to completely vacate such concerns, at least during do-or-die moments. If representational content is crucial for entertaining the very idea of our death and the attitude to take, flow and *mushin* states are most helpful, if elusive, for dispelling such thoughts when actually facing a deadly situation.

Bringing the peril of *imminent* death or serious injury into the equation cuts through the chaff of *explicit* mental content; it excludes strategies that rely on representations cashed out as declarative or propositional content, and concomitant truth or veridicality conditions. This pertains to the practical sense that articulating either worries or possible solutions propositionally is dangerously distracting: thinking to oneself, "I am scared, I can die here!" is likely to make that happen. Getting back on the slackline, self-styled guru Jonathan Hill elaborates, "You have to train the mind like a muscle. Be completely in the present." A slight waver in your focus, a slight inkling of fear, and you'll fall. Highlining is being present taken to the extreme" (Yan 2017). Besides dislodging explicit propositional content, performance when so much is on the line, literally (!), and with such extreme presence of mind, is predicated on being fully present by vacating the sub-personal level also.

To better assess this theoretically, we need to rely on the full range of levels of awareness applicable to skill execution and not just the customary two—otherwise we mischaracterize expert performance and its unique states. Many commentators on either effortless attention (Bruya 2010) or *mushin* (Suzuki 1993; Carter 1997, 2008) struggle with how to conceptualize these states. They waver between endorsing unabated automatism and the need for some sort of agency and awareness. Bruya explains, "A high-level effortless action as purely automated, thereby [would seem] to preclude credit to a subject for creativity, insight, emotional expression, and so forth" (2010, 15). All of them see these as mutually exclusive states wherein performers either act like automata, to echo Suzuki's words, or are fully aware. In keeping with the underlying holism, it is a matter of continuities, in which performers with different skill levels or in different states (sluggish, ill, fully ready) range variously on the continuum of awareness in skill execution.

Three levels interact fluidly in skilled performance. Specified first phenomenologically then psychologically, these are (1) reflective or conscious awareness, (2) the subpersonal or unconscious, and (3), a thick non-tacit pre-reflective bodily self-awareness or Jamesian Background/fringe of consciousness (James 1918). The first two are familiar enough; as for the latter, the non-tacit pre-reflective consciousness (Høffding 2014) or James's background (Mangan 2007) is not a mechanism but a phenomenological structure of our cognition that acts as in-between layer between the other two. It proves advantageous because, being close to sub-personal phenomena, allows judgment, as the tip-of-the-tongue phenomenon (the sensation of being unable to retrieve a word or name that is partially remembered and on the cusp of being retrieved) evinces, and thereby facilitates immediate and effective response in the sort of situations risk sportspersons and swordsmen encounter (Ilundáin-Agurruza 2015, 2016).

By the time sportspeople like Honnold, McNamara, and Potter, and *kenjutsu* masters like Munenori, Musashi, and twelfth-century peerless female samurai Tomoe Gozen, meet the frightful challenges of the moment with equanimity, and with actions in their arms, legs, and body but none in the mind, they have been developing the capacities proper of basic minds through years of training up to that moment. They have built a unique nonrepresentational PKR.[10] The best of them elicit flow or *mushin* states when the need arises. High-stakes, intense action channeled through flow or *mushin* seems to work outside representational content. Where accounts that favor these capsize and wreck, the present REC model gracefully sails onward. Nevertheless, navigating the cultural seascape presents interesting new challenges.

6 The Role of Culture

How does culture affect, if at all, the kinds of cognition, performance states, and activities under discussion? That is, if there is no content connected to the mental states that accompany the high-performance activities of martial artists and risk sportspersons under discussion, how can these states be influenced by culture? Now we aim to provide a theoretical explanation for why the cultural context in which activities arise can create differences even in cases when flow and *mushin* are closest. A sociohistorically situated model of cognition and action is advanced in order to consider the role of culture, specifically Buddhism, and we explore the dynamic boundary between enculturated representation and nonrepresentation. Overall, this shows how enculturation influences practice and experience in deeply constitutive ways that all too often are ignored at the peril of oversimplification.

Cultural and phenomenological accounts help us understand these activities. In simple biological systems, meaningful relationships are often found in organisms' interactions with their immediate environment as required by evolutionary pressures. For humans, meaning arises within narrative accounts in specific cultural contexts. It is peremptory then to examine how the narratives for seventeenth-century *kenjutsu* and contemporary extreme sports differ. A socially situated and extended model helps here.

There is an affinity between situated cognition and enactivist approaches, Shaun Gallagher (2013) details. In a cognitively situated model, social, institutional, historical, and cultural factors can be constitutive or contributory. We endorse a constitutive model. Phenomenologically, the idea is that just as there are embodied, subjective, and intersubjective factors that structure our experience, geo-cultural features such as topology, climate, and political institutions are also structurally constitutive. This view of extended coupling of creatures and environments, such that different worlds, or *ümwelts*, arise, follows pioneer biologist Jacob von Uexküll (2010): the oak tree is a number of different things for those creatures with which it interacts—fox, owl, beetle, hawk, forester. José Ortega y Gasset (2006) adapted this specifically to humans: our cultural and existential history changes a given locale. Skier, photographer, and shepherd experience an escarpment as a radically different environment. The coupling between organism and environment, and how this relates to risk, is something that Dewey captures diaphanously: "At every moment, the living creature is exposed to dangers from its surroundings, and at every moment, it must draw upon something in its surroundings to satisfy its needs. The career and destiny of a living thing are bound up with its interchanges with environment, not externally but in the most intimate needs" (cited in Johnson 2007, 153). Dangers to which sportspeople and swordsmen are or were exposed inform their cognition intimately, and as part of a socially extended cognition.

Gallagher argues for a socially extended model as he develops the idea of what he calls "mental institutions," "in the sense that they are not only institutions with which we accomplish certain cognitive processes, but also are such that without them such cognitive processes would no longer exist" (2013, 6). The legal system provides him with a concrete application to develop his argument. To the extent that we cognitively engage with legal "tools," contracts, and legal institutions—for example, those of property or of rights—we extend and transform our cognitive processes. More importantly and controversially, this gives grounds to extend cognitive processes beyond the heads and brains of jurists, lawyers, juries, and the like, as there are some judgments that "depend on extra-neural practices and process that guide … or that allow the manipulation and management of a large amount of empirical information" (6) The complexity of courtroom legal cases means that these cannot be reduced to processes just in the brain. Rather, such intricacy calls for a distributed cognition across various agents and levels, from jurists to legal repositories. Judgments that could not happen otherwise are possible now. Gallagher states, "If we think of the mind not as a repository of propositional attitudes and information, or in terms of internal belief-desire psychology, but as a dynamic process involved in solving problems and controlling behavior and action—in dialectical, transformative relations with the environment—then we extend our cognitive reach by engaging with tools, technologies, but also with institutions" (2013, 7).

This reaching out and transforming take place in communal settings, in the company of others. If the family may be ontogenetically the first institution (Gallagher 2013, 7), our capacities flourish and are refined in the broader, deeper context of communities that serve as background to institutional practices. These provide the standards of excellence and norms of conduct (MacIntyre 2008) that help develop our cognitive faculties and social engagements. Just as the legal system is a clear example of an extended and socially situated cognition, other institutions and communities mirror this.

The sporting and martial worlds have clear equivalents to all cognitively situated factors Gallagher mentions: institutions, communities, and judgments. At the front lines of performance, the equivalent to legal judgments are the "kinetic judgments" of skills in action: lugers make constant judgments and adjustments as they slide into sharp turns; cutting and parrying need endless fine-tuning and adaptation to the opponent's blade. Such kinetic judgments are part of complex bodies of enactive and enacted performances (refined and passed on within the context of communities). Holistically continuous movements-in-the-moment, kinetic judgments intertwine in complex ways with mental representation and propositional content, often becoming integrated as part of narratives that culture modulates.

Because cultural background extends our cognitive and skillful abilities, it uniquely shapes these: Buddhist tenets or Western secular beliefs subtend and make sense of performers' kinetic judgments very differently. Nonetheless, reflecting the tension between explanatory levels, there is a controversy between universality at the level of skills and "raw experience" and the distinctiveness of cultural expressions. It may be tempting to suppose that non-interpreted and contentless perceptions and actions will result in phenomenological, functional, and structural parity between flow and *mushin* states and, by extension, between risk sports and martial skills. Elsewhere we (Krein and

Ilundáin 2014; Ilundáin-Agurruza 2016, ch. 9) have argued that while *mushin* and flow are extremely close functionally, crucial differences remain. One worth mentioning is that while the West tends to view flow as ancillary by-product to competitive performance goals—a bonus to enjoy should it arise—*mushin* has been expressly cultivated in Japan.

Finding evidence for this is challenging. Reflecting on one's experiences during a high-risk activity is a good way to end up severely injured or dead. This advises against researchers asking athletes to reflectively engage their action when walking a slackline between cliff walls untethered, for instance. Further, when experiencing *mushin* or flow, attempting deliberate analysis or phenomenological reduction will result in the state disappearing along with spontaneous action. Takuan states, "If one puts his mind in the action of his opponent's body, his mind will be taken by the action of his opponent's body. If he puts his mind in his opponent's sword his mind will be taken by that sword" (1986, 29).[11] It is easy to become distracted or caught up by phenomena directly tied to action; all the more so if one tries to think about the thinking itself. Given this, any analysis must be ex post facto. It does not follow, however, that culture does not influence such states. Before considering this, here is Takuan's advice: "The effort not to stop the mind in just one place—this is discipline.... Put nowhere, it will be everywhere. Even in moving the mind outside the body, if it is sent in one direction, it will be lacking in nine others. If the mind is not restricted in one direction, it will be in all ten" (32). After-the-fact reflection means a culturally mediated articulation should performers attempt to understand or explain. That said, an unencumbered mind, as Takuan advises, will be where it needs to be and *also* allow for more clarity and a better grip of the moment.

Two sport psychology studies that ascertained the statistical occurrence of the nine flow characteristics in elite sportspeople (Jackson 1996) and Japanese top athletes (Sugiyama and Inomata 2005) had very similar results across most traits, including those most relatable to *mushin*. The one notable exception was concentration in the task at hand, where 80 percent of Western athletes reported experiencing this while the number for Japanese athletes reached 96 percent. The prevalence of Buddhism, mindfulness, and meditation in Japanese culture may help explain this difference. Even if contemporary Japanese sports are close to Western counterparts, their ethos still carries traditional martial arts values and structural features. As Yoichi Kozuma points out in his cultural psychology study, modern Japanese sport culture's "philosophy of training, practice, and sportsmanship still reflected the samurai culture of the past" (2009, 206). Revealingly, among all possible candidates for being most influential today in Japanese sport culture, Kozuma singles out two swordsmen, Miyamoto Musashi and Yamaoka

Tesshu, and highlights the influence of Zen Buddhism. Since mindfulness and attentional focus are the clear point of departure, mindfulness meditation studies help us see how cultural context may influence states without content.

Mindfulness has been adopted and adapted in many different contexts in the West. Moreover, it has proven popular with current neuroscientific research on brain plasticity and other effects, such as attentional mechanisms (Posner, Rothbart, and Tang 2015) or social cognitive studies (Lee et al. 2012). Examining mindfulness in contemporary psychiatry, and in agreement with our socially situated stance, Kirmayer states, "The effects of meditation on the brain may also depend on the individual's developmental history as well as the challenges and affordances of current social contexts—all of which, in turn, depend on culture" (2015, 451). If this is true, culture influences physiology and changes phenomenal experience. It seems clear that culture fundamentally influences training and practices. Besides regulating normative aspects of sports and martial arts, such as the value ascribed to success, results, and process, culture also affects our phenomenological states at the level of what William James called "pure experience," a "plain, unqualified activity or existence, a simple that" (1976, 13). *Kenjutsu* practice was rigorous and repetitive, with Zen practice influencing it (King 1994; Suzuki 1993). There is some overlap with the various approaches that high-risk sportspersons take, who often embrace certain aspects of Eastern practices, but actual training methods differ considerably. Further, as Kirmayer points out, instructions concerning meditative practices are not neutral. They often provide guidance to understand experiences undergone during meditation. He explains, "Meditative states may reflect ways of being in the world that are based not only on neurophenomenology (that is, the intrinsic structure of our nervous systems) but equally on culturally mediated forms of understanding and action that are conveyed through body practices, narratives, and discourse" (Kirmayer 2015, 459).

Accordingly, cultural context can significantly affect even *mushin* and flow states. The many traits they share (under some descriptions) notwithstanding—attentive mindfulness or reduced or absent internal dialogue—belie underlying structural differences. The most significant one regarding both meditative practices and performance states concerns historical sources and their implementation. Specifically, the fundamental doctrines of Buddhism: the Four Noble Truths, Eightfold Path, and Middle Way, and the three metaphysical elements of ignorance (*avidya*), impermanence (*anicca*), and no-self (*anatta*). Of these, the most significant in *mushin*, and most often ignored in Western adaptations of Buddhist practices, is the doctrine of no-self (Samuel 2015).

No-self, *muga* (無我) in Japanese, is vital in Buddhist soteriology to eliminate attachments, desire, and surmount the fear of death—none of which is involved in Western sport. Through practices such as meditation, the idea is to overcome the delusion of the self (empirical and transcendental) and render it as nothingness in order to discard the desire and attachment that lead to suffering. This realization partially brings freedom from desires and attachments. Our aim is not to idealize Japanese swordsmen as devout Buddhists, but it would be a mistake to ignore that much of the training and understanding of their experiences happened within a Buddhist framework. Sport philosopher and *kendoka* Shinobu Abe confirms that swordsmen had to "overcome fear of death and *delusion*" (Abe 1986, 47; emphasis added). In the context of our discussion, intentional action without contentful representation functionally transmutes into emptiness in the Buddhist framework. Put otherwise, where there is no self, only action remains. In both an enactive account and the context of emptiness in East Asian thought, this is at the foundation of superb performance. Performers, whether risk sportspersons or dueling samurai, do their best when empty of any desires, declarative thinking, and discriminations that might connect with mental content. This leaves room for contentless "thinking in movement" and kinetic judgment in action. Moreover, without self there is no room for death anxiety to abide. Issues such as victory or success are even less significant. Paradoxically, as masters often remark, this is *the* way to succeed and live to see another day. This dialectic also reflects and redresses the basic tension between our proclivity to seek victory or *care* about the result or what happens to us, and how this usually gets in the way. A self-less *muga* person performs in *mushin*, empty of content; she responds and adapts perfectly and instantaneously.

Ignoring the cultural contribution to our cognition misses the forest for the trees. It is convenient but unwisely cherry-picks what *seems* advantageous. There is an informally built culture around the experience of flow in alternative and risk sports. Risk sportspersons often turn to Eastern practices to gain a measure of equanimity, but such attempts rarely compare to fully developed concepts of mindfulness and *mushin* in a Buddhist context. The traditional Buddhist framework provides a foundation for how *mushin* is to be cultivated, attained, and regulated.

In this context the development of *mushin* is, primarily, a means within a soteriology. Mere intellectual comprehension and study, appreciation for various perspectives, or even committed belief, do not suffice. What is needed is lived, embodied, actual self-realization through practice *and* behavioral change. After key lessons, swordsmanship manuals often and variously stress this. Musashi (1983) admonishes regularly, "This should be examined with care," or "You should train these well," and "You must understand these well." By this he means that study alone falls short. Apprentices had to rigorously test these until they made sense "bone-to-bone" (treatises were for in-house trainees). It is the kind of vetting process we can attribute to devoted swordsmen who literally waged their lives on truly embodying their art's innermost secrets. But, such training and reflection are only part of the process of becoming an expert and of understanding the experience accordingly. Takuan Sōhō (1986) and Chozanshi (2006) both emphasize not to confuse the way of the sword, even if steeped in Buddhism, with *the* Way. In a parallel way for us, as Kirmayer notes, "enactivism needs to be taken further to recognize that practices like mindfulness have a history and a social/environmental context" (2015, 453). The point is applicable not just comparatively but also *within* the Western framework.

A situated and cultural lens sensible to corporeality is important for sport psychology. Attentional focus studies are a suitable parallel to *mushin*'s mindful attention. Besides helping to account for the high specificity of sporting and martial skills, minding cultural and situated aspects makes the case for how qualitative studies can supplement a predominantly quantitative methodology. As explained, external focus on task goals seems to make actions more effective (Wulf 2007), while dissociative attention apparently enhances expert performance (Lohse 2015. Hence, external focus and dissociation are often assessed as more "valuable" strategies for training and competition than internal and associative focus. Practically, the focus is on external and quantitative facets of performance, such as VO2 max, watt output, or timing improvements. Benchmarks are established through competitive comparison. But, if interest shifts to qualitative aspects, validating the very experience of how X *feels* kinesthetically or kinetically (often hallmarks of flow states)—for example, how *well* one is gliding on the luge track or how swimming in the open water *feels*—an internal focus is preferable. This is the case in particular for nature and risk sports, where the conditions of success are different from competitive ones, which instrumentalize qualitative aspects as means to winning results. This concerns perceptual dynamics. How these impinge on culture is the next and last waypoint.

If internal representations are required for some types of understanding, such as how actions play a role in a larger cultural framework, and if the best performances in swordsmanship and risk sports include actions that are independent of contentful representations, then there is a seeming tension between enculturated and representational cognitive expressions and the nonrepresentational model defended here. It is requisite to explain, however briefly, how they relate to each other under pain of opacity if not incongruence. Does the effect of culture go all the way down, influencing the very contentless engagements of performers? Does the nonrepresentational level affect culture? In essence, this is a two-way process that goes bottom up and top down. As Chozanshi elucidates, "Principle is explained from the top down, while training is sought after from the bottom up, and this is just the way things are" (2006, 59).

This bidirectionality is a pervasive feature of the enactive and situated perspective. When discussing mental institutions, Gallagher corroborates this, for we do not and cannot keep "in the head" the legal system in toto, and its many elements effectively extend the mind. Gallagher argues that this "also suggests that cognition does not simply extend from the brain outward to incorporate tools, technologies, and institutions, but that it sometimes works from the outside in; tools, technologies and institutions often shape our cognitive processes, make our brains work in certain ways, and may even elicit plastic changes in neuronal structure" (2013, 7). Likewise, our perceptual and skillful engagements go inside out and vice versa. That is, at the interface between our skillful worldly interactions and our narrative expressions thereof, we find that, congruent with the continuity hypothesis, the nonrepresentational and the representational interact richly at their points of surface tension.

In trying to get a handle on what Western athletes can say about their experiences, it is important to note two ideas. First, an enactive cognition does not entail lack of phenomenal content in human performance and experience. Such cognition may be nonrepresentational, but it can have phenomenological content endowed with intentionality and phenomenality. It could be argued that this *is* content, but this is not within the bounds of mainstream representational views, and has a higher burden of proof. Perhaps it could be theorized as Jamesian "pure experience" or raw sensation. Second, at the higher order of enculturation, narratives articulate what this is about. Sensations become *interpreted* perceptions: the feeling of uncontrolled skidding on a slope becomes "slippery" or "scary." But, for risk sportspeople, the rich supply of intense experiences needs a more robust framework for narratives with which to better describe and understand such experiences.

7 Conclusion

Dire scenarios like those found in adventure sports or *kenjutsu* place performers at the outer boundaries of human skill and experience. Their richer PKRs enable them to take on bigger challenges than others while distributing attentional resources better. Because of this, they can live experiences foreclosed to those less skilled and can notice more fine-grained qualities in the experiences. Just as wine experts can distinguish a palette of aromas and flavors beyond most people's capabilities, experts-on-the-edge can read rock, water, wind, and their bodies as easily as the reader makes out these words in what otherwise would be invisible meanings and blurry lines for the illiterate. To make reference to Sutton and McIlwain's exposition on sport experts, they think "in more thorough, more varied, and more fine-grained terms about current conditions … and about specific actions and responses" (2015, 101). Such superior skills, discriminatory capabilities, and richer experiences, however, result in harder articulation and comprehension challenges.

Extreme circumstances starkly highlight the challenge of "languaging" the nonrepresentational deployment of skillful ways and resultant phenomenal experience. Clearly, we can have phenomenal experience without representation. The experiences of some sportspeople in flow states and martial artists in *mushin* are quite rich phenomenologically, but defy both articulation and representation. Performers may vaguely speak of feelings of oneness with something larger than themselves, as Potter does; they may cryptically talk about egolessness as Munenori does. Zimmermann and Saura detail how "adventurers summarize their experiences by using metaphors, interjections, one-word utterances: breath-taking, awesome, extreme, exciting, amazing, adrenaline. All of these indicate a corporeal engagement that is better experienced than explained" (2017, 166). These are but nebulous approximations to ostensibly ineffable experiences. Free-diver Eric Fatthah avows, "No words can ever describe what dives over 80 [meters] feel like—the experience is so otherworldly, dreamlike, transcendent, and exhausting, that the only way you can really understand the experience is to experience it yourself" (Fattah 2010). Generally, they cannot rely on those who might provide suitable theoretical or semantic frameworks (not many researchers line up their ranks).

It is clear that the experiences of risk sportspersons are profound, yet many struggle to understand and verbalize them. This points to a disconnection between encultured and nonrepresentational levels, especially in the West. Comparatively, the centuries-old traditional Buddhist context in Japan and its sophisticated analyses, accompanying *dō* practices, and express cultivation of *mushin* provide a robust cultural framework in which the experiences can occur and be understood and articulated.

When it comes to making sense of such experiences as descending a 60-degree slope or deflecting a blade shy of one's neck, it is no wonder performers resort to platitudes, clichés, or dumbstruck silence. The concepts may not be there to capture sensorial input and phenomenological gestalt quality of such intense experiences. Yet, speechlessness does not (have to) mean meaninglessness. It may mean finding keener, deeper, better cognitively situated ways that may bridge the nonrepresentational and content. To cite Kirmayer, "The idea that we can get beyond culture ignores the extent to which we need to be encultured in both bodily and discursive ways to have our most complex thoughts and feelings" (2015, 459). As well as actions, we might add.

If the original disclosure of the world as *aletheia* happens through poetry for Heidegger (1971), there may be need for the advent of kinetic poets of risk capable of performing in the empty gaps where contentless cognition operates in lethal situations but who *still* manage to "silver tongue" the mystery. It may also mean that such experiences are unique to those capable of achieving them. As Laozi said, "The way that can be spoken of is not the constant way" (Laozi 1963, 5). Those who seek to comprehend such experiences may need to just do them.

Acknowledgments

This work was supported by the Australian Research Council Discovery Project Minds in Skilled Performance (DP170102987).

Notes

1. It is telling that Japan is the only country in military history to have relinquished more advanced technology to return to more traditional ways of fighting, notably with the sword. The reasons are complex (Perrin 197), but for our purposes, what is of interest is that swordsmanship and its importance for the Japanese psyche played a key role in the sword's evolution from lethal weapon to tool of self-flourishing.

2. This followed a much broader and deeper pattern, too intricate to fully explain here, wherein certain practices, e.g., *kendō* or *chadō*, 茶道, the way of tea, became *dō* 道, ways or paths designed to express and refine character. See Carter (2008).

3. Automatism and spontaneity differ in that the former is completely sub-personal whereas the latter allows for awareness and a measure of control.

4. There has been much debate about the actual rotation degrees of Slater's jump. See http://www.surfinglife.com.au/news/sl-news/12395-when-kelly-slater-s-540-was-a-720.

5. We have bracketed "heart-mind" as a more accurate rendition of the original Japanese in lieu of the translator's choice of "mind."

6. See endnote 5.

7. See endnote 5.

8. See endnote 5.

9. With the proviso that their analysis includes representation at a higher level of operationalization, this is compatible with an analysis of action-representation in the context of Dreyfus's background.

10. Of course, the role of community in such development should not be underestimated in this process.

11. See endnote 5.

References

Abe, Shinobu. 1986. "Zen and Sport." *Journal of the Philosophy of Sport* 13 (1): 45–48.

Araújo, Duarte, Keith Davids, and Robert Hristovski. 2006. "The Ecological Dynamics of Decision Making in Sport." *Psychology of Sport and Exercise* 7 (6): 653–676.

Beilock, Sian L. 2008. "Beyond the Playing Field: Sport Psychology Meets Embodied Cognition." *International Review of Sport and Exercise Psychology* 1 (1): 19–30.

Bennett, Max R., and Peter Michael Stephan Hacker. 2003. *Philosophical Foundations of Neuroscience*. Hoboken, NJ: Blackwell.

Birch, Jens E. 2010. "The Inner Game of Sport: Is Everything in the Brain?" *Sport, Ethics and Philosophy* 4 (3): 284–305.

Bisharat, Andrew. 2016. "Why Are So Many BASE Jumpers Dying?" *National Geographic*, August 30. http://www.nationalgeographic.com/adventure/features/why-are-so-many-base-jumpers-dying/.

Breivik, Gunnar. 2007. "Skillful Coping in Everyday Life and in Sport: A Critical Examination of the Views of Heidegger and Dreyfus." *Journal of the Philosophy of Sport* 34 (2): 116–134.

Breivik, Gunnar. 2013. "Zombie-Like or Superconscious? A Phenomenological and Conceptual Analysis of Consciousness in Elite Sport." *Journal of the Philosophy of Sport* 40 (1): 85–106.

Brooks, Rodney A. 1991. "Intelligence without Representation." *Artificial Intelligence* 47 (1–3): 139–159.

Bruya, Brian. 2010. *Effortless Attention: A New Perspective in the Cognitive Science of Attention and Action*. Cambridge, MA: MIT University Press.

Brymer, Eric, and Robert Schweitzer. 2013. "Extreme Sports Are Good for Your Health: A Phenomenological Understanding of Fear and Anxiety in Extreme Sport." *Journal of Health Psychology* 18 (4): 477–487.

Caesar, E. D. 2013. "It's More Like a Suicide Than a Sport." *New York Times*, July 26. http://www.nytimes.com/2013/07/28/magazine/its-more-like-a-suicide-than-a-sport.html?pagewanted=all.

Cappuccio, Massimiliano, and Michael Wheeler. 2012. "Ground-Level Intelligence: Action-Oriented Representation and the Dynamics of the Background." In *Knowing without Thinking: Mind, Action, Cognition, and the Phenomenon of the Background*, edited by Zdravko Radman, 13–36. London: Palgrave Macmillan.

Carter, Robert Edgar. 1997. *Nothingness beyond God: An Introduction to the Philosophy of Nishida Kitaro Second Edition*. St. Paul, MN: Paragon House.

Carter, Robert Edgar. 2008. *The Japanese Arts and Self-Cultivation*. Albany: SUNY Press.

Chemero, Anthony. 2009. *Radical Embodied Cognitive Science*. Cambridge, MA: MIT Press.

Chozanshi, Issai. 2006. *The Demon Sermon on the Martial Arts and Other Tales*. Tokyo: Kodansa International.

Christensen, Wayne, John Sutton, and Doris J. F. McIlwain. 2016. "Cognition in Skilled Action: Meshed Control and the Varieties of Skill Experience." *Mind & Language* 31 (1): 37–66.

Csíkszentmihályi, Mihaly. 1990. *Flow: The Psychology of Optimal Experience*. New York: Harper and Row.

Davids, Keith, Duarte Araújo, Ludovic Seifert, and Dominic Orth. 2015. "Expert Performance in Sport: An Ecological Dynamics Perspective." In *Routledge Handbook of Sport Expertise,* edited by Joseph Baker and Damian Farrow, 130–144. London: Routledge.

Dewey, John. 1988. Human Nature and Conduct: An Introduction to Social Psychology. New York: Henry Holt.

Drestke, Fred. 1995. *Naturalizing the Mind*. Cambridge, MA: MIT Press

Dreyfus, Hubert. 1992. *What Computers Can't Do: A Critique of Artificial Reason*. Cambridge, MA: MIT Press.

Dreyfus, Hubert. 1999. The Primacy of Phenomenology over Logical Analysis. *Philosophical Topics* 27 (2): 3–24.

Erickson, Karl, Daniel Warren, Jennifer Agans, and Richard Lerner. 2015. "Young Athlete Development in High Performance Sport Organizations: The Case of USA Luge." Presented at North American Society for the Psychology of Sport and Physical Activity (NASPSPA) Annual Conference, Portland, OR, June.

Ericsson, K. Anders. 2006. "The Influence of Experience and Deliberate Practice on the Development of Superior Expert Performance." In *The Cambridge Handbook of Expertise and Expert Performance*, edited by K. A. Ericsson, N. Charness, P. J. Feltovich, and R. R. Hoffman, 683–704. Cambridge: Cambridge University Press.

Eriksen, Jørgen W. 2010. "Mindless Coping in Competitive Sport: Some Implications and Consequences." *Sport, Ethics and Philosophy* 4 (1): 66–86.

Fattah, Eric. 2010. "Eric Fattah Sets a New Canadian Record." http://liquivision.com/eric.php.

Fodor, Jerry, A. 1987. *Psychosemantics: The Problem of Meaning in the Philosophy of Mind*. Cambridge, MA: MIT Press.

Fodor, Jerry A., and Zenon Pylyshyn. 2014. *Minds without Meanings: An Essay on the Content of Concepts*. Cambridge, MA: MIT Press.

Gallagher, Shaun. 2005. *How the Body Shapes the Mind*. Oxford: Oxford University Press.

Gallagher, Shaun. 2009. "Philosophical Antecedents to Situated Cognition." In *Cambridge Handbook of Situated Cognition*, edited by Philip Robbins and Murat Aydede, 35–50. Cambridge: Cambridge University Press.

Gallagher, Shaun. 2012. *Phenomenology*. Basingstoke, UK: Palgrave Macmillan.

Gallagher, Shaun. 2013. "The Socially Extended Mind." *Cognitive Systems Research* 25 (December): 4–12.

Gwin, Peter. 2011. "Battle for the Soul of Kung Fu." *National Geographic Magazine* (March): 94–113.

Heidegger, Martin. 1962. *Being and Time*. New York: Harper and Row.

Heidegger, Martin.1971. "The Origin of the Work of Art." In *Poetry, Language, Thought*. New York: Harper and Row.

Høffding, Simon. 2014. "What is Skilled Coping? Experts on Expertise." *Journal of Consciousness Studies* 21 (9/10): 49–73.

Honnold, Alex, and David Roberts. 2015. *Alone on the Wall*. New York: W.W. Norton.

Hutto, Dan, and Erik Myin. 2013. *Radicalizing Enactivism: Basic Minds without Content*. Cambridge, MA: MIT Press. doi:9780262018548.001.0001.

Hutto, Daniel D. 2012. "Exposing the Background: Deep and Local." In *Knowing without Thinking: Mind, Action, Cognition, and the Phenomenon of the Background*, edited by Zdravko Radman, 37–56. New Directions in Philosophy and Cognitive Science. London: Palgrave Macmillan.

Ilundáin-Agurruza, Jesús. 2007. "Kant Goes Skydiving: Understanding the Extreme by Way of the Sublime." In *Philosophy, Risk and Adventure Sports*, edited by Mike McNamee, 149–167. London: Routledge.

Ilundáin-Agurruza, Jesús. 2015. "From Unskilled Failure to Skillful Fluency: A Phenomenological Analysis of an Eastern Solution to Sport's Choking Effect." *Phenomenology and the Cognitive Sciences* 14 (2): 397–421.

Ilundáin-Agurruza, Jesús. 2016. *Skillful Striving: Holism and the Cultivation of Excellence in Sports and Performative Endeavors*. London: Routledge.

Ilundáin-Agurruza, Jesús. 2017. "A Different Way to Play: Holistic Sporting Experiences." In *Philosophy: Sport*, edited by R. Scott Kretchmar, 319–343. Macmillan Interdisciplinary Handbooks. Farmington Hills, MI: Macmillan.

Jackson, Susan. 1996. "Toward a Conceptual Understanding of the Flow Experience in Elite Athletes." *Research Quarterly for Exercise and Sport* 67 (1): 76–90.

James, William. 1918. *Principles of Psychology*. New York: Dover.

James, William. 1976. *The Works of William James: Essays in Radical Empiricism*. Cambridge, MA: Harvard University Press.

Johnson, Mark. 2007. *The Meaning of the Body: Aesthetics and Human Understanding*. Chicago: University of Chicago Press.

King, Winston L. 1994. *Zen and the Way of the Sword: Arming the Samurai Psyche*. Oxford: Oxford University Press.

Kirmayer, Laurence J. 2015. "Mindfulness in Cultural Context." *Transcultural Psychiatry* 52 (4): 447–469.

Kotler, Steven. 2014. *The Rise of Superman*. New York: Houghton Mifflin Harcourt.

Kozuma, Yoichi. 2009. "Samurai and Science: Sport Psychology in Japan." In *Cultural Sport Psychology*, edited by Robert Schinke and Stephanie Hanrahan, 205–217. Champaign, IL: Human Kinetics.

Krein, Kevin. 2007. "Nature and Risk in Adventure Sports." *Philosophy, Risk and Adventure Sports*, edited by Mike McNamee, 80–93. London: Routledge.

Krein, Kevin, and Jesús Ilundáin-Agurruza. 2014. "An East-West Comparative Analysis of *Mushin* and Flow." In *Philosophy and the Martial Arts*, edited by Graham Priest and Damon Young, 139–164. London: Routledge.

Krein, Kevin J. 2014. "Nature Sports." *Journal of the Philosophy of Sport* 41 (2): 193–208.

Laozi. 1963. *Dao de Jing*. London: Penguin.

Lee, Tatia M., Mei-Kei Leung, Wai-Kai Hou, Joey C. Y. Tang, Jing Yin, Kwok-Fai So, Chack-Fan Lee, and Chetwyn C. H. Chan. 2012. "Distinct Neural Activity Associated with Focused-Attention Meditation and Loving-Kindness Meditation." *PLoS One* 7 (8): e40054.

Lohse, Keith. 2015. "On Attentional Control." In *Routledge Handbook of Sport Expertise*, edited by Joseph Baker and Damian Farrow, 38–49. London: Routledge.

MacIntyre, Alasdair. 2008. *After Virtue*. Notre Dame, IN: Notre Dame University Press.

Mangan, Bruce. 2007. "Cognition, Fringe Consciousness, and the Legacy of William James." In *The Blackwell Companion to Consciousness*, edited by Max Velmans and Susan Schneider, 673–685. Malden, MA: Blackwell.

Masters, Rich, and Jon Maxwell. 2008. "The Theory of Reinvestment." *International Review of Sport and Exercise Psychology* 1 (2): 160–183.

Masters, Richard, John van der Kamp, and Catherine Capio. 2013. "Implicit Motor Learning by Children." In *Conditions of Children's Talent Development in Sport*, edited by Jean Côté and R. Lidor, 21–40. Morgantown, WV: Fitness Information Technology.

Millikan, Ruth Darrett. 1984. *Language, Thought, and Other Biological Categories*. Cambridge, MA: MIT Press.

Moe, Vegard Fusche. 2005. "A Philosophical Critique of Classical Cognitivism in Sport: From Information Processing to Bodily Background Knowledge." *Journal of the Philosophy of Sport* 32 (2): 155–183.

Moe, Vegard Fusche. 2007. "Understanding the Background Conditions of Skilled Movement in Sport: A Study of Searle's 'Background Capacities.'" *Sports, Ethics and Philosophy* 1 (3): 299–324.

Musashi, Miyamoto. 1983. *The Book of Five Rings*. Translated by T. Cleary. Boston, MA: Shambhala.

Noë, A. 2004. *Perception in Action*. Cambridge, MA: MIT Press.

Ortega y Gasset, José. 2006. "Corazón y Cabeza, in Teoría de Andalucía y Otros Ensayos." *Obras Completas* 6:208–211. Madrid: Taurus.

Perrin, Noel. 1979. *Giving Up the Gun: Japan's Reversion to the Sword, 1543–1879*. Boston, MA: David R. Godine.

Posner, Michael I., Mary K. Rothbart, and Yi-Yuan Tang. 2015. "Enhancing Attention through Training." *Current Opinion in Behavioral Sciences* 4 (August): 1–5.

Potter, Dean. 2011. *Eiger Unroped*. June 14. Video, 1:26. https://www.outsideonline.com/1862536/eiger-unroped.

Pursell, Robert. 2016. "Big Mountain Skier Matilda Rapaport Dies after Avalanche." GrindTV.com. July 18. http://www.grindtv.com/skiing/big-mountain-skier-matilda-rapaport-dies-avalanche/.

Russell, John S. 2005. "The Value of Dangerous Sport." *Journal of the Philosophy of Sport* 32 (1): 1–19.

Samuel, Geoffrey. 2015. "The Contemporary Mindfulness Movement and the Question of Non-self." *Transcultural Psychiatry* 52 (4): 485–500.

Schack, Thomas, Kai Essig, Cornelia Frank, and Dirk Koester. 2014. "Mental Representation and Motor Imagery Training." *Frontiers in Human Neuroscience* 8:328. http://doi.org/10.3389/fnhum.2014.00328.

Shapiro, Larry. 2011. *Embodied Cognition*. London: Routledge.

Sheets-Johnstone, Maxine. 2010. "Thinking in Movement: Further Analyses and Validations." In *Enaction: Toward a New Paradigm for Cognitive Science*, edited by John Stewart, Olivier Gapenne, and Ezequiel A. Di Paolo, 165–181. Cambridge, MA: MIT Press.

Sheets-Johnstone, Maxine. 2011. *The Primacy of Movement*. 2nd ed. Amsterdam: John Benjamins.

Sōhō, Takuan.1986. *The Unfettered Mind: Writings of the Zen Master to the Sword Master*. Tokyo: Kodansha.

Sugiyama, Takuya, and Kimihoro Inomata. 2005. "Qualitative Examination of Flow Experience among Top Japanese Athletes." *Perceptual and Motor Skills* 100 (3 Pt 2): 969–982.

Suits, Bernard. 2005. *The Grasshopper: Games, Life and Utopia*. Peterborough, ON: Broadview Press.

Sutton, John. 2007. "Batting, Habit and Memory: The Embodied Mind and the Nature of Skill." *Sport in Society* 10 (5): 763–786.

Sutton, John. 2014. "Remembering as Public Practice: Wittgenstein, Memory, and Distributed Cognitive Ecologies." In *Mind, Language, and Action: Proceedings of the 36th Wittgenstein Symposium*, edited by D. Moyal-Sharrock, V. A. Munz, and A. Coliva, 409–443. New Brunswick, NJ: Ontos-Verlag.

Sutton, John, and Doris McIlwain. 2015. "Breadth and Depth of Knowledge in Expert versus Novice Athletes." In *The Routledge Handbook of Sport Expertise*, edited by Damion Farrow and Joe Baker, 95–105. London: Routledge.

Suzuki, D. 1993. *Zen and Japanese Culture*. New York: Princeton University Press.

Thelen, Esther, and Linda Smith. 1994. *A Dynamic Systems Approach to the Development of Cognition and Action*. Cambridge, MA: MIT Press.

Thompson, Evan. 2007. *Mind in Life: Biology, Phenomenology, and the Sciences of the Mind*. Cambridge, MA: Harvard University Press.

Ueshiba, Morihei. 1992. *The Art of Peace*. Translated by John Stevens. Boston: Shambhala.

Uexküll, Jakob V. 2010. *A Foray into the Worlds of Animals and Humans: With A Theory of Meaning*. Minneapolis: University of Minnesota Press.

Varela, Francisco, Eleanor Rosch, and Evan Thompson. 1991. *The Embodied Mind*. Cambridge, MA: MIT Press.

Wingsuitfly.com. 2017. "Wingsuiting Death and Risk Statistics: Infographic Danger Percentage." http://www.wingsuitfly.com/risk/4572000812.

Wrathall, Mark A. 2014. "Introduction: Hubert Dreyfus and the Phenomenology of Human Intelligence." In *Skillful Coping*, edited by Mark Wrathall, 1–21. Oxford: Oxford University Press.

Wulf, Gabriele. 2007. *Attention and Motor Skill Learning*. Champaign, IL: Human Kinetics.

Yagyu, Munenori. 2003. "The Life-Giving Sword: Secret Teachings for the House of the Shogun." Translated by William Scott Wilson. Tokyo: Kodansha.

Yamamoto, Tsunetomo. 1979. *Hagakure [The Book of the Samurai]*. Tokyo: Kodansha.

Yan, Laura. 2017. "Never Die." *Victory Journal*. http://victoryjournal.com/stories/never-die/.

Yuasa, Yasuo. 1987. *The Body: Toward an Eastern Mind-Body Theory*. Albany: SUNY Press.

Zimmermann, Ana, and Soraia Saura. 2017. "Body, Environment and Adventure: Experience and Spatiality." *Sport, Ethics and Philosophy* 11 (2): 155–168. doi:10.1080/17511321.2016.1210207.

Zhuangzi. 1968. *The Complete Works of Chuang Tzu*. Translated by A. C. Graham. New York: Columbia University Press.

17 Stereotype Threat and the Female Athlete: Swimming, Surfing, and Sport Martial Arts

Michele Merritt, Audrey Yap, Cassie Comley, and Caren Diehl

1 Introduction

It has long been documented that there is an inconsistency in the way female and male athletes are treated. From the way they are received by the public to the way they are coached, this disparity reflects an essentialist ideology that sees the differences between female and male physiology as absolute determinants of performance. Such thinking also tends to treat *gender*—the way a person presents and performs in the world as a man, woman, or any other socially constructed role—as a natural offshoot of *sex*—the biological markers that classify bodies as male or female. Such thinking has been criticized from several fronts. For instance, this so-called natural attitude (Garfinkel 1957) has been criticized in trans studies, for instance by Talia Bettcher (2007, 2009).

From the perspective of this natural attitude, "throwing like a girl," is just what girls naturally do, which is to say, throw poorly, awkwardly, and much less effectively than their "boy" counterparts. In fact, to be male and to be accused of throwing like a girl, or to perform in any way whatsoever like a girl, is an insult, whereas to be like Sarah Hudek, one of the top pitchers in all of college softball *and* baseball (Axisa 2016), is viewed as a miraculous feat, bordering on freakish. Her performance is certainly not treated as "normal" or natural, despite evidence that female pitchers can perform nearly if not equally as well as males (Mirsky 2015). And, as we discuss below, this phenomenon is by no means confined to throwing sports; we find it in many other places.

The source of this unequal treatment of athletes of different genders comes from stereotypes about the inherent abilities of female athletes. These stereotypes are tied to the idea that one's athletic abilities are inextricably linked to one's biological sex, and that biology, as it were, is destiny. Further compounding the problem is the commonly held social view that not only is it unnatural for women to be good at sports, but also the behaviors required to exhibit good athletic performance are unfeminine—inappropriate ways for women to behave in the world.

With respect to the biological perspective, females, it is argued, are naturally weaker, slower, and have less muscle mass than males. As such, they are less exciting to watch, they are too fragile to play rough, and they will never outperform male athletes. These stereotypes have unfortunate negative consequences, such as the underrepresentation of female athletes in the media or the near-bankruptcy of an entire organization like the Women's National Basketball Association (WNBA), which also provides an example of the ever-present pay gap between female and male athletes (Berri 2015). The US women's soccer team, for example, collected $2 million in 2015, while the men's team collected $9 million in 2014, despite the fact that the women's team won the World Cup while the men only advanced to the second stage of the competition. Negative stereotypes, unsurprisingly, also lead to sexist and misogynist attacks on women, such as recent slurs against Serena Williams and, by proxy, all female tennis stars who dare threaten to eclipse the popularity of their male counterparts (Dator 2016). Stereotypes can also hinder athletic performance itself; an internalized sense that the world sees them as physically incapable can lead to diminished performance, if not all-out failure, for many women and girls. The internalization of these stereotypes and the associated effects of *stereotype threat* on athletic performance is the main focus of this chapter.

We do not deny that physiological differences exist between male and female athletes, nor do we deny that these physiological differences affect the ways certain sports are performed. For instance, women are, on average, shorter than men, and as such, the heights of basketball nets in the NBA and WNBA reflect this biological statistic, which is arguably a reasonable accommodation. What we argue, though, is that these physiological differences do not necessitate the aforementioned negative assumptions about the abilities of female athletes. So what we will be exploring and ultimately critiquing are ways that negative stereotypes surrounding female athletes psychologically affect the athletes, their embodied subjectivity, and their athletic performance. Furthermore, by looking at not only the effects of the stereotyping, but also at the *source*—namely, from whence the stereotypes arise—we hope to offer some insights into ways to improve the conditions affecting the psychology, phenomenology, and training of female athletes. First, we provide a brief overview of stereotype threat in competitive sports. While stereotype threat is prevalent in nearly all sports, we concentrate on swimming, surfing, and martial arts, as these three sports are sufficiently dissimilar to represent a broad spectrum, and yet there are interesting commonalities among them in terms of the role that gendered norms play in performance, coaching, and competition. Next, we look at the potential sources of these gender stereotypes and how gender itself is constructed, utilized, and sustained in practices surrounding coaching and training of female athletes. To this end, we draw from a rich history of gender theory and analysis that demonstrably indicates the fluid and socially constructed nature of most stereotypes surrounding feminine versus masculine embodiment. Where our argument takes a novel turn is in also drawing from some of the current trends in the philosophy of cognitive science, particularly the *enactivist* view of the mind, which sees cognition as a dynamically interactive process between organisms and environment, including the social environment (cf. Varela, Thompson, and Rosch 1991; Thompson 2007; Krueger 2013). We argue that gender is a socially and dynamically enactive process that emerges from and is maintained by interactions among participants and that, depending on context, gender norms can appear quite differently, and therefore be applied quite differently. Stereotypes, in this view, are not static representations or ideals, but are shared and collective experiences that serve to shape and reinforce the psychological framework of not only the athletes participating in a given sport, but their coaches, spectators, and fans as well. And all of these participants participate in and are influenced by a myriad of other social systems, such as the media, that play important roles in constructing and maintaining stereotypes. The phenomenon of stereotype threat, it turns out, is wholly intersubjective and socially dynamic.

2 Stereotype Threat in Competitive Sports

Stereotype threat is a phenomenon through which salient negative stereotypes about a group can adversely affect the performance of its members (Chalabaev, Sarrazin, et al. 2013; Steele and Aronson 1995). Although physiological factors may play a role in explaining the differences in performance between genders, Eagly (1995) has shown that only 5 percent of variance in physical ability is due to gender. Therefore in this section, we examine how gender stereotypes function in sports in order to demonstrate the validity of this construct in the sociological sciences (Messner 2000; Musto 2014). Besides showing up in sports, stereotype threat is also documented to affect performance on math, science, and spatial reasoning tasks, such that it is often the case that negative biases about women and girls within STEM (science, technology, engineering, math) fields lead to poor performance within and even avoidance of those domains entirely (Shapiro and Williams 2012; Ambady et al. 2001; Spencer, Steele, and Quinn 1999). Analogous negative stereotypes persist in many sports and can impede performance of female athletes. These implicit biases serve to create an atmosphere in which the preconceived attitude that women and girls bring to their sport or activity is often already a sense of "I cannot," in Iris Marion Young's (2005) sense. In male participants, on the other hand, positive stereotypes create an atmosphere of "I can." Performance is affected either way. Stereotypes, it turns out, can function like self-fulfilling prophecies.

In the United States, sport is an arena that has historically been constructed as a male domain (Cahn 1994; Messner 1988; Riemer and Visio 2003), which plays a critical role in naturalizing essentialist differences between the genders (Kimmel 1996; Messner 2011; Musto 2014). Within the past century, the institution of sport has played a key role in the construction and stabilization of a "male-dominant, hetero-sexist system of gender relations" (Messner 1995, 16) that favors competition, aggressiveness, and violence. This system of gender relations typically excludes women, working-class men, men of color, and immigrants (Dworkin and Messner 2002; Kimmel 1990). Sport has become a major "testing ground" on which men enact and defend their masculinity (Kimmel 1996; Messner and Sabo 1990). Despite the fact that the arena of sport routinely and systematically creates and reinforces an ideology of male superiority (Messner 1995), women continue to pursue and participate in sports. Within the past half century, large numbers of women have been participating in a variety of sports.

During the 1970s, there was an explosion of female athletic participation across the United States (Messner 1988; Hargreaves 1994; Messner 2011). With the passing of Title IX—an antidiscrimination portion of the 1972 US Education Amendments—during this era, sport opportunities for women and girls in the United States dramatically increased, especially in sports that have been traditionally associated with men (Pelak 2002). Increases in participation can be seen in both organized team sports such as basketball and baseball, and in more alternative and highly individualized sports such as surfing, skateboarding, and snowboarding. These monumental increases in participation led scholars to start examining sport as a "terrain of contradictory and contested gender meanings and relations" (Messner 2011, 151; see also Messner 1988). Although arguably more women are participating in sports post-Title IX (Heywood and Dworkin 2003; Sabo and Veliz 2008), sporting women continue to struggle with earning respect from their male peers (Roy and Caudwell 2014), being seen as authentic members of the culture (Atencio, Beal, and Wilson 2009; Olive, McCuaig, and Phillips 2015), navigating essentialist and categorical beliefs about gender relations (Messner 2011), and receiving appropriate quantity and quality of televised coverage of professional sports (Cooky, Messner, and Musto 2015). Some of these obstacles can be explained in part by an individual's shared beliefs about natural differences that exist between boys and girls and the salience of gender.

Research has found that stereotype threats have a negative impact on performance, especially if the belief is internalized (Chalabaev, Brisswalter, et al. 2013). Chalabaev, Brisswalter, and colleagues (2013) conducted a study exploring stereotype threats on a simple strength task and found that velocity of force production was decreased when the negative stereotype threat was introduced for female participants. Similar results were also present in other sporting tasks such as golf putting (Beilock et al. 2006; Beilock and McConnell 2004), soccer dribbling (Chalabaev et al. 2008), and free throw in basketball (Krendl, Gainsburg, and Ambady 2012).

Sport scholars have recently started to document the ways in which gender varies in salience across sport contexts and what factors impact the salience of gender within interactions (Messner 2000; Musto 2014). In order to understand shifts in salience, Musto (2014) and Messner (2000) examined how individuals enact different patterns of gender relations within and across contexts. In her study of a coed youth swim team, Musto discovered that during focused (structured) aspects of swim practice gender was less salient. It was during these aspects of swim practice that Musto observed the athletes interacting in ways that were not antagonistic. Instead of focusing on how they differ across genders, the swimmers followed their coach's instructions and compared race times with one another regardless of their gender. By focusing on time (performance) and following their coach's instructions, the swimmers were able to compare themselves in terms of overall ability. During unfocused (unstructured) aspects of swim practice, gender was highly salient, and swimmers interacted with each other in antagonist ways. It was also during unfocused aspects of swim practice that boys and girls engaged in "borderwork" (Musto 2014; see also Messner 2000; Thorne 1993). Borderwork happens when "individuals draw on and affirm group boundaries between the genders," such that during this aspect of swim practice, one of the ways boys engaged in borderwork was by physically separating themselves from the girls (Musto 2014, 372). Parents and coaches play a crucial role in reinforcing gender boundaries between the boys and girls (Messer 2000). When the salience of gender is low and the given context allows for individuals to interact with each other in ways that showcase similarities between the genders (overall race times), individuals are able to construct gender relations without hegemonic beliefs (Musto 2014). These studies are an important reminder for scholars to consider the ways in which gender relations and the meanings individuals attach to gender can shift across contexts. Examining which situations and which conditions activate gender boundaries—for example paying attention to what roles coaches and parents play—will aid scholars in further understanding how individuals (de)construct gender beliefs.

Similar engagements in borderwork and gender construction more generally have been studied in martial arts contexts as well. In their study of the interactions between adolescent judokas both on and off the mat, Guérandel and Mennesson (2007) found several ways in which the athletes reaffirmed gender stereotypes and gender boundaries. Interactions between athletes of the same gender often take place in ways that fit nicely with stereotypical male and female interests and modes of interaction, with girls talking about relationships and displaying physical affection toward each other, while boys often discuss sports and display a "virile camaraderie" even when not engaged in athletic activity (Guérandel and Mennesson 2007, 173–174).

During practice itself, gender hierarchies nevertheless remained, with girls being perceived (even by other girls), as being less challenging opponents. The internalized expectation in mixed-gender matches is that the boys will be stronger opponents than the girls. This manifests in boys throwing the girls more softly, retying their belts if they fall off, and other such behavior that might be described as gentlemanly. That this kind of behavior manifests, of course, assumes that boys and girls will even be allowed to fight each other in the first place. Sisjord (1997) notes in her study of adolescent wrestlers that many girls did not even practice with boys, unless those boys were relatively young, in order to ensure even matches of size and skill. Swimming training, at least at the Olympic level in the United States, is perhaps an exception to this rule, as team USA notoriously hosts mixed-gender practices, but more importantly, male swimmers do not tend to view their female counterparts as inherently easy to beat. The recent surge in fame of swimmers like Katie Ledecky, for example, has prompted questions pertaining to how elite swimmers train, and more often than not, Ledecky is described as a "pace-setter" and a strong competitor, even by Michael Phelps, the most decorated Olympic swimmer of all time. Ledecky has tied him on the 400-meter freestyle during practice. However, swimmers like Ledecky are few and far between, and despite the ever-decreasing gap between male and female swimmers' performances, there is still a marked tendency to view male swimmers as innately better at the sport, in part, because they tend to be taller than females. Even Phelps has commented that Ledecky "swims like a guy." Ironically, Ledecky, unlike many top male swimmers, *does not* in fact possess great height, large hands, or big feet, so it is odd that Phelps describes her in this way: "I've watched her stroke so much, really, over the last couple of years. Really, she swims almost like a guy. Her long, loping stroke [gets] … stronger and stronger throughout the race. I think her stroke is so different from all the other females that she swims against" (Zaccardi 2015).

But, it can be gleaned from the above quote that Phelps is chalking this uncanny ability of Ledecky's to a masculine technique she has mastered. It is the only way to make sense of her superhuman speed. In marathon swimming, similar stereotypes persist, despite the fact that female swimmers in this sport are not only closing the gap in performance levels, but oftentimes exceed their male counterparts. And when a female swimmer does tie or outperform a male, such as Diana Nyad's record-breaking distance of 110 miles from Cuba to Florida, it is often the case that the performance is questioned or the swimmer is even accused of cheating (Holpuch 2013). In short, even in swimming, stereotypes about male and female ability persist and influence training, which in turn influences the way the athletes themselves view one another (Wainer, Nju, and Palmer 2000). These stereotypes extend to the way coaches are perceived as well, with male coaches dominating swimming and being viewed as more capable (Medwechuk and Crossman 1994).

Even though nontraditional sport spaces can offer sporting women a greater promise for the "realization of alternative and resistant sport forms" (Birrell and Theberge 1994, 371), women participants in nontraditional sport contexts still face obstacles that are in part influenced by negative salient stereotypes. Within alternative physical cultures like surfing or snowboarding, women are often marginalized or excluded from the sporting space through "cultural understandings and expectations" of how the activities should be performed or the assumptions about male and female performances (Olive, McCuaig, and Phillips 2015). For example, some female snowboarders believe their abilities are often measured using "the boy's scale" (Thorpe 2005, 93), and young male skaters believe the lack of female involvement in skateboarding culture is tied to the ideology that "girls don't like to get hurt" (Beal and Wilson 2004, 47). Some participants believe there are female- and male-appropriate ways of engaging in physical activities, so that even when women do well or show commitment to their sport, their performance is still demarcated by gender, such as, they are still only good "for a girl" (Booth 2001; Atencio, Beal, and Wilson 2009; Sisjord 2009). Surfing is a valuable site for understanding how women navigate salient beliefs about gender because even though a growing number of women and girls enter the sport every year (Ford and Brown 2006), surfing is an arena typically dominated by masculine gender norms (Thorpe 2009; Stoddart 2011).

Women surfers' experiences of the sporting space are varied, with some sporting women feeling patronized and differentiated by male surfers out in the lineup (Olive, McCuaig, and Phillips 2015; Comley 2016) and others feeling empowered to the extent that they use surfing as a space to contest traditional discourses of both femininity and motherhood (Knijnik, Horton, and Cruz 2010; Spowart, Burrows, and Shaw 2010). Recreational surfing is not bound by any particular system of rules, which means this activity is not necessarily articulated in terms of sex/gender teams or leagues (Olive, McCuaig and Phillips 2015). Thus, recreational surfing can be conceptualized as a situation/condition that is unstructured/unfocused free time, which means gender should be more salient. Findings from studies about women surfers' experiences support this claim, in that some male surfers are engaging in practices that marginalize and differentiate women. For example, women surfers report receiving extra levels of attention, support, and encouragement from male surfers (Olive, McCuaig and Phillips 2015) and feeling as if they have to "represent" all women (Comley 2016). Many women surfers discuss the importance of catching that first wave of the session and how they feel added pressure to perform well (Fendt and Wilson 2012, Comley 2016). Although male surfers believe their actions are altruistic and supportive, women surfers perceive their behaviors as patronizing and differentiating. Patronizing behaviors can make women feel as if they were not "authentic" surfers (Olive, McCuaig, and Phillips 2015). By differentiating women in the water, male surfers reinforce and maintain the idea that women surfers are just "women that surf" instead of "surfers" (Olive, McCuaig, and Phillips 2015, 265). Even when women surfers felt patronized and were being differentiated, they could still be agentic by refusing the advice and help they received in the lineup. By refusing to accept being differentiated, women surfers have the potential to "carve out alternative ways of operating within the power relations that circulate in the waves" (Olive, McCuaig, and Phillips 2015, 273).

3 Sources of Stereotypes: The Construction of Gender Essentialism

Here we discuss more generally the way sex and gender are assumed, tracked, and applied. Our aim here is to reveal the ways current theories and practices of gender are at odds with or have at least not filtered into the domain of competitive sports, especially not in the coaching or mentoring of young athletes in swimming, surfing, and sport martial arts. The idea of an absolute binary between male and female—assumed to be exclusive and exhaustive—is rarely, if ever, questioned in professional sports. Cases involving female athletes with atypically high levels of endogenous testosterone, and the forced genetic testing that is imposed on such athletes (such as the South African runner, Caster Semenya), have given professional sport committees and directors reason to at least reconsider some of these practices (Karkazis et al. 2012).

Furthermore, in certain sports, such as marathon swimming, for instance, it is arguably the case that gender difference in technique and performance is negligible at best (Eichenberger et al. 2012); women like Diana Nyad have attempted and succeeded at distances far greater than any male long-distance swimmer. But, perhaps unsurprisingly, when a swimming performance like Nyad's is achieved, instead of rethinking the attitudes toward gender differences, the reaction has been to question the validity of her performance and assume she was somehow cheating (Holpuch 2013).

It is unfortunate, however, that the assumption of this dichotomy remains in athletic settings, given that it has long been challenged by scientists, philosophers, and sociologists, to name a few disciplines. Fausto-Sterling (2000), Fine (2010), and Roughgarden (2004) are a few who have challenged various aspects of conventional social views about sex, gender, and innate differences between men and women. For instance, Fine (2010) argues that implicit social assumptions about gender differences are already presupposed in many psychology studies that purport to discover differences between male and female brains. Such studies often result in popular articles arguing that men and women are inherently "wired differently," explaining why women are better suited to some tasks and men to others (Connor 2013). This "neurosexism," as Fine calls it, can be debunked if we pay closer attention to the details and methodology of the research involved. The more significant source of cognitive gender differences, she argues, is cultural.

One popular belief about gendered cognition is that women tend to have more emotional intelligence than men; women, some say, are hardwired for empathy, while men are typically hard-pressed to understand the feelings of others (Baron-Cohen 2003). This has been measured through the use of Baron-Cohen's Empathy Quotient (EQ) test, on which women tend to score higher than men. One striking fact, however, about the test, is that it is unclear whether it measures empathy or one's self-perception as empathetic, given questions such as "I can easily tell if someone else wants to enter a conversation." Further, Eisenberg and Lennon (1983), in an extensive literature survey of tests used to measure empathy, found that the extent to which tests found women to be more empathetic than men were very strongly correlated to the method of testing used. And self-assessment tests such as the EQ were those most strongly favoring women.

Further, studies that prime gender tend to show more stereotypical behavior, in the sense that subjects that were thinking about gender differences in empathy had a stronger tendency to exhibit them. As a result, Klein and Hodges (2001) suggest an alternative explanation for gendered differences in empathic ability: rather than women being innately better empathizers than men, women are more often *motivated* to be good empathizers. When placed in circumstances in which they were well motivated to have good empathic accuracy, such as when there were monetary rewards for correct answers, there were no significant gender differences between men and women. And in general, when we look at the range of studies, the conclusion is that empathic ability and motivation cannot be separated from the social circumstances in which they are deployed. Social views about gender are intertwined with the salience of our gender identities (Fine 2010, 19–26). Our argument in this chapter is analogous to Fine's, in that we outline mechanisms through which women internalize norms and stereotypes of feminine weakness and lack of athleticism, just as women internalize norms and stereotypes of feminine caring and empathy. And just as these gendered norms about emotional aptitude are closely connected to the ways in which that aptitude manifests itself, gendered norms about athletic ability are closely connected to athleticism in practice. Thus negative stereotypes about women and athleticism are part of what results in women *being* weaker and less athletic.

4 Inhibited Intentionality and Gender Construction

One result of gendered socialization is the internalization of norms for men's and women's bodily comportment, some of which have a purported basis in biology. Iris Marion Young's (2005) article "Throwing Like a Girl" explicitly addresses shortcomings in Erwin Straus's analysis of the difference between men and women's movement when throwing. Straus attributes women's throwing style to biological (though not purely anatomical) differences, but Young points out that this neglects to account for the basic modalities of feminine bodily existence. While her analysis is limited to women living in a relatively narrowly circumscribed set of industrialized Western cultures, it nevertheless addresses many preconceptions held in those cultures about women's movement and abilities.

The three modalities of feminine movement that Young outlines are *ambiguous transcendence, inhibited intentionality*, and a *discontinuous unity* with its surroundings. All of these are related to the idea that women relate to their bodies in distinct and conflicting ways: both as an object (sometimes burdensome) that must be dealt with and as a source of intentionality. The second of these—inhibited intentionality—is the main focus of our discussion in this chapter. In order to understand how intentionality can be *inhibited*, we can contrast it with *uninhibited* intentionality: bodily movement exemplifying uninhibited intentionality is smoothly goal-directed, with an unbroken directedness between the aim of the action and its enactment. In much feminine movement, this directedness is broken, and women find themselves simultaneously attempting to carry out the act in question and stiffening against its easy performance. Stereotypical "throwing like a girl" exemplifies this inhibited movement, in which women perform the action, but still fail to take advantage of their full range of bodily possibilities. Whether inhibited intentionality is still experienced by women to the same extent it was when Young's essay was originally written is, to some extent, controversial (Young 1998; Chisholm 2008; Foster 2009). But even if diminished, the stereotypes about women in sport nevertheless remain, and as the studies discussed above show, many of us have certainly internalized views of feminine weakness, which seem to impair women's ability to participate in sport. And, at least in the case of fighting sports, some component of this inhibited intentionality may yet remain (Yap 2016). Part of the mechanism for this might be explained by Butler's (1999) idea of gender as *performative*, such that gender is not a static attribute that a person has; rather, one's gender identity is constituted by the historically and socially contingent ways in which it is expressed. Gender identity, then, is not best understood as a fixed source from which one's behavior follows—it is not *because* someone is a woman that they conform to feminine modes of bodily comportment, whatever those might be in the historical and cultural location in which they are situated. Although the stylized repetition of acts through which one conforms to gendered norms of behavior, appearance, and the like may create the illusion of a stable gender identity prior to and grounding those acts, Butler claims that it is the acts themselves that ground our gender identity—or at least create the appearance of such a ground.

Given that women's athletic inferiority is a popular and deeply embedded stereotype within our culture, skilled female athletes face a challenge when it comes to possessing an intelligible gender—one that coheres and sustains gendered norms within one's culture. If exceptional athletic excellence is not seen as compatible with being a woman, then female athletes might end up possessing what Merritt (2014) calls "nonsensical gender," meaning that they cannot be sensibly understood as women in our society. Given the idea we have assumed of gender as performative, women who do not behave in accordance with our common sociocultural understanding of women's behavior are in some sense not actually women. We shall see in the discussion that follows how this applies in the case of women athletes.

5 The Female/Athlete Paradox

Female athletes face a double challenge, in which they are expected to perform with excellence at their sport while also maintaining their "proper place" behind male athletes when it comes to overall performance. Often, when a woman threatens to surpass a man in terms of strength, speed, or power, she is questioned, denounced, and vilified. Part of this suspicious attitude toward female athletes, we argue, stems from what scholars have referred to as the "female/athlete paradox," which is the notion that a female athlete must simultaneously appear strong, confident, and adept at her sport, but must also retain all the trappings of a "feminine" and "normal" woman (Krane 2001; Kolnes 1995; Meân and Kassing 2008; Ross and Shinew 2008). This has also been found to discourage adolescent girls from participating in athletic activities in the first place. A fear of masculinization and the additional pressure of the male gaze can also explain adolescent girls' anxiety about participation in sports in mixed gender contexts (Evans 2006).

The pressure to conform to typical norms of femininity can be seen in media coverage of female athletes across several different sports. It applies to women in swimming—Nyad, for example, and also the recently acclaimed Katie Ledecky, who has been touted as the next Michael Phelps, if not a superior version of him (*Time* 2015). In surfing, Maya Gabeira, for example, was criticized for being "reckless" when she had a near-death experience attempting to ride the biggest wave ever surfed by a woman, despite such reckless behavior being undertaken by men on numerous occasions without the same critique (Skenazy 2014). This pressure also applies in sport martial arts. The popularity of mixed martial arts leagues such as the UFC and Strikeforce gives us a clear view of how the media treats successful female fighters such as Ronda Rousey and Cristiane Justino. Rousey, despite a feminine and conventionally sexy public image, has nevertheless been subject to more than her share of media scrutiny related to her body size. It is typical in mixed martial arts for fighters to have a natural weight that is significantly higher than the weight class in which they compete, but media commentary on Rousey's appearance led her to comment publicly on reasons why she takes pride in her body (Cepeda 2015). Arguably worse yet, though, have been sexist and transphobic comments about another dominant fighter, Cristiane Justino, nicknamed "Cris Cyborg," who has never maintained an especially feminine image (Guillan 2015).

Though swimming, surfing, and sport martial arts are all individual sports, the mechanisms for competition are different in each one. In swimming, the winner is the first to swim the requisite distance; in surfing, points are awarded by judges based on the maneuvers performed; and in sport martial arts, points are awarded for successful strikes or throws performed on an opponent. While some gender segregation may happen in training, it is nevertheless very common for young athletes in all these sports to train together. This makes the sports interesting in terms of observing the ways group dynamics and biases shape performance. In these three sports, like many others, gendered stereotypes are applied, much to the detriment of many female athletes. For instance, many adolescent girls in sport martial arts have already internalized the idea that girls are inherently weaker competitors than boys (Sisjord 1997; Guerandel and Menneson 2007). What is compelling to us, especially in swimming, surfing, and sport martial arts, is that the mechanism by which these stereotypes emerge and are sustained is not a wholly internal process, but is rather a collective, dynamic, and interactive one.

6 Enacting and Embodying Stereotypes: The Construction of Inhibited Intentionality

In our view, it is best to conceive of the internalization of stereotypes by athletes as a process that emerges and is maintained by socially interactive dynamics. In other words, rather than assuming that the phenomenology underpinning how stereotypes are embodied is a solely *subjective* experience, it is better, we argue, to think of this process as *intersubjective* in nature. As it turns out, the enactivist view of the mind, a theory recently developed and defended in the philosophy of cognitive science, provides an excellent framework for explaining how stereotype threat is developed and sustained and, furthermore, how it shapes the embodied phenomenology of female athletes.[1] In particular, arguments that emphasize shared meaning-making through dynamic coupling (Varela, Thompson, and Rosch 1991; Fuchs and De Jaegher 2009; De Jaegher and Di Paolo 2007) make a convincing case for a distributed and externalized account of the ways that stereotypes influence the psychology of athletes and ultimately alter their performance, in both positive and negative ways.

To get an idea of how the enactivist approach is unique as well as useful in accounting for stereotype threat, it is helpful to contrast it with what can be labeled "standard" cognitive science. Often synonymous with *cognitivism*, standard accounts of cognition treat thought as an internal, representational, and rational process. There is disagreement as to exactly how much of cognition is representational, whether it is entirely brain-bound or extended into the central nervous system, and so on, and we will not rehearse those variations here. It suffices to generally understand the cognitivist paradigm as one that sees thought as a result of receiving data from the world and processing it much like a computer processes information—symbolically, and guided by internal norms of representational content.

Like many nonstandard approaches to cognitive science (cf. Clark 2008; Varela, Thompson, and Rosch 1991; Hutto and Myin 2012), enactivism abandons the idea that cognition is an entirely internal process. Drawing from the work of Gibson (1977), for example, enactivists claim that the world affords us with potentials to act, and it is in this interplay among brains, bodies, and environment that thought emerges. It is important to note, however, that the way cognition emerges is not haphazard, nor the result of just any interaction. Instead, organisms and their environments are "structurally coupled" (Maturana 1987), insofar as only certain interactions are afforded by the organization of each. Consider, for example, the bluefin tuna, whose body weight and shape would seem to preclude efficient hydrodynamics (Triantafyllou and Triantafyllou 1995). Nevertheless, by exploiting features of the environment—namely, the vortices and eddies that form as a result of propulsion through the water—the fish are able to move much faster than simple physics would deem possible. Notice, however, that in this case, the fish must have a particular structural organization (the tail fin strength to manipulate the wake) and the environment must also be primed and ready for such interaction (the perturbation of the water by the fins of the fish, which in turn give the fish just enough power to stir up even more propulsive force).

The example above parallels the way cognition is argued to "co-emerge" when humans interact with their environments. To be sure, we sometimes exploit features of the world—such as when we use technological devices like smartphones to store memories—but the environment also places demands on us, forcing us to think and behave in context-specific ways, such as when we make assumptions and predictions about whole objects despite their not being presented to us as such.[2] Humans and their specific environments, therefore, form a tightly coupled system that we can call cognitive in its own right. For instance, the removal of a part of my brain responsible for, say, language processing, would be expected to result in the loss of certain linguistic abilities; similarly, if I were to remove features of the environment from this coupled system of which I am a part, I should also expect whatever cognitive task in which I am engaged to be altered drastically, if not be altogether eliminated. As Maturana (1987) describes this co-emergence,

> If I have a living system ... then this living system is in a medium with which it interacts. Its dynamics of state result in interactions with the medium, and the dynamics of state within the medium result in interactions with the living system. What happens in interaction? Since this is a structure determined system ... the medium triggers a change of state in the system, and the system triggers a change of state in the medium. What change of state? One of those which is permitted by the structure of the system. (75)

When it comes to *meaning* and how sense is made in these human-environment interactions, enactivism rejects the cognitivist argument that signification occurs wholly within the confines of the human organism, let alone her brain. While the body is crucial, as it must be structured in such a way that features of the environment show up as meaningful in the first place (I cannot, for example, make sense of some noises that my dog can, because my tympanic membrane and auditory cortex are not nearly as sensitive as that of my canine friend), the way the world is set up is also essential for meaning-making. Gibson (1977) explained this quite well with his theory of affordances: objects don't show up to me as "able to be acted upon' if they don't already conform in some way to my body and its structure. As DiPaolo and Thompson (2014) argue, regarding sense-making under an enactivist framework,

> From this perspective, the body is not just the means but also an end of being a cognitive system. To put the point another way, basic cognition is more a matter of adaptive self-regulation in precarious conditions than abstract problem solving. The point here is not to deny that we can and do engage in high-level problem solving. Rather, it is to say that this kind of narrow cognition presupposes the broader and more basic cognition that we call sense-making. (73)

This brief overview of the enactivist paradigm is meant to provide a basis for interpreting stereotypes and female athletic embodiment through a much more dynamic and interactive lens than most traditional theories of cognitive science would permit. If we think of the ways in which stereotypes, as features of the environment, shape the thoughts and ultimately serve to structure the bodily comportment of athletes, while the performance of those athletes in turn feeds back into the stereotypes themselves, the phenomenon of stereotype threat begins to look a lot more like Maturana's picture of a coupled system, whose identity is sustained by mutual interdependence. In the case of female athletes internalizing and performing on the basis of stereotypes, the system at play is one in which meaning is made by the stereotypes influencing and being influenced by the athlete's embodied cognition and performance within that system.

Before going further with this analysis, it is worth noting that the enactivist framework has also been extended to include the affective dimensions of embodied cognition (von Scheve and Salmela 2014; Krueger 2014). Whereas traditional theories of emotions treat them as internal "feelings" (Lang 1994), perceptions (Kraut 1986; Prinz 2004), or appraisals (Nussbaum 2003), proponents of a more enacted view of cognition tend to view affect in the same way they view cognition generally, namely, as a dynamically interactive process. Emotions, in this view, emerge during exchanges between organisms and their environment, and in the case of humans, this environment is often social in nature. Especially if we consider emotions beyond the primary feelings of sadness, anger, and the like and broaden our view to include social emotions (shame, pride, etc.) and background emotions (long-term moods like depression, anxiety, etc.), then it becomes clear why it is better to think of many forms of affect as intersubjective. Take, for example, the "Still Face" experiment (Tronick et al. 1978), wherein caregivers cease responding to the facial expressions and gestures of their infants, and instead offer an expressionless stare. In very little time, the infants become distressed, their moods change from happy to angry or upset, and they begin to seek out attention and interaction by making loud noises, flailing limbs, and so forth. In other words, their detachment from the other—the lack of synchrony—is what constitutes the change in emotion.

Krueger (2014) also points out that the same structures that synchronously regulate infant-caregiver relationships are present in adult emotional interactions and can serve to extend and enhance the affective background. My anger, for example, can be charged and heightened by talking to others who are angry at the same set of events. At a sporting event, my excitement will feed off of the crowd of other fans. In fact, it has been documented that emotional expression by professional athletes is actually *drawn out* by the excited faces of others, such as when a bowler makes a strike and does not appear to care much about the success until he or she turns to a group of proud and smiling spectators (Kraut and Johnston 1979). The smiles of others, to put it simply, can be contagious, as can negative emotions, such as fear, anger, and sadness. As adults, these affective states occur and co-occur over much longer periods of time and are therefore often components of much more complicated systems of thought, relationships to others, and transactions within institutions.

Affect almost certainly plays a key role in the way stereotypes are internalized and thereby alter cognition and bodily phenomenology. As the discussion of Young's work above illustrates quite nicely, emotions help shape our bodily comportment: positive affect allows for an "I can" sense of embodied capability, whereas negative affect yields an "I cannot." But the development of the "I can" or "I cannot" is not wholly subjective, and cannot be separated from the individual's environment. Indeed, as Fine's studies on emotional intelligence indicate, background assumptions are already at play in stereotypes—such as "boys just don't have empathy" or "women are so emotional"—and that background is intersubjectively constituted. In other words, the belief that women are naturally less capable at this or that sport is developed and maintained through social transactions that serve to reiterate the idea and imbue it with more reality (cf. Butler ...), and in the process, new forms of affect that would not be possible without these interactions emerge. Shame, for example, at being the only woman on a hiking excursion and feeling the weight of one's body as an impediment, which subsequently slows one down, manifests itself as a relational phenomenon—that is, this social emotion is made possible only insofar as I compare myself to others, the stereotypes surrounding them versus me, and so forth.

7 Conclusion

Our argument that stereotypes are internalized dynamically through social interaction has important consequences for the training and mentoring of female athletes. As we have seen already, there is no reason to think that women are inherently weak as athletes. To name just a few female athletes with groundbreaking achievements, Serena Williams holds more major singles, doubles, and mixed doubles titles combined than any other player (male or female). With twenty-one Grand Slam titles, she is also the only tennis player to have ever won singles titles at least six times in three of four Grand Slam tournaments. Mia Hamm, an American football (soccer) player, held the record for having scored the most goals at an international level, for any player, male or female, with 159 goals. She held this record until 2013, when it was beaten by Abby Wambach, who has now scored 184 goals and is the current world-record holder (Capatides 2016). Kelly Kulick (bowling), in 2010, was the first woman to win a national tournament. She beat out sixty-two of the top US male bowlers to win (McManus 2011). There is a great deal of evidence, then, that women can perform extremely well in sports at very high levels, in some cases outperforming men. Given that women do have this capacity for high performance, we should look at and attempt to eliminate the gendered factors in their training that might inhibit them.

Schmalz and Kerstetter (2006) found in their study that "children as young as eight are aware of and are affected by gender stereotypes" (551). Parents and coaches need to be educated as well about the words they employ, and the way they react and behave toward all genders should be similar (Chalabaev, Sarrazin, et al. 2013). Therefore, coaches and trainers should take a closer look at the way they speak to and treat their athletes, since, according to our view, these interactions can play a significant role in their female athletes internalizing a sense of inhibited intentionality and stereotypes about female weakness. Instead, coaches should try to create an environment in which athletes of all genders avoid internalizing potentially damaging stereotypes. After all, part of what makes the underperformance effect of stereotype threat so difficult to counteract is that it is to some extent a self-fulfilling prophecy. A person exposed to salient stereotypes predicting their poor performance will often exemplify those stereotypes.

One step toward helping women at the present moment is to educate them about this phenomenon of stereotype threat (Johns, Schmader, and Martens 2005) and ensure they are aware of other women in sports who have outperformed their male counterparts, such as the women mentioned above. Interventions need to start at a young age to create an environment in which girls internalize an "I can" rather than an "I cannot," in which they are encouraged to embody norms of athleticism and strength rather than more restrictive norms of feminine bodily comportment. This means that they need to be able to see their bodies as capable of free action and movement rather than as encumbrances; and they need to be able to see themselves as acting subjects rather than as things objects that are acted upon. This means actively discouraging stereotypes of female weakness and incapacity. However, even if the training environment does not contribute to the internalization of these stereotypes in young female athletes, it would be naïve to think that they would be able to avoid exposure to them in the media and in society at large. Therefore, measures still need to be taken to counteract the effects of stereotype threat, given the prevalence of negative stereotypes about female athletes.

One way that coaches can counteract the effects of stereotype threat is by employing insights from the growth mind-set literature. Yeager and Dweck (2012), for instance, discuss implicit theories, which are assumptions about personal characteristics that people have, such as intelligence or athletic ability. Fixed, or entitative, theories can be contrasted with malleable, or incremental, theories. Those with more of an entitative theory of intelligence, for example, tend to see intellectual ability as something people have a fixed amount of—some are just naturally smarter than others—whereas those with an incremental theory tend to see it as something that can be grown and developed over time.

At least in the area of intellectual ability, researchers have found that the adoption of a growth mind-set can help counteract the effects of stereotype threat (Dweck 2007). Good, Dweck, and Rattan (2005) compared the experiences of female students in a calculus course who held entitative views of mathematical ability with those who held incremental views (see Dweck 2007). While many students in the class were well aware of negative stereotypes about women's mathematical ability, this view had much less influence on the students who held incremental theories of learning. Those who, in contrast, viewed mathematics as a gift were more vulnerable to setbacks and developed reduced confidence and sense of belonging.

To generalize these insights to the realm of athletics, coaches should foster a growth mind-set by de-emphasizing the contribution of natural ability to athletic success, focusing instead on the importance of consistent training and hard work. They might also share stories of high-level athletes who were not initially thought to have significant talent and promise but developed their skills through time and perseverance.

Also in line with the enactivist model that we have adopted here, some researchers argue that stereotype threat is situationally triggered, and that lower social status is not necessarily a precondition for it to occur (Leyens et al. 2000). Hively and El-Alayli (2014) found that if the task was easy, then even when pressure was added, stereotype threats did not hinder performance; this idea could be implemented in interventions to boost the confidence of female athletes. Gradual, incremental increases in task difficulty could also reinforce the development of a growth mind-set about training.

In general, our argument is that we should take very seriously the idea that social dynamics are equally, if not more, responsible in shaping the embodied capability of an individual than her own sense of ability. Coaches, trainers, and parents responsible for training athletes of different genders should pay careful attention to potential conflicts between stereotypes and norms of athletic performance. And when possible, they should foster a growth mind-set in their athletes in order to counteract the effects of the stereotypes they will almost inevitably encounter. This would result in positive changes to the way that female athletes are trained in swimming, surfing, sport martial arts, and many other embodied practices.

Notes

1. There are several strands of enactivism, to be sure, but our focus is limited to the general thesis that cognition is not a passive and internal thing that happens to us or inside us, but is something we *do*—a process we engage in when we are meaningfully coupled to the environment (cf. Noë 2010).

2. As I walk down a busy downtown street, I might, for example, see a church steeple and think to myself, "St. Paul's Cathedral is approximately five blocks away." But my estimation is not simply the result of inputting a set of complete data as to the whereabouts of the cathedral to my brain and performing the requisite computational analysis. In fact, I don't even see the whole building—just a small fraction of it. And yet, it is given to me in experience as a whole object. This is what Merleau-Ponty (1962) has referred to as having presence in absence, or the idea that objects are never actually wholly presented to us, and yet, they are experienced as such even in their lack of wholeness.

References

Ambady, Nalini, Margaret Shih, Amy Kim, and Todd L. Pittinsky. 2001. "Stereotype Susceptibility in Cchildren: Effects of Identity Activation on Quantitative Performance." *Psychological Science*, 12 (5): 385–390.

Atencio, Matthew, Becky Beal, and Charlene Wilson. 2009. "The Distinction of Risk: Urban Skateboarding, Street Habitus and the Construction of Hierarchical Gender Relations." *Qualitative Research in Sport and Exercise* 1 (1): 3–20.

Axisa, Mike. 2016. "Female Pitcher Sarah Hudek Picks Up First Collegiate Win." CBS Sports, February 13. Accessed May 31, 2016. http://www.cbssports.com/mlb/eye-on-baseball/25482728/female-pitcher-sarah-hudek-picks-up-first-collegiate-win.

Baron-Cohen, Simon. 2003. *The Essential Difference: Male and Female Brains and the Truth about Autism*. New York: Basic Books.

Beal, Becky, and Charlene Wilson. 2004. "'Chicks Dig Scars': Commercialisation and the Transformations of Skateboarders' Identities." In *Understanding Lifestyle Sport: Consumption, Identity and Difference*, edited by Belinda Wheaton, 31–54. New York: Routledge.

Beilock, Sian L., William A. Jellison, Robert J. Rydell, Allen R. McConnell, and Thomas H. Carr. 2006. "On the Causal Mechanisms of Stereotype Threat: Can Skills That Don't Rely Heavily on Working Memory Still Be Threatened?" *Personality and Social Psychology Bulletin* 32 (8): 1059–1071.

Beilock, Sian L., and Allen R. McConnell. 2004. "Stereotype Threat and Sport: Can Athletic Performance Be Threatened?" *Journal of Sport and Exercise Psychology* 26 (4): 597–609.

Berri, David. 2015. "Basketball's Gender Wage Gap Iis Even Worse Than You Think." Vice Sports, August 12. https://sports.vice.com/en_us/article/basketballs-gender-wage-gap-is-even-worse-than-you-think.

Bettcher, Talia. 2007. "Evil Deceivers and Make-Believers: On Transphobic Violence and the Politics of Illusion." *Hypatia* 22 (3): 43–65.

Bettcher, Talia. 2009. "Trans Identities and First-Person Authority." In *You've Changed: Sex Reassignment and Personal Identity*, edited by Laurie Shrage, 98–120. Oxford: Oxford University Press.

Birrell, Susan, and Nancy Theberge. 1994. "Feminist Resistance and Transformation in Sport." In *Women and Sport: Interdisciplinary Perspectives*, edited by D. Costa and Sharon Ruth Guthrie, 361–376. Champaign, IL: Human Kinetics.

Booth, Douglas. 2001. "From Bikinis to Boardshorts: Wahines and the Paradoxes of Surfing Culture." *Journal of Sport History* 28 (1): 3–22.

Butler, Judith. 1999. *Gender Trouble*. New York: Routledge.

Cahn, Susan K. 1994. *Coming on Strong: Gender and Sexuality in Twentieth-Century Women's Sport*. New York: Free Press.

Capatides, Christina. 2016. "Greatest Female Athletes of All Time." *CBS News*. Accessed March 13, 2016. http://www.cbsnews.com/pictures/greatest-female-athletes-of-all-time/.

Cepeda, Elias. 2015. "Ronda Rousey: 'I'm Not a Do-Nothing B****.'" Fox Sports, July 29. http://www.foxsports.com/ufc/story/ronda-rousey-i-m-not-a-do-nothing-bitch-072915.

Chalabaev, Aïna, Jeanick Brisswalter, Rémi Radel, Stephen A. Coombes, Christopher Easthope, and Corentin Clément-Guillotin. 2013. "Can Stereotype Threat Affect Motor Performance in the Absence of Explicit Monitoring Processes? Evidence Using a Strength Task." *Journal of Sport and Exercise Psychology* 35 (2): 211–215.

Chalabaev, Aïna, Philippe Sarrazin, Paul Fontayne, Julie Boiché, and Corentin Clément-Guillotin. 2013. "The Influence of Sex Stereotypes and Gender Roles on Participation and Performance in Sport and Exercise: Review and Future Directions." *Psychology of Sport and Exercise* 14 (2): 136–144.

Chalabaev, Aina, Philippe Sarrazin, Jeff Stone, and François Cury. 2008. "Do Achievement Goals Mediate Stereotype Threat? An Investigation on Females' Soccer Performance." *Journal of Sport and Exercise Psychology* 30 (2): 143–158.

Chisholm, Dianne. 2008. "Climbing Like a Girl: An Exemplary Adventure in Feminist Phenomenology." *Hypatia* 23 (1): 9–40.

Clark, Andy. 2008. *Supersizing the Mind: Embodiment, Action, and Cognitive Extension*. Oxford: Oxford University Press.

Comley, Cassie. 2016. "'We Have to Establish Our Territory': How Women Surfers 'Carve Out' Gendered Spaces within Surfing." *Sport in Society* 19 (8/9): 1289–1298.

Connor, Steve. 2013. "The Hardwired Difference between Male and Female Brains Could Explain Why Men Are 'Better at Map Reading.'" *The Independent*, December 3. http://www.independent.co.uk/life-style/the-hardwired-difference-between-male-and-female-brains-could-explain-why-men-are-better-at-map-8978248.html.

Cooky, Cheryl, Michael A. Messner, and Michela Musto. 2015. "'It's Dude Time!' A Quarter Century of Excluding Women's Sports in Televised News and Highlight Shows." *Communication and Sport* 3 (3): 261–287.

Dator, James. 2016. "Serena Williams Sends Powerful Message to Indian Wells CEO over Sexist Comments." SBNation, March 20. http://www.sbnation.com/2016/3/20/11273222/serena-williams-press-conference-sexist-comments-indian-wells-ceo.

De Jaegher, Hanne, and Ezequiel Di Paolo. 2007. "Participatory Sense-Making: An Enactive Approach to Social Cognition." *Phenomenology and the Cognitive Sciences* 6 (4): 485–507.

Di Paolo, Ezequiel, and Evan Thompson. 2014. "The Enactive Approach." In *The Routledge Hhandbook of Embodied Cognition,* edited by Lawrence Shapiro, 68–78. London: Routledge.

Dweck, Carol S. 2007. "Is Math a Gift? Beliefs that Put Females at Risk." In *Why Aren't More Women in Science? Top Researchers Debate the Evidence,* edited by Stephen J. Ceci and Wendy M. Williams, 47–55. Washington, DC: American Psychological Association.

Dworkin, Shari L., and Michael A. Messner. 2002. "Gender Relations in Sport." *Sociological Perspectives: Official Publication of the Pacific Sociological Association* 45 (4): 347–352.

Eagly, Alice H. 1995. "The Science and Politics of Comparing Women and Men." *American Psychologist* 50 (3): 145–158.

Eichenberger, Evelyn, Beat Knechtle, Christoph Alexander Rüst, Patrizia Knechtle, Romuald Lepers, and Thomas Rosemann. 2012. "No Gender Difference in Peak Performance in Ultra-Endurance Swimming Performance: Analysis of the 'Zurich 12-H Swim' from 1996 to 2010." *Chinese Journal of Physiology* 55 (5): 346–351.

Eisenberg, Nancy, and Randy Lennon. 1983. "Sex Differences in Empathy and Related Capacities." *Psychological Bulletin* 94 (1): 100–131.

Evans, Bethan. 2006. "'I'd Feel Ashamed': Girls' Bodies and Sports Participation." *Gender, Place and Culture* 13 (5): 547–561.

Fausto-Sterling, Anne. 2000. *Sexing the Body*. New York: Basic Books.

Fendt, Laura Sophia, and Erica Wilson. 2012. "'I Just Push through the Barriers Because I Live for Surfing': How Women Negotiate Their Constraints to Surf Tourism." *Annals of Leisure Research* 15 (1): 4–18.

Fine, Cordelia. 2010. *Delusions of Gender: How Our Minds, Society, and Neurosexism Create Difference.* New York: W.W. Norton.

Ford, Nick, and David Brown. 2006. *Surfing and Social Theory: Experience, Embodiment and Narrative of the Dream Glide.* New York: Taylor and Francis.

Foster, Susan Leigh. 2009. "Throwing Like a Girl, Dancing Like a Feminist Philosopher." In *Dancing with Iris: The Philosophy of Iris Marion Young,* edited by Ann Ferguson and Mechthild Nagel, 69–78. Oxford: Oxford University Press.

Fuchs, Thomas, and Hanne De Jaegher. 2009. "Enactive Intersubjectivity: Participatory Sense-Making and Mutual Incorporation." *Phenomenology and the Cognitive Sciences* 8 (4): 465–486.

Garfinkel, Harold. 1957. *Studies in Ethnomethodology*. Oxford: Polity.

Gibson, James J. 1977. "The Theory of Affordances." In *Perceiving, Acting, and Knowing: Toward an Ecological Psychology,* edited by Robert Shaw and John Bransford, 67–83. Mahwah, NJ: Lawrence Erlbaum.

Guérandel, Carine, and Christine Mennesson. 2007. "Gender Construction in Judo Interactions." *International Review for the Sociology of Sport* 42 (2): 167–186.

Guillen, Adam, Jr. 2015. "Cris Cyborg Erupts after 'Disrespectful' Joe Rogan Jokes She Has a Penis." SBNation, November 17. http://www.mmamania.com/2015/11/17/9749762/ufc-cris-cyborg-blasts-dana-white-and-joe-rogan-for-hurtful-dick-jokes-mma.

Hargreaves, Jennifer. 1994. *Sporting Females: Critical Issues in the History and Sociology of Women's Sports*. New York: Routledge.

Heywood, Leslie, and Shari L. Dworkin. 2003. *Built to Win: The Female Athlete as Cultural Icon.* Minneapolis, MN: University of Minnesota Press.

Hively, Kimberly, and Amani El-Alayli. 2014. "'You Throw Like a Girl': The Effect of Stereotype Threat on Women's Athletic Performance and Gender Stereotypes." *Psychology of Sport and Exercise* 15 (1): 48–55.

Holpuch, Amanda. 2013. "Skeptics Debate the Conditions of Diana Nyad's Record Swim from Cuba." *Guardian,* September 9. http://www.theguardian.com/world/2013/sep/09/diana-nyad-skeptics-record-swim-cuba.

Hutto, Daniel D., and Erik Myin. 2012. *Radicalizing Enactivism: Basic Minds without Content.* Cambridge, MA: MIT Press. https://doi.org/10.7551/mitpress/9780262018548.001.0001.

Johns, Michael, Toni Schmader, and Andy Martens. 2005. "Knowing Is Half the Battle: Teaching Stereotype Threat as a Means of Improving Women's Math Performance." *Psychological Science* 16 (3): 175–179.

Karkazis, Katrina, Rebecca Jordan-Young, Georgiann Davis, and Silvia Camporesi. 2012. "Out of Bounds? A Critique of the New Policies on Hyperandrogenism in Elite Female Athletes." *American Journal of Bioethics: AJOB* 12 (7): 3–16.

Kimmel, Michael. 1996. *Manhood in America: A Cultural History*. New York: Free Press.

Kimmel, Michael S. 1990. "Baseball and the Reconstitution of American Masculinity, 1880–1920." In *Sport, Men and the Gender Order: Critical Feminist Perspectives,* edited by Michael A. Messner and Donald F. Sabo, 55–65. Champaign, IL: Human Kinetics.

Klein, Kristi J. K., and Sara D. Hodges. 2001. "Gender Differences, Motivation, and Empathic Accuracy: When It Pays to Understand." *Personality and Social Psychology Bulletin* 27 (6): 720–730.

Knijnik, Jorge Dorfman, Peter Horton, and Lívia Oliveira Cruz. 2010. "Rhizomatic Bodies, Gendered Waves: Transitional Femininities in Brazilian Surf." *Sport in Society* 13 (7/8): 1170–1185.

Kolnes, Liv-Jorunn. 1995. "Heterosexuality as an Organizing Principle in Women's Sport." *International Review for the Sociology of Sport* 30 (1): 61–77.

Krane, Vikki. 2001. "We Can Be Athletic and Feminine, but Do We Want To? Challenging Hegemonic Femininity in Women's Sport." *Quest* 53 (1): 115–133.

Kraut, Robert. 1986. "Love De Re." *Midwest Studies In Philosophy* 10 (1): 413–430.

Kraut, Robert E., and Robert E. Johnston. 1979. "Social and Emotional Messages of Smiling: An Ethological Approach." *Journal of Personality and Social Psychology*, 37 (9): 1539–1553.

Krendl, Anne C., Izzy B. Gainsburg, and Nalini Ambady. 2012. "The Effects of Stereotypes and Observer Pressure on Athletic Performance." *Journal of Sport and Exercise Psychology* 34 (1): 3–15.

Krueger, Joel. 2013. "Ontogenesis of the Socially Extended Mind." *Cognitive Systems Research* 25 (December): 40–46.

Krueger, Joel. 2014. "Emotions and the Social Niche." In *Collective Emotions*, edited by Christian von Scheve and Mikko Salmela, 156–171. New York: Oxford University Press.

Lang, Peter J. 1994. "The Varieties of Emotional Experience: A Meditation on James–Lange Theory." *Psychological Review* 101 (2): 211–222.

Leyens, Jacques-Philippe, Michel Désert, Jean-Claude Croizet, and Catherine Darcis. 2000. "Stereotype Threat: Are Lower Status and History of Stigmatization Preconditions of Stereotype Threat?" *Personality and Social Psychology Bulletin* 26 (10): 1189–1199.

Maturana, Humberto. 1987. "Everything Said Is Said by an Observer." In *Gaia: A Way of Knowing*, edited by William Thompson, 65–82. New York: Lindisfarne Press.

McManus, Jane. 2011. "Can Women Play with the Men?" ESPN, May 9. http://espn.go.com/espnw/news/article/6495612/women-pro-sports-women-play-men.

Meân, Lindsey J., and Jeffrey W. Kassing. 2008. "'I Would Just Like to Be Known as an Athlete': Managing Hegemony, Femininity, and Heterosexuality in Female Sport." *Western Journal of Speech Communication* 72 (2): 126–144.

Medwechuk, Nicole, and Jane Crossman. 1994. "Effects of Gender Bias on the Evaluation of Male and Female Swim Coaches." *Perceptual and Motor Skills* 78 (1): 163–169. doi:10.2466/pms.1994.78.1.163.

Merritt, Michele. 2014. "Making (Non)Sense of Gender." In *Enactive Cognition at the Edge of Sense-Making: Making Sense of Non-Sense*, edited by Massimiliano Cappuccio and Tom Froese, 285–306. New Directions in Cognitive Science. London: Palgrave-MacMillan.

Messner, Michael. 2011. "Gender Ideologies, Youth Sports, and the Production of Soft Essentialism." *Sociology of Sport* 28 (2): 151–170.

Messner, Michael A. 1988. "Sports and Male Domination: The Female Athlete as Contested Ideological Terrain." *Sociology of Sport Journal* 5 (3): 197–211.

Messner, Michael A. 1995. *Power at Play*. Boston: Beacon Press.

Messner, Michael A. 2000. "Barbie Girls versus Sea Monsters: Children Constructing Gender." *Gender and Society* 14 (6): 765–784.

Messner, Michael A., and Donald F. Sabo. 1990. *Sport, Men, and the Gender Order: Critical Feminist Perspectives*. Champaign, IL: Human Kinetics.

Mirsky, Steve. 2015. "First Woman MLBer Will Probably Pitch." *Scientific American*. May 19. http://www.scientificamerican.com/podcast/episode/first-woman-mlber-will-probably-pitch/.

Musto, Michela. 2014. "Athletes in the Pool, Girls and Boys on Deck: The Contextual Construction of Gender in Coed Youth Swimming." *Gender and Society* 28 (3): 359–380.

Merleau-Ponty, Maurice. 1962. *Phenomenology of Perception*, trans. C. Smith. London: Routledge and Kegan Paul.

Noë, Alva. 2010. *Out of Our Heads: Why You Are Not Your Brain, and Other Lessons from the Biology of Consciousness*. New York: Farrar, Straus and Giroux.

North, Anna. 2012. "7 Sports in which Women Have Beaten Men." Buzzfeed, August 3. http://www.buzzfeed.com/annanorth/7-sports-in-which-women-have-beaten-men#.plx6y1J9n.

Nussbaum, Martha C. 2003. *Upheavals of Thought: The Intelligence of Emotions*. Cambridge: Cambridge University Press.

Olive, Rebecca, Louise McCuaig, and Murray G. Phillips. 2015. "Women's Recreational Surfing: A Patronising Experience." *Sport, Education, and Society* 20 (2): 258–276.

Pelak, Cynthia Fabrizio. 2002. "Women's Collective Identity Formation in Sports: A Case Study from Women's Ice Hockey." *Gender and Society* 16 (1): 93–114.

Prinz, Jesse J. 2004. *Gut Reactions: A Perceptual Theory of Emotion*. Oxford: Oxford University Press.

Riemer, Brenda A., and Michelle E. Visio. 2003. "Gender Typing of Sports: An Investigation of Metheny's Classification." *Research Quarterly for Exercise and Sport* 74 (2): 193–204.

Ross, Sally R., and Kimberly J. Shinew. 2008. "Perspectives of Women College Athletes on Sport and Gender." *Sex Roles* 58 (1/2): 40–57.

Roughgarden, Joan. 2004. *Evolution's Rainbow: Diversity, Gender, and Sexuality in Nature and People*. Oakland: University of California Press.

Roy, Georgina, and Jayne Caudwell. 2014. "Women and Surfing Spaces in Newquay, UK." In *Routledge Handbook of Sport, Gender and Sexuality*, edited by Jennifer Hargreaves and Eric Anderson, 235–244. New York: Routledge.

Sabo, Donald F., and Phil Veliz. 2008. *Go Out and Play: Youth Sports in America*. East Meadow, NY: Women's Sports Foundation.

Schmalz, Dorothy L., and Deborah L. Kerstetter. 2006. "Girlie Girls and Manly Men: Children's Stigma Consciousness of Gender in Sports and Physical Activities." *Journal of Leisure Research* 38 (4): 536–557.

Shapiro, Jenessa R., and Amy M. Williams. 2012. "The Role of Stereotype Threats in Undermining Girls' and Women's Performance and Interest in STEM Fields." *Sex Roles* 66 (3): 175–183.

Sisjord, Mari-Kristin. 1997. "Wrestling with Gender: A Study of Young Female and Male Wrestlers' Experiences of Physicality." *International Review for the Sociology of Sport* 32 (4): 433–438.

Sisjord, Mari-Kristin. 2009. "Fast-Girls, Babes and the Invisible Girls: Gender Relations in Snowboarding." *Sport in Society* 12 (10): 1299–1316.

Skenazy, Matt. 2014. "Maya Gabeira Takes a Breath." *Outside*, September 3. http://www.outsideonline.com/1925936/maya-gabeira-takes-breath.

Spencer, Steven J., Claude M. Steele, and Diane M. Quinn. 1999. "Stereotype Threat and Women's Math Performance." *Journal of Experimental Social Psychology* 35:4–28.

Spowart, Lucy, Lisette Burrows, and Sally Shaw. 2010. "'I Just Eat, Sleep and Dream of Surfing': When Surfing Meets Motherhood." *Sport in Society* 13 (7/8): 1186–1203.

Steele, Claude M., and Joshua Aronson. 1995. "Stereotype Threat and the Intellectual Test Performance of African Americans." *Journal of Personality and Social Psychology* 69 (5): 797–811.

Stoddart, Mark C. J. 2011. "Constructing Masculinized Sportscapes: Skiing, Gender and Nature in British Columbia, Canada." *International Review for the Sociology of Sport* 46 (1): 108–124.

Thompson, Evan. 2007. *Mind in Life: Biology, Phenomenology, and the Sciences of Mind*. Cambridge, MA: Harvard University Press.

Thorne, Barrie. 1993. *Gender Play: Girls and Boys in School*. New Brunswick, NJ: Rutgers University Press.

Thorpe, Holly. 2005. "Jibbing the Gender Order: Females in the Snowboarding Culture." *Sport in Society* 8 (1): 76–100.

Thorpe, Holly. 2009. "Bourdieu, Feminism and Female Physical Culture: Gender Reflexivity and the Habitus-Field Complex." *Sociology of Sport Journal* 26 (4): 491–516.

Time. 2015. "The 30 Most Influential Teens of 2015." October 27. http://time.com/4081618/most-influential-teens-2015/.

Triantafyllou, Michael S., and George S. Triantafyllou. 1995. "An Efficient Swimming Machine." *Scientific American* 272 (3): 64–70.

Tronick, Edward Z., Heidelise Als, Lauren Adamson, Susan Wise, and T. Berry Brazelton. 1978. "The Infant's Response to Entrapment between Contradictory Messages in Face-to-Face Interaction." *Journal of the American Academy of Child Psychiatry*, 17 (1): 1–13.

Varela, Francisco, Evan Thompson, and Eleanor Rosch. 1991. *The Embodied Mind: Cognitive Science and the Human Experience*. Cambridge, MA: MIT Press.

von Scheve, Christian, and Mikko Salmela. 2014. *Collective Emotions: Perspectives from Psychology, Philosophy, and Sociology*. Oxford: Oxford University Press.

Wainer, Howard, Catherine Njue, and Samuel Palmer. 2000. "Assessing Time Trends in Sex Differences in Swimming and Running." *Chance* 13 (1): 10–17.

Yap, Audrey. 2016. "(Hip) Throwing Like a Girl: Martial Arts and Norms of Feminine Body Comportment." *IJFAB: International Journal of Feminist Approaches to Bioethics* 9 (2): 92–114.

Yeager, David Scott, and Carol S. Dweck. 2012. "Mindsets That Promote Resilience: When Students Believe That Personal Characteristics Can Be Developed." *Educational Psychologist* 47 (4): 302–314.

Young, Iris Marion. 1998. "'Throwing Like a Girl': Twenty Years Later." In *Body and Flesh: A Philosophical Reader*, edited by Donn Welton, 259–273. Malden, MA: Blackwell.

Young, Iris Marion. 2005. "Throwing Like a Girl: A Phenomenology of Feminine Body Comportment, Motility, and Spatiality." In *On Female Body Experience: "Throwing Like a Girl" and Other Essays*, edited by Iris Marion Young, 27–45. New York: Oxford University Press.

Zaccardi, Nick. 2015. "Michael Phelps Jokingly Challenges Katie Ledecky to Race." NBC Sports, April 18. http://olympics.nbcsports.com/2015/04/18/michael-phelps-katie-ledecky-race-swimming-mesa-olympics/.

18 Ethnomethodological Respecifications of Cognition in Sport

Raúl Sánchez-García, Giolo Fele, and Kenneth Liberman

1 Introduction

Research in sport and skill acquisition is monopolized by psychology-based analysis, not taking into account explanations about cognition coming from the social sciences. In social activities such as sports, cognitive processes cannot be reduced to individual minds and must be understood as part of the complex and dense embedded interactional work that participants maintain through embodied interaction. Such a praxeological view of cognition can be developed through ethnomethodology's (EM) research program. The general aim of this chapter is to develop the social dimension of the embodied cognition in sport. To do so, we provide an ethnomethodological respecification of some cognition-related topics through the empirical analysis of specific cases in sport settings. We use the EM approach as an alternate for some of the pitfalls and limitations regarding the social dimension of cognition presented by the main paradigms for analyzing skill acquisition and sport performance: information processing and ecological dynamics. Regarding these two paradigms, EM is more critically opposed to information processing than it is to ecological dynamics. An EM research program can contribute to an ecological approach by developing a more well-rounded analysis of the social dimension.

First, we briefly present an ethnomethodological approach to cognition; then we criticize the information-processing approach to decision making and rule-based reasoning by presenting an EM analysis of street-crossing and surfing and the information-processing approach to imagery through an EM analysis of climbing. We continue with an improvement of ecological dynamics approaches through EM's introduction of the social dimension to solve the selection of affordance problem in Krav Maga; to better explain functional variability in defense against screening in basketball; and to make a more appropriate characterization of instructions as augmented information through an EM analysis of instructed action in aikido.

2 Ethnomethodology's Study of Cognition as Practical Reasoning

Ethnomethodology (EM) is a research program developed by Harold Garfinkel (1967, 1996, 2002, 2006; Garfinkel and Sacks 1986) that proposes to study and report on practical methods (ethnomethods) that occur in the concerted actions among actors. Ethnomethods provide habitual ways of doing things as part of the routine grounds for action. They do not belong to a particular subject (in the sense of someone owning some ethnomethods) but to the social dimension of practice among members. Thus, EM offers a research program to study the social dimension of cognition. EM offers a way to study practical reasoning and practical actions embodied and embedded *in* and *as* ethnomethods of members engaged in concerted actions. By and through these ethnomethods, a common understanding related to normal patterns of action is produced among the parties. These practical methods imply a certain kind of practical reasoning, which must be studied as domain-specific phenomena; no universal reason, but domain-specific reasons (Livingston 2008).

EM's understanding of practical reasoning is a direct critique of info-processing theories and a defense of the embodied and embedded features of cognition. In a nutshell: if cognition is embedded and embodied, as EM maintains, then info-processing theories fail to explain cognition. EM considers the body as a constitutive element of cognition, precluding the possibility of conceiving cognition as something that exists only inside the subject's brain.[1] EM considers thinking as non-separable from the perceiving and acting of a subject embedded in a specific activity. According to Livingston (2006), "A pervasive prejudice in academic work is that reasoning is a mental operation: it is something that goes on in the brain. Once separated from embodied perception and embodied action, and from the temporal circumstances and contingencies of immediately present situations, all reasoning is made equivalent and all reasoning is accountable to formal inference" (423).

Livingston (2008, 39) advocates for a research on reasoning in the concrete practices, a "midenic reasoning" (in the middle of doing things), in contrast to first modelling what reason is about and then applying the model top-down to specific tasks. Thus, the EM research program avoids experimental settings that lack a "representative experimental design" (Brunswik 1956) of real situations. The research should "examine connections between lived-reasoning and action and between reasoning, skill, embodiment and perception" (Livingston 2008, 29). EM proposes an analysis of human interaction based not just on talking but also on variegated and multiple modes such as gesture, gaze, posture, talk, materials, and so on (LeCouter and Feo 2011; Streeck, Goodwin, and LeBaron 2011).

The other dominant paradigm in the study of skill acquisition and sport, ecological dynamics, offers a much more promising research program than information processing to understand embodied and embedded cognition. Nonetheless, it also presents some limitations referred to the social dimension that can be remedied through an EM approach. Garfinkel (2002) offered an ethnomethodological remedy—what he dubbed "ethnomethodological alternates"—to the mere formal analyses that sociology offers about the social phenomena. In the same vein, ecological dynamics renders formal analysis but misses the "interaction order" (Goffman 1983). Such order is constituted by the dense interaction work to which agents are continuously attending, constituting true "environments for each other" (McDermott 1976, 36) through embodied communicative interaction in variegated and multiple modes.

In this chapter we present ethnomethodological respecifications ("EM alternates") of some cognition-related topics that have been already analyzed, either by information-processing or ecological dynamics approaches. By doing so, we aim to provide a more adequate analysis of cognition's social dimension in sport.

3 Information Processing (1): Cognitive Decisions and Rule Following

The main assumption of the information-processing paradigm is to define cognition as a computation of symbolic representations and the brain as some kind of computer doing this computation. Cognitive processes are present not only in the decision-making phase; they also heavily influence the perception and action phases: sensory inputs coming from the environment are cognitively transformed (thanks to memory) in order to gain information for the agent who makes decisions on what kind of responses to take and, afterward, control motor responses by cognitive motor programs that imply some kind of rule-based reasoning.

In the fields of skill acquisition and sport performance, information processing still maintains a predominant position. It has been specifically applied to sport thanks to an "expertise approach," placing special importance on the comparison of the differences between novices and experts and on how the strategies and knowledge of experts are acquired in real-life sport domains (Summer 2004, 13). This paradigm has been applied in a research program that emphasizes the phenomenon of decision making, affected by cognitive systems such as working memory and attention. Some cognitive abilities determining decision making are stored in the memory and can be understood as a set of rules to follow in order to solve different problems. Information coming from the actual situation (via perception) and blended with already stored knowledge about the activity will produce certain response in the game. Expert players not only have superior cognitive abilities affecting perception, but also have better tactical knowledge (a rule-based reasoning) of the game, that is to say, they have stored knowledge about the game that allows them to anticipate and make better decisions during the game than do novices (Starkes, Helsen, and Jack 2001; Williams, Davids, and Williams 1999).

The EM approach to cognition discards processing of information and rule-based reasoning as valid concepts to account for the intelligent behavior of players and places a direct critique of information-processing views that over-cognitivize the phenomenon of cognition and decision making. Information processing is an idealized version that captures in a distorted way a sliver of what might be going on during social interactions. EM proposes an alternative understanding of cognitive phenomena as embedded and embodied practical reasoning.

Let us start with the basic activity of crossing the street. Liberman (2013) analyzed the ethnomethods used by different actors potentially involved in the activity (bus drivers, car drivers, skateboarders, pedestrians). Such ethnomethods comprised a variegated corpus of strategies that kept the traffic flow running. The crossing was a matter of local orderliness for the actors. That is, actors' practical reasoning provided adequate solutions to what they encountered there. What they did to maintain this local orderliness was not as formally rational as information-processing models propose. Without relief, new problems must be confronted on each next occasion. Actors needed neither a general theory of traffic flow to be applied in this particular place and time nor any internalized set of rules that must be applied to solve the problem. As Liberman (2013) remarks, "The bulk of the actions are responses to one or another *salience* of a gestalt contexture and are largely unavailable to rational planning" (20; emphasis original). A salience is an opportunity that is segregated from the phenomenal field and seized upon.

The case of local orderliness and practical reasoning developed through ethnomethods and their relation to rules was also rendered visible in surfing (Sánchez-García and Liberman 2015). We were interested in analyzing the naturally occurring phenomena of surfers taking turns in the lineup as they wait for ocean waves. Even though certain basic rules for deciding rights over the next wave—such as outside rider (the one closest to the peak, which implies the longest run in the wave) and first to stand up (first surfer to stand up on the board)—are known to competent members of the surfing community, surfers did not move through the phenomenal field acting as rational actors with rules in their mind. We argue that the basic rules of surfing are not mental contents in the heads of surfers. Rules of surfing are just glosses for ethnomethods used on local situations to render actions legitimate or illegitimate. The rules of "outside rider" and "first to stand up" are just glosses for a myriad of behaviors that we can encounter in certain circumstances when two or more surfers are getting ready to ride a wave. Some of these behaviors are considered as correct and some others as wrong, but all of them are subject to serendipitous contingencies that are rendered orderly by the surfers' ethnomethods.

But how does one distinguish what is correct behavior? A quick answer would be to go to the rule to interpret what is going on. Since rules are only glosses, in order to interpret what is taking place we need to rely on legitimate and illegitimate habitual ways of doing surfing, acting as a context for the interpretation of the ongoing activity. But we would be mistaken if we accepted the rules as a stock of knowledge that rests in the heads of the surfers (that would be the default perspective of a cognitivist view of rules). Rather, we examine how the ethnomethods, habitual embodied ways of interacting with the environment we call surfing, are developed and employed. That is why level of expertise (implying more or less previous experiences) affects a correct application of rules and a correct interpretation of what is going on in the water; the application of rules and interpretations by novices would be hindered by their having a very small stock of previous experiences. Nevertheless, this is not to say that expert surfers always interpret everything right or that the rules they keep adapting are legitimate.

The breaking of basic rules carries moral implications, the adequacy of which depends on the breaking of those rules being made publicly witnessable, which is part of the constant interactive work that participants must take up. Besides, in some circumstances there is competition among different basic rules that can be made applicable to a situation. For instance, as we can observe in the images in figure 18.1, when an inside surfer is already up and riding the wave when the outside person stands up, this can undermine the claim that the outside rider has an exclusive right to the wave.

Basic rules are just another kind of resource used by surfers to decide who gets the ride in different circumstances. The precarious situation in which surfers make judgments (moving fast, with a limited field of vision and sound, threatened by the risk of crashing waves or crashing participants) makes rule application a complex but necessary matter. Such complexity is increased by the possibility of different rules competing during the same occasion. Besides, the risky essence of the activity implies that security matters can prevail over rights to obtain the ride.

In fact, surfers were paddling around and making circumspect inspections that maintained some orientation within the developing scene. They were waiting for adequate saliences to catch the wave in the swarm of competing surfers, using basic rules as just one kind of resource for acting in concert with the activity of others but also taking into account the many risks involved; on days when the swell is large, simply surviving the waves is the limited aim. Ethnomethods of expert surfers encompass all

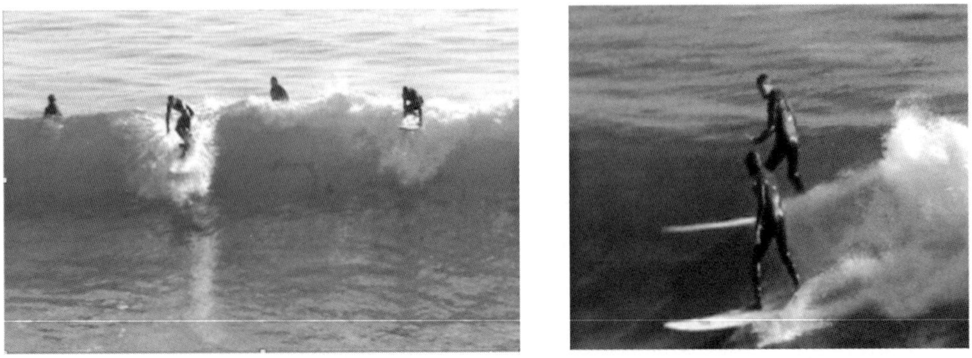

Figure 18.1
The inside rider was witnessably the first to stand up (left), disallowing the outside rider's claim to hold sole rights to the wave (right).

of these matters (rules being just one of them). Because rules can be used by social theorists to devise a decision-making process that is more rational than is actually the case, their status as stable objects are inflated. Many hours in the water with other surfers are needed (A) to acquire rules and (B) to learn how to adapt them flexibly and reflexively to local circumstances.

Those ethnomethods are observable-reportable (accountable): this means that what actors do makes sense (i.e., one can see it and can talk about it) to those with whom they interact, because otherwise social interaction would not be possible. This implies, in turn, that these are phenomena that can be studied and transmitted through the elaboration of the episodes or courses of action in which ethnomethods are generated.

4 Information Processing (2): The Topic of Imagery

Even if the notion of "imagery" is controversial, it still holds a vast currency in the sciences of sport, especially from the perspective of the information-processing paradigm.

Thus, we consider it useful to first introduce the notion as it is commonly used in the sport literature, and then propose an ethnomethodological analysis of a real case of imagery in climbing as part of the ongoing concerted actions deployed in real time in a specific setting.

In English there are idiomatic ways of talking about visual mental imagery, as "visualizing," "seeing in the mind's eye," "having a picture in one's head," "picturing," "having/seeing a mental image/picture," and so on. By "imagery" is commonly implied a process of internal representation of some kind of scenario. Visual mental imagery (MI) typically occurs “when a representation of the type created during the initial phase of perception is present but the stimulus is not actually being perceived; such representations preserve the perceptible properties of the stimulus and ultimately give rise to the subjective experience of perception” (Kosslyn, Thompson, and Ganis 2006, 4). According to Ganis, Thompson, and Kosslyn (2004) mental imagery consists of different functions that can be located in different neural networks through the use of brain scanning techniques such as fMRI.

The concept of imagery has been particularly successful in sport psychology (Vealey and Greenleaf 2006; Morris, Spittle, and Perry 2004). The concept of imagery in sport has helped researchers in focusing on the techniques athletes use to prepare for a motor performance. It is suggested that athletes can anticipate the progressive steps of their performance, at a slower pace, in a controlled, imaginary atmosphere. In this way, athletes can cognitively control the correct execution of the action and can psychologically control the emotional strain of the performance. Focusing on the physical gestures and keeping psychological tensions under control as a result of effective mental imagery results in improving the performance and regulating arousal and anxiety, increasing the athlete’s self-confidence. The notion of (mental) imagery has been proven to be the basis of peak performances and has been analyzed in several sport disciplines, such as rowing (Barr and Hall 1992), golf (Bernier and Fournier 2010), netball (Callow and Hardy 2001), skiing (Callow, Roberts, and Fawkes 2006), softball (Calmels et al. 2004), rugby (Evans, Jones, and Mullen 2004), basketball (Guillot, Nadrowska, and Collet 2009), tennis (Malouff et al. 2008), and karate (Weinberg, Seabourne, and Jackson 1981), among others.

Imagery in climbing (Boyd and Munroe 2003) has been used as the practice of fictionally rehearsing the path of the climb, in which the climbers, before actually starting the ascent, visually inspect the wall or the crag in search of the most effective approach. The use of imagery, that is, a mental dry run of the actual exercise, is seen as a key aspect to better accomplishing the real ascent in terms of efficacy or performance optimization (Sanchez et al. 2012) and can enhance the pleasure experienced by the athlete during the performance.

Many are the possible criticisms of the idea of imagery. First, there is the problem of accessing a mental state. In order to characterize such an inner condition of athletes, researchers have largely used tools reconstructing ex post facto the condition to be analyzed: in research papers we find athletes filling out a Sport Imagery Questionnaire (Boyd and Munroe 2003) or subjects seated in front of a PC (Smyth and Waller 1998). Although research conducted in laboratory-like settings has flourished, fewer studies have been done in real-world settings with a naturalistic paradigm: that is, observing what the climbers do and say in actual, naturally occurring situations and not in made-up conditions (see for instance Barratt 2012; Dutkiewicz 2015; Jenkings 2013). Asking questions after the fact impedes the access to the actual event of route planning.

The notion of imagery also implies disregarding the careful analysis of how the route preview works (or, in other words, what it means to *imagine* a route), in favor of assessing this imaginative work through the results obtained by this act of preparation. Sanchez et al. (2012) assess the performance of climbers in terms of route completion and the number and duration of moves and stops during the ascent. The authors note "expert climbers benefiting most from route preview. The ability to visually inspect a climb before its ascent may represent an essential component of performance optimization" (Sanchez et al. 2012, 67). In this way, however, we still ignore what it really means to "visually inspect a climb," and whether any role in this inspection is played by imagery.

If we examine closely what happens in the moment previous to the actual climbing, we can appreciate how the concept of visual (contrasted with auditory, olfactory, gustatory) imagery as a mental notion, made of ideal, abstract, or fictional rehearsal, often overlooks a series of actual, practical, overt bodily activities called "marking" (Kirsh et al. 2009). Marking accompanies any acts of anticipating the route to be taken, the ways the path should be executed, and the very concrete ways the various holds should be approached and held. Marking is a form of gestured action that the performer does with her hands, feet, or any part of the body and that stands in for a completed movement or step (Muntanyola and Kirsh 2010). Instead of being an act of mentally reconstructing a fictional picture in the obscure inside of a performer, the route preview or the pre-ascent climbing route visual inspection is better approached as a publicly accessible and socially observable sequence of action in which marking is a paramount feature of the interaction.

The following data are taken from video recordings of climbers preparing to climb at the base of a climbing wall during the IFSC Climbing World Championship 2011 (in Arco, Italy, July 15–24, 2011). The rules of the International Federation of Sport Climbing state that prior to each on-sight rock climbing competition, climbers are given the opportunity to preview the route.[2] In the modality of on-sight competition, no previous knowledge of the wall is allowed, and information regarding holds and paths is kept carefully hidden. Competitors are allowed to enter the competition space only minutes before the commencement of a round. Climbing on the wall is not permitted, but a collective observation period is allowed. The rules state that competitors may also use binoculars to observe the route, or make hand-drawn sketches and notes, but no recording equipment is permitted. When admitted to the competition space,

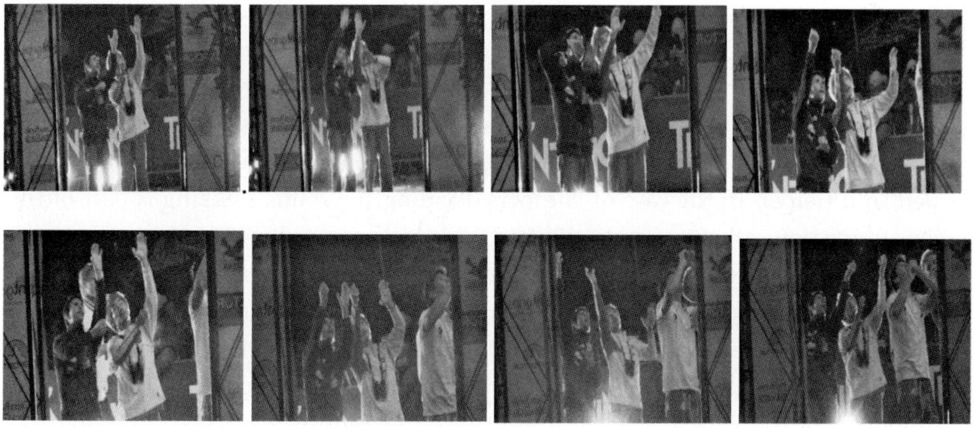

Figure 18.2
Sequence of gestures at the bottom of the climbing wall by competitors before the competition.

competitors are allowed to touch only the marked starting holds, without leaving the ground with any of their feet.[3] These rules shape the experience of being in the competition field for the first time and organize the ways in which knowledge of the wall can be acquired and climbers can plan their ascent.

If we observe what happens in those preliminary moments, we can see how climbers make sense of the task at hand. It seems that climbers do not rely on hidden mental skills but proceed through peculiar configurations of their bodies and verbal descriptions in a rather collaborative and interactional context.

As we can see from the sequence of pictures in figure 18.2, the climbers simulate the progression on the wall in an overt bodily configuration, step by step. The progression on the wall is rehearsed with movements of the body, reaching of the arms, the ways the hand is shaped depending on the kind of hold reached. If any "mental" process is involved in this preliminary marking, what is striking is the visible, open, and public process of corporal enacting of the actual movements as if they were already engaged with the material effort of vertically progressing up the wall.

Although these performers' bodily work has already been pointed out by some researchers (see, for instance Pezzullo et al. 2010, 69), less attention has been paid to the fact that this planning behavior is not an isolated, subjective, and individual activity: it is a social and shared chain of anticipatory actions. The performers act not as isolated individuals in front of an individual task; instead it appears that each climber exhibits in a public manner what for him is the way to approach each single step, and that "interpretation" is open for scrutiny by his fellow teammate. His teammate, in turn, does the same, with the same import. The result is a kind of dynamic bodily configuration, a sort of synchronized dance, a shared choreography of steps, which are jointly performed and practically displayed. In fact, as Muntanyola (2015) showed in the case of corrections in synchronized swimming, marking is a "socially organized skill," taking the place of speech, or co-occurring, in the communication between the athlete and trainer. In the case of climbers deciding the route, marking is part of this social interaction, allowing each climber to see the movements of the other, to be able to contribute to the "interpretation" of the ascent step by step. In this sense, the cognitive notion of imagery (in sport psychology), intended as the individual creation or re-creation of an experience generated from memorial information, can be respecified as the active and concrete bodily work of marking, in which some future action is projected for the sake of sharing a joint interpretation of the situation with other teammates.

5 Ecological Dynamics (1): Selection of Affordances

Ecological dynamics is the term used in sport sciences to study skill acquisition by blending dynamical systems theory and Gibson's ecological psychology (Vilar et al. 2012). The human movement system constitutes a self-organizing open system, affected by constant interaction between subject-environment in recurrent perception-action loops where affordances, understood as opportunities for action (Gibson 1979), emerge within a goal-directed activity. According to ecological dynamics, decision making appears as an emergent process in the continuous interaction of an individual with certain abilities and the surrounding environment with certain energy flows presented as invariants that are perceived by the individual as opportunities for action (affordances). Therefore, decision making can be conceived as "a goal-directed process of acting on the affordances available in the performance environment" (Correia et al. 2012, 306). But, which is the goal? Is it perfectly clear in every occasion for the subject who is immersed in the activity? Beek dealt with such problems more specifically in what he dubbed the "selection of affordance" problem. As the author stated, "The first issue that will have to be addressed is that of the selection of affordances. In virtually all research on affordances the goal of the performed action, and thus the actor's intention, is either explicitly given or unambiguously implicit in the experimental set-up" (Beek 2009, 147).

The selection of affordances occurs in the course of action, related to the intending-perceiving-acting cycle affected by task and organismic and environmental constraints (Newell 1986). Organismic constraints are present at the biochemical, biomechanical, neurological, and morphological levels; environmental constraints can be ambient/

global to action (gravity, temperature) or local/focal to action (use of tools); and task constraints include the goals of the action as well as any socially agreed-upon rules (Newell 1996, 404), either implicit or explicit (Newell and Valvano 1998, 53). For Araújo, Davids, and Hristovski (2006), intentional rules for action are not computational; they are to be found at an ecological scale. It is our claim that the constraints caused by these intentional rules for action imply a truly social dimension; they are constituted *in* and *as* ethnomethods (Garfinkel 1967) that represent a truly embodied, embedded normativity (what Rietveld 2008 considers situated normativity). Ethnomethods constitute embedded/embodied habitual patterns that function as routine grounds of social interaction and make possible the selection of affordances, that is to say, decision making. Ethnomethods are bound to the level of expertise. Thus, the "acquisition" of more expert ethnomethods appears as a consequence of the history of interactions between learners and the environment. The normativity of distinguishing a reasonable (good, correct) from a nonreasonable action (bad, incorrect) cannot be predefined by an external rule but only by the action's relation to the normal, habitual pattern of occurrence (Camus 2009, 103) for expert members; that is to say, it is the burden of expert ethnomethods to express reasonable actions in certain situations, and here "reasonable" includes making publicly witnessable one's own good sense of the game.

Ethnomethods imply an intrinsic social dimension. We do not talk about the ethnomethods of John or Carla (even though personal styles do exist) but about ethnomethods as the habitual pattern of occurrence shared by members of a community. Moreover, the differences among novice, intermediate, or expert ethnomethods can be distinguished only by attending to this social dimension of the community of practice.

Nonetheless, saying that ethnomethods represent habitual patterns does not imply a rigid or mechanical response. Bernsteins's (1967) conceptualization of "dexterity" as a way to solve a task in innovative, creative ways can bring some light to this point. In a well-known Bernsteinian formula, dexterity is achieved by solving a problem again and again (iteration as "repetition without repetition"). This is precisely what happens in the process of "acquiring" certain ethnomethods. Members learn to navigate in situations that maintain certain "family resemblance" (Wittgenstein 2001 [1953]). They are never facing the very same situation; it is like solving a problem with certain variations again and again. This variability is indispensable for providing enough flexibility to adapt to rich and diverse performance contexts. Nonetheless, this kind of variability does not resemble the noise displayed by novices. Expert ethnomethods feature stable adaptability in order to respond to the contingencies of the situations. The combination of stability and flexibility is the hallmark of skilled performance (Warren

2006); it is precisely what ecological dynamics consider the core of functional variability (Davids, Button, and Bennett 2008). That is why, from a nonlinear pedagogy, the encouragement of change and adaptation during learning is key, avoiding narrow idealized solutions. The fostering of creative solutions is achieved through the suitable introduction of constraints.

In a study of Krav Maga (a comprehensive self-defense system), Sánchez-García, Villaroya-Gil, and Elrio-López (2016) developed further the social dimension of the constraints-led model by stating that ethnomethods were a crucial feature of the task constraints. They generated a manipulation of task constraints in order to understand—among other things—how the ethnomethods, related to the level of expertise, were accountable for response adaptability. Following Garfinkel's (1967) recommendation on "breaching experiments," the attack included unexpected actions to which Krav Maga practitioners had to respond. In both groups, novices, intermediates, and experts were included. For group 1, the attacker wore full boxing equipment and the attack consisted in two consecutive jabs (direct punches) followed by morote gari, a technique wherein the attacker aims for the legs of the opponent (an action known as shoot) in order to throw him to the ground; for group 2, the attacker wore full judo equipment and the attack consisted in a short approach to the participant showing grappling intentions and then executing a jab to the helmet of the participant. Every participant, regardless of their level of expertise, was surprised by the unexpected action. Nonetheless, the efficiency of performance (the problem solving) depended on the level of expertise (see figure 18.3). That is why, when novices tried to react after the breaching action, the tactical situation posed an unsolvable problem for them; the novices could not make sense of the attack (they did not know how to defend themselves, how to react properly). Also, the comparison of two specific case studies suggested that adaptability to the challenging situation of the experiment was possible only for experts, and not for novices.

6 Ecological Dynamics (2): Functional Variability

The idea of variability as a functional solution for the contingencies of the situation that only experts in Krav Maga achieved in the previous example was also made visible in research on screening in basketball (Sánchez-García and Muntanyola, under review). An EM-based analysis of dyadic defensive actions against direct screenings was conducted to detect different key features of the game in real time that affected variation from the prearranged defensive plan. Such key features were part of complex multimodal interactions among players that would remain invisible if applying just the formal analysis advocated by the standard ecological dynamics approach.

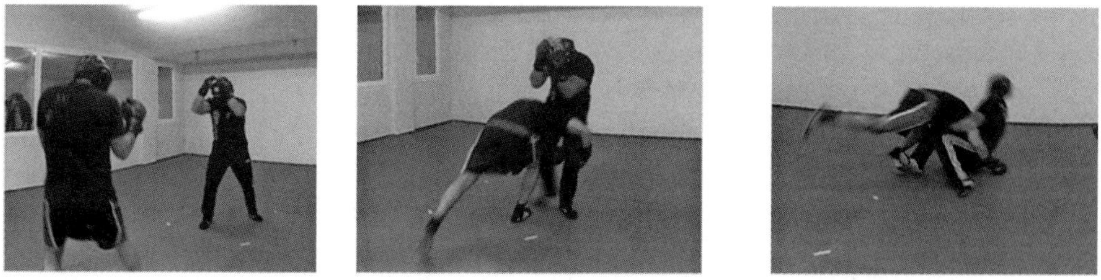

Figure 18.3
An expert is surprised by the unexpected attack. Nonetheless he is able to land in an advantageous position for ground work. Reprinted from Sánchez-García, Villaroya-Gil, and Elrio-López (2016), 133–154.

The high complexity of team sports such as basketball affects the decision making of players heavily. Trainers try to reduce such complexity by giving strategic orientations before competition, but they cannot exhaust the myriad of problems that appear and must be solved locally in each situation of the game (Araújo and Esteves 2009). Lucy Suchman (1987) analyzed this specific relationship between plans and situated actions: the plan acts as an "orienting device for situated action," a guide for local interactions. In her example of canoeing, the plan "I'll get as far over to the left as possible, try to make it between those two large rocks, then backferry hard to the right to make it around that next bunch" (Suchman 1987, 72) allowed the canoe to encounter the best conditions to deal with the situated actions when facing different rapids but did not tell how to perform in these situated actions. Thus, to explain decision making, we should take into account not only the preestablished plan offered by trainers acting as a constraint (e.g., how to defend screens in specific situations) but also all the contingent conditions that constrain the decision making of the players in each situation. These contingent conditions can include unexpected circumstances that influence players to abandon the preestablished plan in order to solve the situation. In this fashion, Sánchez-García and Muntanyola (under review) avoided seeing variations of the strategy simply as errors. In fact, some variations of the plan were really functional and implied an expert understanding of the game to adapt to unexpected features during specific play. For instance, during a handoff screening, solved usually by applying "push" (the defender of the screener physically pushes his opponent, forming a compact block, and the defender of the ball passes behind the block of screener/defender to follow his opponent), defenders changed the defense to two-on-one and succeeded (see figure 18.4). Because of (1) the specific position of the attacker with the ball, located in an area of the field that was very close to the sideline and to the division line

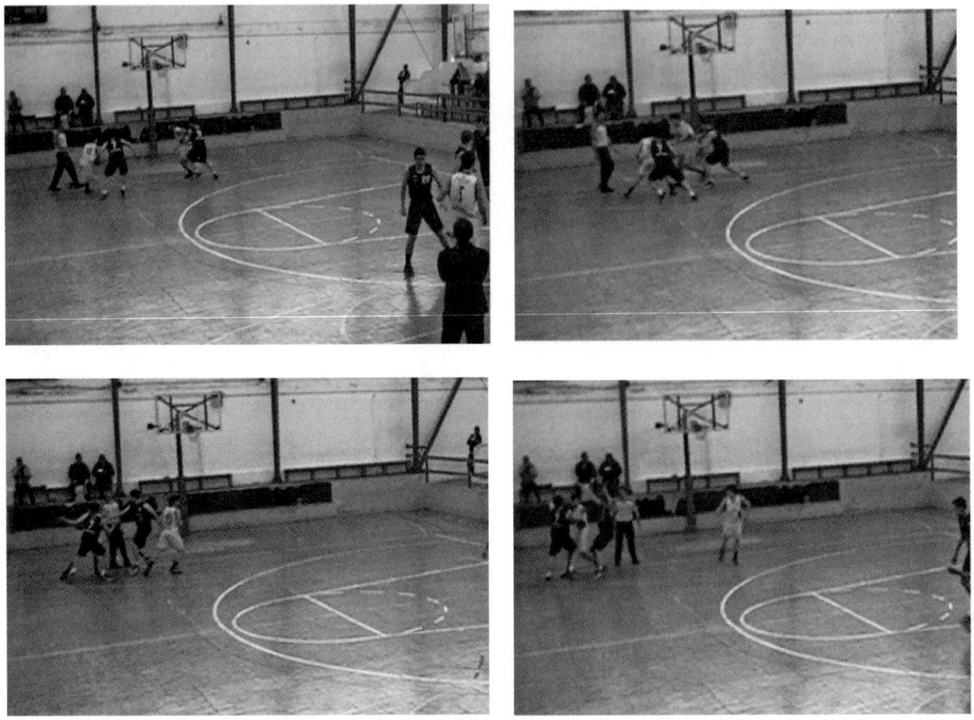

Figure 18.4
Because of the area of the field and the attacker's (the one playing the ball) orientation, defenders change to a two-on-one situation to force error. Reprinted from R. Sánchez-García and D. Muntanyola (under review).

and (2) to his specific body posture and orientation, facing backward, the defenders coordinate their actions to generate a two-on-one situation, forcing a bad pass and recovering the ball.

From an EM standpoint, the idea of variability or improvisation is tightly related to habitual patterns of action. Variability is only possible against some habitual pattern. Garfinkel (2006) described routine grounds as preconditions for improvisation. If we step back to the previous discussion about how ethnomethods are "acquired," we see that members learn to navigate in situations with a loose connection of resemblance. That is why, to become an expert, you have to solve the same kinds of problems again and again. Nonetheless, if we take the plan stated in the strategy as the only ideal solution, and we train our players to act always according to this plan, we are not enriching the players' ethnomethods for defending screening; they are not solving problems in vivo but following an ideal script. Their routine grounds for defending screening become too narrow, and improvisation is not fostered. The problem is that the ideal solution must be tailored for each occasion of the game. The strategy or plan is a resource for mutual orientation and coordination that can be varied if the conditions of the situation demand so. In order to respond with positive functional variability, improvisation must be fostered through training.

7 Ecological Dynamics (3): Instructions as Augmented Information

According to ecological dynamics, the self-organizing behavior of the subject-environment system can be affected or "channeled" (Araújo and Davids 2004, 50) by different kinds of constraints. As we have seen above, Newell (1986) identified three sources of constraints affecting the behavior of the system on a short time scale (decision making while performing a skill) or a longer time scale (the learning process of a skill): organism, environment, and task constraints. According to the constraints-led approach—a didactic approach based on ecological dynamics (Renshaw et al. 2016)—the introduction of the right constraints becomes a paramount issue. By introducing relevant constraints, we can help learners become perceptually attuned to those relevant affordances to perform the specific skill. This is a common phenomenon in sport activities. Davids, Button, and Bennet (2008) and Renshaw et al. (2010) have proposed a nonlinear pedagogical approach based on introducing and modifying constraints in the learning environment. One of the main concerns of teachers is to be able to offer a constrained setting to facilitate the self-exploratory activity.

This is not to say that the role of the teacher is just to set the proper field and then leave the student to explore. The didactic setting is much more interactive between teacher and students. For instance, a common didactic strategy used by teachers/trainers is to convey relevant information through instructions. Newell (1996) dubbed the term augmented information to refer to a subcategory of environmental constraints that treats supplementary didactic information not normally available to "free-range" learners in their self-exploratory activities. Augmented information comes in a variety of modalities, including speech and gesture but also direct physical contact. Augmented information itself breaks down into three different types that are thus subcategories of environmental constraints: (1) prescriptive information refers to the multimodal specification of the target action (e.g., information coming from the modeling performance of the teacher); (2) information feedback is what the performer receives from her own movement, whether during the action (concurrent) or as its result (terminal); and (3) transition information is any kind of external input that reacts to the agent's performance of an action by way of offering qualifying instructions toward the prospective reenactment of that action (e.g., "Turn more energetically this time!").

Categories (1) and (3) properly represent what Newell and Ranganathan (2010) characterized as instruction: a forward-looking category that acts as a nonphysical, informational constraint. The information conveyed in instructions can be about the goal of the task and about the movement pattern (Newell and Ranganathan 2010, 21–22). Valuable as these categorizations of instructions are, these authors are conscious of the need of taking into account contextual and social features of the settings where instructions are used:

> A caveat as background is the recognition that is difficult to consider a particular instructional strategy in isolation of other instructional strategies. Thus, for example, instructions cannot be considered independent of demonstrations which often are used to convey the *same* information. Furthermore, instructions and specifically the information to be conveyed through the instructions, cannot be considered independently of *what* is to be learned, the particular practice strategy in place (e.g. distribution of practice), the motor skill at hand (e.g. tennis forehand), and the skill level of learner/performer. (Newell and Ranganathan 2010, 18; emphasis original)

Nevertheless, even though the authors point to the potential flaw, they do not present a methodological remedy for it. Thus, to deal with these potential problems and improve the ecological dynamics approach, we propose an EM respecification of information and instructions as the in vivo practices of instructed actions (Garfinkel 2002). EM defends a praxeological analysis of information within social practices. According to Garfinkel, we must conceive information not as something stored and transmitted from mind to mind, inside the subjects' heads, but as pertaining to embodied/embedded practices of concerted actions among social actors: "I would prefer ... to regard information as something not recalled but re-created out of the resources of the available order of possibilities of experience, available sensory materials, actions, etc. Thus preferred usage would be to talk of a communicant as knowledge*able* rather than talking of his knowledge" (Garfinkel 2008, 158; emphasis original).

In the specific case of educational context, such as PE or sport training, the embodied/embedded practices of concerted actions are referred to as instructed actions. Instructed actions highlight the fact that instructions are not just a trade of information but a matter of interaction between students and teacher. By the same logic, a goal should not be considered as an idea or value conveyed by instructions but as an orientation toward ordered sequences of events among actors (Garfinkel 2008). Whereas the former is static, the latter is dynamic and renders a much more congruent account of how social activities such as sports unfold. In didactic interactions, student and teacher try to get to the same page in order to obtain a clear idea about how to proceed.

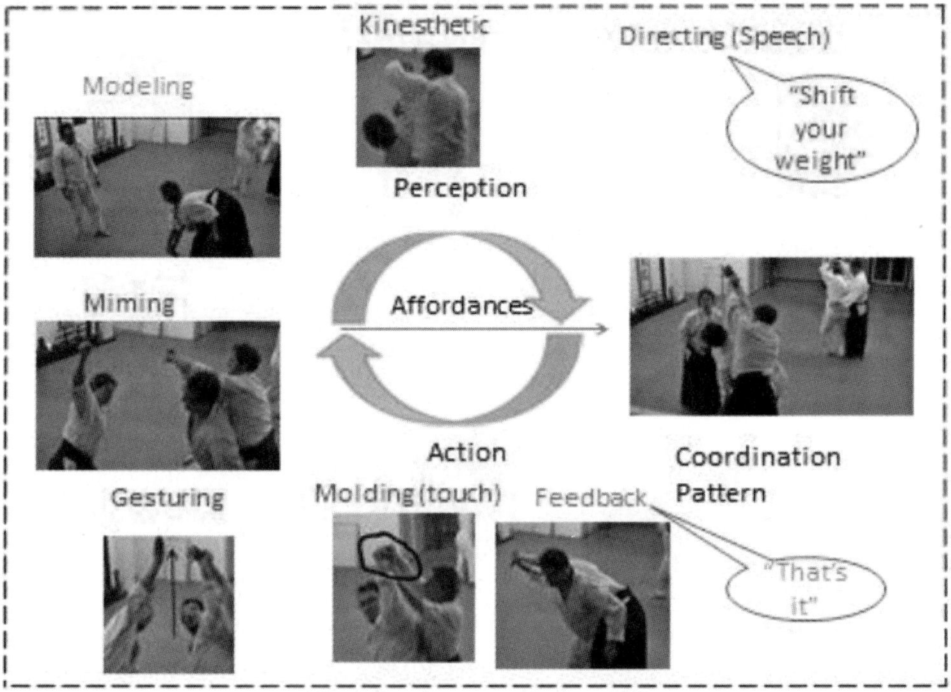

Figure 18.5
Different types of augmented information to convey the right execution of an aikido technique.

The key to didactic success lays in their joint effort of listening (not only with ears but with all the senses) to each other, staying together along the way. These didactic interactions unfold as an iterative process hindered by "execution gaps": gaps between instruction and the actual performance. The fact that the student cannot understand and/or perform flawlessly what the trainer is describing prevents them from being on the same page all the time; in these occasions, some "repair work" must be deployed as part of their concerted actions addressed to making the didactical activity successful.

In order to gain further insight on these matters, let us explore an ethnomethodological perspective on the specific analysis of instructed actions in aikido (Muntanyola and Sánchez-García, in press).[4] We include an ethnomethodological analysis on the use of augmented information through different didactical strategies (modeling, verbally guiding, gesturing, molding by guiding through direct physical manipulation of the learner's body, and so on), as shown in figure 18.5.

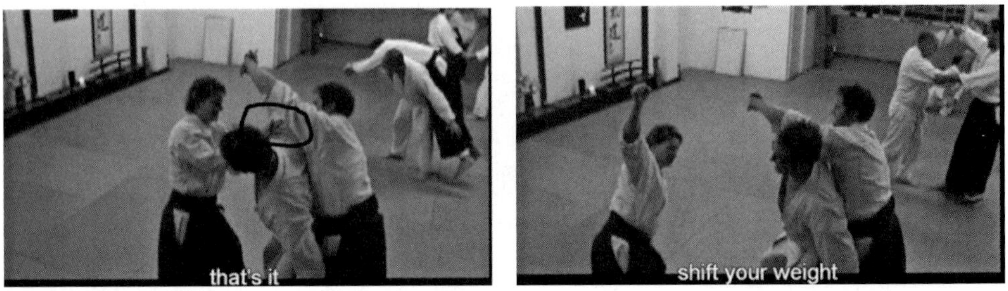

Figure 18.6
Multimodal transcription on the use of augmented information during didactical interactions in aikido. Reprinted from D. Muntanyola and R. Sánchez-García (in press).

The excerpt we transcribe and analyze in detail refers to a typical episode of pedagogical interaction: one junior student (man wearing white jacket and trousers) and one senior student (man wearing black hakama [pleated semi skirt] and white jacket) are practicing the technique. The instructor or sensei (woman wearing black hakama and white jacket) approaches the couple, observes how they are performing, and then chooses to give some augmented information. Let us pay a close look at the concerted actions depicted in figure 18.6.

This excerpt represents a successful episode of iteration in instructed actions: the fragment starts with both students conceding instructor's actions by stopping the execution of the technique and allowing being molded. The delivering of instructions and their receipt are choreographed by the parties as a collaborative exercise. The molding action of the instructor is reinforced by the utterance "That's it" as a way to remark the action of the molding as clearly relevant. After this, the junior student executes the technique and the instructor gives verbal feedback. Then the instructor self-selects, giving augmented information both with the utterance "Shift your weight" and through miming the action. We refer to miming when the technique is performed in the absence of the tool, implement, or partner (Abrahamson 2013). When the instructor ends the instruction, the junior student executes the technique again and the instructional exchange continues in subsequent fragments not included here.

8 Conclusion

This chapter demonstrates what EM can offer to the study of embodied cognition in sport. EM provides a detailed analysis of cognition's social dimension. Cognitive processes cannot be reduced to individual minds (as the information-processing paradigm does). Cognitive processes are essentially social. But this social dimension cannot be accounted for solely by defining social factors—such as motivational strategies settled by the coach or behavior by the audience (Carvalho, Correia, and Araújo 2013)—to be introduced unproblematically within "elaborate formal (mathematical) models of tactical behavior" (Araújo, Travassos, and Vilar 2010, 1087), as ecological dynamics claims. EM can truly enhance the ecological dynamics approach to the social dimension: (1) by rendering visible a truly social situated normativity (ethnomethods) within task constraints that was obviated by ecological dynamics and (2) by providing what Garfinkel (2002) dubbed "ethnomethodological alternates" to the formal analytic reductions that ecological dynamics offers to substitute the real phenomena. Ecological dynamics renders formal analysis but misses the full scope of interactional work to which the agents are continuously attending, constituting true "environments for each other" (McDermott 1977, 36) through multimodal embodied communicative interaction. Cognitive processes must be understood as part of the ethnomethods that subjects use during concerted actions. To do so we must take into account the complex and dense interactional work that participants maintain through embodied interaction.

This chapter has presented a praxeological view of cognition, which has been suitably rendered visible and publicly accessible in this chapter through the audiovisual analysis of different topics in different sports: rules and decision making in street-crossing and surfing; imagery in climbing; selection of affordances in Krav Maga and basketball; and instructions within an aikido lesson. These cases have been helpful for opening a debate between EM and other research programs that may produce more adequate and fruitful approaches (particularly when combining EM/ecological dynamics) to the study of embodied cognition's social dimension in sport.

Notes

1. The EM approach to cognition clearly resonates and aligns with enactive approaches. For a REC (radical enactive cognition) analysis of cognition in sport, see Hutto, Kirchhoff, and Renshaw (this volume) and Hutto and Sánchez-García (2015).

2. See http://www.indoorclimbing.com/comp_preview.html.

3. See https://www.ifsc-climbing.org/index.php/world-competition/event-regulation.

4. See Okada (2013) for an interactional analysis of instructions in boxing and Lefebvre (2016) for an EM-inspired analysis of aikido training.

References

Abrahamson, Dor. 2013. Personal communication at the EDRL seminar at Berkeley School of Education, February 27.

Araújo, Duarte, and Keith Davids. 2004. "Embodied Cognition and Emergent Decision-Making in Dynamical Movement Systems." *Junctures: The Journal for Thematic Dialogue* 2:45–57.

Araújo, Duarte, Keith Davids, and Robert Hristovski. 2006. "The Ecological Dynamics of Decision Making in Sport." *Psychology of Sport and Exercise* 7 (6): 653–676.

Araújo, Duarte, and Pedro Esteves. 2009. "The Irreducible Variability of Decision Making in Basketball." In *Aportaciones Teóricas Y Prácticas Para El Baloncesto Del Futuro*, edited by A. Lorenzo, S. J. Ibáñez, and E. Ortega, 11–30. Madrid: Wanceulen SL.

Araújo, Duarte, Bruno Travassos, and Luis Vilar. 2010. "Tactical Skills Are Not Verbal Skills: A Comment on Kannekens and Colleagues." *Perceptual and Motor Skills* 110 (3C): 1086–1088.

Barr, Kathryn, and Craig Hall. 1992. "The Use of Imagery by Rowers." *International Journal of Sport Psychology* 23 (3): 243–261.

Barratt, Paul. 2012. "'My Magic Cam': A More-than-Representational Account of the Climbing Assemblage." *Area* 44 (1): 46–53.

Beek, Peter J. 2009. "Ecological Approaches to Sport Psychology: Prospects and Challenges." *International Journal of Sport Psychology* 40 (1): 144–151.

Bernier, Marjorie, and Jean F. Fournier. 2010. "Functions of Mental Imagery in Expert Golfers." *Psychology of Sport and Exercise* 11 (6): 444–452.

Bernstein, Nikolai A. 1967. *The Co-ordination and Regulation of Movements*. Oxford: Pergamon.

Boyd, Jean, and Krista J. Munroe. 2003. "The Use of Imagery in Climbing." *Athletic Insight: The Online Journal of Sport Psychology* 5 (2): 15–30.

Brunswik, Egon. 1956. *Perception and the Representative Design of Psychological Experiments*. Berkeley: University of California Press.

Callow, Nichola, and Lew Hardy. 2001. "Types of Imagery Associated with Sport Confidence in Netball Players of Varying Skills." *Journal of Applied Sport Psychology* 13 (1): 1–17.

Callow, Nichola, Ross Roberts, and Joanna Z. Fawkes. 2006. "Effects of Dynamic and Static Imagery on Vividness of Imagery Skiing Performance, and Confidence." *Journal of Imagery Research in Sport and Physical Activity* 1 (1): 1–15. doi:10.2202/1932-0191.1001.

Calmels, Claire, Paul Holmes, Christelle Berthoumieux, and Robert N. Singer. 2004. "The Development of Movement Imagery Vividness through a Structured Intervention in Softball." *Journal of Sport Behavior* 27 (4): 307–322.

Camus, Laurent. 2009. "Action instruite et coordination." Unpublished master's diss., Ecole des Hautes Etudes en Sciences Sociales, Paris.

Carvalho, João H., Vanda Correia, and Duarte Araújo. 2013. "A Constraints Led Approach to Skill Enhancement in Tennis." *ITF Coaching and Sport Science Review* 60 (21): 10–11.

Correia, Vanda, Duarte Araújo, Alan Cummins, and Cathy M. Craig. 2012. "Perceiving and Acting upon Spaces in a VR Rugby Task: Expertise Effects in Affordance Detection and Task Achievement." *Journal of Sport and Exercise Psychology* 34 (3): 305–321.

Davids, Keith W., Chris Button, and Simon J. Bennet. 2008. *Dynamics of Skill Acquisition: A Constraints-Led Approach.* Champaign, IL: Human Kinetics.

Dutkiewicz, Jan. 2015. "Pretzel Logic: An Embodied Ethnography of a Rock Climb." *Space and Culture* 18 (1): 25–38.

Evans, Lynne, Leigh Jones, and Richard Mullen. 2004. "An Imagery Intervention during the Competitive Season with an Elite Rugby Union Player." *Sport Psychologist* 18 (3): 252–271.

Ganis, Giorgio, William L. Thompson, and Stephen M. Kosslyn. 2004. "Brain Areas Underlying Visual Mental Imagery and Visual Perception: An fMRI Study." *Brain Research: Cognitive Brain Research* 20 (2): 226–241.

Garfinkel, Harold. 1967. *Studies in Ethnomethodology.* Cambridge: Prentice-Hall.

Garfinkel, Harold. 1996. "Ethnomethodology's Program." *Social Psychology Quarterly* 59 (1): 5–21.

Garfinkel, Harold. 2002. *Ethnomethodology's Program: Working Out Durkheim's Aphorism.* Lanham, MD: Rowman and Littlefield.

Garfinkel, Harold. 2006. *Seeing Sociologically.* Boulder, CO: Paradigm.

Garfinkel, Harold. 2008. *Toward a Sociological Theory of Information.* Boulder, CO: Paradigm.

Garfinkel, Harold, and Harvey Sacks. 1986. "On Formal Structures of Practical Actions." In *Ethnomethodological Studies of Work,* edited by Harold Garfinkel, 160–193. London: Routledge and Kegan Paul.

Gibson, James J. 1979. *An Ecological Approach to Visual Perception.* Norwood, NJ: Psychology Press.

Goffman, Erving. 1983. "The Interaction Order: American Sociological Association, 1982 Presidential Address." *American Sociological Review* 48 (1): 1–17.

Guillot, Aymeric, Edyta Nadrowska, and Christian Collet. 2009. "Using Motor Imagery to Learn Tactical Movements in Basketball." *Journal of Sport Behavior* 32 (2): 189–206.

Hutto, Daniel D., and Raúl Sánchez-García. 2015. "Choking RECtified: Embodied Expertise beyond Dreyfus." *Phenomenology and the Cognitive Sciences* 14 (2): 309–331.

Jenkings, K. Neil. 2013. "Playing Dangerously: An Ethnomethodological View upon Rock-Climbing." In *Ethnomethodology at Play,* edited by P. Tolmie and M. Rouncefield, 191–210. Surrey, UK: Ashgate Surrey.

Kirsh, David, Dafne Muntanyola, R. Joanne Jao, Amy Lew, and Matt Sugihara. 2009. "Choreographic Methods for Creating Novel, High Quality Dance." In *Proceedings, DESFORM: 5th International*

Workshop on Design and Semantics and Form: 188–195. https://pure.tue.nl/ws/files/4421285/770736.pdf.

Kosslyn, Stephen M., William L. Thompson, and Giorgio Ganis. 2006. *The Case for Mental Imagery*. New York: Oxford University Press.

LeCouteur, Amanda, and Rebecca Feo. 2011. "Real-Time Communication during Play: Analysis of Team-Mates' Talk and Interaction." *Psychology of Sport and Exercise* 12 (2): 124–134.

Lefebvre, Augustin. 2016. "The Pacific Philosophy of Aikido: An Interactional Approach." *Martial Arts Studies* 2:91–109.

Liberman, Kenneth. 2013. *More Studies in Ethnomethodology*. Albany: SUNY Press.

Livingston, Eric. 2006. "Ethnomethodological Studies of Mediated Interaction and Mundane Expertise." *Sociological Review* 54 (3): 405–425.

Livingston, Eric. 2008. *Ethnographies of Reason: Directions in Ethnomethodology and Conversation Analysis*. Aldershot, UK: Ashgate.

Malouff, John M., John A. McGee, Helen T. Halford, and Sally E. Rooke. 2008. "Effects of Pre-Competition Positive Imagery and Self-Instructions on Accuracy of Serving in Tennis." *Journal of Sport Behavior* 31 (3): 264–275.

McDermott, Raymond Patrick. 1977. Kids Make Sense: An Ethnographic Account of the Interactional Management of Success and Failure in One First-Grade Classroom. Unpublished PhD diss., Department of Anthropology, Stanford University, CA.

Morris, Tony, Michael Spittle, and Clark Perry. 2004 "Mental Imagery in Sport." In *Sport Psychology: Theory, Applications and Issues*, 2nd ed., edited by T. Morris and J. Summers, 344–387. Brisbane: Wiley.

Muntanyola, Dafne. 2015. "Distributed Marking in Sport Corrections: A Conversation Analysis of Synchronized Swimming." *Journal of Cognitive Science* 16 (3): 337–353.

Muntanyola, Dafne, and David Kirsh. 2010. "Marking as Physical Thinking: A Cognitive Ethnography of Dance." *Proceedings of the IWCogSc-10 ILCLI International Workshop on Cognitive Science*, Donosti: 339–355.

Muntanyola, Dafne, and Raúl Sánchez-García. In press. "Distributed Attention: A Cognitive Ethnography of Instruction in Sports Settings." *Journal for the Theory of Social Behaviour.*

Newell, Karl M. 1986. "Constraints on the Development of Coordination." In *Motor Development in Children: Aspects of Coordination and Control* 34, edited by M. G. Wade and H. T. A. Whiting, 341–361. Amsterdam: Martinus Nijhoff.

Newell, Karl M. 1996. "Change in Movement and Skill: Learning, Retention and Transfer." In *Dexterity and Its Development*, edited by M. Latash and M. Turvey, 393–429. Mahwah, NJ: LEA.

Newell, Karl M., and Rajiv Ranganathan. 2010. "Instructions as Constraints in Motor Skill Acquisition." In *Motor Learning in Practice: A Constraints-Led Approach*, edited by I. Renshaw, K. Davids, and J. P. Savelsbergh, 17–32. Florence, KY: Routledge.

Newell, Karl M., and Joanne Valvano. 1998. "Movement Science: Therapeutic Intervention as a Constraint in Learning and Relearning Movement Skills." *Scandinavian Journal of Occupational Therapy* 5 (2): 51–57.

Okada, Misao. 2013. "Embodied Interactional Competence in Boxing Practice: Coparticipants' Joint Accomplishment of a Teaching and Learning Activity." *Language and Communication* 33 (4): 390–403.

Pezzulo, Giovanni, Laura Barca, Alessandro Lamberti Bocconi, and Anna M. Borghi. 2010. "When Affordances Climb into Your Mind: Advantages of Motor Simulation in a Memory Task Performed by Novice and Expert Rock Climbers." *Brain and Cognition* 73 (1): 68–73.

Renshaw, Ian, Duarte Araújo, Chris Button, Jia Yi Chow, Keith Davids, and Brendan Moy. 2016. "Why the Constraints-Led Approach Is Not Teaching Games for Understanding: A Clarification." *Physical Education and Sport Pedagogy* 21 (5): 459–480.

Renshaw, Ian, Jia Yi Chow, Keith Davids, and John Hammond. 2010. "A Constraints-Led Perspective to Understanding Skill Acquisition and Game Play: A Basis for Integration of Motor Learning Theory and Physical Education Praxis?" *Physical Education and Sport Pedagogy* 15 (2): 117–137.

Rietveld, Erik. 2008. "Situated Normativity: The Normative Aspect of Embodied Cognition in Unreflective Action." *Mind: A Quarterly Review of Psychology and Philosophy* 117 (468): 973–1001.

Sánchez-García, Raúl, and Kenneth Liberman. 2015. "Turn-Allocation in the Surfing Line-Up." Oral presentation at the Congress of the International Association for Ethnomethodology and Conversational Analysis, held in Kolding, Denmark, August 4–7.

Sánchez-García, Raúl, and Dafne Muntanyola. Under review. "A Cognitive Ethnography of Basketball: Variability in Interpersonal Coordination during Defense against Direct Screenings." *International Journal of Sport Psychology*.

Sánchez-García, Raul, Á. Villaroya-Gil, and Alejandro Elrio-López. 2016. "Manipulating Task Constraints of Situated Normativity to Study Decision Making in Krav Maga." *International Journal of Sport Psychology* 47 (2): 133–154.

Sanchez, X., Ph Lambert, G. Jones, and D. J. Llewellyn. 2012. "Efficacy of Pre-Ascent Climbing Route Visual Inspection in Indoor Sport Climbing." *Scandinavian Journal of Medicine and Science in Sports* 22 (1): 67–72.

Smyth, Mary M., and Adam Waller. 1998. "Movement Imagery in Rock Climbing: Patterns of Interference from Visual, Spatial and Kinaesthetic Secondary Tasks." *Applied Cognitive Psychology* 12 (2): 145–157.

Starkes, J. L., W. Helsen, and R. Jack. 2001. "Expert Performance in Sports and Dance." In *Handbook of Sport Psychology*, 3rd ed., edited by R. N. Singer, H. A. Hausenblas, and C. M. Janelle, 174–201. New York: John Wiley & Sons.

Streeck, Jürgen, Charles Goodwin, and Curtis LeBaron. 2011. "Embodied Interaction in the Material World: An Introduction." In *Embodied Interaction: Language and Body in the Material World*, edited by J. Streeck, C. Goodwin, and C. Lebaron, 1–28. Cambridge: Cambridge University Press.

Suchman, Lucy A. 1987. *Plans and Situated Actions: The Problem of Human*-Cambridge. Cambridge: Cambridge University Press.

Summer, Jeffery J. 2004. "A Historical Perspective in Skill Acquisition." In *Skill Acquisition in Sport: Research, Theory and Practice*, edited by A. Williams and N. J. Hodges, 1–26. London: Routledge.

Vealey, Robin, and Christy Greenleaf. 2006. "Seeing Is Believing: Understanding and Using Imagery in Sport." In *Applied Sport Psychology: Personal Growth to Peak Performance*, 2nd ed., edited by J. M Williams, 220–224. Mountain View, CA: Mayfield.

Vilar, Luís, Duarte Araújo, Keith Davids, and Ian Renshaw. 2012. "The Need for 'Representative Task Design' in Evaluating Efficacy of Skills Tests in Sport: A Comment on Russell, Benton and Kingsley (2010)." *Journal of Sports Sciences* 30 (16): 1727–1730; author reply 1731–1733.

Warren, William H. 2006. "The Dynamics of Perception and Action." *Psychological Review* 113 (2): 358–389.

Weinberg, Robert S., Thomas G. Seabourne, and Allen Jackson. 1981. "Effects of Visuo-Motor Behavior Rehearsal, Relaxation, and Imagery on Karate Performance." *Journal of Sport Psychology* 3 (3): 228–238.

Williams, Mark A., Keith Davids, and John G. Williams. 1999. *Visual Perception and Action in Sport*. London: Taylor & Francis.

Wittgenstein, Ludwig. 2001 [1953]. *Philosophical Investigations*. Translated by G. E. M. Anscombe. Hoboken, NJ: Blackwell.

VI Affordances and Action Selection

19 The Irreducible Embeddedness of Action Choice in Sport

Duarte Araújo, Keith Davids, and Patrick McGivern

1 Introduction

The capacity of humans to choose and coordinate actions with environmental events during goal-directed behavior has been a long-standing topic of investigation in the behavioral sciences. This capacity is predicated on the organization of stable, adaptive behaviors. It implicates the coordination of action, when the degrees of a freedom of an organism (i.e., its muscles, joints, neurons, etc.) become temporarily organized into ordered movement patterns or when coordinated states emerge from interpersonal dynamics of performers in social systems such as team sports. Perception is needed because information about the world and the body enables adaptive, functional behaviors in performers to satisfy changing environmental constraints (Warren 2006). Fundamentally, therefore, the problem of performers' decision making is continuous with the problem of perception and action (Araújo, Davids, and Hristovski 2006).

A prevailing assumption in psychological science has been that decision making implies the existence of a centralized controller—a type of pattern generator, action plan, knowledge structure, or internal model responsible for behavior organization and regulation (e.g., Rosenbaum et al. 2007; Schmidt 1975). As an alternative, Warren (2006) proposed that the structure and physics of the environment, biomechanics of the body, perceptual information about the state of the agent-environment system, and specific task demands serve to constrain behavioral outcomes. Adaptive behavior, rather than being imposed by a preexisting structure, emerges from this confluence of constraints under the boundary conditions of a particular performance task or goal. Distinct from being localized in an internal structure, control is actually distributed over the performer-environment (P-E) system (Gibson 1979).

In line with this idea, Kelso and Engström (2006) argued that transitions among stable behavioral states emerge as a result of dynamic instability, providing a universal decision-making process for switching between polarized states. If more functional movement solutions exist to satisfy performance circumstances and context, fluctuations will help the P-E system discover, explore, and harness them. System bifurcations act as a selection mechanism platform to "decide" when a particular mode of behavior may no longer be functional, supporting a switch to another mode (see Kelso and Engström 2006). Such stabilities do not exist a priori in the performers' structure, but are co-determined by the confluence of individual and task constraints, exemplifying how control lies in the P-E system (Gibson 1979; Warren 2006).

From an ecological point of view, cognition, perception, and action should be understood in direct connection with the hypothesis of the reciprocal fit between living things and their terrestrial surroundings (see Turvey and Carello 2012). Living things and their ecosystems are not logically independent of each other. Nervous system, body, and environment are all continuously evolving and simultaneously influencing one another during an individual's goal-directed behaviors (van Gelder and Port 1995).

Dynamics is a large and diverse set of concepts and methods, and consequently there are many different ways that cognitive phenomena can be understood dynamically. Modeling of some aspects of cognitive performance has been one of the ultimate goals of a dynamical analysis. The modeling process is a matter of distilling the phenomena to be understood, obtaining the time-series data, developing a model, and interpreting whether the model has captured a significant proportion of the data. When conducted successfully, the modeling process yields not only precise descriptions of existing data, but also predictions that can be used in evaluating the model (see Haken, Kelso, and Bunz 1985). However, every human behaves in different ways, and is embedded in a rich, constantly changing environment, making it challenging for science to apply to cognition the kinds of explanatory techniques that have worked so successfully in studying other natural dynamical systems (Tschacher and Dauwalder 2003).

As argued by Araújo, Davids, and Hristovski (2006), in goal-directed behavior,

> With each step closer to the goal the information detected and used for action must become ever more specific, narrowing the possible action paths available for the movement system, until ultimately, at the moment of goal accomplishment, the emergent path becomes uniquely defined (Kugler et al. 1990; Shaw 2001). Given this view, decision-making is viewed as a functional and emergent process in which a selection is made among converging paths for an intended goal. Choices are made at bifurcation points where more specific information becomes available, constraining the environment-athlete system to switch to the most functional path. (661)

Here, we elaborate on these ideas, describing two examples of the emergence of such behaviors, and discuss the key features of the concept of emergence illustrated by these examples.

2 Dynamic Models of Action Choice in Sport

Emergent behavioral patterns can be formally modeled using differential equations and potential functions to describe the long-range dynamics underlying interactions of system components (e.g., Haken, Kelso, and Bunz 1985; Scholz, Kelso, and Schöner 1987). The potential functions can describe an attractor landscape, in which the wells function as attractors and exemplify relatively stable behavioral states. The landscape changes as attractors disappear or originate and, because of system multi-stability, transitions between different modes of behavior can be induced. Two types of system parameter are important in such descriptions. *Control parameters* represent variable factors that drive the system through different behavioral patterns. *Order parameters*—the temporal behavior of which is described by a gradient equation—represent collective variables that capture the overall state of a system.

Despite great complexity of the integrated components of a social system, such as attacker-defender dyadic subsystems in team sports, research by Araújo, Davids, and Hristovski has revealed that these agent interactions can also be described in terms of low-dimensional order parameter dynamics (Araújo, Davids, and Hristovski 2006). They have shown how, in such sport systems, decision making can be considered to emerge from continuous interactions of team players. For example, inter-performer coordination has been studied in 1vs1 subphases of team games like basketball and rugby union (Araújo et al. 2004; Davids et al. 2006; Passos et al. 2008). In these social systems, attackers and defenders form closely interacting dyads in which both individuals do not deliberately seek to coordinate actions, since an attacker needs to avoid stable dyadic organization with a marking defender. Individual cooperating and competing performers in sport systems do not share a common neuronal system, and so coordination processes solely emerge from the task constraints present in specific performance environments.

Specifically, related to action choice, part of the attractiveness of dynamic models is derived from the fact that they can explain different decisions by means of the same underlying process of originating and decaying attractors. For example, a model proposed by Tuller et al. (1994) was established to study the perceptual judgement between the words "say" and "stay," when an acoustic parameter was varied. This same dynamical model has also accounted for the study of decision-making behaviors in other tasks such as the walk-run transition (Diedrich and Warren 1998), or the decision to start from right or left position in a sailing regatta (Araújo et al. 2015). In the model of Tuller et al. (1994), it is assumed that the system's state changes over time under the influence of the attractor landscape. In the study of Araújo et al. (2015), the system's state was the decision, expressed by the place on the starting line where the sailors started, and the angle between the wind direction and the starting line was the control parameter.

3 Action Choice in Sailing

In agreement with predictions of Tuller et al.'s (1994) model, Araújo, Davids, and Hristovski (2006) and Araújo et al. (2015) observed properties such as qualitative changes, abrupt jumps, critical fluctuations, and multi-stability. Importantly, by manipulating the control parameter, they changed the dynamics of the action choice (the place chosen to start the regatta). Moreover, the starting positions possessed a significant amount of variability, especially in the region around the neutral influence of the control parameter. Therefore, the decisions were a juxtaposition of deterministic and stochastic influences that produced system variability: the larger the absolute value of the control parameter, the easier it was to predict which decision would emerge. Interestingly, in the crucial pre-start period, there is no single "valid" course for each boat to follow, so the boats engage in an intensive pre-start competition, in which each continuously tries to gain a positional advantage over the other. Analysis of sailors' displacement of boats during the pre-start period reveals that, although decisions regarding the discrete optimal starting place could be made in advance, this tactic is inherently misleading because of the need to consider and interact with instantaneously changing task (e.g., movements of opposing boats) and environmental (e.g., ocean currents) constraints (Araújo, Davids, and Serpa 2005; Pluijms et al. 2013).

To understand this different (nonoptimizing) view of decision making, it is necessary to take into account the interactive effects between environmental and individual constraints that influence emergent behaviors in a sailing regatta (Araújo, Davids, and Hristovski 2006; Pluijms et al. 2013). The implication is that decision making in sport should be considered as a temporally extended process that is constrained by the intertwined relations among intention, perception, and action in a continuous way (Araújo, Davids, and Hristovski 2006). Indeed, time-extended analyses of pre-start periods in match-race sailing have revealed unexpected structure in actions observed (Araújo, Davids, and Hristovski 2006). This is because sequences of linked decisions in a dynamic task reveal conditional coupling, a property of complex, dynamical systems in nature (Van Geert 1994).

Each separate decision in activities like sailing should not be viewed as functionally independent (i.e., categorically separate) from other decisions emerging during performance. Behavior that is conditionally coupled occurs because the state of a dynamical system (i.e., a match-race regatta) at any one moment remains dependent on previous states of the system. For example, interactions with an adversary during the pre-start period clearly constrain the choice of start line locations for each competing sailor. Understanding the momentary accuracy of snapshot decisions (e.g., a decision to approach or avoid the adversary in each local interaction) may be less important than understanding a performer's accumulated accuracy of decision-making behaviors. The latter emerge from continuous interactions within the performance context geared toward achieving an overarching goal (e.g., acquiring an advantageous position in the starting line when a regatta commences; Araújo et al. 2005).

Araújo et al. (2015) showed that, since both boats in a race wanted to achieve an advantageous start, their interactions created a self-sustained competitive system in which coadaptations between members were sensitive to environmental, task, and individual influences (Gopalsamy 1982), thus revealing emergent decision-making behaviors. Importantly, decisions clearly emerged under interacting constraints, and were not determined by one single source of constraint, such as a mental representation of a start in a competitor. They observed that, in match-race sailing performance, coadaptive competitive behaviors between boats (the cycles and their oscillations), exemplified interpersonal self-sustaining, and thus self-organizing, processes during continuous decision-making behaviors. This process of decision making (the selection of a path to the optimal starting point) clearly cannot be based on mental comparisons between optimal and actual states represented internally, because they emerge under the interaction of constraints such as an adversary's actions, wind changes, ocean currents, and personal preferences. Because of the high computation load required, it would be highly infeasible to be able to precisely calculate the exact state of each source of constraint such as the adversary, wind, tide, and own personal/boat movements, then predict their changes, and plan how to act accordingly, on a moment-to-moment basis (figure 19.1).

By tracing the spatiotemporal displacements of the boats, time-series analyses (autocorrelations, periodograms, running correlations) revealed that trajectories of match-racing boats are coupled more than 88 percent of the time during a pre-start race, via continuous, competing coadaptions between boats. Araújo et al. (2015) argued that both the continuously selected trajectories of the sailors and their categorical starting point locations are examples of emergent choices. In this dynamical conception of action mode choice, strategic positioning at the start of a regatta emerged as a function of interacting task, personal, and environmental constraints. They considered that phase transitions in decision making would emerge from manipulation of key information sources for competitive sailors, demonstrated as the angle between the wind direction and the line (in line with previous data reported by Araújo, Davids, and Hristovski 2006). They

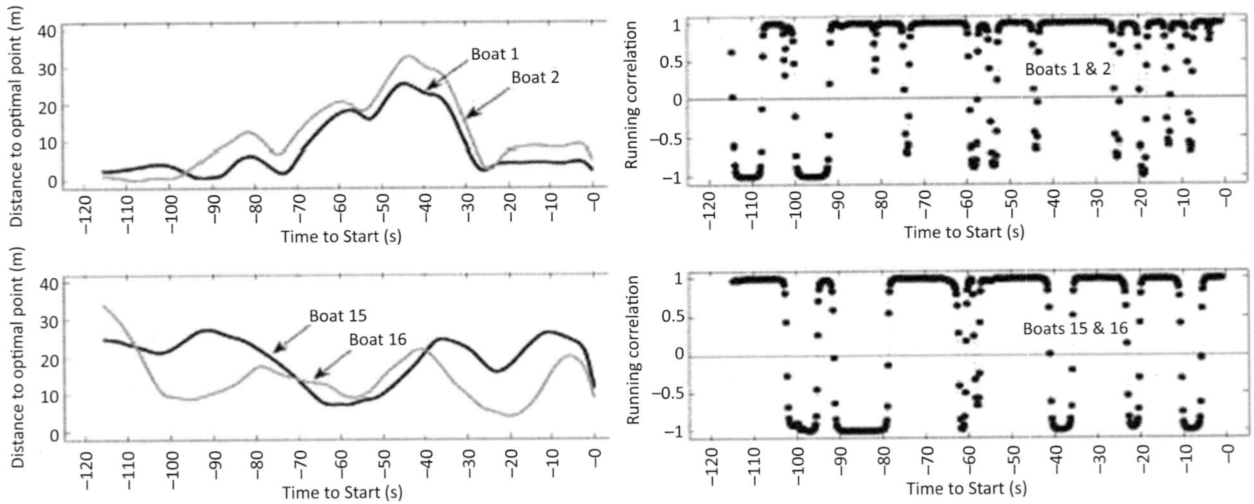

Figure 19.1
Two exemplars of time series referent to the distance (left), in meters, and their running correlations (right), from pairs of boats to the optimal starting position with higher running correlation (top) and lower correlation (bottom), relative to specific boats' match races.
Source: Araújo et al. (2015), 198–199.

observed sudden jumps in categorical decisions in successive match-race starts, because sailors seek to align local continuous decisions, emerging from their active exploration of situational constraints (e.g., the continuous interactions with the other boat in a competitive environment), with distal decisions about optimal start locations.

It seems that practice attunes performers to the perceptual variables that reliably specify states of affairs relevant to performance in a specific task (Araújo, Rocha, and Davids 2011). In this way, athletes can use the current performance situation as its own best model (Brooks 1991) and actively explore it, sampling it in detail at specific locations according to the particular needs of the moment. This process can be enhanced by using technological support to record and analyze sport performance pre- and post-competition. This performance-review process can be enhanced by framing decision making in sport environments in terms of the interactions of multiple local constraints (e.g., location of the yachts and of the starting line, their speed, sailors' cognitions, age and morphology, the currents, wind directions in a regatta). Performers' situated cognitions are a fundamental means of using active strategies to focus on emergent information in the performance environment, and practicing to enhance the use of real-time sequences of body-context interactions to solve problems in a robust and flexible way (Clark 1997). The model of decision making promoted here is predicated on conceptualizing performance as a coupled complex system, at the person-environment scale of analysis (e.g., a sailor and the regatta context), in which joint activity leads to emergent solutions.

4 Emergent Route Selection in Rugby Union

The descriptions of choice behaviors need to be systematically modeled and extended, although some extant models of social system transitions (Schmidt, Carello, and Turvey 1990; Schmidt et al. 2011) have tended to explain task dynamics as characterized by two attractors. Araújo et al. (2014), however, formally modeled a three-attractor task for an attacker-defender dyadic system. This model is considered to exemplify a social sport system in the dynamic performance context of rugby union.

Regardless of the different trajectories that a dyadic system in a team sport like rugby union might take, because of slight differences in initial performance conditions, empirical demonstrations have shown that three possible coordination patterns characterized as attractor states can emerge from attacker-defender interactions (Passos et al. 2008, 2009): (1) physical contact occurs in an effective tackle and an attacker does not pass a defender (system stability maintained: no phase transition); (2) physical contact occurs in a tackle but an attacker passes a defender (system destabilized: phase transition physically constrained); and (3), the attacker passes the defender without physical contact to score a clean try (system destabilized: phase transition informationally constrained).

In previous work, Passos and colleagues identified a collective variable that described space-time relations of attacker-defender dyads characterizing behavior in social neurobiological systems like team sports (e.g., Passos et al. 2008, 2009). Attackers were required to run past defenders with the ball starting from a position 10 meters from the try line. Collective variable values were calculated based on an angle between the defender-attacker vector and an imaginary horizontal line parallel to the try line, with its origin located in the defender's position. This analysis method revealed an angle close to +90 degrees before the attacker reached the defender's location, and close to −90 degrees after the attacker successfully passed the defender, with a zero crossing point emerging precisely when the attacker passed the defender (Passos et al. 2009). Behavioral information contributes to the emergence of pattern dynamics that attract a social neurobiological system to a required coordinated state (e.g., successful tackle; clean try). In line with this insight, Araújo et al. (2014) hypothesized that a specific coordinated state may function as an attractor. Despite the potentially huge variability of behavioral trajectories that both players might undertake, the dyadic system will always be attracted to one of the three coordinated states previously mentioned.

An attacker-defender dyadic system can be described by the angle *x* between a vector connecting the participants and the try line. This variable was proposed as an order parameter of the system and could be dynamically expressed by integrating a potential function. Empirical evidence has revealed that this kind of system has three stable attractors, with a potential function of the form $V(x) = -k_1\,x + k_2\,a\,x^2/2 - b\,x^4/4 + x^6/6$, where k_1 and k_2 are two control parameters. Random fluctuations were also observed in system behavior, modeled as white noise e_t, leading to the motion equation $dx/dt = -dV/dx + Q^{0.5}\,\varepsilon_t$, where Q is the noise variance (Araújo et al. 2014).

This model differs from generic statistical and mathematical models or empirical curve-fitting models, because it is derived from theoretical principles of the functioning of neurobiological systems (e.g., qualitative changes, instabilities, bifurcations), not from general statistical assumptions (e.g., linearity, normality). More to the point, the model starts from the well-established HKB (Haken, Kelso, Bunz; named after its authors) model in neurobiology and extends the initial model proposed by Tuller and colleagues, already applied in sport coordination tasks (e.g., sailing). These models have already accommodated the basic facts of neurobiological system functioning.

With the empirical demonstrations previously undertaken by Passos et al. (2008, 2009), revealing that these particular social neurobiological systems (dyadic systems in team sports) share the same properties of previously modeled systems (qualitative changes, abrupt jumps, fluctuations, bifurcations and so on), Araújo et al. (2014) have simply extended insights of those theoretical models to a three-attractor model.

To incorporate the potential effects of random influences and noise inherent in the dyadic system, the trajectory toward the attractor can be considered a random walk (Busemeyer and Diedrich 2010). This involves assuming, in general, that the mean drift in the random walk at *x* is a function of $V'(x)$, such that the drift is negative for $V'(x) > 0$ and positive for $V'(x) < 0$. The characteristic nature of the attractor states for $V(x)$ is such that, for all states within an attractor well, the system will tend to be pulled toward the minimum of the well. Once the system is caught in an attractor well, the system will tend to drift toward the minimum (where $V'(x) = 0$), and then meander stochastically around this minimum. The system is considered to have settled when this situation occurs (i.e., when the system is stabilized in an attractor well). It is assumed that a decision has been made as soon as the system has settled. The system is assumed to start in some initial state, x_0, and stochastically change over time until it settles and a new pattern is initiated. Random fluctuations in the behavior of the social neurobiological system can be modeled as white noise ε_t (Schoner, Haken, and Kelso 1986).

This modeling work implicated the value of interpersonal distance between dyadic system performers (attacker and defender in team sports) as a system-control parameter, verified by empirical evaluation (e.g., see Passos et al. 2006; Passos et al. 2008). The data from this research program revealed the influence on interpersonal dynamics of another candidate control parameter: the relative velocity between participants in a dyad. Figure 19.2 shows the graphical representation of the potential function and the motion equations of this model.

For the potential function plotted in figure 19.2(a), the attractor well displays a displacement to the left. The motion equation plotted in figure 19.2(b) shows that when the first derivative reaches zero, the dyadic system moves to $-\pi/2$ attractor state. This finding means that, with an increase in relative velocity, the dyadic system is attracted to a state characterized by a clean try scored. For the potential function plotted in figure 19.2(c), the attractor well remains at the center. The motion equation plotted in figure 19.2(d) shows that when the first derivative reaches zero, the dyadic system moves to the 0 attractor state. In this state, both players can annihilate each other's actions. When that happens, relative velocity undergoes small fluctuations ($k_1 = 0$) and at the 0 (zero) attractor, the interpersonal coordination dynamics that emerged were characterized by a tackle, wherein the attacker passed the defender, but fell down nearby. The potential function plotted in figure 19.2(e) displays a displacement of the attractor well to the right. The motion equation plotted in figure 19.2(f) shows that when the first derivative reaches zero, the dyadic system moves to the $\pi/2$ attractor state. This observation

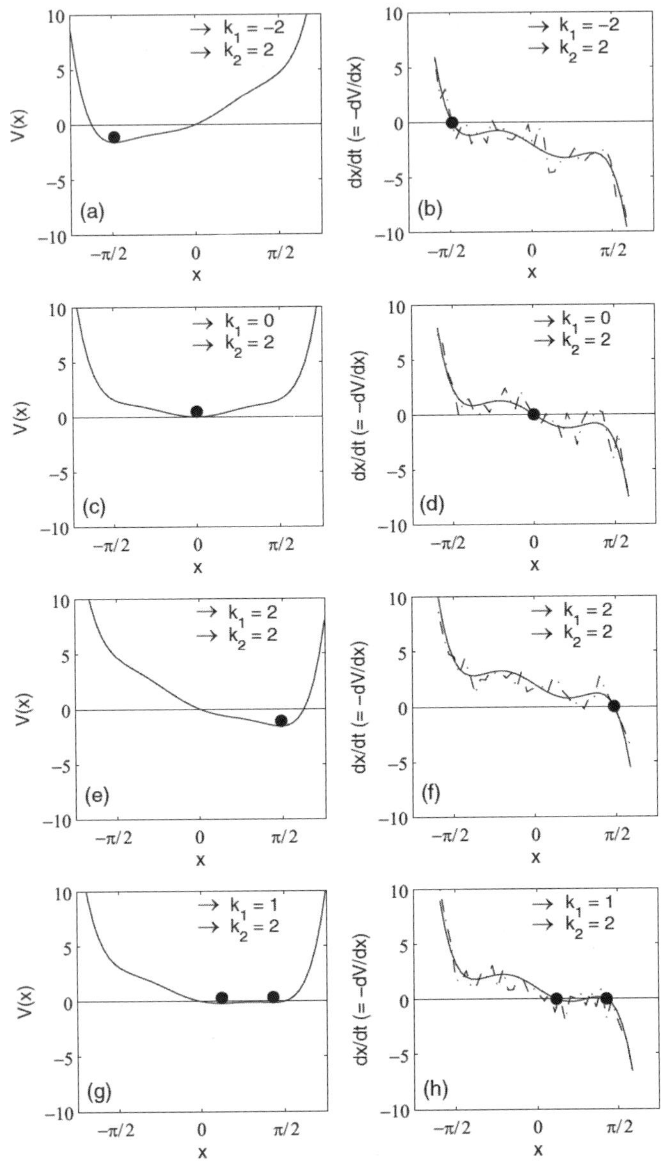

Figure 19.2

Graphical representation of the potential function (the left-hand side) and the motion equation (the right-hand side). (a) and (b): Clean try; (c) and (d): tackle but the attacker passes the defender; (e) and (f): effective tackle; (g) and (h): bi-stability between "tackle but the attacker passes the defender" and "effective tackle."

Source: Araújo et al. (2014).

means that because of changes in relative velocity, the dyadic system is attracted to a state characterized by an effective tackle. Importantly, the model successfully mirrored dyadic system performance outcomes in which attackers dominated (scoring a clean try) and when defenders were successful (performing an effective tackle).

5 The Concept of Emergence

In what sense do the preceding examples illustrate cases of *emergence*, and how does emergence in this sense relate to concepts of emergence in other areas?

Philosophical discussions of emergence have ranged across a variety of ontological categories, ascribing emergence to properties, entities, levels, or phenomena more generally. For the most part, especially within the literature in contemporary metaphysics and philosophy of mind, philosophical analyses of emergence have tended to focus on emergent *properties* and *entities* (see, among many other examples, Bedau 2008, Kim 2006, O'Connor and Wong 2005, and Wilson 2010 for a variety of influential accounts of emergence in these senses). So one distinctive feature of the foregoing examples is the focus on *behavior* as the product of emergence. Emergent action choice in these cases involves dynamically unfolding behaviors rather than static properties fully instantiated at a moment in time. This is most closely related to philosophical accounts of emergence in physics that also stress the role of dynamical concepts in characterizing emergence, such as Newman's (1996) account of emergence in terms of "strange attractors" in chaotic nonlinear dynamical systems, or McGivern and Rueger's (2010) account in terms of topological relations between dynamical portraits. Though the details of these dynamical accounts of emergence are distinct, the underlying idea is quite similar: in each case, we recognize behavior as emergent by considering how it is best modeled in terms of dynamical systems, and it is the features of the overall dynamical portrait—rather than just the specific, localized description of behavior—that determines whether or not a system's behavior is emergent.

Aside from the emphasis on dynamical behavior, though, we can distill four distinct features of the examples described here. Collectively, these four features form the basis of the idea of emergence in these examples. Some of these features overlap with features found in standard philosophical characterizations of emergence, but others have not been emphasized in those accounts.

The first feature involves the *coupling* of activities against a background of environmental constraints. For instance, this involves coupling between rival competitors engaged in sporting activities, against a set of constraints determined both by the environment and by the nature of the sporting task. Of course in some sense *all* activities take place against a background of constraints. These particular activities involve the exploration of possible modes of action, ultimately leading to a choice of action. This exploration and choice is best represented as the joint activity of a collection of coupled agents rather than as the result of choices discovered and made by individual agents acting separately. Representing behavior as a joint exploration of the range of possible actions allows investigators to adequately represent it in dynamical terms. By representing action ranges in this way, investigators can capture the similarities in behavior among systems that are superficially very distinct.

The idea that coupling is a central feature of emergent behavior, in performance contexts like sport, overlaps with one of the features most commonly associated with emergence—the idea that emergence involves activities of composite systems or "wholes" (e.g., teams), whose properties or behaviors do not reduce or resolve in some sense to the properties or behaviors of their parts (e.g., an individual team player). While the philosophical literature on emergence has explored a wide variety of ways in which this irreducibility might be understood, the key point for our examples is simply that our best models of a competitor's actions are ones that model the group of competitors as a single system exploring the range of strategic possibilities, rather than as individuals trying to negotiate a fixed background of constraints. The immediate concern is with the structure of the dynamical models that are most effective in capturing that behavior. In these cases, those are models that treat the actions of the competitors as engaged in a joint exploration of possible courses of action.

The second feature is an important outcome of the approach to modeling suggested by the first feature, and that is the *universality* of the dynamical patterns of action choice that are revealed when we model systems as collections of coupled and interacting agents. Even if we admit that this type of modeling is distinct from an approach wherein each agent is treated as an independent actor, we might wonder why the kinds of coupled models described here should be regarded as *better than* decoupled ones. In order for the kind of coupling associated with the first feature to be significant, there needs to be something that we would miss or fail to recognize unless we modeled our systems in this way. That is the feature of universality. The dynamical models described earlier support impressive generalizations of behavioral transitions across a wide range of modes of behavior—for instance, from sailing to rugby union to the walk-run transition. This is analogous to the kind of universality associated with emergence in other contexts. For example, philosophers of science have emphasized the significance of universality in physical system and the relationship between universality and concepts of emergence (Batterman 2000, 2001). These cases involve explanations of universalities in the description of phenomena such as critical point phenomena in thermodynamics, where systems with very different molecular structures display very similar patterns of behavior near so-called critical points of pressure and temperature. Those explanations involve techniques such as the "renormalization group" that allow us to establish formal connections between models that are superficially quite distinct. Doing *that* allows physicists to explain why systems composed of entirely different types of molecules will exhibit the same critical points behaviors (see Pfeuty and Toulouse 1977 for an overview of the renormalization group and the explanation of critical phenomena). The mathematical details of the examples described here are different, but the underlying point is very similar: the explanation of behavior in terms of a dynamical process of originating and decaying attractors allows not only for the explanation of individual cases, but also for a common explanation of action choice across a wide range of situations, involving actions (and actors) that are very different in detail.

The third important feature of these examples also relates to their dynamical nature. This is the *self-sustaining* nature of the interactive coupling. As with universality, part of the importance of this feature has to do with the way that it indicates that the dynamical coupling between agents is significant, rather than being transitory or accidental. Universality reveals this significance by relating the dynamics of one coupled system to the similar dynamics of a disparate variety of other systems. The fact that a coupled system is self-sustaining reveals this significance in more local ways: being a self-sustaining system gives us some reason for recognizing a collection as the kind of thing that could have its own behavioral dynamics, rather than as an aggregate of elements that only momentarily interact.

Note that it is common in philosophical discussions to distinguish between *synchronic* and *diachronic* accounts of emergence, and both dimensions are important for the examples described here. Synchronic accounts of emergence are concerned with relationships between "emergent" and "base" properties instantiated at the same moment in time, while diachronic accounts focus on the emergence of phenomena at one time from some other phenomena at another time (presumably, an earlier moment in time). The idea that emergent behaviors must be self-sustaining involves a combination of the synchronic dependence between the coupled activity of the system and the individual contributions of its components, and the diachronic dependence between the system at later moments in time and the same system at earlier (i.e., its self-sustaining activity).

The fourth important feature of these examples is the sense in which they involve behavior that is not preplanned, preprogrammed, or prearranged in some way. As Warren (2006) writes, describing similar accounts of emergent dynamical action, "Adaptive behavior, rather than being imposed by a pre-existing structure, emerges from [a] confluence of constraints under the boundary condition of a particular task or goal" (Warren 2006, 358). Furthermore, this emergent behavior involves "a pattern of behavior that does not reside a priori in the individual components of the system but is a consequence of their interdependence and interaction" (Warren 2006, 362). In part, this point is directed at the distributed nature of the systems that are engaging in the behavior: rather than the behavior being directed by a particular individual unit, the direction of behavior is determined by the collaborative interactions in a variety of units. However, since that idea is really what is already captured by the idea of *coupling,* the distinctive aspect of this fourth feature is better described in terms of the lack of preexisting structure—whether that structure is distributed or localized.

In some ways, the idea that there is no preexisting control structure is relatively trivial once we recognize the role of coupling. If the system's behavior is determined jointly be the interactions of it components, then there is clearly a sense in which that controlling structure does not exist prior to the system being formed. But there are two other, more interesting, senses in which a system's behavior could arise without being determined by a preexisting structure.

In the first of these, a system's behavior might be determined by the contributions made by each component, wherein each component is effectively following the same rules or patterns of behavior it followed prior to becoming coupled within the system, and where those coupled behaviors then generate a distinctive kind of behavior. This would be similar to standard examples of "weak emergence" such as those illustrated by the Game of Life, in which individual cells always follow the same set of simple rules, but where arrangement of such cells generate complex units—such as gliders and other phenomena—whose behavior can be described by other rules (see Bedau 2008 for a discussion of "weak emergence" in this context). From this view, there is no change in the underlying behavior of the couple components, though there is some sense in which the complex coupled system is characterized by laws or regularities that apply to it only as a whole.

The second sense of a lack of preexisting structure would be a stronger one wherein the behavior of components within a coupled system was not related to any underlying behaviors or rules that the system's components followed before becoming coupled. From this perspective, the lack of preexisting structure would mean that whatever structure was controlling those components before they became coupled ceases to exist—or ceases to be relevant—once they are coupled. Similarly, whatever structure controls the coupled system only comes into existence—or only becomes relevant—once those components come together. Emergent behaviors in this sense could be characterized by shifts in the governing dynamics of a system, in which the behavior of system in one region of its space of possible configurations is entirely distinct from the behavior of the system in other regions. Meehl and Sellars (1956) argued for a dynamical account of emergence along these lines, suggesting that emergent behaviors could be associated with particular regions of state space. They argued that the kind of "qualitative shifts" associated with traditional accounts of emergence could be captured by a change in a system's governing equations as it passed from one area of state space to another.

Philosophical discussions of emergence often dismiss weaker varieties as uninteresting, but in cases like the ones described in this chapter, we can see a clear reason why emergence in the weaker sense would still be interesting and important to recognize. The emergent actions in the sport performance contexts described earlier may well arise from individual patterns of behavior that remain stable before and during coupling. However, it is the patterns of *coupled* emergent actions that are universal in the sense described earlier—not the more specific actions performers considered separately. So it is only by focusing on those actions that we can see the common patterns across many different types of interaction. Furthermore, and perhaps more significantly, emergent behaviors of the sort we have described are patterns of behavior that we often think *could* be preexisting, programmed, represented or planned within an individual agent. As we have argued, in these cases, the explanations are unnecessarily overcomplicated. This is an important point about the value of recognizing emergent behaviors. If those patterns or actions were *obviously* not the sorts of things that could be preplanned by an individual agent, then the fact that they arise from the collaborative interaction of a collection of individuals would be relatively unsurprising. But since they are the kinds of actions, plans, and decisions we often associate with individual agents, we might have no hesitation in attributing them separately to the individual agents involved in that system. However, that is the mistake that understanding emergent action in the sense described here can help us correct: we can have a system that explores options, finds advantageous paths, and makes choices—all things we expect individual agents to do—without the agents in that system individually exploring, finding, and choosing in an identical way.

Note that these four features of emergence—coupling, universality, being self-sustaining, and being "unprogrammed" (or not preexisting)—are all distinct: we could have coupled systems that do not display universal behavior, we could have universal behavior that is not self-sustaining, we could have self-sustaining behavior that *is* preprogrammed or preplanned, and so on. It is the combination of these four different features that is being highlighted as characteristic of emergence in these cases. This type of emergence does not come down to a simple matter of unpredictability or irreducibility, or some manner in which features of systems are distinct from the features of components. Instead, emergence involves a cluster of features that together make a significant difference to how the behaviors of systems can best be modeled and understood.

6 Conclusion

This chapter has elucidated dynamical models showing how action choice is an emergent feature of coordination in sport systems. In support of this theoretical modeling we interpreted empirical data from interpersonal interactions in experimental tasks representative of performance in the team sport of rugby union and in regatta sailing. Extant models of transitions in neurobiological system behaviors have explained task dynamics as characterized by two and three attractors. The model predictions were supported by empirical research that demonstrated that (1) within multi-stable regions of sport system state space, switches in action choice can occur as a consequence of random disturbances; and (2), as multi-stable regions narrow (toward the region of an unstable critical point), there is a smaller chance of observing switches to one of the performance solutions modeled as one of three possible system states. Importantly, the models successfully captured the behavioral dynamics of performer in a sport system, both for players in rugby union and sailors in match racing.

Understanding the significance of these models and the sense in which the behaviors involved can be described as emergent has drawn attention to four key features: the systems involve behavior that is *coupled*, *universal*, *self-sustaining*, and *not preexisting*. We have tried to clarify these features, their significance, and their relationship to concepts of emergence. Focusing on dynamic social contexts, such as the understanding of behavior in sport, is crucial for developing an appropriate theoretical understanding of concepts such as emergent action.

Acknowledgments

This work was partly supported by the Fundação para a Ciência e Tecnologia, with the Grant UID/DTP/UI447/2013 to CIPER—Centro Interdisciplinar para o Estudo da Performance Humana (unit 447).

References

Araújo, Duarte, Keith Davids, Simon J. Bennett, Chris Button, and Graham Chapman. 2004. "Emergence of Sport Skills under Constraints." In *Skill Acquisition in Sport: Research, Theory and Practice*, edited by A. Mark Williams and Nicola J. Hodges, 409–433. London: Taylor and Francis.

Araújo, Duarte, Keith Davids, Ana Diniz, Luís Rocha, João Coelho Santos, Gonçalo Dias, and Orlando Fernandes. 2015. "Ecological Dynamics of Continuous and Categorical Decision-Making: The Regatta Start in Sailing." *European Journal of Sport Science* 15 (3): 195–202.

Araújo, Duarte, Keith Davids, and Robert Hristovski. 2006. "The Ecological Dynamics of Decision Making in Sport." *Psychology of Sport and Exercise* 7 (6): 653–676.

Araújo, Duarte, Keith Davids, and Sidónio Serpa. 2005. "An Ecological Approach to Expertise Effects in Decision-Making in a Simulated Sailing Regatta." *Psychology of Sport and Exercise* 6 (6): 671–692. doi:10.1016/j.psychsport.2004.12.003.

Araújo, Duarte, Ana Diniz, Pedro Passos, and Keith Davids. 2014. "Decision Making in Social Neurobiological Systems Modeled as Transitions in Dynamic Pattern Formation." *Adaptive Behavior* 22 (1): 21–30.

Araújo, Duarte, Luís Rocha, and Keith Davids. 2011. "The Ecological Dynamics of Decision-Making in Sailing." In *Motor Learning in Practice: A Constraints-Led Approach*, edited by Ian Renshaw, Keith Davids, and Geert J. P. Savelsbergh, 131–143. London: Routledge.

Batterman, Robert W. 2000. "Multiple Realizability and Universality." *British Journal for the Philosophy of Science* 51 (1): 115–145.

Batterman, Robert W. 2001. *The Devil in the Details: Asymptotic Reasoning in Explanation, Reduction, and Emergence.* New York: Oxford University Press.

Bedau, Mark A. 2008. "Is Weak Emergence Just in the Mind?" *Minds and Machines* 18 (4): 443–459.

Brooks, Rodney A. 1991. "Intelligence without Representation." *Artificial Intelligence* 47 (1–3): 139–159. doi:10.1016/0004-3702(91)90053-M.

Busemeyer, Jerome R., and Adele Diedrich. 2010. *Cognitive Modeling.* Thousand Oaks, CA: SAGE.

Clark, Andy. 1997. *Being There: Putting Brain, Body, and World Together Again.* Cambridge, MA: MIT Press.

Davids, Keith, Chris Button, Duarte Araújo, Ian Renshaw, and Robert Hristovski. 2006. "Movement Models from Sports Provide Representative Task Constraints for Studying Adaptive Behavior in Human Motor Systems." *Adaptive Behavior* 14 (1): 73–95. doi:10.1177/105971230601400103.

Diedrich, Frederick J., and William H. Warren. 1998. "Dynamics of Human Gait Transitions." In *Timing of Behavior: Neural, Psychological, and Computational Perspectives*, edited by David A. Rosenbaum and Charles E. Collyer, 323–343. Cambridge, MA: MIT Press.

Gibson, James J. 1979. *An Ecological Approach to Visual Perception.* Boston, MA: Houghton-Mifflin.

Gopalsamy, K. 1982. "Exchange of Equilibria in Two Species Lotka-Volterra Competition Models." *Journal of the Australian Mathematical Society B: Applied Mathematics* 24 (2): 160–170. doi:10.1017/S0334270000003659.

Haken, Hermann, Scott Kelso, and Herbert Bunz. 1985. "A Theoretical Model of Phase Transitions in Human Hand Movements." *Biological Cybernetics* 51 (5): 347–356.

Kelso, Scott, and David A. Engstrøm. 2006. *The Complementary Nature*. Cambridge, MA: MIT Press.

Kim, Jaegwon. 2006. "Emergence: Core Ideas and Issues." *Synthese* 151 (3): 547–559.

McGivern, Patrick, and Alexander Rueger. 2010. "Emergence in Physics." In *Emergence in Science and Philosophy*, edited by Antonella Corradini and Timothy O'Connor, 213–232. New York: Routledge.

Meehl, P. E., and Wilfrid Sellars. 1956. "The Concept of Emergence." In *The Foundations of Science and the Concepts of Psychology and Psychoanalysis,* edited by Herbert Feigl and Michael Scriven, 239–252. Minneapolis: University of Minnesota Press.

Newman, David V. 1996. "Emergence and Strange Attractors." *Philosophy of Science* 63 (2): 245–261.

O'Connor, Timothy, and Hong Yu Wong. 2005. "The Metaphysics of Emergence." *Noûs* 39 (4): 658–678. doi:10.1111/j.0029-4624.2005.00543.x.

Passos, Pedro, Duarte Araújo, Keith Davids, Luís Gouveia, João Milho, and Sidónio Serpa. 2008. "Information Governing Dynamics of Attacker-Defender Interactions in Youth Level Rugby Union." *Journal of Sports Sciences* 26 (13): 1421–1429. doi:10.1080/02640410802208986.

Passos, Pedro, Duarte Araújo, Keith Davids, Luís Gouveia, and Sidónio Serpa. 2006. "Interpersonal Dynamics in Sport: The Role of Artificial Neural Networks and Three Dimensional Analysis." *Behavior and Research Methods* 38 (4): 683–691. doi:10.3758/BF03193901.

Passos, Pedro, Duarte Araújo, Keith Davids, Luís Gouveia, Sidónio Serpa, João Milho, and Sofia Fonseca. 2009. "Interpersonal Pattern Dynamics and Adaptive Behavior in Multi-Agent Neurobiological Systems: A Conceptual Model and Data." *Journal of Motor Behavior* 41 (5): 445–459. doi:10.3200/35-08-061.

Pfeuty, Pierre, and Gerard Toulouse. 1977. *Introduction to the Renormalization Group and to Critical Phenomena*. London: John Wiley and Sons.

Pluijms, Joost P., Rouwen Cañal-Bruland, Serge Kats, and Geert J. P. Savelsbergh. 2013. "Translating Key Methodological Issues into Technological Advancements When Running In-Situ Experiments in Sports: An Example from Sailing." *International Journal of Sports Science and Coaching* 8 (1): 89–103.

Rosenbaum, David A., Rajal G. Cohen, Steven A. Jax, Daniel J. Weiss, and Robrecht van der Wel. 2007. "The Problem of Serial Order in Behavior: Lashley's Legacy." *Human Movement Science* 26 (4): 525–554. doi:10.1016/j.humov.2007.04.001.

Schmidt, Richard A. 1975. "A Schema Theory of Discrete Motor Skill Learning." *Psychological Review* 82 (4): 225–260.

Schmidt, Richard C., Claudia Carello, and Michael T. Turvey. 1990. "Phase Transitions and Critical Fluctuations in the Visual Coordination of Rhythmic Movement between People." *Journal of Experimental Psychology and Human Perception and Performance* 16 (2): 227–247.

Schmidt, Richard C., Paula Fitzpatrick, Robert Caron, and Joanna Mergeche. 2011. "Understanding Social Motor Coordination." *Human Movement Science* 30 (5): 834–845. doi:10.1016/j.humov.2010.05.014.

Scholz, John P., J. A. Scott Kelso, and Gregor Schöner. 1987. "Nonequilibrium Phase Transitions in Coordinated Biological Motion: Critical Slowing Down and Switching Time." *Physics Letters A* 123 (8): 390–394. doi:10.1016/0375-9601(87)90038-7.

Schöner, Gregor, Hermann Haken, and J. A. Scott Kelso. 1986. "A Stochastic Theory of Phase Transitions in Human Hand Movement." *Biological Cybernetics* 53 (4): 247–257. doi:10.1007/BF00336995.

Tschacher, Wolfgang, and Jean-Pierre. Dauwalder. 2003. *The Dynamical Systems Approach to Cognition: Concepts and Empirical Paradigms Based on Self-Organization, Embodiment, and Coordination Dynamics*. Singapore: World Scientific.

Tuller, Betty, Pamela Case, Mingzhou Ding, and J. A. Scott Kelso. 1994. "The Nonlinear Dynamics of Speech Categorization." *Journal of Experimental Psychology: Human Perception and Performance* 20 (1): 3–16. doi:10.1037/0096-1523.20.1.3.

Turvey, Michael T., and Claudia Carello. 2012. "On Intelligence from First Principles: Guidelines for Inquiry into the Hypothesis of Physical Intelligence (PI)." *Ecological Psychology* 24 (1): 3–32. doi:10.1080/10407413.2012.645757.

van Geert, Paul. 1994. *Dynamic Systems of Development: Change between Complexity and Chaos*. New York: Harvester Wheatsheaf.

van Gelder, Timothy, and Robert F. Port. 1995. *Mind as Motion: Explorations in the Dynamics of Cognition*. Cambridge, MA: MIT Press.

Warren, William H. 2006. "The Dynamics of Perception and Action." *Psychological Review* 113 (2): 358–389. doi:10.1037/0033-295X.113.2.358.

Wilson, Jessica. 2010. "Non-Reductive Physicalism and Degrees of Freedom." *British Journal for the Philosophy of Science* 61 (2): 279–311. doi:10.1093/bjps/axp040.

20 Selecting among Affordances: A Basis for Channeling Expertise in Sport

Duarte Araújo, Matt Dicks, and Keith Davids

1 Introduction

During sport performance, an athlete's actions generate perceptual information, which, in turn, constrains the emergence of further movements. For example, in climbing, Seifert and colleagues (2014) observed how skilled climbers perceived different properties of ice surface structures to adapt their actions with ice tools and crampons. When they detected holes in the ice surface left by previous climbers, hooking actions emerged. Conversely, when the ice was smooth and dense, climbers used swinging actions to create holes needed for a safe and rapid traversal. In turn, a climber's movements continuously change his or her relationship with the ice surface and the reciprocal search for information that offers subsequent opportunities for action. Seifert and colleagues (2014) reported that skilled climbers used a large range of actions, including limbs crossing the body midline, leading them to detect different sources of kinesthetic information and supporting different body positions on the ice to maintain stability on the surface while traversing. During sport, different surfaces, texture, and objects present opportunities for action (known as affordances) for performers to realize specific behaviors. These actions, in turn, reveal information that supports further functional behaviors in a cyclical fashion. The concept of affordances provides a powerful tool for coupling perception and action in human behavior, since "within the theory of affordances, perception is an invitation to act, and action is an essential component of perception" (Gibson 1979, 46). In order to couple perception-action subsystems to successfully regulate behaviors in achieving performance outcomes, individuals need to be able to become perceptually attuned to information in a performance environment as well as acquire the ability to scale information to their own action capabilities (i.e., calibration) (Fajen, Riley, and Turvey 2009). Studies such as those of Seifert et al. (2014) have shown, in climbing, how affordances are perceived in relation to the relevant properties of each individual, including the scale of key body dimensions (e.g., limb length) or action capabilities (e.g., flexibility and strength of fingers).

Data from such studies provide rich insights into the importance of detecting information during the control of actions and of actions in revealing information (Gibson 1979). Specific to the domain of sport, such ideas offer a means for explaining how selection of a course of action is based on the relationship between each athlete and a performance environment. In contrast with these ideas, traditionally, decision-making research in behavioral sciences has been predicated on *rational normative* models of decision making, founded on classical utility theory used to analyze behaviors of economic systems (e.g., Wolpert and Landy 2012; O'Brien and Ahmed 2015). In rational theories, forms of optimization (such as performance maximization) replace determinism and assumptions of unlimited computational power are center stage. Optimization of decision-making performance, here, refers to an individual's capacity to find a *putative single* best option within a set of potential courses of action (Gigerenzer 2006).

2 The Fallacy of Optimizing Decision Making

For many sport scientists and practitioners, the goal of a rational optimization of technique and tactics commonly provides a gold standard for empirical research (Glazier and Davids 2009; O'Brien and Ahmed 2016). Rationality works in a closed system, where, given certain assumptions, optimal solutions can always be derived if a rational process is followed. In contrast, Gigerenzer (2006) proposed that the ecology, not a rational model of optimization, frames the reference for functional decisions and actions in humans. Decisions and actions are functional ("correct") if they achieve an intended goal, not if they are performed according to what is prescribed by a putative optimal performance model.

In sport, performance environments provide athletes with the most powerful feedback about the functionality of their behaviors, thus providing a criterion for rationality, in response to a concern such as "How good was a particular decision?" In this way, Gigerenzer's views (2006) followed Brunswik's (1956) emphasis on the need to include the ecology as a reference for evaluating behaviors. Brunswik advocated the value of understanding the ecological, rather than putatively normative, aspects of rationality (e.g., Bayesian theory) by considering the informational "texture" of an environment. This view contrasts with normative models, which define a priori what is a putative "optimal" solution without referencing the ecology, even when it is not effective.

Instead of having an optimal decision as a point of reference, Gigerenzer (2006) argues for the relevance of an achieved decision or the degree of effectiveness of a specific action (see Hammond 2007, for a discussion). For Gigerenzer, behavior is successful if it is adapted to the structure of the information in the environment in which it is realized (Gigerenzer, Todd and The-ABC-research-group 1999). That is, the ecology is the reference point for the observation of a behavior. This view is contrasted with traditional optimal reference points in sport research, for which correct decisions are typically defined a priori by a group of coaches (e.g., Vaeyens et al. 2007) or an optimal movement technique is seen as the "best" solution, even when utilization of supposed nonoptimal techniques are no less effective in achieving an intended goal (Dicks et al. 2016). This idea can be exemplified in methods for training the reproduction of a classical sport technique, such as shooting at the basket in basketball. The performer may display an optimal technical movement pattern, even if the shot misses the basket (the aim is to repeat a specific—"optimal"—movement pattern, not to ensure that the throw is successful).

Unbounded rationality (assuming that athletes have developed the internal machinery to evaluate costs and benefits of every single solution made in performance), therefore, ignores the ecological constraints imposed on performers by a particular task environment (Davids and Araújo 2010). In this chapter, in contrast to models of performance optimization, we discuss how some explanations of decision-making behaviors in sport, such as ecological dynamics (Araújo, Davids, and Hristovski 2006), have focused on how decisions emerge from continuous interactions within a performer-environment system. We explain how this process can occur without proposing the involvement of additional inference mechanisms or mediating rules located within each performer.

Araújo and colleagues (Araújo, Davids, and Hristovski 2006; Davids and Araújo 2010) have previously explained that decision-making behavior during performance takes place in a landscape of attractors (stable system states), as potential task solutions. From this viewpoint, athletes search an attractor landscape of performance possibilities to arrive at a stable, functional solution. A viable option selected is the *strongest* attractor for an individual at a given moment, with other options having less strength of attraction. With increasing expertise, skilled individuals in sport learn how to become attuned to sources of information that specify goal achievement. Decision making is explained within an integration of intentions, actions, and perceptions, since selected options are the realization of *affordances*, or opportunities for functionally relevant actions (Gibson 1979; see also Rietveld and Kiverstein 2014, for the similar concept of landscape of affordances). This selection emerges only from the continuous interactions of an individual and a performance environment. Ignoring other options (that perhaps exist, as such, only from a third-person's perspective) is a dynamical consequence, since if a system relaxes to one attractor, it concomitantly ignores remaining options (attractors). The fact that there is a stronger attractor does not eliminate the influence of other attractors in the dynamic landscape of action possibilities (e.g., Araújo et al. 2013). Under dynamic performance conditions, other attractors (i.e., other options) may emerge and exert their attraction, emphasizing the performer-environment reciprocity. These ideas have powerful implications for understanding decision-making behaviors in sport, particularly for the design of practice environments to enhance performance.

This explanation of decision making and action choice in ecological dynamics (Araújo, Davids, and Hristovski 2006; Davids and Araújo 2010) theoretically captures the organism-environment symmetry in some current explanations of performance in sport. The approach proposes how action choice can emerge from a dynamic performance landscape composed of various performance opportunities or affordances for a specific performer. Conceptualizing such landscapes of action possibilities for sport performers shows how difficult it is to prescribe the existence in advance of "the optimal" decision for a particular performer. This is because affordances are dynamic and differ in stability (i.e., they emerge and dissolve momentarily in landscapes within dynamic performance environments), dependent on interactions of intrinsic dynamics of an individual performer, as well as task dynamics and environmental constraints (Fajen, Riley, and Turvey 2009).

3 Affordances and Goal-Directed Behaviors

As noted, affordances are possibilities for action in a particular setting (Gibson 1979); they are what an arrangement of surfaces, texture, and objects offers to a performer. Whether a hurdle, for example, is a "running over" obstacle or a "jumping over" obstacle is not determined by its absolute size or shape but by how it relates to an individual performer, including particularities such as size, limb dimensions, agility, and style of locomotion. The assumptions central to Gibson's (1979) theory of affordances are that (a) actor-scaled properties of the environment afford given behaviors for a performer; (b) informational invariants in energy arrays closely relate to a calibrated action; and finally (c), provided observers have a perceptual system sensitive to this information, they are able to perceive an affordance (Gibson 1979; Warren 1984; Withagen and Michaels 2005). The concept of affordances presupposes that the environment is directly perceived in terms of what actions a performer can achieve within a performance environment (i.e., it is not dependent on a perceiver's expectations; Richardson et al. 2008). Moreover, to perceive an affordance is to perceive how one could act with respect to an environmental layout. From this viewpoint, affordances are neither external properties of an environment, nor are they representational properties of mind; they are relational properties of a performer-environment system, which captures the dynamic between the individual and environment and are perception-action system specific (Fajen, Riley, and Turvey 2009). Thus, in sport, affordances capture the action-specific relations that exist between the skills/capacities of an individual performer and the action-relevant properties of a task, including social interactions (Heft 1989; Withagen et al. 2012). The theory of affordances is based on the dual interdependence of perception and action, wherein affordances are the primary objects of perception and action is the realization of affordances (Richardson et al. 2008).

Inspired by Gibson's (1979) ecological psychology and the work of Bernstein (Bernstein 1967), Reed (1996) argued that skilled behavior requires subtle resource usage, asserting that it is not intrinsically mechanical, but functional. He argued that in the course of evolution, selection pressures gave rise to different action systems, enabling performers to establish new functional relationships with their performance environments (see also Withagen and Michaels 2005). Whereas Gibson's theorizing on affordances was primarily concerned with how they are perceived, Reed addressed how affordances are realized. During performance in sport, resources can emerge from the performer (e.g., height, movement velocity, limb length) or from the environment (e.g., friction of the floor, jumpable obstacle, traversable surface). From this perspective an action should not be considered as a simple displacement of anatomical parts of the body (Withagen and Michaels 2005), because humans and other animals exhibit the capacity for stable and unstable patterned relationships to emerge between system parts through self-organization (Davids et al. 2001).

The empirical studies described by Araújo, Davids, and McGivern (this volume), clarify that, as a performer moves with respect to his or her surroundings, opportunities for action persist, emerge, and dissolve, even though the surroundings analyzed as objects, and the relations among them, remain stable. Subtle changes in action can give rise to multiple and marked variations in opportunities for subsequent actions. Decision making from this perspective is considered a complex, dynamic, temporally extended process that does not characterize an individual as having made a decision prior to its behavioral expression (Araújo, Davids, and Hristovski 2006). Indeed, decision-making behavior is considered at the level of the performer-environment relationship and is viewed as emerging from the interactions of individuals with environmental constraints over time on the path toward specific goals. In the context of team sports such as basketball, rugby, and hockey, a player in possession of the ball is required to, for example, decide whether she should pass or run with the ball. With every unfolding moment, information in the environment (e.g., co-positioning of teammates and opponents; appearance and disappearance of gaps in the playing area) will alter, inviting a new set of possible actions. For achieving task goals, some affordances are clear invitations, informing the performer how to proceed (Withagen et al. 2012). Therefore, an important question needs to be discussed: How are affordances selected by an individual performer?

4 Selecting among Affordances

Reed (1996) argued that affordances create selection pressure on the behavior of individuals, and consequently, behavior is regulated with respect to the affordances of an environment for a given individual. Therefore, behavior is not caused by the environment, since affordances are possibilities for action and, in some cases, invitations for action (Withagen et al. 2012; see also Bruineberg and Rietveld 2014; Heft 2010; Dreyfus and Kelly 2007; Käufer and Chemero 2015; Rietveld 2008). This performer-environment basis of conceptualizing behavior indicates that affordances can be used, motivating an organism to act, but they are not to be viewed as causes of behavior, because a person may not act on a perceived affordance. Affordances favor certain behaviors and select against others. This selection pressure occurs across all time scales, from the behavioral (for a discussion on emerging and decaying affordances see Fajen, Riley, and Turvey 2009), through the developmental, up to the phylogenetic time scale (Reed 1996).

The factors underlying the tendency for favored behaviors to be realized are multiple. For example, as considered at the outset of this chapter, a rock surface may be traversable for an individual climber in a specific way, depending on the availability and spatial organization of surface texture properties (holes, nodules, cracks, crevices offering stability, instability, gripping, and balancing) (Seifert et al. 2014). Indeed, each surface property has many affordances, and it is from this selection, of which affordance to act on, that it is possible to understand the dynamics of behavior in different climbers. Whether the individual takes up these possibilities or not is a separate matter (e.g., opportunities are not cast in stone: one can decline or accept an invitation to act in a specific way) (see Withagen et al. 2012).

Goal-directed behaviors emerge in performance contexts in which individuals face multiple affordances. Since affordances do not select themselves, the intention to use an affordance, as Reed (1993) put it, like other biological phenomena, emerges out of a process of variation and selection. Reed's (1993, 1996) ecological approach includes an account of intention (the selection of an affordance among those that can be picked up by an individual) that is rooted in Gibson's (1979) concept of affordances and information, thereby giving rise to an alternative conception of intention. As mentioned above, earlier psychological approaches have generally assumed that meaning is internally attributed and putatively originates in a representation somewhere in the human brain. Hence, any account of goal-directed intentionality rooted in this premise tends to focus on the regulation of behaviors like decision making by these internal states (see Reed 1996). By starting with the assumption that the animal's environment consists of values (affordances) and meaning (information), Reed (1993, 1996) developed an alternative, ecological account, arguing that what animals are seeking are not internal mental states, but rather values and meanings in a performance environment.

Reed argued that these intentional patterns of behavioral organization emerge in situations in which animals have choices of behavior, that is, in which different affordances can be utilized. Examples of choices of behavior in sport contexts include which strategic positions to adopt—on field—in an upcoming football fixture, or seeking the appropriate moment to begin an attack in a cycling race. Importantly, Reed contextualized intentions, suggesting that they should be interpreted at the level of the individual-environment system (Reed 1993, 68). Indeed, Reed stressed that *animals* are in charge of their own activity—"they *make their way in the world*" (Reed 1996, 19; emphases original)—placing the ideas of environmental *in*determinism and self-regulation at the center of his ecological approach. Reed asserted that in a dynamic performance environment that offers multiple affordances, perception-action cycles compete with each other, and the selection to use a specific affordance, and consequently goal-directed behavior, emerge out of this competitive behavioral process (Reed 1993; for a more recent and neuroscientific view based on this theory, see Cisek 2006, 2007; Cisek and Kalaska 2010; Pezzulo and Cizek 2016).

4.1 Selecting among Affordances in Sport Tasks

Our work has revealed that sport is a rich performance context for seeking empirical evidence for instantiations of affordance selection described above (Correia et al. 2012; Carvalho et al. 2014; Esteves, de Oliveira, and Araújo 2011). For example, Esteves, de Oliveira, and Araújo (2011) studied one-on-one basketball subphases and showed that a decision made by an attacker to drive to the left or right of a marking defender was based on selection of a specific affordance predicated on values of interpersonal distance between the two performers. As figure 20.1 shows, the specific body position adopted by a defender can guide the decisional behaviors of the attacker. Both novice

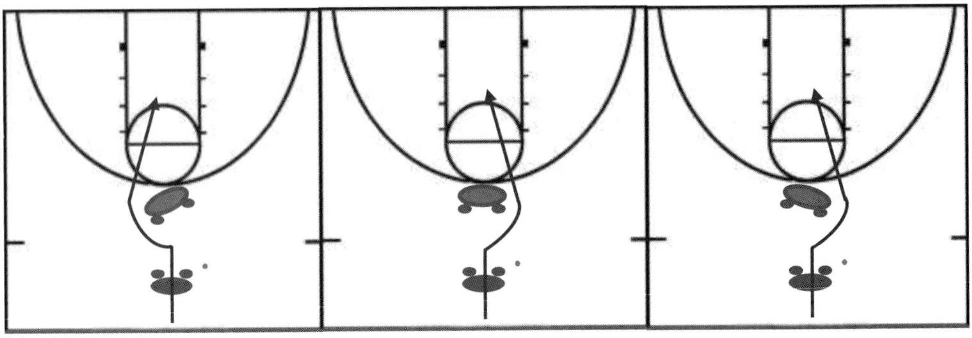

Figure 20.1
Schematic of a defender's positioning on a basketball court. Positioning was defined as the angle between the line passing both feet (taking left foot as reference), and the line parallel to the midfield. In the left-hand figure, the defender has the right foot advanced (300°), while in the right-hand figure, the defender has the left foot advanced (240°).

and intermediate attackers made the same affordance-based decisions by driving to the side of the defender's most advanced foot, but only at small values of interpersonal distances.

Leftward drives by attackers occurred when the defender had his right foot advanced and rightward drives occurred when the defender had his left foot advanced (figure 20.2). The use of this information by attackers was not prescribed by experimenters and emerged when participants dribbled toward the basket, without differing between levels of expertise. This finding indicates that the selection of an affordance (e.g., body position of the defender relative to the attacker with the ball) was expressed through the behaviors of participants, a finding in line with data reported in other studies (e.g., Cordovil et al. 2009). By acting on an affordance, the attackers were able to rely on information about a future state of the player-environment system, an effective means for controlling ongoing actions and achieve task goals.

The interesting fact is that it was also possible to pass a defender's back foot. So, why was there a preference to drive past a defender by the side of his most advanced foot? Interestingly, the affordance invited by the defender's body position gave an advantage to achieve a next subgoal: to dribble toward the basket. By acting on this first affordance, performers could rely on information about a future state of the player-environment system, a future affordance, in a functional way to control ongoing actions and achieve multiple task subgoals. The perception of affordances depends on the level of attunement of an individual to relevant properties of the environment, acquired through experience and learning (Fajen, Riley, and Turvey 2009). The fact that all participants

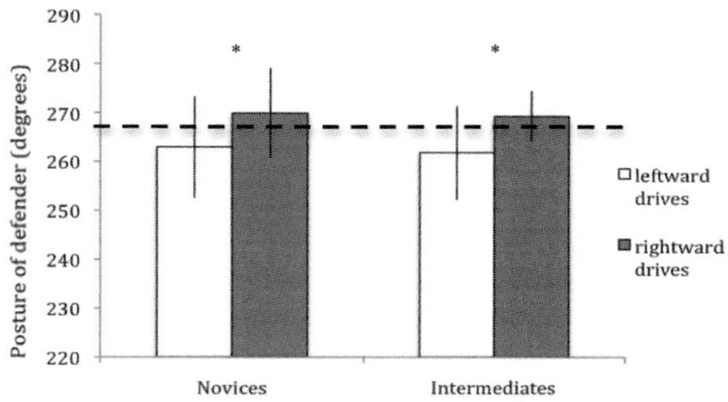

Figure 20.2
Average angles of feet positioning (posture) of the defenders at which the leftward and rightward drives of the attackers took place. Angles lower than 270° mean that the defender had the right foot advanced, and angles higher than 270° means that the defender had the left foot advanced.
Source: Esteves, de Oliveira, and Araújo (2011).

acted on a defender's body position information in a similar way indicated that novices may have picked up this specific affordance because it has an advantage for achieving the final task goal: shooting at the basket.

An ecological explanation for sequential behaviors (the link among affordances) suggests that the exploratory activities of a novice basketball player, observed by Esteves, de Oliveira, and Araújo (2011) might have led to the search and creation of information, which supported further actions to ensure goal achievement. One could construe the (small) trial-to-trial variations in the way that basketball players implemented the leftward and rightward drives as mere "noise" (figure 20.3 shows that half of the attackers' drives are directed to each side of the defenders). But it is quite possible that such variations highlighted the exploratory activities by the players for picking up affordances of each side of the defender for different purposes. That is, for driving to the left or right of the defender, given his more advanced foot position.

These observations fit with Gibsonian (1979) ideas of exploratory actions to pick up specific affordances of the available contextual information (defender's body position). It was only after passing the defender that the attacker could attempt to score (shoot at the basket) in the study by Esteves, de Oliveira, and Araújo (2011). The exploitation of an initial affordance of the defender's position was used to achieve a remote goal (to score) and has to be combined with a second affordance of the space near the basket. This outcome suggested that the ongoing behavior of the players comprised sequences of action (sub)goals, defined by three concatenated affordances: dribble past defender→ approach the basket→ shoot to score.

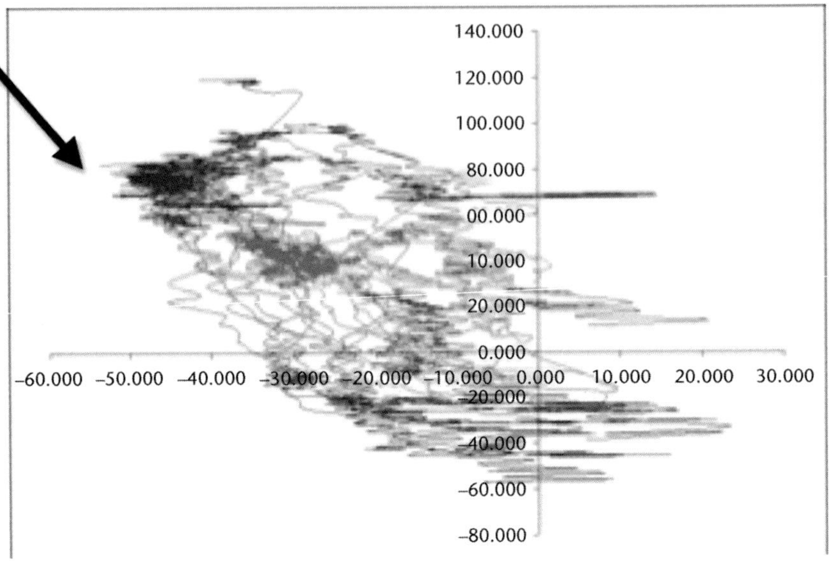

Figure 20.3
Trajectories of basketball players in a one-on-one task near the basket. Upper and lower lines correspond to the attackers' trajectories and central lines correspond to the defenders' trajectories. The point of the arrow corresponds with the attackers' starting position on each trial.

One possible explanation for how a particular affordance is selected among many other affordances is that each action on the selected affordance corresponded to a nested dynamic state of organization. This idea was developed by Keijzer (2001) on the basis of coupled multi-scale dynamics that generates behavioral sequences, such as "dribble past defender→ approach the basket→ shoot to score." Keijzer (2001) proposed that a behavioral sequence is generated by modulating the individual-environment system dynamics at appropriate points to yield a trajectory that transits closer to the final task goal. The short time-scale dynamics are modulated by the individual (Araújo, Davids, and Hristovski 2006). In turn, these dynamics are coupled to larger time-scale dynamics, guiding the formation of the behavioral trajectory over longer time scales. Reciprocally, the longer-term dynamics could influence the short-term interactions (thus highlighting specific affordances), for example, by altering environmental conditions. Because a behavioral trajectory is assembled anew on each occasion, the action sequence is historically contingent and variable, allowing for the flexibility observed in ordinary action sequences. Self-organized order is thus extended over larger spatiotemporal scales so that distal goals can be achieved. Therefore, the selection of an intention is not simply related with a selection between what the individual can or cannot do, but it is concerned with the explanation about why he or she engaged in a basketball task. By conceiving nested affordances in multi-scale dynamics, sequential behaviors need not be explained with recourse to a priori structures fixed in advance within the organism's central nervous system (Davids and Araújo 2010). Even though the same behaviors could be achieved through different processes, empirical research shows that even nonneural organisms (e.g., slime molds) display decision-making behaviors evidenced by approach or avoidance, predicated on selection, learning, and use of information to regulate such actions (Boisseau, Vogel, and Dussutour 2016).

Sequential affordances, as considered above, may imply an understanding of the perception of affordances in multi-scale dynamics. In the basketball example of Esteves, de Oliveira, and Araújo (2011), a novice player's exploratory activities appear to create information, which supports further actions to enable goal achievement. Trial-to-trial variations in the way that basketball players implement the leftward and rightward drives serve as exploratory activities by the players for picking up affordances of each side for different purposes: that is, for driving to the left or right of the defender, given the defender's more advanced foot. It is only after passing the defender that the attackers can realize affordances to score.

These observations also suggest that nested affordances are not internalized hierarchical plans. Instead, their dynamic assembly is based on information exploited during the control of action (Gibson 1979). In the same way that it is possible to detect information *for* learning (Jacobs and Michaels 2007), here we suggest that one important way to explain how affordances are selected is based on information for the next affordance. This is the informational basis for perception of affordances in multi-scale dynamics. This means that affordances are conditionally coupled (van Geert 1994), allowing a dynamic assembly of overall behavioral sequences.

4.2 Information for the Next Affordances and Skill

An important notion is that of skilled intentionality (Kiverstein and Rietveld 2015), which is defined as "the individual's selective openness and responsiveness to a rich landscape of affordances" (701). This definition indicates that the everyday environment offers a range of more or less inviting affordances (Withagen et al. 2012). However, these affordances are only accessible to individuals with the necessary skills to act on them, which reflects the invitational status of the athlete-environment relationship. For example, during sport, in the exact *same* situation, the affordances will vary from one player to the next depending on his abilities. For example, where one soccer player with an excellent passing ability may perceive an opportunity to play a long pass to a teammate, another player who is highly skilled at running with the ball may perceive an opportunity to dribble past an opposing defender. Thus, sport people interact with a surrounding environment through skilled engagement with the concrete affordances that a specific environment offers them because of their unique skills. From this viewpoint, the process of perceptual attunement through skill levels brings an "openness" to affordances that, without skill, would not be accessible, since it is skill that opens possibilities for action to an individual.

Moreover, individuals act behaviorally relative to multiple relevant affordances simultaneously, or to what Kiverstein and Rietveld (2015) call a whole "field of affordances," each of which is of greater or lesser significance to the animal. The significance of an affordance manifests in the urgency with which the affordance is currently moving the individual to ready her- or himself for action. For Kiverstein and Rietveld (2015), this idea justifies why an individual is open to and ready to act on multiple affordances at the same time. They define the landscape of affordances as the possibilities for action available in a particular "form of life" (equivalent to a distinct social/physical/psychological context in a specific sport like climbing or basketball) because of the patterned and coordinated activities that members of this form of life are *able* to partake in. However, the field of affordances reflects the multiple possibilities for action that stand out as relevant for each individual in a particular situation because of her specific needs, skills, experience, and concerns. In sum, skilled intentionality is based on the selective responsiveness to a landscape of affordances and in the openness to a field of affordances understood as different degrees of readiness of an individual to act on multiple affordances because of her skills.

The relationship between information for the next affordance and skill is exemplified through the analysis of behaviors in tennis rallies. Carvalho and colleagues (2014) showed how decision making is expressed by transitions in the player-environment system state, during goal-directed activity. These investigators developed the *goal-directed displacement index*, a measure that simultaneously considered the distance of the players in relation to two on-court reference points during competitive performance. The graphical representation of this index enabled identification of different patterns of action and rally break situations that expressed the successive affordances that guided the players' behavior (figure 20.4).

Figure 20.4 exemplifies the different functional relations that can be established between skilled players attuned, open, and responsive to match affordances. In their interactions, the players try to gain an advantage. This also signifies that a player with an advantage is perceiving and creating affordances for the other (see Fajen, Riley, and Turvey 2009, for a discussion about affordances for others in sport), where the other is invited to act on such affordances, since he is open and responsive to play in the

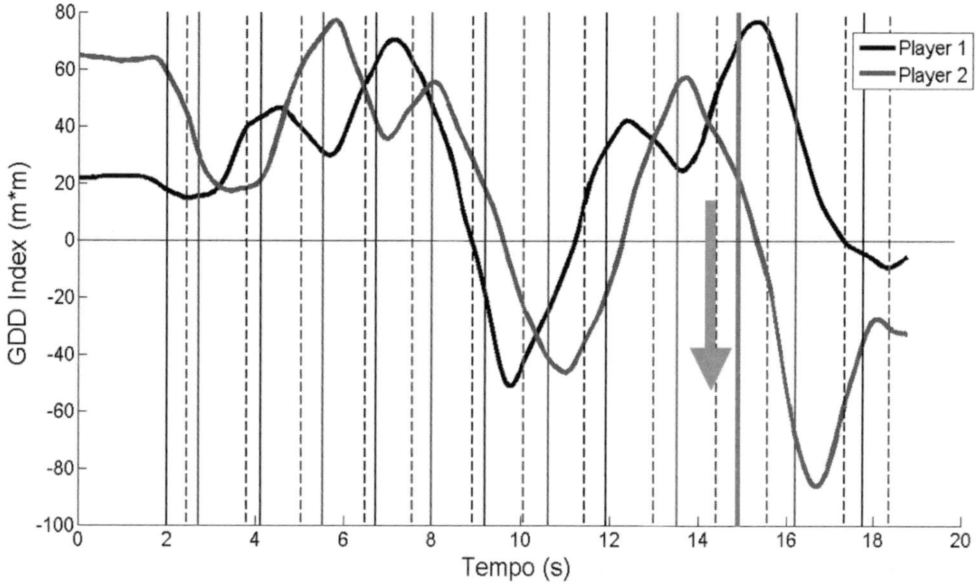

Figure 20.4

Exemplar data of goal-directed displacement index representing the position of the players during a rally. The vertical lines represent the strokes (thick line) and of the bounces of the ball (dotted). If the players' lines are on the same side, both players are positioned on the same side of the court playing a cross-court rally. If the lines are on different sides, the players are positioned facing each other (i.e., one on the right-hand side and the other on the left-hand side of their court). In this example, in the sixth shot, player 1 makes a parallel variation with a backhand down-the-line that invites player 2 to make a major move from the left-hand side to the right-hand side of the court. After this time, both players are playing facing each other, and when player 1 hit the next shot, he was closer to the center of the court.

rally. On the other hand, the stability of the interactions between players is highly constrained by the coadaptations (co-positioning) of the players (near or away from the central line of the court) and the pattern of interactions developed during play (cross-court or down-the-line rallies). In such landscape of affordances, a player with an advantage needs to create a successively more unstable situation for the other player, stroke after stoke, affordance after affordance, in an effort to destabilize the existing spatiotemporal coordination between them. When one player moves away from the central line of the court to hit the ball, the other player may approach the central line of the court to defend her court. Assuming a reference of two coordinate systems, if the players were playing a cross-court rally they would be moving in opposite directions (anti-phase mode of coordination). If they were playing a down-the-line rally, they would be moving in the same direction (in-phase mode of coordination). Conversely, if both players were approaching or moving away from the central line of the court, this relationship would signify the existence of instability in the game context. Whenever the players were moving away from the more stable modes of coordination, a system perturbation or rally break may emerge. This is exactly what a player with an advantage seeks to do, and what the player at a disadvantage tries to avoid or adapt to. Therefore, the advantage in a rally is a process that is developed though successive actions, where nested affordances are dynamically assembled and imply perceptual attunement to information for the next affordance.

5 Affordances and the Development of Expertise

The perspective outlined in this chapter until now considers that expertise is constituted by an individual's ability to detect special relationships among affordances and to act on those relationships to achieve particular functional outcomes. Complementary to this view, we have previously proposed that the adaptive variability of a performer can be enhanced through training to facilitate exploration of dynamic performance landscapes, with rich patterns of behavior emerging in metastable regions (when conditions are equally poised to facilitate system stability and instability) (e.g., Araújo, Davids, Chow, et al. 2009). Learning designs in sport that place individuals in a metastable region (exemplified through tasks with several performance solutions) can enhance decision making through experience of different action possibilities. For example, it has been shown that trainee boxers located at a specific scaled distance to a punch bag explored a rich variety of punching actions, including jabs, uppercuts, and hooks, which they had learned during training (Hristovski, Davids, and Araújo 2006). Without specific instructions on when to use a specific punch, boxers used different punch combinations that were highly varied when distance to target was scaled to their arm length at a mid-range. In contrast, when the boxers were either very close to or at arms-length from the punch bag, only a limited number of performance solutions emerged. Thus, designing sport practice task constraints in a way that invites a range of exploratory activities and adaptive behaviors of athletes may prove particularly beneficial, in contrast to prescriptive coaching instructions and feedback.

During the development of expertise, performers become attuned to affordances as invitations to support achievement of performance goals in specific circumstances. The ability to perceive an affordance is predicated on an individual's ability to detect information in a performance environment relative to his existing action capabilities (e.g., whether a hold on a rock affords a vertical pinch hand-grasp or horizontal crimp hand-grasp action for a climber during a traversal) (Orth, Davids, and Seifert 2014). The modification of practice tasks for different individual learners may therefore help them probe the boundaries between affordances. To exemplify, on a tennis court, the development of skill in the backhand volley might be facilitated by designing different affordances into a practice rally between a player and coach/training partner. Different types of feeds by a coach offer the performance of different shots by a specific athlete. In some feeds, a specific ball trajectory relative to the practicing player will lead to the emergence of a backhand or forehand drive from a tennis player. Specific strokes emerge as a developing expert gains knowledge of a performance environment through perceiving an affordance of a ball in flight and acting on it (Araújo, Davids, Cordovil, et al. 2009; Carvalho et al. 2013). As expertise in a sport is enhanced, a player becomes attuned to a wider range of spatial and temporal perceptual variables and gains a greater sensitivity to the contextual consequences of her actions (Araújo, Davids, and Hristovski 2006). For example, later in learning, cricketers begin to converge on more useful information from a bowler, such as body orientation, arm position, and hand adjustments prior to ball release (Pinder et al. 2011).

Following this reasoning, the ecological dynamics approach inspired by Bernstein's (1996) theorizing on motor learning and Jacobs and Michaels (2007) on perceptual learning elaborated a three-stage (search, discover, exploit) model of expertise development (Araújo, Davids, Chow, et al. 2009; Davids et al. 2012; Renshaw et al. 2016).

5.1 Search: Exploring Degrees of Freedom to Achieve a Task Goal

Many perceptions and actions are possible in a given performance environment. In specific performance situations, certain opportunities for action are more functional than others and, with experience, individuals improve on selecting the affordances they realize. Different intentions are presumed to organize perceptual-motor systems in different ways. As Turvey defines it, intentionality is predicated on directedness toward objects, places, people, or events (1986). Indeed, Gibson pursued a perceptual theory that was fundamentally intentional rather than one that is made intentional as an afterthought (i.e., added by mental representations).

Educating the intention of performers might have an important influence on which affordance needs to be perceived by a performer. In understanding the development of expertise, one needs to consider how and when intentions arise, as well as how they manifest themselves in the activities of the performer (Arzamarski et al. 2010). Iberall's (1977; Iberall and McCulloch 1969) ideas about intentions suggest that living systems cycle among their associated action modes—competing in soccer, training, watching games, and so on—and that these modes entail goal-directed actions: belonging to a team, a club, a competitive league, a veritable form of life. In this form of life (Rietveld and Kiverstein 2014), one can learn about match competition, tactics, conventions, and rules, and the education of intention is about establishing such task goals, according to skill. The education of intention is also an information-guided process. Intention plays its role by setting up a perceptual system to be sensitive to information appropriate for a to-be-perceived property or for a to-be-undertaken action. In other words, intention directs attention. Appreciating the circular causality of perception-action makes this more concrete: intentions motivate explorations that constrain perception, which further constrains action, and so on.

These considerations of the co-implication of intention, information, and exploration indicate that initial exploratory actions entailed by the intention to perceive some environmental property are expected to reveal information about that property (Turvey, Carello, and Kim 1990). In a one-on-one basketball game close to the basket, for instance, it can be assumed by observers that attackers with the ball intend to dribble past the defender and to shoot at the basket in order to score, rather than to simply maintain possession of the ball. Assuming a particular intention is a crucial aspect of practice design in sport, which is required to define and identify what informational variables are relevant at any moment (Jacobs and Michaels 2007). This aspect of practice design is also influenced by Bernstein's (1967) insights. As is well known by now, he raised the problem of how the large number of individual degrees of freedom to be regulated during learning and performance has to be reorganized in order to make control possible. When the intention of a performer corresponds to the task goal, there is a need to coordinate the redundant degrees of freedom of her movement system. Control may be obtained by "freezing" solutions that may facilitate goal achievement (Vereijken et al. 1992; Savelsbergh and van der Kamp 2000) or by realizing exploratory actions to find a solution that gets the job done (Araújo, Davids, and Serpa 2005).

It is not surprising that different people may rigidly stabilize different solutions (i.e., stable movement patterns and/or use informational variables) to achieve the same goal. At this stage, movement may be using information (in the above described Gibsonian sense) "that works," but that does not mean it specifies the property of the environment that the performer intended to perceive (i.e., it may be a nonspecifying variable). The term *specifying variable* is used only for a variable that specifies a property (i.e., the informational variable) that a perceiver intends to perceive (e.g., the focus of expansion of the ball on a performer's retina when catching a pass), and the term *nonspecifying variable* only for a variable that does not specify the property that a perceiver intends to perceive (e.g., a player attempting to judge the flight path of a ball from the deceptive movements of an opponent projecting it), regardless of whether a so-called nonspecifying variable might specify other properties of the environment

(Jacobs and Michaels 2007). When performers increase their exploratory actions, this is due to the difficulty in discriminating which properties of the environment constitute information to achieve task goal and which do not. Exploration of what is available in a performance situation can reveal what environmental properties are informative in relation to a specific intention (Araújo, Davids, and Serpa 2005). In sum, by exploring a landscape of affordances, the intentions of a performer become aligned with a task goal. Information and action couplings emerge and synergistically coordinate the system degrees of freedom needed to (attempt to) realize the task.

5.2 Discover: Exploring Task Solutions and Strengthening Them

In a subsequent phase, the performer identifies tentative performance solutions and attempts to reproduce them when performing the sport task. With the irreducible variability of the initial conditions to perform the task, information-movement couplings start to become more regular. A way to stabilize a movement solution is to "free" the previously exaggerated constriction of degrees of freedom. This means that the most relevant degrees of freedom for achieving the task goal are identified, and also that the conditions *when* an informational variable is useful are also identified and acted on. Therefore, new action possibilities start to be identified.

During this stage, the same intention might lead to the detection of other variables. The process of attending to more useful variables is referred to as the education of attention, or perceptual attunement (Gibson 1966, 1979). Perceptual attunement refers to changes in the informational variables on which one relies to guide movement (Fajen, Riley, and Turvey 2009). Thus, even if an intention does not change, with experience, performers can use perceptual variables in a more functional way, or can attend to more useful variables. Perceptual attunement is the process of learning which sources of information to attend to in which situations and when to attend to them (Jacobs and Michaels 2007). With practice, performers converge from sources of information that may be only partly useful in one particular situation (i.e., nonspecifying) to sources of information that are more useful (i.e., specifying), under a variety of performance circumstances. In sum, in this phase there is a strengthening of discovered solutions, as well as an exploration of the limits of these solutions, and consequent search for new information-action couplings.

5.3 Exploit: Exploiting Perceptual-Motor Degrees of Freedom

Specifying information sources tend to be regularly used when performing a task, and the fluidity of movement (i.e., the mastering of motor degrees of freedom) is supported by the use of external forces (passive dynamics), contrasting with previous opposition or elimination of these forces. The exploitation of motor and perceptual degrees of freedom (Savelsbergh and van der Kamp 2000) supports adaptation to situational demands and goal achievement. An important point at this stage is the attunement to wider spatial and temporal variables and higher sensitivity to the contextual consequences of one's actions (Araújo, Davids, and Serpa 2005); although more action variability occurs, this variability is functional (i.e., it is constrained and convergent to goal achievement). This means that degeneracy, or the ability of elements that are structurally different to perform the same function or yield the same output, is an essential feature of this process (Davids et al. 2006).

A relevant process at this stage is that of calibration, or the scaling of action to information (Withagen and Michaels 2005). Body dimensions and action capabilities are not fixed, but often change across both short and long time scales. When body dimensions and action capabilities change, actions that were once possible may become impossible (or vice versa; see Fajen, Riley, and Turvey 2009). In perception-action, calibration and recalibration are necessary to establish and update the mapping between the units in which the relevant properties of the world are perceived and the units in which the action is realized (Warren 1984). Calibration in practice makes it possible for performers to perceive the world in intrinsic units even after changes in body dimensions and action capabilities. For a properly calibrated performer, body-scaled and action-scaled affordances can be directly and reliably perceived by simply detecting the relevant sources of information (Fajen, Riley, and Turvey 2009). Although recalibration occurs quite rapidly, it is likely that continued experience leads to further improvements in calibration. Importantly, an athlete can be properly attuned—in the sense that he or she is relying on an informational variable that invariantly specifies the relevant property—but not properly calibrated. Thus, to reliably perceive affordances, both attunement and calibration are necessary (Fajen, Riley, and Turvey 2009).

These ideas illustrate the importance of recognizing individual differences in the way that skilled performers achieve functional task solutions. For example, Dicks, Davids, and Button (2010) reported that experienced goalkeepers scaled the timing of their actions relative to their agility when attempting to save penalty kicks. The more agile the goalkeeper, the later the diving action was likely to be initiated. Analyses of the movement kinematics of penalty takers have revealed that the kinematic information that unfolds in the final moments of the action has a high congruency with the final kicking direction (Lopes et al. 2014). Specific to the study of Dicks, Davids, and Button (2010), the slower goalkeepers who moved earlier exploited kinematic information from the penalty taker's action that led to a fewer number of saves and a greater likelihood of being deceived. Thus, being able to calibrate movements to later information appeared to support more successful performance. Moreover, as young adults, tennis players can reach passing ball trajectories to volley rather than having to wait for the ball to bounce to drive it. With aging, system reorganization in older adult players might signify that letting a ball bounce for a drive is a more functional shot than striving to volley a passing ball early. This example also highlights how athletes' effective body dimensions can be mediated by using equipment in sport such as racquets, roller blades, bats, and sticks. This is so because a number of affordances can be described primarily in terms of the relation between some dimension of a player's body, such as arm length, and a complementary property of the environment, such as the distance to a passing ball. Body-scaled affordances can be measured on a scale that is intrinsic to the perceiver (e.g., in units of arm length), rather than according to an extrinsic measurement system such as inches or centimeters. Perceiving the environment in body-scaled units thus relates the environment directly to the perceiver's action capabilities. An avenue for future research concerns the use of implements that modify an athlete's capabilities, such as by extending an athlete's effective body dimensions (e.g., by extending reach, such as using a racquet to intercept a ball) (Araújo et al. 2004).

6 Conclusion

In this chapter we have considered how ecological dynamics views intentions, perceptions, and actions as intertwined processes that can be harnessed to utilize affordances in specific sport performance environments. This process can benefit from the education of intention, attunement to information, and calibration as the performer-environment system changes because of processes such as learning, development, and maturation. These ideas suggest that learning environments need to be carefully designed in order to continuously facilitate appropriate interactions between intentions, perception, and action to support ever-increasing functionality of performance behaviors in athletes (Araújo and Davids 2015). A key practical implication is that the emphasis on the importance of exploration as a strategy to enhance performance can facilitate skill channeling and adaptation of an athlete to a specific form of life in sport.

References

Araújo, Duarte, and Keith Davids. 2015. "Towards a Theoretically-Driven Model of Correspondence between Behaviours in One Context to Another: Implications for Studying Sport Performance." *International Journal of Sport Psychology* 46 (6): 268–280.

Araújo, Duarte, Keith Davids, Simon J. Bennett, Chris Button, and G. Chapman. 2004. "Emergence of Sport Skills under Constraints." In *Skill Acquisition in Sport: Research, Theory and Practice*, edited by Nicola Hodges and A. Mark Williams, 409–433. London: Routledge.

Araújo, Duarte, Keith Davids, Jia Yi Chow, Pedro Passos, and Markus Raab. 2009. "The Development of Decision Making Skill in Sport: An Ecological Dynamics Perspective." In *Perspectives on Cognition and Action in Sport*, edited by Duarte Araújo, Hubert Ripoll, and Markus Raab, 157–169. Hauppauge, NY: NOVA Science.

Araújo, Duarte, Keith Davids, Rita Cordovil, João Ribeiro, and Orlando Fernandes. 2009. "How Does Knowledge Constrain Sport Performance? An Ecological Perspective." In *Perspectives on Cognition and Action in Sport*, edited by Duarte Araújo, Hubert Ripoll, and Markus Raab, 119–131. Hauppauge, NY: Nova Science.

Araújo, Duarte, Keith Davids, and Robert Hristovski. 2006. "The Ecological Dynamics of Decision Making in Sport." *Psychology of Sport and Exercise* 7 (6): 653–676.

Araújo, Duarte, Keith Davids, and Sidónio Serpa. 2005. "An Ecological Approach to Expertise Effects in Decision-Making in a Simulated Sailing Regatta." *Psychology of Sport and Exercise* 6 (6): 671–692. doi:10.1016/j.psychsport.2004.12.003.

Araújo, Duarte, Ana Diniz, Pedro Passos, and Keith Davids. 2013. "Decision Making in Social Neurobiological Systems Modeled as Transitions in Dynamic Pattern Formation." *Adaptive Behavior* 22 (1): 21–30. doi:10.1177/1059712313497370.

Arzamarski, Ryan, Robert W. Isenhower, Bruce A. Kay, Michael T. Turvey, and Claire F. Michaels. 2010. "Effects of Intention and Learning on Attention to Information in Dynamic Touch." *Attention, Perception, and Psychophysics* 72 (3): 721–735. doi:10.3758/APP.72.3.721.

Bernstein, Nikolai. 1967. *The Co-ordination and Regulation of Movements*. Oxford: Pergamon.

Bernstein, Nikolai. 1996. "On Dexterity and Its Development." In *On Dexterity and Its Development*, edited by Mark L. Latash and Michael T. Turvey, 3–24. Mahwah, NJ: Erlbaum.

Boisseau, Romain P., David Vogel, and Audrey Dussutour. 2016. "Habituation in Non-neural Organisms: Evidence from Slime Moulds." *Proceedings of the Royal Society B: Biological Sciences* 283 (1829): 20160446. doi:10.1098/rspb.2016.0446.

Bruineberg, Jelle, and Erik Rietveld. 2014. "Self-Organization, Free Energy Minimization, and Optimal Grip on a Field of Affordances." *Frontiers in Behavioral Neuroscience* 8 (August): 599. doi:10.3389/fnhum.2014.00599.

Brunswik, Egon. 1956. *Perception and the Representative Design of Psychological Experiments*. 2nd ed. Berkeley: University of California Press.

Carvalho, João, Duarte Araújo, Bruno Travassos, Pedro Esteves, Luís Pessanha, Fernando Pereira, and Keith Davids. 2013. "Dynamics of Players' Relative Positioning during Baseline Rallies in Tennis." *Journal of Sports Sciences* 31 (14): 1596–1605. doi:10.1080/02640414.2013.792944.

Carvalho, João, Duarte Araújo, Bruno Travassos, Orlando Fernandes, Fernando Pereira, and Keith Davids. 2014. "Interpersonal Dynamics in Baseline Rallies in Tennis." *International Journal of Sports Science and Coaching* 9 (5): 1043–1056. doi:10.1260/1747-9541.9.5.1043.

Cisek, Paul. 2006. "Integrated Neural Processes for Defining Potential Actions and Deciding between Them: A Computational Model." *Journal of Neuroscience* 26 (38): 9761–9770. doi:10.1523/JNEUROSCI.5605-05.2006.

Cisek, Paul. 2007. "Cortical Mechanisms of Action Selection: The Affordance Competition Hypothesis." *Philosophical Transactions of the Royal Society of London B: Biological Sciences* 362 (1485): 1585–1599. doi:10.1098/rstb.2007.2054.

Cisek, Paul, and John. F. Kalaska. 2010. "Neural Mechanisms for Interacting with a World Full of Action Choices." *Annual Review of Neuroscience* 33:269–298. doi:10.1146/annurev.neuro.051508.135409.

Cordovil, Rita, Duarte Araújo, Keith Davids, Luís Gouveia, João Barreiros, Orlando Fernandes, and Sidónio Serpa. 2009. "The Influence of Instructions and Body-Scaling as Constraints on Decision-Making Processes in Team Sports." *European Journal of Sport Science* 9 (3): 169–179. doi:10.1080/17461390902763417.

Correia, Vanda, Duarte Araújo, Alan Cummins, and Cathy M. Craig. 2012. "Perceiving and Acting upon Spaces in a VR Rugby Task: Expertise Effects in Affordance Detection and Task Achievement." *Journal of Sport and Exercise Psychology* 34 (3): 305–321.

Davids, Keith, and Duarte Araújo. 2010. "The Concept of 'Organismic Asymmetry' in Sport Science." *Journal of Science and Medicine in Sport / Sports Medicine Australia* 13 (6): 633–640.

Davids, Keith, Duarte Araújo, Robert Hristovski, Pedro Passos, and Jia Yi Chow. 2012. "Ecological Dynamics and Motor Learning Design in Sport." In *Skill Acquisition in Sport: Research, Theory and Practice,* edited by Nicolas Hodges and Mark Williams, 112–130. London: Routledge.

Davids, Keith, Chris Button, Duarte Araújo, Ian Renshaw, and Robert Hristovski. 2006. "Movement Models from Sports Provide Representative Task Constraints for Studying Adaptive Behavior in Human Movement Systems." *Adaptive Behavior* 14 (1): 73–95. doi:10.1177/105971230601400103.

Davids, Keith, Damian Kingsbury, Simon Bennett, and Craig Handford. 2001. "Information—Movement Coupling: Implications for the Organization of Research and Practice during Acquisition of Self-Paced Extrinsic Timing Skills." *Journal of Sports Sciences* 19 (2): 117–127. doi:10.1080/026404101300036316.

Dicks, Matt, Chris Button, Keith Davids, Jia Yi Chow, and J. Van der Kamp. 2016. "Keeping an Eye on Noisy Movements: On Different Approaches to Perceptual-Motor Skill Research and Training." *Sports Medicine* 47 (4): 575–581. doi:10.1007/s40279-016-0600-3.

Dicks, Matt, Keith Davids, and Chris Button. 2010. "Individual Differences in the Visual Control of Intercepting a Penalty Kick in Association Football." *Human Movement Science* 29 (3): 401–411. doi:10.1016/j.humov.2010.02.008.

Dreyfus, Hubert, and Sean D. Kelly. 2007. "Heterophenomenology: Heavy-Handed Sleight-of-Hand." *Phenomenology and the Cognitive Sciences* 6 (1): 45–55. doi:10.1007/s11097-006-9042-y.

Esteves, Pedro, Rita F. de Oliveira, and Duarte Araújo. 2011. "Posture-Related Affordances Guide Attacks in Basketball." *Psychology of Sport and Exercise* 12 (6): 639–644. doi:10.1016/j.psychsport.2011.06.007.

Fajen, Brett R., Michael A. Riley, and Michael T. Turvey. 2009. "Information, Affordances, and the Control of Action in Sport." *International Journal of Sport Psychology* 40 (1): 79–107.

Gibson, James J. 1966. *The Senses Considered as Perceptual Systems.* Boston: Houghton Mifflin.

Gibson, James J. 1979. *The Ecological Approach to Visual Perception.* Mahwah: NJ: Lawrence Erlbaum.

Gigerenzer, Gerd. 2006. "Bounded and Rational." In *Contemporary Debates in Cognitive Science,* edited by R. J. Stainton, 115–133. Oxford: Blackwell.

Gigerenzer, Gerd, Peter M. Todd, and The-ABC-Research-Group. 1999. *Simple Heuristics That Make Us Smart.* Oxford: Oxford University Press.

Glazier, Paul S., and Keith Davids. 2009. "Constraints on the Complete Optimization of Human Motion." *Sports Medicine* 39 (1): 15–28. doi:10.2165/00007256-200939010-00002.

Hammond, Kenneth R. 2007. *Beyond Rationality: The Search for Wisdom in a Troubled Time.* Oxford: Oxford University Press.

Heft, Harry. 1989. "Affordances and the Body: An Intentional Analysis of Gibson's Ecological Approach to Visual Perception." *Journal for the Theory of Social Behaviour* 19 (1): 1–30. doi:10.1111/j.1468-5914.1989.tb00133.x.

Heft, Harry. 2010. "Affordances and the Perception of the Landscape: An Environmental Perception and Aesthetics." In *Innovative Approaches to Researching Landscape and Health: Open Space: People Space 2,* edited by Catharine Ward Thompson, Peter Aspinall, and Simon Bell, 9–32. Abingdon, UK: Routledge.

Hristovski, Robert, Keith Davids, and Duarte Araújo. 2006. "Affordance-Controlled Bifurcations of Action Patterns in Martial Arts." *Nonlinear Dynamics, Psychology and Life Sciences* 10 (4): 409–444.

Iberall, Arthur S. 1977. "A Field and Circuit Thermodynamics for Integrative Physiology. I. Introduction to the General Notions." *American Journal of Physiology: Regulatory, Integrative, Comparative Physiology* 233 (5): R171–180.

Iberall, Arthur S., and Warren S. McCulloch. 1969. "The Organizing Principle of Complex Living Systems." *ASME: Journal of Basic Engineering* 91 (2): 290–294. doi:10.1115/1.3571099.

Jacobs, David M., and Claire F. Michaels. 2007. "Direct Learning." *Ecological Psychology* 19 (4): 321–349. doi:10.1080/10407410701432337.

Käufer, Stephan, and Anthony Chemero. 2015. *Phenomenology: An Introduction.* Hoboken, NJ: John Wiley and Sons.

Keijzer, Fred A. 2001. *Representation and Behavior.* Cambridge, MA: MIT Press.

Kiverstein, Julian, and Erik Rietveld. 2015. "The Primacy of Skilled Intentionality: On Hutto & Satne's The Natural Origins of Content." *Philosophia* 43 (3): 701–721. doi:10.1007/s11406-015-9645-z.

Lopes, José E., David M. Jacobs, David Travieso, and Duarte Araújo. 2014. "Predicting the Lateral Direction of Deceptive and Non-Deceptive Penalty Kicks in Football from the Kinematics of the Kicker." *Human Movement Science* 36 (August): 199–216. doi:10.1016/j.humov.2014.04.004.

O'Brien, Megan K., and Alaa A. Ahmed. 2015. "Threat Affects Risk Preferences in Movement Decision Making." *Frontiers in Behavioral Neuroscience* 9 (June): 150. doi:10.3389/fnbeh.2015.00150.

O'Brien, Megan K., and Alaa A. Ahmed. 2016. "Rationality in Human Movement." *Exercise and Sport Sciences Reviews* 44 (1): 20–28. doi:10.1249/JES.0000000000000066.

Orth, Dominic, Keith Davids, and Ludovic Seifert. 2014. "Hold Design Supports Learning and Transfer of Climbing Fluency." *Sports Technology* 7 (3/4): 159–165. doi:10.1080/19346182.2014.968167.

Pezzulo, Giovanni, and Paul Cizek. 2016. "Navigating the Affordance Landscape: Feedback Control as a Process Model of Behavior and Cognition." *Trends in Cognitive Sciences* 20 (6): 414–424. doi:10.1016/j.tics.2016.03.013.

Pinder, Ross A., Keith Davids, Ian Renshaw, and Duarte Araújo. 2011. "Representative Learning Design and Functionality of Research and Practice in Sport." *Journal of Sport and Exercise Psychology* 33 (1): 146–155.

Reed, Edward S. 1993. "The Intention to Use a Specific Affordance: A Conceptual Framework for Psychology." In *Development in Context: Acting and Thinking in Specific Environments*, edited by Robert M. Wozniak and Kurt W. Fischer, 45–76. Hillsdale, NJ: Erlbaum.

Reed, Edward S. 1996. *Encountering the World: Toward an Ecological Psychology*. Oxford: Oxford University Press.

Renshaw, Ian, Duarte Araújo, Chris Button, Jia Yi Chow, Keith Davids, and Brendan Moy. 2016. "Why the Constraints-Led Approach Is Not Teaching Games for Understanding: A Clarification." *Physical Education and Sport Pedagogy* 21 (5): 459–480. doi:10.1080/17408989.2015.1095870.

Richardson, Michael J., Kevin Shockley, Brett R. Fajen, Michael A. Riley, and Michael T. Turvey. 2008. "Ecological Psychology: Six Principles for an Embodied-Embedded Approach to Behavior." In *Handbook of Cognitive Science: An Embodied Approach*, edited by Paco Calvo and Toni Gomila, 161–187. New York: Elsevier.

Rietveld, Erik. 2008. "Situated Normativity: The Normative Aspect of Embodied Cognition in Unreflective Action." *Mind: A Quarterly Review of Psychology and Philosophy* 117 (468): 973–1001. doi:10.1093/mind/fzn050.

Rietveld, Erik, and Julian Kiverstein. 2014. "A Rich Landscape of Affordances." *Ecological Psychology* 26 (4): 325–352. doi:10.1080/10407413.2014.958035.

Savelsbergh, Geert J. P., and John van der Kamp. 2000. "Information in Learning to Co-ordinate and Control Movements: Is There a Need for Specificity of Practice?" *International Journal of Sport Psychology* 31 (4): 476–484.

Seifert, Ludovic, Léo Wattebled, Romain Herault, Germain Poizat, David Adé, Nathalie Gal-Petitfaux, and Keith Davids. 2014. "Neurobiological Degeneracy and Affordance Perception Support Functional Intra-Individual Variability of Inter-Limb Coordination during Ice Climbing." *PLoS ONE* 9 (2): e89865. doi:10.1371/journal.pone.0089865.

Turvey, Michael T. 1986. "Intentionally: A Problem of Multiple Reference Frames, Specificational Information, and Extraordinary Boundary Conditions on Natural Law." *Behavioral and Brain Sciences* 9 (1): 153–155.

Turvey, Michael T., Claudia Carello, and Nam-Gyoon Kim. 1990. "Links between Active Perception and the Control Action." In *Synergetics of Cognition*, edited by Hermann Haken and Michael Stadler, 269–295. Berlin: Springer.

Vaeyens, Roel, Matthieu Lenoir, A. Mark Williams, Liesbeth Mazyn, and Renaat M. Philippaerts. 2007. "The Effects of Task Constraints on Visual Search Behavior and Decision-Making Skill in Youth Soccer Players." *Journal of Sport and Exercise Psychology* 29 (2): 147–169.

van Geert, Paul. 1994. *Dynamic Systems of Development: Change between Complexity and Chaos.* New York: Harvester Wheatsheaf.

Vereijken, Beatrix, Richard E. van Emmerik, H. T. A. Whiting, and Karl M. Newell. 1992. "Free(z)ing Degrees of Freedom in Skill Acquisition." *Journal of Motor Behavior* 24 (1): 133–142. doi:10.1080/00222895.1992.9941608.

Warren, William H. 1984. "Perceiving Affordances: Visual Guidance of Stair Climbing." *Journal of Experimental Psychology: Human Perception and Performance* 10 (5): 683–703.

Withagen, Rob, Harjo J. de Poel, Duarte Araújo, and Gert-Jan Pepping. 2012. "Affordances Can Invite Behavior: Reconsidering the Relationship between Affordances and Agency." *New Ideas in Psychology* 30 (2): 250–258. doi:10.1016/j.newideapsych.2011.12.003.

Withagen, Rob, and Claire F. Michaels. 2005. "On Ecological Conceptualizations of Perceptual Systems and Action Systems." *Theory and Psychology* 15 (5): 603–620. doi:10.1177/0959354305057265.

Wolpert, Daniel M., and Michael S. Landy. 2012. "Motor Control Is Decision-Making." *Current Opinion in Neurobiology* 22 (6): 996–1003. doi:10.1016/j.conb.2012.05.003.

21 Affordances and the Ecological Approach to Throwing for Long Distances and Accuracy

Andrew D. Wilson, Qin Zhu, and Geoffrey P. Bingham

1 Introduction

All organisms are capable of producing behavior that is exquisitely tied to their current task demands. We can quickly and effectively adapt our actions as these demands change, which matters because of the dynamic and shifting nature of our environments. We see this level of sophistication and skill in high-performance situations (e.g., elite sporting activities such as the Olympics), but, if you look, you can also see it in your own day-to-day activity. We walk efficiently and effectively from place to place, effortlessly avoiding obstacles and preserving our balance. We reach and grasp for objects around us and manipulate them with great dexterity. Skilled performance is the rule, not the exception. So the big question facing psychology is, what kind of mechanism underpins this level of success? How, exactly, do we behave so effectively for so much of the time?

Skilled, functional behavior is behavior that forms a suitable complement to the task demands. This means that to understand a given behavior, we must first understand the task it is complementing and how we come to know about it. To rephrase slightly, what properties of the environment are action-relevant, and how do we perceive them? These two questions are at the heart of the ecological approach to perception and action (Gibson 1979; Turvey et al. 1981). The ecological hypothesis is that there are action-relevant properties of the world called *affordances* (Gibson 1979; Scarantino 2003; Turvey 1992; Turvey et al. 1981) and that we perceive these directly via *specifying information* in energy media (e.g., the optic array, Warren 2008; the acoustic array, Gaver 1993). Skilled behavior emerges as we perceive these affordances and use this perception to shape our behavior to meet their opportunities and demands.

This chapter explains affordances and the perception of affordances in the context of throwing for distance and accuracy. We begin with the idea of *task dynamics* (Bingham 1988; Bingham and Muchisky 1995; Saltzman and Kelso 1987) and describe how these dynamics can produce *ecological perceptual information* about themselves. We then take a task-dynamical approach to characterizing and studying the affordances for throwing, which has led to numerous experiments about how humans select projectiles and launch those for distance, accuracy, or both. This fascinating skill is a unique human specialty (other animals have been known to throw, but none can do so with the speed and precision of a trained human), and it has played a major part in our evolutionary success (e.g., Bingham 1999; Calvin 1983; Darlington 1975; Isaac 1987; Knusel 1992; Martin 2005; Meltzer 2009; Shea 2006). It is the perfect test bed for studying affordances and the perception of affordances, and we review our work on these questions here. This research program stands as a developing exemplar of the kind of research program required to study affordances, and to therefore understand the nature of the ecological world that we perceive and act in.

We also propose for the first time here that our task-dynamical affordances provide the ideal specification of "task goal" required for modern movement variability analyses derived from the motor abundance hypothesis (Latash 2008, 2012). There are four basic flavors of analysis: uncontrolled manifold analysis (UCM) (e.g., Scholz and Schöner 1999); stochastic optimal control theory (e.g., Todorov and Jordan 2002); nonlinear covariation (e.g., Müller and Sternad 2003); and the goal equivalent manifold (e.g., Cusumano and Cesari 2006). These motor control methods evaluate movement variability with respect to a task goal, but none come with a theory about what those task goals are or how they are perceived. The ecological, perception-action, task-dynamical approach to affordances is just such a theory. With all these pieces in hand, we can move toward unveiling the dynamic causal mechanisms (Bechtel and Abrahamsen 2010; Craver 2007) that underpin skilled, functional behavior more generally.

2 Task Dynamics

Organisms produce functional behavior by temporarily ("softly") assembling ourselves into *smart* solutions to the task at hand (Runeson 1977). Smart solutions differ from general purpose rote solutions the way heuristics differ from algorithms; they take advantage of things that are locally true and use those as reliable shortcuts to solve particular problems, instead of trying to come up with longer, more complex solutions that can be successfully applied to all situations.

Why do we think perception-action systems are smart rather than rote? There are two reasons. First, for tasks you do often that contain reliable shortcuts, smart solutions are faster, more efficient and more stable than rote solutions (Runeson 1977). These are good things. Second, smart solutions are often the *only* way to solve a given problem (Bingham 1988). Human bodies have a large number of redundant degrees of freedom

(Bernstein 1967), which means that we can in principle solve a given task in many different ways. The only way to reliably pick one solution is to allow yourself to be constrained by the task dynamics, because otherwise there are too many possible ways to move and we would be frozen by indecision.[1] So you identify the task and then pick a solution, which means solutions are *task-specific*. Understanding the solution requires understanding the task.

Tasks (events involving objects and organisms in the world) unfold over time in particular ways that have to do with the composition and organization of the event. This unfolding can be completely characterized and uniquely identified only at the level of *dynamics* (Bingham 1995). The formal language of dynamics provides all the elements required to describe the components, the organization of those components (in the form of a particular equation of motion), the form of the change over time (the kinematics), and the forces that caused that particular motion (the kinetics). Kinematic variables include time, position, and all the temporal derivatives of position (velocity, acceleration, jerk, and so on). Kinetic variables are all of these as well as mass. A given dynamical system description of an event in the world uses some combination of these variables and arranges them in a particular way, in an equation (via addition, multiplication, and other operations). These equations then fully describe how the given event type unfolds over time, and why, and setting the parameters on the variables (say, making the movement faster or slower) creates a specific instance of this event type. Finally, two or more dynamical systems can be coupled if some of the terms in one equation reflect terms from another, and vice versa.

This gives us a principled and valid way to classify the tasks facing an organism. Two different events are different tasks if they are unfolding according to different dynamics—that is, if they are described using different equations (different combinations and arrangements of dynamical variables). The physics of something in free fall and something being propelled are described by different equations, and thus attempts to intercept them are two different tasks. Two different events are the same task if the dynamics are the same, even if the parameters of those dynamics are different. Things fall differently on the Moon and on the Earth, but this is due to varying parameters on gravity rather than the addition of an additional source of energy.

3 Affordances

Gibson's (1979) definition of affordances is notoriously annoying:

> The affordances of the environment are what it offers the animal, what it provides or furnishes, either for good or ill. The verb to afford is found in the dictionary, but the noun affordance is not. I have made it up. I mean by it something that refers to both the environment and the

> animal in a way that no existing term does. It implies the complementarity of the animal and the environment. (119)

There have been many attempts to cash this out more formally. Turvey et al. (1981) and Turvey (1992) described affordances as *dispositional properties*, and Scarantino (2003) expanded and improved on this analysis thanks to Mumford's (1998) book-length treatment of dispositions (see also Bingham and Muchisky 1995). Others have formalized them as relational properties created by interactions in the organism-environment system (e.g., Chemero 2003, 2009; Rietveld and Kiverstein 2014; Stoffregan 2003). These relational accounts are popular, but currently suffer from one fatal problem—none of them include a mechanism for how such relations can create information and thus be perceived. Given the strong positive case for dispositions and the major negative against the relational accounts, we begin our analysis of affordances by treating them as dispositional properties of tasks (see Scarantino 2003 for an excellent analysis of what this means in practice).

Affordances are the perceptible, action-relevant subset of the dispositional properties of a task: tasks are defined dynamically; affordances must therefore be defined dynamically. A *dynamical task analysis* involves characterizing the task to be solved by the organism in terms of the dynamics. This can provide a finite list of candidate affordance properties to work with (Wilson and Golonka 2013)—a given task has a limited number of properties, and only some of these are affordances. It's then a matter of empirical investigation to identify which properties are action-relevant and therefore constitute the affordance. We elaborate on this research program below in the context of throwing for long distances and accuracy.

4 The Perception of Affordances

> The central question for the theory of affordances is not whether they exist and are real but whether information is available in ambient light for perceiving them.
>
> —Gibson, *The Ecological Approach to Visual Perception*, 1979

Affordances are dynamical properties of the environment. Perception must therefore be about these dynamics, but perception has a problem. Perceptual systems have no direct access to these dynamics; instead, they interact with energy media such as light, which support only a kinematic projection of the dynamics (Bingham 1988). In order to perceive a dynamical affordance, that affordance must create a kinematic pattern in an energy media that an organism can use to make perceptual contact; the pattern must be able to be used as *information* for the affordance. That information cannot be identical to the underlying dynamics, but it must specify (map 1:1 to) those dynamics.

Let's focus on the optic array for a moment, although this analysis applies to all the media that perceptual systems interact with. Briefly, the interaction of light and a surface is governed by the laws of physics, which means that a given dynamical property will lead to the same optical consequences every time it occurs. There will be some variation; for example, if the light level is lower the second time, the intensity of the light will be different, or you may see the world from a different vantage point. But higher order relations (*invariants-over-transformation*) will still be preserved over these transformations. These invariants are, by definition, specific to the task-dynamical property that created them; they map 1:1 onto the dynamics of the world. These invariants are ecological information.

Ecological information was first described in detail in Gibson (1966) and then Gibson (1979). Turvey et al. (1981) then formalized the ecological laws of perceiving and acting that dictate how dynamical properties are projected into, for example, light, in a way that makes the pattern informative. (Gaver 1993 has also produced an equivalent analysis for the acoustic array.) Then Runeson and Frykholm (1983) demonstrated several concrete examples of this kinematic specification of dynamics (KSD) and showed that people's perceptions were clearly attuned to them. There is now a variety of evidence that perception depends on these specifying patterns (e.g., Fink, Foo, and Warren 2009; Gibson et al. 1969; Kaplan 1969; McBeath, Shaffer, and Kaiser 1995; Scholl and Tremoulet 2000; Wilson and Bingham 2008).

The ecological hypothesis is therefore that dynamical properties of the world can interact with energy media in such a way as to create higher-order kinematic patterns that specify those dynamics. These patterns are not identical to the world, but because of specification, they can be used by an organism to stand in for the world. If an organism detects and uses these patterns as information, it is described ecologically as perceiving the world.

The ecological research program is therefore tasked with (a) dynamically characterizing the action-relevant properties of a given task; (b) kinematically characterizing the information created by those properties, and (c) empirically testing whether organisms are using that information to perceive those dynamics. The ecological approach is doing well to the extent that the answer to (c) is "yes."[2]

The rest of this chapter describes our ecological research program that has investigated the affordances and perception of the affordances for throwing to maximum distance.

5 Throwing

5.1 The Task Dynamics of Throwing

Throwing is an example of projectile motion. The dynamics of projectile motion describe how an object moves through space after being given an initial push and then being left alone, other than the effects of gravity and friction (drag)—no additional propulsion. That initial push can be anything (being thrown, being shot out of a gun or cannon, being hit by a baseball bat, and so on). The trajectory of the projectile and the distance it travels depends on the object size and weight; the release height, angle, and velocity; drag, air density, and gravity. The goal of the dynamics of throwing is to therefore produce a task-appropriate instance of a projectile motion.

Embodied perception-action research must always remember that it has to also analyze the task from the first-person perspective of the organism (Barrett 2011). As far as the organism is concerned, the task-dynamic variables listed above must be sorted in the following way:

- *Things to be perceived*: object size, object weight, distance traveled (or distance to be traveled, in the case of targeted throwing)
- *Things to be controlled*: release height, release velocity, release angle
- *Things outside your control*: drag, air density, gravity

Implementing a given throw requires implementing the dynamics of throwing based on perceived size, weight, and distance, and coupling those dynamics to the dynamics of projectile motion. You couple two dynamical systems together by having the output of one feed into the other, and sometimes vice versa. Throwing is a one-way coupling, achieved by having the dynamics of throwing put the body into a state that can be described with three values (release angle, release velocity, and release height), which are used as parameters on the relevant variables making up the dynamics of projectile motion.

The parameters chosen depend on the task at hand, and the affordances that help select the right parameters vary from task to task as well. We have so far researched three cases; throwing for maximum distance, throwing to hit a target, and throwing to inflict damage in hunting. We now review the maximum-distance data, as this is the most developed thread of the program, and then briefly discuss the two papers relevant to targeted and effective throwing.

5.2 Throwing for Maximum Distance

Bingham, Schmidt, and Rosenblum (1989) began the study of affordances for throwing by examining how the human perceptual system, specifically haptic perception, is able to identify the best object for maximum-distance throwing. Given objects of varying size, participants happily indicated the weight they preferred for throwing after hefting each object in their throwing hand. The preferred objects increased in weight as they increased in size, and the preferred objects were indeed subsequently thrown the farthest by the participants. People were both therefore confident and accurate in their judgments. Bingham, Schmidt, and Rosenblum (1989) suggested that hefting might provide information about the affordance via a similarity between hefting and throwing dynamics and motions.

Zhu and Bingham (2008) replicated and extended these findings. They found that this affordance (size/weight/distance relation) can be perceived only by hefting with the skilled throwing hand (as opposed to elbow or foot). They also found that when they had people throw the objects, only object weight affected distance via the throwing dynamics (and then, only release speed but not release angle). Object size has its effect on maximum distance during the projectile motion. Therefore, although hefting to perceive the affordance requires perceiving both object weight and size in relation to throwing distance, only the weight directly affects the throwing motions (both size and weight affect the projectile motion). Zhu and Bingham (2008) therefore showed that Bingham's original hypothesis about how hefting provided access to the throwing affordance was incorrect; size matters for distance, but not for the throwing motion. The source of information about the affordance therefore remained unknown.

The next set of experiments concerned learning to perceive the affordance. Zhu and Bingham (2010) and Zhu, Dapena, and Bingham (2009) investigated how the ability to perceive the affordance for throwing is acquired through perceptual learning. At baseline, unskilled throwers were asked to select objects for throwing and subsequently throw all objects. Their preferences were random, and the preferred objects were not thrown the farthest. Hence, unskilled throwers cannot perceive the affordance for throwing.

Next, Zhu and Bingham (2010) investigated the process of learning to perceive the affordance using an experimental design to contrast two alternative hypotheses about the form of the learning. The first hypothesis was an associative process of function learning that entails both interpolation and extrapolation along the function from experienced exemplars (e.g., McDaniel and Busemeyer 2005). This account predicted that learning and transfer would be restricted by the nature of the training set. The second hypothesis was the ecological process of becoming attuned to specifying information (e.g., Gibson 1969; Gibson and Pick 2000). This account predicted that learning would generalize to the entire space over which the information is defined, regardless of training set.

Unskilled throwers practiced throwing over the period of a month, with each thrower assigned to one of four groups: group 1 threw with vision using a subset of objects of varying size but constant weight; group 2 threw with vision using a subset of objects of varying weight but constant size; group 3 threw with vision using a subset of objects varying in both size and weight, but of constant density; group 4 threw without vision using the same set of objects used by group 3. After training, all participants significantly improved throwing distances. Groups 1–3 also improved their perception of the affordance; they were now able to pick the optimal throwing object from the full set that varied in both size and weight, regardless of which set they trained with. Interestingly, throwers in group 4 (who did not see the distance to which object were thrown during practice) did not improve on the affordance perception task until they received an extra throwing session with vision of the throw allowed. They then immediately improved on the perception task. Based on these results, Zhu and Bingham concluded that the learning process was one of attuning to information about the size-weight relation in the objects and calibrating which specific relation to use by perceiving the distance thrown. The question remained, to what invariant did this enable the throwers to become attuned? What is the information for the size-weight relation?

5.3 The Information for the Maximum-Distance Affordance

The affordance for maximum-distance throwing consists of a specific relation between object sizes and weights, with larger weights for larger sizes. Bingham, Schmidt, and Rosenblum (1989) noted that the specific relation was similar to that for equal "heaviness" according to the classic size-weight illusion. The illusion is that object weights are misperceived; equal felt heaviness requires that larger objects weigh more. Perhaps it is a specific felt heaviness that is invariant with optimality for maximum-distance throws. Zhu and Bingham (2011) examined this hypothesis.

Skilled throwers were initially asked to identify the best weighted objects for throwing in various sizes. Then, among the preferred objects, either the smallest or the largest object was selected as the reference object (unbeknownst to the participants) for a judgment of equal felt heaviness. In a second task, the throwers compared the reference object with the remaining objects to judge those that felt equally heavy to the reference object. The throwers selected the same objects at each weight that they had chosen as best for throwing. The results supported the hypothesis that all objects preferred for throwing were those that felt of a specific equal heaviness. Learning the affordance entails learning about equal heaviness in the throwing context, and distance traveled must be perceived so as to pick out the specific heaviness. Once this heaviness is identified, learning can generalize across untrained objects.

In all of these studies on the affordance for throwing, it was consistently found that optimal objects for throwing increased in weight with increasing size in the same way as for equal heaviness in the size-weight illusion. Therefore, the illusion in fact has an ecological function, namely, it enables throwers to reliably detect the best object for throwing. The illusion is not an illusion or misperception of weight at all; instead, it is a functionally effective and accurate perception of an affordance (Zhu and Bingham 2011).

Felt heaviness has been shown to vary as a function of the rotational inertia (e.g., Shockley, Carello, and Turvey 2004; see Turvey 1996 for an overview of this notion of dynamic touch). Since the felt heaviness is also used for detecting the affordance for throwing, the obvious question was whether the rotational inertia would change the felt heaviness and, thus, perception of the affordance. Zhu et al. (2013) systematically manipulated the rotational inertias of objects and asked skilled throwers to judge both throw-ability and equal heaviness while hefting the objects. The results showed that the perceived affordance for throwing did not vary with the rotational inertias; dynamic touch is not the basis of the perception of this particular affordance.

Another ecological question concerning perception of this affordance is whether the *relative* optimality of objects for throwing can be perceived. When selecting objects to throw in the world, the actually optimal object is not necessarily present; can people select the best object from a given set? Zhu, Mirich, and Bingham (2014) investigated this question using a magnitude-estimation task. Skilled throwers were asked to rate each object on its throw-ability by comparing it to a reference object that was previously selected as preferred for throwing. The results showed a good match between the mean magnitude estimation and mean distances of throwing, suggesting that the relative optimality objects for throwing can be detected if the optimal object is not available.

5.4 Summary of Maximum-Distance Throwing

Projectiles afford throwing for maximum distance to the extent that their size-weight relation falls on a specific function. This function is one of many that describe when objects of different sizes and weights feel equally heavy to humans (the size-weight illusion). Learning to perceive the affordance requires learning the specific felt heaviness that matches the specific function that identifies objects that will travel the farthest when thrown by a human. This requires experience with variation in size, weight, or density (size and weight) plus visual perception of the distance traveled by those varied objects.

5.5 Throwing for Accuracy

The second type of throwing task is throwing to hit a target. It is the same kind of task as above because the dynamics are the same; only the parameters change. The goal of the throwing dynamics is still to produce a particular release angle, release speed, and release height. However, which combination is best now depends on the target's size and location in space (distance, height, and orientation) relative to the thrower, rather than the goal of maximizing distance. In other words, the relevant affordance in this task, given a projectile, is the affordance of the target to be hit.

Wilson, Weightman, et al. (2016) had experts from three sports (male baseballers and cricketers, female softballers) throw tennis balls to hit a vertically oriented 4-foot-by-4-foot Perspex target. In Experiment 1, the target was set at one of three distances (5m, 10m, 15m) and three heights (centered at 1m, 1.5m, 2m; roughly eye height +/- 0.5m). The results showed that all the experts scaled their release parameters to the target location; changes in distance led to changes in release angle and speed, while changes in height led to changes in angle. Experts liked to "throw a rope," that is, fast and flat (this minimizes flight time, often a pressure in a sporting context).

A projectile motion can also cover a given distance by flying slow and high. In a second experiment, we forced male cricket experts into this mode by changing the target orientation from vertical to horizontal and varying the distance. The experts readily changed their throwing from fast and flat to slow and high and maintained near perfect accuracy in all conditions. This remained true even under monocular viewing conditions.

To identify why throwers were choosing the release parameters that they were, we ran extensive simulations of the projectile motion of a tennis ball thrown toward our target. For each target location and orientation condition, we ran the equations within two loops, one for variation in release angle (ranging from -30° to 90°; this range emerged from the simulations as necessary to map the complete affordance structure for all target locations) and one for variation in release speed (here ranging from $0ms^{-1}$ to $45ms^{-1}$; our highest observed release speed across the two experiments reported below was $45.01ms^{-1}$). The results revealed a set of parameter combinations that led to a hit. This set changed with distance, height, and orientation, and this set is the affordance of a given target to be hit by throwing. We now refer to the plots of these sets as *affordance maps* (refer to figure 21.1 for an example; see Wilson, Weightman, et al. 2016 for details).

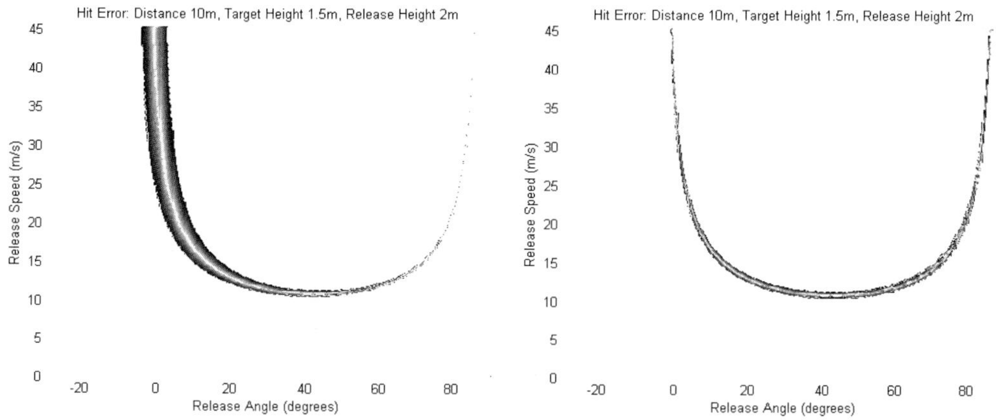

Figure 21.1
Affordance maps for throwing to hit a vertical (a) and horizontal (b) target, both located 10m away and at a height of 1.5m. See text and Wilson, Weightman, et al. (2016) for more details.

Expert performance fell into the identified sets, and variability in performance was also shaped by the form of the sets. Fast and flat throws reside in a stable location in the map for vertical targets (small errors in either speed or angle often still produce throws that lead to hits). This stability goes away when the target changes orientation, and when it is horizontal the slow and high throws are in the most stable region. The target affordance analysis accounted for the expert release parameter selection nicely; they clearly acted as if they perceived it. How they perceive it (the information for the target affordance) remains to be explored.

6 The Affordances of Prehistoric Objects

Throwing, it turns out, is a human specialization. Other animals have been known to throw things, but none can match the speed, distance, and accuracy of a trained human. Physical adaptations to support throwing have been evolving in the human lineage for two million years (Roach et al. 2013) and the relationship between the size-weight illusion and the perception of throwing affordances suggests we have psychological adaptations as well (Zhu and Bingham 2011).

One of the most common early technologies found at sites of prehistoric human activity is the spheroid, a rock shaped by either nature or hand to be fairly spherical. Their exact function is unknown. One hypothesis, however, is that they served as projectiles for hunting (e.g., Isaac 1987; Mason 1988). We recently tested this hypothesis using our affordance analyses, in collaboration with Lawrence Barham and Ian Stanistreet (Wilson, Zhu, et al. 2016).

We examined a spherical subset of spheroids from the Cave of Hearths, a site in South Africa (Mason 1988; McNabb and Sinclair 2009). These objects are at most 500,000 years old and were formed by natural weathering processes in a river about 2 kilometers from the cave. The evidence suggests that these objects were selected and transported by the humans living at the cave for some purpose. We know from the work above that modern humans can perceive the relatively optimal objects for throwing from a set that varies in size and weight such as might be found in a riverbed (Bingham, Schmidt, and Rosenblum 1989; Zhu and Bingham 2008, 2010; Zhu, Dapena, and Bingham 2009; Zhu, Mirich, and Bingham 2014). If the spheroids were intended to be projectiles, they should all ideally afford throwing.

We first simulated the projectile motions these spheroids would undergo if thrown by a modern human, using parameters from the maximum-distance work cited above (e.g., Zhu and Bingham 2008; Zhu, Dapena, and Bingham 2009; throwing for maximum distance involves maximizing release speed, which also then maximizes impact forces). We found the objects could be thrown 20–40 meters and at release speeds of around $17ms^{-1}$. At various points in the trajectory, we then computed the damage each object would do to a medium-sized prey animal (an impala). We used the blunt criterion (BC) (Sturdivan, Viano, and Champion 2004), which is an energy ratio of the energy imparted by the impact divided by the target's ability to absorb that energy. Sturdivan, Viano, and Champion also regressed BC scores with measured injury damage, and that equation enabled us to estimate the probability of a given amount of damage for each object.

We found that 81 percent of the spheroids tested were in the ideal range to optimize damage when thrown, and that if they hit the target, they had a better than even chance of breaking a bone, even at maximum distance. No single spheroid could kill an impala, but given that humans hunted in groups, even a few hits would have substantially slowed the animal down, making it much easier prey. The spheroids show every sign of having been selected to be thrown for impact by prehistoric humans.

7 Affordances as Perceived Task Goals

Finally, we want to identify for the record a soon-to-be-tested relationship between our affordance analysis and movement variability analyses such as the uncontrolled manifold analysis (e.g., Scholz and Schöner 1999).

As described above, the cardinal feature of the perception-action system is the degrees of freedom problem (Bernshteĭn 1967). Our bodies have more elements that can change their state than are typically ever required for any given movement. This means that there are an indefinite number of solutions to each and every task demand. This poses an extraordinarily complex control problem—out of all the movement trajectories we *can* make, how and why do we select and implement the ones that we *do* make? Theories of motor control must therefore provide solutions to both the problem of *action selection* and *action control*.

Traditional solutions to this problem replace the indefinitely large set of possible movement trajectories with a single "desired" action trajectory, either by imposing a cost function (e.g., minimizing jerk; Flash and Hogan 1985) or by assembling a synergy in which multiple degrees of freedom can be controlled as a single device to produce a single outcome (e.g., Turvey 1990). However, these solutions are underconstrained themselves (Which cost function? Which synergy? Why?) and do not fit the typical data, in which trajectory variability remains the rule and not the exception.

A more recent framing of the problem is the *motor abundance hypothesis* (Latash 2008, 2012). From this perspective, there is no single optimal movement. Instead, because there are always many movement trajectories that can satisfy a task goal, the goal of motor control must be to preserve the outcome, not a specific implementation. In other words, the human action system must exhibit *degeneracy* (e.g., Whitacre and Bender 2010).

All movements show variability, but not all variability is equal. Some will prevent you from achieving the goal state, some will not. In the motor abundance framework, the job of the action control system changes from selecting optimal trajectories to the strategic deployment of control. The system only applies active control if the current variability will cause failure to preserve the required outcome. This will sometimes entail changing trajectories partway through movements, but this is, first, possible because the system is not having a single trajectory imposed on it and, second, still functional because of the degeneracy. The motor abundance hypothesis is that this arrangement enables an organism to continuously have access to movement options to preserve flexibility, while still simplifying the control problem to the point where it is solvable.

This approach is embodied in several formal data analysis techniques, which all focus on analyzing the structure of the variability in movements relative to a task demand (a *performance variable*). These analyses include the uncontrolled manifold (UCM) (e.g., Scholz and Schöner 1999); stochastic optimal control theory (e.g., Todorov and Jordan 2002); nonlinear covariation (e.g., Müller and Sternad 2003); and the goal-equivalent manifold (e.g., Cusumano and Cesari 2006). These techniques all have different origins and motivations, but all embody the key ideas of the motor abundance hypothesis and generally converge on the same kind of solution to the problem of motor control, specifically on-line feedback control relative to a task goal.

All these analyses assume that the system is working to achieve a task goal, but none of them include a theory about what that goal is or how it is perceived. In fact, Todorov and Jordan (2002) explicitly identify that there are as yet no principled ways to independently identify how people perceive the task. The general solution is to simply set the goal to be the task instructions from the experimenter. From the first-person perspective of the organism, however, task goals must create information and be perceived in order to be able to affect behavior. We need a method for characterizing the perception of action-relevant task goals in terms that would enable the goal-oriented deployment of control processes by an actual organism.

It should come as no surprise at this point that we believe our affordance methods to be exactly the methods required by the analyses. For example, the affordance maps identify the set of release parameters leading to a hit. This quantifies the affordance of the target to be hit by throwing, or, in other words, it quantifies the action-relevant task goal/performance variable. We therefore hypothesize, first, that the strategic deployment of control processes described by motor abundance analyses is driven by the real-time perception of task-dynamically defined affordances.

This relationship can be seen in the affordance maps from the targeted throwing paper (Wilson, Weightman, et al. 2016). The set of release parameters (action variables) that lead to a hit is a multi-valued subset of the total parameter space: a manifold. Variation within this manifold does not need to be controlled away; the combinations all lead to hits. We saw clear signs that end-point variability across trials was being organized with respect to this manifold, but we did not collect the necessary full-body motion-capture data required for, say, UCM analysis. We will be running this study shortly.

Another feature of our analysis is that the affordance manifolds vary in their stability. All values within the manifold led to hits, but not all regions of the manifold tolerated error to the same degree, and the most stable regions shifted around with, for example, changes in orientation (Wilson, Weightman, et al. 2016). Building manifolds from the bottom up, based on real parts and processes, enables us to quantify the internal structure of the manifold itself in a way that does not yet really feature in the literature.

There is another intriguing hypothesis we believe we can test using these methods. Motor abundance analyses all assume that the system is primarily a feedback control system; in fact, Todorov and Jordan (2002) explicitly show that this is the optimal control architecture when possible, and detail the criteria for when it is possible. On-line feedback control for a throw is not always possible at every moment in an action; for example, the movement may be too fast (although see data on extremely late corrections in Urbin 2013) or the hand may not be in view. If control is only exerted when the relation between the limb and the task goal can be perceived, then changes in the various variability measures across a trial should index the onset and offset of perceptual control. We believe this strong interpretation would be licensed by the fact our manifolds are defined with respect to real parts and processes (affordances and the perception of affordances).

Uncontrolled manifold analysis can be performed at various stages of a movement (e.g., Yang and Scholz 2005). Changes in the relative amounts of acceptable variability that leave you on the manifold (V_{UCM}) and problematic variability that takes you it (V_{ORT}) can be tracked over time within a movement. If V_{ORT} begins to increase and is not immediately reduced by a control process, this suggests the real-time feedback control system is not currently active. When V_{ORT} begins to get removed, feedback control has come back on-line. For us, the feedback control system is using information about performance relative to the perceived task affordances. Therefore our second hypothesis is that changes in the way V_{UCM} and V_{ORT} shrink and grow over a movement indexes the onset and offset of affordance-based feedback control (cf. Fajen 2005, 2007). This will provide information about what is being perceived, when, and how (e.g., if control of the arm requires vision of the arm).

All of this remains to be explicitly tested, but there is clear conceptual overlap between the motor abundance hypothesis and the ecological approach to perception and action. If these hypotheses are supported, our affordance analysis will close a gap in motor abundance analyses and provide a way of formally defining the task, the task goals, and the resulting pattern of control used to achieve that goal, all in the same dynamical framework and language. This upgraded *perception-action abundance* framework enables truly causal mechanistic *explanations* of the process of perception-action control (explanations grounded in reference to real parts and processes; Bechtel and Abrahamsen 2010; Craver 2007).

8 Conclusion

Functional behavior is that which successfully complements the demands of the current task. Tasks can be formally characterized in terms of their dynamics, and each task offers opportunities for actions to different organisms—tasks have affordances. Affordances can be quantified by using the task dynamics in the context of specific actions and behaviors, and the research we have described here has had great success in explaining, rather than simply describing, why people do what they do in the presence of the different affordances that support various parts of throwing for distance and accuracy.

Throwing itself is a fascinating task for many reasons. It is a unique human specialization, and there is growing evidence for the crucial role it has played in our evolutionary success by enabling our weak bipedal ape ancestors to hunt a variety of prey animals. The act itself is also a beautiful example of the exquisite timing and control the human perception-action system is capable of, and best of all, the tools now exist to study it rigorously in the lab in its natural form. Modern motion-capture technology, coupled to the new motor abundance style analyses shaped and guided by our task-dynamical affordance framework, will allow us to continue to make big strides in understanding and explaining the mechanisms underpinning throwing performance, and this research program will stand as an exemplar to guide research on other actions.

Notes

1. This is a very similar motivation to Latash's motor abundance hypothesis, which is one reason we believe task dynamical affordances will fit that framework nicely.

2. See Fajen's *affordance-based control* framework for a good example of this program in action; Fajen (2005, 2007).

References

Barrett, Louise. 2011. *Beyond the Brain: How Body and Environment Shape Animal and Human Minds*. Princeton, NJ: Princeton University Press.

Bechtel, William, and Adele Abrahamsen. 2010. "Dynamic Mechanistic Explanation: Computational Modeling of Circadian Rhythms as an Exemplar for Cognitive Science." *Studies in History and Philosophy of Science* 41 (3): 321–333.

Bernshteĭn, Nikolaĭ Aleksandrovich. 1967. *The Co-Ordination and Regulation of Movements*. London: Pergamon.

Bingham, Geoffrey P. 1988. "Task-Specific Devices and the Perceptual Bottleneck." *Human Movement Science* 7 (2–4): 225–264.

Bingham, Geoffrey P. 1995. "Dynamics and the Problem of Visual Event Recognition." In *Mind as Motion: Dynamics, Behavior and Cognition*, edited by R. Port and T. van Gelder, 403–448. Cambridge, MA: MIT Press.

Bingham, Geoffrey P., and Michael M. Muchisky. 1995. "Center of Mass Perception: Affordances as Dispositions Determined by Dynamics." In *Global Perspectives on the Ecology of Human-Machine Systems*, edited by J. Flach, P. Hancock, J. Caird, and K. Vicente, 359–395. Hillsdale, NJ: LEA.

Bingham, Geoffrey P., R. C. Schmidt, and L. D. Rosenblum. 1989. "Hefting for a Maximum Distance Throw: A Smart Perceptual Mechanism." *Journal of Experimental Psychology: Human Perception and Performance* 15 (3): 507–528.

Bingham, Paul M. 1999. "Human Uniqueness: A General Theory." *Quarterly Review of Biology* 74 (2): 133–169.

Calvin, W. H. 1983. "A Stone's Throw and Its Launch Window: Timing Precision and Its Implications for Language and Hominid Brains." *Journal of Theoretical Biology* 104 (1): 121–135.

Calvin, William H. 2010. *The Throwing Madonna: Essays on the Brain.* Lincoln, NE: iUniverse.

Chemero, A. 2009. *Radical Embodied Cognitive Science.* Cambridge, MA: MIT Press.

Chemero, Anthony. 2003. "An Outline of a Theory of Affordances." *Ecological Psychology* 15 (2): 181–195.

Craver, Carl F. 2007. *Explaining the Brain: Mechanisms and the Mosaic Unity of Neuroscience.* Oxford: Clarendon Press.

Cusumano, Joseph P., and Paola Cesari. 2006. "Body-Goal Variability Mapping in an Aiming Task." *Biological Cybernetics* 94 (5): 367–379.

Darlington, P. J., Jr. 1975. "Group Selection, Altruism, Reinforcement, and Throwing in Human Evolution." *Proceedings of the National Academy of Sciences of the United States of America* 72 (9): 3748–3752.

Fajen, Brett R. 2005. "Perceiving Possibilities for Action: On the Necessity of Calibration and Perceptual Learning for the Visual Guidance of Action." *Perception* 34 (6): 717–740.

Fajen, Brett R. 2007. "Affordance-Based Control of Visually Guided Action." *Ecological Psychology* 19 (4): 383–410.

Fink, Philip W., Patrick S. Foo, and William H. Warren. 2009. "Catching Fly Balls in Virtual Reality: A Critical Test of the Outfielder Problem." *Journal of Vision* 9 (13): 14.1–8.

Flash, T., and N. Hogan. 1985. "The Coordination of Arm Movements: An Experimentally Confirmed Mathematical Model." *Journal of Neuroscience* 5 (7): 1688–1703.

Gaver, William W. 1993. "What In the World Do We Hear? An Ecological Approach to Auditory Event Perception." *Ecological Psychology* 5 (1): 1–29.

Gibson, Eleanor Jack. 1969. *Principles of Perceptual Learning and Development.* East Norwalk, CT: Appleton-Century-Crofts. http://doi.apa.org/psycinfo/1969-35014-000.

Gibson, Eleanor Jack, and Anne D. Pick. 2000. *An Ecological Approach to Perceptual Learning and Development.* Oxford: Oxford University Press.

Gibson, J. J., G. A. Kaplan, H. N. Reynolds, and K. Wheeler. 1969. "The Change from Visible to Invisible." *Perception & Psychophysics* 5 (2): 113–116.

Gibson, James Jerome. 1966. *The Senses Considered as Perceptual Systems.* Boston: Houghton Mifflin.

Gibson, James Jerome. 1979. *The Ecological Approach to Visual Perception.* Boston: Houghton Mifflin.

Isaac, Barbara. 1987. "Throwing and Human Evolution." *African Archaeological Review* 5 (1): 3–17.

Kaplan, G. A. 1969. Kinetic Disruption of Optical Texture: The Perception of Depth at an Edge." *Perception and Psychophysics* 6 (4): 193–198.

Knüsel, C. J. 1992. "The Throwing Hypothesis and Hominid Origins." *Human Evolution* 7 (1): 1–7.

Latash, Mark L. 2008. *Synergy*. Oxford: Oxford University Press.

Latash, Mark L. 2012. "The Bliss (Not the Problem) of Motor Abundance (Not Redundancy)." *Experimental Brain Research* 217 (1): 1–5.

Martin, Paul S. 2005. *Twilight of the Mammoths*. Berkeley: University of California Press. http://www.ucpress.edu/book.php?isbn=9780520252431.

Mason, R. J. 1988. *Cave of Hearths, Makapansgat, Transvaal*. Johannesburg: Archaeological Research Unit Occasional Paper No. 21, University of the Witwatersrand.

Mason, Revil J., and Charles Kimberlin Brain. 1988. *Cave of Hearths, Makapansgat, Transvaal*. Archaeological Research Unit, University of the Witwatersrand.

McBeath, M. K., D. M. Shaffer, and M. K. Kaiser. 1995. "How Baseball Outfielders Determine Where to Run to Catch Fly Balls." *Science* 268 (5210): 569–573.

McDaniel, Mark A., and Jerome R. Busemeyer. 2005. "The Conceptual Basis of Function Learning and Extrapolation: Comparison of Rule-Based and Associative-Based Models." *Psychonomic Bulletin and Review* 12 (1): 24–42.

McNabb, J., and A. Sinclair. 2009. *The Cave of Hearths: Makapan Middle Pleistocene Research Project: Field Research by Anthony Sinclair and Patrick Quinney, 1996–2001*. Oxford: Archaeopress.

Meltzer, David J. 2009. *First Peoples in a New World: Colonizing Ice Age America*. Berkeley: University of California Press.

Müller, Hermann, and Dagmar Sternad. 2003. "A Randomization Method for the Calculation of Covariation in Multiple Nonlinear Relations: Illustrated with the Example of Goal-Directed Movements." *Biological Cybernetics* 89 (1): 22–33.

Mumford, S. 1998. *Dispositions*. Oxford: Oxford University Press.

Rietveld, Erik, and Julian Kiverstein. 2014. "A Rich Landscape of Affordances." *Ecological Psychology* 26 (4): 325–352.

Roach, Neil T., Madhusudhan Venkadesan, Michael J. Rainbow, and Daniel E. Lieberman. 2013. "Elastic Energy Storage in the Shoulder and the Evolution of High-Speed Throwing in Homo." *Nature* 498 (7455): 483–486.

Runeson, S., and G. Frykholm. 1983. Kinematic Specification of Dynamics as an Informational Basis for Person-and-Action Perception: Expectation, Gender Recognition, and Deceptive Intention." *Journal of Experimental Psychology* 112 (4): 585.

Runeson, Sverker. 1977. "On the Possibility of 'Smart' Perceptual Mechanisms." *Scandinavian Journal of Psychology* 18 (1): 172–179.

Saltzman, E., and J. A. Kelso. 1987. "Skilled Actions: A Task-Dynamic Approach." *Psychological Review* 94 (1): 84–106.

Scarantino, Andrea. 2003. "Affordances Explained." *Philosophy of Science* 70 (5): 949–961.

Scholl, B. J., and P. D. Tremoulet. 2000. "Perceptual Causality and Animacy." *Trends in Cognitive Sciences* 4 (8): 299–309.

Scholz, J. P., and G. Schöner. 1999. "The Uncontrolled Manifold Concept: Identifying Control Variables for a Functional Task." *Experimental Brain Research* 126 (3): 289–306.

Shea, John J. 2006. "The Origins of Lithic Projectile Point Technology: Evidence from Africa, the Levant, and Europe." *Journal of Archaeological Science* 33 (6): 823–846.

Shockley, Kevin, Claudia Carello, and M. T. Turvey. 2004. "Metamers in the Haptic Perception of Heaviness and Moveableness." *Perception and Psychophysics* 66 (5): 731–742.

Stoffregen, Thomas A. 2003. "Affordances as Properties of the Animal-Environment System." *Ecological Psychology* 15 (2): 115–134.

Sturdivan, Larry M., David C. Viano, and Howard R. Champion. 2004. "Analysis of Injury Criteria to Assess Chest and Abdominal Injury Risks in Blunt and Ballistic Impacts." *Journal of Trauma* 56 (3): 651–663.

Todorov, Emanuel, and Michael I. Jordan. 2002. "Optimal Feedback Control as a Theory of Motor Coordination." *Nature Neuroscience* 5 (11): 1226–1235.

Turvey, M. T. 1990. "Coordination." *American Psychologist* 45 (8): 938.

Turvey, M. T. 1992. "Affordances and Prospective Control: An Outline of the Ontology." *Ecological Psychology* 4 (3): 173–187.

Turvey, M. T. 1996. "Dynamic Touch." *American Psychologist* 51 (11): 1134–1152.

Turvey, M. T., R. E. Shaw, E. S. Reed, W. M. Mace. 1981. "Ecological Laws of Perceiving and Acting: In Reply to Fodor and Pylyshyn." *Cognition* 9 (3): 237–304.

Urbin, M. A. 2013. "Visual Regulation of Overarm Throwing Performance." *Experimental Brain Research* 225 (4): 535–547.

Warren, W. H. 2008. "Optic Flow." In *The Senses: A Comprehensive Reference*, 219–230. Amsterdam: Elsevier.

Whitacre, James, and Axel Bender. 2010. "Degeneracy: A Design Principle for Achieving Robustness and Evolvability." *Journal of Theoretical Biology* 263 (1): 143–153.

Wilson, A. D., and G. P. Bingham. 2008. "Identifying the Information for the Visual Perception of Relative Phase." *Perception and Psychophysics* 70 (3): 465–476.

Wilson, Andrew D., and Sabrina Golonka. 2013. "Embodied Cognition Is Not What You Think It Is." *Frontiers in Psychology* 4 (February): 58.

Wilson, Andrew D., Andrew Weightman, Geoffrey P. Bingham, and Qin Zhu. 2016. "Using Task Dynamics to Quantify the Affordances of Throwing for Long Distance and Accuracy." *Journal of Experimental Psychology: Human Perception and Performance* 42 (7): 965–981.

Wilson, Andrew D., Qin Zhu, Lawrence Barham, Ian Stanistreet, and Geoffrey P. Bingham. 2016. "A Dynamical Analysis of the Suitability of Prehistoric Spheroids from the Cave of Hearths as Thrown Projectiles." *Scientific Reports* 6 (August): 30614. doi:10.1038/srep30614.

Yang, J.-F., and J. P. Scholz. 2005. "Learning a Throwing Task Is Associated with Differential Changes in the Use of Motor Abundance." *Experimental Brain Research* 163 (2): 137–158.

Zhu, Qin, and Geoffrey P. Bingham. 2008. "Is Hefting to Perceive the Affordance for Throwing a Smart Perceptual Mechanism?" *Journal of Experimental Psychology: Human Perception and Performance* 34 (4): 929–943.

Zhu, Qin, and Geoffrey P. Bingham. 2010. "Learning to Perceive the Affordance for Long-Distance Throwing: Smart Mechanism or Function Learning?" *Journal of Experimental Psychology: Human Perception and Performance* 36 (4): 862–875.

Zhu, Qin, and Geoffrey P. Bingham. 2011. "Human Readiness to Throw: The Size-Weight Illusion Is Not an Illusion When Picking the Best Objects to Throw." *Evolution and Human Behavior* 32 (4): 288–293.

Zhu, Qin, Jesus Dapena, and Geoffrey P. Bingham. 2009. "Learning to Throw to Maximum Distances: Do Changes in Release Angle and Speed Reflect Affordances for Throwing?" *Human Movement Science* 28 (6): 708–725.

Zhu, Qin, Todd Mirich, and Geoffrey P. Bingham. 2014. "Perception of Relative Throw-Ability." *Experimental Brain Research* 232 (2): 395–402.

Zhu, Qin, Kevin Shockley, Michael A. Riley, Michael T. Tolston, and Geoffrey P. Bingham. 2013. "Felt Heaviness Is Used to Perceive the Affordance for Throwing but Rotational Inertia Does Not Affect Either." *Experimental Brain Research* 224 (2): 221–231.

22 Affordances and the Anticipatory Control of Action

Wayne Christensen and Kath Bicknell

1 Introduction[1]

Picture this: you're riding your bike along an unfamiliar dirt road. It's sunny, it's warm, you're feeling good, and you have another hour before you need to return home. Suddenly, the weather changes. The skies open up and the ground becomes wet and muddy; the surface feels thick, slippery, and slow. You become cold and start to shiver a little. You pull on the brakes and notice they are no longer as fast and reliable as they were twenty minutes ago. The track ahead slopes downhill. You see water running over the trail and can't quite tell what lies underneath it. Another cyclist rides past you. They descend the hill quickly, yelling happily like a small, excited child and ride away.

What do you do next? Do you ride down the hill and hope for the best? Do you observe the flow of the water over different parts of the trail and use this as a guide for directing the bike? Are you as skilled as that other rider? Do you turn around and head home a different way? Do you get off your bike and walk? What would most other people you know do? If you choose to ride down the trail, what precautions do you take so you have more chance of staying on the bike than falling to the ground? How do you process these multiple options for action afforded by the environment, your equipment, and your skills?

In this chapter we explore the relation between affordances and anticipatory control. Specifically, we examine the nature of awareness of the qualities of the environment around us and our own abilities: how we select options from the range of possibilities available, factors that influence our perception of these, and how different disciplinary and theoretical approaches account for this. We argue that representational mechanisms are likely to play a role in the ability to skillfully and flexibly cope with situations that are complex, difficult, and sometimes unfamiliar, such as successfully descending down that mud-covered hill in the rain. But we will suggest that responsiveness to affordances is multifaceted, and that many mechanisms, including some that are nonrepresentational, probably make a contribution. Indeed, such is the complexity of affordance sensitivity and awareness that many research approaches are needed to develop a full understanding.

We begin by outlining the ways affordances are understood in the psychological literature. We then describe how the concept has been developed and extended in other disciplines, including neuroscience, philosophy, anthropology, and performance studies. Next, we describe a case study from the sport of mountain bike riding that demonstrates technological, physiological, and skillful and sociocultural aspects of affordance perception and raises questions about the nature of awareness of action possibilities and anticipation control. These include the problem of understanding how high-level athletes demonstrate both high flexibility and specificity of action awareness in dynamic, novel situations, taking into account multiple interacting factors.

2 The Gibsonian Approach to Affordances

The term *affordances* was invented by James Gibson, who described them as what the environment "*offers* the animal, what it *provides* or *furnishes*, either for good or ill" (1979, 127; italics original). For example, the ground affords walking, stairs afford climbing, a nearby cup affords reaching, a Facebook button affords liking (or, by 2017, other reactions such as surprise, sadness, or love). There have been a number of different approaches to understanding affordances, many of which depart from Gibson's work without paying explicit attention to the strict parameters of this initial conceptualization. We start with the Gibsonian approach, and look at examples of how it has been used to think about braking in a car, and catching a ball, before reviewing some of the other approaches to affordance perception and how they relate to anticipation.

The Gibsonian account of affordances is part of an ambitious and radical theory of perception, one that seeks to ground meaning in action and takes an anti-representationalist view of perception. We can understand this approach in terms of three key claims:

Affordances are action possibilities. Thus, a cup affords grasping and a chair, sitting.

Perception is primarily concerned with affordances. Thus, Gibson says, "what we perceive when we look at objects are affordances, not their qualities.... The special combination of qualities into which an object can be analyzed is ordinarily not noticed."

Affordances are perceived directly rather than represented. Gibson's idea is that there are no distinct states in the head (neural or mental "pictures") that count as representations of the affordances perceived. Direct perception involves

> "information pickup" through exploratory activities that detect patterns of light that correspond to action possibilities and that can be used to guide those activities (134, 147).

Some examples can help elucidate these ideas. One way to think about animal behavior, which Gibson rejects, is representational: an animal represents its current state (such as being near a prey animal), goal states (such as catching the prey), and engages in behaviors that aim to bring about the goal states (such as stalking and pouncing). The Gibsonian approach conceptualizes the control of behavior in a way that dispenses with representations. For instance, an animal might remain still in the face of disturbances (such as wind) by acting so as to cancel any changes in the optic array (Warren 1988, discussed in Fajen 2005). Note here that there is no representation of self or world, simply a particular kind of optical pattern that generates a behavior that affects the animal's situation in the world. A number of human activities have been studied along similar lines. According to one account of the way that a fielder catches a fly ball, the fielder must run backward or forward so as to cancel the optical acceleration of the tangent of the angle subtended by the ball and the horizon (Chapman 1968). Lee (1976) gives a similar account of braking to avoid an obstacle. As an obstacle is approached, it expands optically, and a certain high-order optical variable (referred to as "tau-dot") can be used to adjust movement in a way that produces smooth braking. That is, when tau-dot is less than a certain value, deceleration is too slow, and when it is greater than that value, deceleration is sufficient to stop before the object.

Fajen (2005) gives a somewhat more complicated account of braking to avoid an obstacle, which he argues solves some problems with Lee's account (726–728). Specifically, on Lee's model, tau-dot is used to directly adjust braking through feedback control in a way that produces optimally smooth deceleration, but humans do not usually brake in this way. Rather, they tend to brake relatively late to minimize the time spent braking, and individuals can be quite variable in the way that they brake. Fajen suggests instead that perceivers may make adjustments to keep their actual state within a safe region consistent with successfully braking, with the specific deceleration being determined on a situation-by-situation basis. One issue that then arises is to understand how this safe region could be perceived, and Fajen proposes that for braking this is based on the maximum deceleration that is possible. Fajen (2005) further proposes that we can understand the perception of affordances in terms of perception of the boundaries of the individual's action abilities: an action is possible when it is possible to remain within these boundaries (731).

These examples illustrate the idea that perception of affordances is direct rather than based on representations. Just as in the case of the animal maintaining its position,

Fajen's account of braking involves no representations—there is no representation of the object as such or distance to the object, merely the detection of a certain pattern of optical expansion that is used to modify behavior in such a way that the individual stops before colliding with the object.

2.1 Ambiguity in Perception

Gibson's idea that perception is direct has been interpreted by some Gibsonians as implying that the perception of affordances is generally unambiguous. The standard view is that perceptual information is often ambiguous, meaning that the information that arrives at the senses, such as light striking the retina, might correspond to more than one state of the world. In order for the perceiver to determine what the state of the world is, it must employ inferential processes, and these can include integrative processes that draw on further information in order to reduce the ambiguity. To use an analogy with language, words often have multiple meanings—the word "bank" for instance can mean the land alongside a river or a financial institution, among other things—and during comprehension we resolve these ambiguities by drawing on contextual information. For instance, the sentence fragment "Sarah ran to the bank" is ambiguous, but the meaning of "bank" might be specified by taking into account the sentence as a whole, for example, "Sarah ran to the bank to deposit money before it closed" or "Sarah ran to the bank to stop her little brother from jumping into the water."

Gibson believed that the idea that perceptual information is often ambiguous is based on a flawed conception of the perceiver as passive and of perception as a process of interpreting a static picture on the retina. But people are often moving through their environment, and by doing so they gain access to much richer information. This idea is illustrated in the accounts of catching a fly ball and braking we've just described, wherein the movement of the perceiver plays an essential role in acquiring the information about the action possibility. In effect, rather than compensating for ambiguous perceptual information by means of integrative processes in the head, the idea is that the perceiver can eliminate the ambiguity of instantaneous perceptual information through movement, which acquires more perceptual information. Some Gibsonians have claimed that this generally eliminates ambiguity in affordance perception—in other words, moving perceivers can typically acquire perceptual information that corresponds perfectly to the action possibilities perceived (e.g., Turvey 1990). This is a very strong assumption, and it has been criticized by Withagen and Chemero (2009) as being incompatible with an evolutionary view of animal perception. This is because modern evolutionary theory posits that variability is the norm, implying that different animals within a species will perceive their affordances in different ways. We agree with Withagen and Chemero but think their critique doesn't go far enough. There are numerous biological phenomena that are based on perceptual ambiguity, including camouflage, masquerade, warning coloration, mimicry, deception, and cuckoldry (Davies, Krebs, and West 2012).[2]

Withagen and Chemero believe that the theory of the direct perception of affordances can be preserved even while recognizing that perception can be ambiguous, but we are skeptical about this. The examples of sentence comprehension we gave provide a simple illustration of the way that cognitive integration processes "in the head" can reduce ambiguity, and we think it is very plausible that such processes are often involved in affordance perception. The affordances of objects can often be variable and context-sensitive, with the consequence that perceptual information is ambiguous. For instance, a pen can look like it affords writing, but the ink may have run dry; a cup of tea can look like it affords drinking, but may still be too hot. In the example we gave at the start, water running over the trail surface obscures the shapes and textures of the ground beneath, making it unclear to the rider what line she should take, or whether she should ride down the slope at all. In many cases, when perceptual information about affordances is ambiguous, this ambiguity can be reduced or eliminated by drawing on wider information. You may not be able to *see* that the pen has no ink but you can *remember* this information from the last time you tried to use it.

The problem of perceptual ambiguity has implications for understanding anticipatory action control. One of the advantages claimed for the Gibsonian approach is that it provides an anticipatory account of action control. This is evident in the fly ball and braking examples, where perceptual information is used to produce action that anticipates an outcome (catching the ball or stopping before the obstacle). But anticipation here is limited by perception—the individual can't anticipate future states for which there is no immediate perceptual information. It is plausible, however, that action control often employs forms of anticipation that go beyond immediate perception. When a mountain biker picks a good line around a corner, they may take into account not only what they can see as they approach the corner but also what they know lies beyond it but can't see in the present moment, like a drop, boulder, mud bog, series of slippery tree roots or another corner. This could be termed "strategic remembering."

The Gibsonian approach is austere by design, and it has yielded insights into perception and action that are not readily apparent from a representational point of view. Specifically, it has shown how the perceptual control of action might exploit movement and associated perceptual patterns. But, as we've just suggested, there are reasons to think that the restrictive assumptions it employs might not yield a complete account of action control, and it is important therefore to consider other approaches to affordances. Before we turn to this, we raise a final concern that applies not only to the Gibsonian approach but also to most other work on affordances. This problem lies with the very definition of affordances as action possibilities. Gibson's original definition describes affordances as what the environment offers the animal, for good or ill, but there are many things that the environment offers that are not action possibilities as such. The presence of prey in the environment can afford hunting and nutrition for a predator, but while hunting is an action, nourishment is not. A marathon can afford running for a competitor, pride or disappointment at the outcome, and a sense of social belonging. Only the first is an action; the last two are not, although they might lead to further actions.

Michaels (2003, 138) is aware of this issue, but she argues that the term "affordances" should be restricted to action possibilities on the grounds that including nonaction affordances would undermine the Gibsonian approach. To appreciate the point, note that many nonaction affordances are outcomes that actions function to bring about. The coffee on the table is reachable and drinkable, and will also provide a warm, delicious experience and a caffeine buzz. Intuitively it seems that we often reach for a coffee *in order* to have the experience that drinking it will bring. But this invites a representational view of action control in which the reaching is based not only on the reachability of the cup but also on awareness of the outcome. Specifically, the intentional control of instrumental action seems to involve representation of the relation between the action and the outcome. It is this idea that Michaels wants to avoid. In our view, though, it is plausible that a great deal of action control *does* take into account instrumental structure. Thus, a mountain bike rider may take a slower approach going into a corner in order to set herself up properly for the obstacle that follows. That is, people often perform actions for *reasons*. Some approaches to affordances have not taken up the anti-representationalism of Gibson, but they have adopted the view that affordances are action possibilities—which can also be problematic. Before we turn to representational accounts, however, we briefly examine efforts to extend the anti-representationalist approach to affordances to accommodate phenomena usually thought of as representational.

2.2 Recent Extensions of the Nonrepresentational Approach

Rietveld and colleagues (Bruineberg and Rietveld 2014; Rietveld and Kiverstein 2014) recently proposed that a more expansive understanding of affordances can be obtained if we develop the idea that the affordances available to an animal are based on its way of life. In the case of humans this includes the full set of abilities provided by human sociocultural practices, meaning affordance responsiveness is not limited to the kind of movement-based activities that the Gibsonian approach has primarily focused on. Indeed, Rietveld and Kiverstein (2014) claim that nonrepresentational affordance responsiveness can include phenomena associated with higher cognition, such as capacities for making perceptual judgments and the giving and asking of reasons (343).

Given that humans do confront extremely rich possibilities for action, a question that arises is how they manage to respond selectively to some affordances rather than others. Drawing on work by Withagen and colleagues (Withagen et al. 2012), Rietveld and Kiverstein suggest that this can understood in terms of "solicitation"; some affordances solicit or invite responses more strongly than others, and this solicitation is dependent on the current interests of the individual and the specific structure of the situation. Rietveld and Kiverstein (2014) further claim that, in the case of skilled individuals, this selective responsiveness is not reflective—there is no explicit comparison of options with choice based on reasons; rather, "experts develop a 'nose' that enables them to immediately sniff out which possibilities for action are better or worse in a specific situation" (341). Bruineberg and Rietveld (2014) address the question of what mechanisms might underlie this selectivity by appealing to the concept of self-organization. In essence, they suggest that dynamical self-organization drives the system toward the achievement of optimal grip on a field of affordances (3).

In assessing Rietveld's view, we cannot delve very far into the larger issues at play in debates between representationalism and anti-representationalism. However, it is important to observe that the account is not yet developed in enough detail to make a strong case against representationalist approaches. There are many detailed, empirically based representational models of cognitive phenomena, and a powerful case for anti-representationalism can be made only by providing equally detailed nonrepresentational models that are more plausible.

Broadly speaking, a representational model proposes a mechanism that incorporates representations whose function is to track certain kinds of information. A distinctive feature of many of these models is that they describe ways that multiple representations can combine to form complex representations whose content reflects the content of the source representations. In some cases complex representations represent structured relations amongst multiple elements. One area of representational research that is relevant to our current concerns is work that has distinguished multiple memory systems in the brain (Squire 1992). Specifically, declarative memory (memory for events and facts) has been found to be functionally and anatomically distinct from a variety of forms of implicit memory (including motor adaptations and habits).

Although its name suggests that declarative memory is language-based, recent theories propose instead that it is based on relational processing performed by the hippocampus and is found in nonhuman animals (Eichenbaum 2000). To give a specific example, in a certain kind of radial-arm maze problem, the maze consists of arms that radiate out from a central location. Each arm is baited with food, and the rat should visit each arm only once if it is to find all the food efficiently. Rats are good at learning to do this, and they do so without using a simple rule such as "visit each arm in sequence." The standard interpretation is that they represent where they have been in the maze and plan where they should go next (Matzel and Kolata 2010).

This example provides us with a case wherein we have a detailed specification of a behavioral problem and a representational model for how it is solved. Per se, the claim that selective response is based on solicitations whose structure is shaped by dynamical self-organization doesn't provide a satisfactory explanation for how rats (or people) solve problems like this, and while a more detailed nonrepresentational model might be constructed, we cannot assess its plausibility in advance. More broadly, the example illustrates the way that declarative memory might contribute to action awareness by bringing to bear information about the larger situation. Above we suggested that awareness of whether a pen affords writing might incorporate awareness that you have recently tried to use the pen and it has no ink. This is also a case where affordance awareness draws on declarative memory, and we discuss a case study in detail below that similarly implicates declarative memory.

In view of this, we should regard cautiously Rietveld and Kiverstein's (2014) claim that higher cognition can be understood nonrepresentationally in terms of skilled engagement with affordances. Their suggestion that perceptual judgments and reason-giving can be understood this way raises questions that need more extended discussion. For instance, minimally, to give a reason for an action is to give a description that cites a cause of the action, and this description is, on the face of it, representational. A possible nonrepresentational model of reason-giving might be that the situation solicits the individual to make a verbal utterance, and the individual does so without cognitively taking into account the content of the utterance, while the listener is solicited to accept the utterance as a reason without cognitively taking into account the content of the utterance. This does not seem plausible to us, however.

3 Cognitive Approaches to Affordance Perception

Most neuroscientific and psychological approaches to affordance perception start from the view that the brain represents the world. The standard neuroscientific view is that perception involves successively more complex and abstract representations starting at the sensory periphery and proceeding through multiple stages of processing that extract particular kinds of information. In the case of vision, this includes motion, color, and form (Reid 2003). Research on affordances from this perspective has investigated some of the specific kinds of brain areas and representations that may be involved in affordance perception and selection. There is an extensive body of work that we cannot hope to review here, but we note some relevant highlights. In particular, some of the key points follow.

According to the two-systems theory of Milner and Goodale (Milner and Goodale 1995, 2008), the visual system divides into two major streams, one ventral and one dorsal, with the ventral stream being responsible for visual awareness of scenes—objects spatially related to each other—and the dorsal stream being responsible for the "on-line" control of action.

Affordance perception incorporates a distinction between the space within which one can reach (peripersonal space) and the space beyond (extrapersonal space) (Brain 1941; di Pellegrino and Làdavas 2015). Moreover, these regions can be rapidly remapped as a result of experience. For example, using a long tool can cause the area of space within range of the tool to be remapped from far to near space (Berti and Frassinetti 2000).

Some research suggests that perception of action possibilities is influenced by the agent's current physical state. Test subjects wearing a backpack, for instance, perceived a hill as being steeper than those who were not carrying extra weight (Bhalla and Proffitt 1999).[3] In another test, as people became fatigued, their estimates of action ability appeared to track actual changes in ability caused by fatigue (Pijpers et al. 2007).

Differences in action ability among individuals can give rise to different strategies that affect affordance perception. In a study of goalkeepers, faster keepers waited longer before moving than slower keepers, which allowed them to gain more information about the kicker and the path of the ball (Dicks, Davids, and Buttons 2010).

Taken together, these lines of research suggest that affordance perception involves some quite complex forms of information integration that take into account diverse features of the external world such as distance and equipment, as well as bodily changes in physiology and ability (including fatigue). The flexibility of these processes suggests that they play an important role in adjusting to the specificity of performance situations.

Above we discussed Rietveld's approach to the problem of understanding how, of all the many affordances present at any given time, only one comes to guide action. A theory by Cisek (2007; Cisek and Kalaska 2010), called the *affordance competition hypothesis*, provides another account of how this filtering might take place, developed within the framework of representational neuroscience. According to Cisek's proposal, the dorsal visual stream, together with a parietal network, identifies action possibilities and also specifies the structure of action execution. When there are multiple possibilities for action, each option generates activity in the network, and there is competition between the options. Other brain systems, including the prefrontal cortex, process information about the structure of the task and influence action control by biasing activity in the affordance network.

If we take into account the theories of both Milner and Goodale and Cisek, it raises the possibility that there may be at least two distinct kinds of affordance perception. This is because the representations of the dorsal system don't reach consciousness, according to Milner and Goodale (2008), whereas the representations of the tasks that bias affordance selection on Cisek's account must also include representations of action possibilities. If the ventral (conscious) visual system also represents action possibilities (and surely it does, since we are consciously aware of at least some of them), this would help explain forms of affordance perception that do not easily fit Cisek's theory. Wagman (2012) found that perception of maximum reach height can take into account changes in posture or use of a tool, such as a chair. This is intriguing because the dorsal system is only responsive to immediate perceptual information, whereas affordance perception here involves anticipated changes.

Recall that in part 2 we argued that affordance perception can sometimes take into account anticipations of the future that go beyond what can be immediately perceived. Wagman's experiment provides an example of this, and suggests that higher cognition isn't simply helping to select between affordances, it is influencing which affordances are perceived.

4 Social, Cultural, and Historical Specificity

We saw above that Rietveld has drawn attention to sociocultural aspects of affordances. In the humanities, as one might expect, several scholars have been examining cultural, social, historical, and context-specific aspects of the relationships among people, affordances, and their environments. Just as a cup affords grasping only when it is in reach of a person who is able to grasp it, a road that affords driving does so only in eras since the car was invented. From a contemporary, physical perspective, an empty road affords driving on either side equally, or indeed down the middle, but local culture dictates that you should drive down one particular side. Likewise, a road will signify different things to people who have learned how to drive as compared with those who have not, to women in Saudi Araba who (until 2018) were not legally permitted to drive, and to someone living in the 1500s who traveled with a horse and cart. Put simply, what a road affords is culturally, historically, and socially specific. Research in the humanities on affordances has been concerned with these kinds of factors.

Tim Ingold, an anthropologist, has developed an extension of the Gibsonian approach that is intended to serve as a framework for understanding culture. His focus is on the way that objects and features of the environment become significant through human action and interaction. He claims, "Meanings are not attached by the mind to objects in the world, rather these objects take on their significance—or in Gibson's terms, they afford what they do—by virtue of their incorporation into a characteristic pattern of day-to-day activities. In short, far from being inscribed upon the bedrock of physical reality, meaning is immanent in the relational contexts of people's practical engagement with their lived-in environment" (2011, 168).

Ingold proposes a concept of his own, the taskscape: "Every task exists as part of what I have called a *taskscape*," he writes, "understood as the totality of tasks making up the pattern of activity of a community" (325). He is concerned with the way patterns of movement are developed socially, not just by individuals acting in isolation with their environments.

While Ingold remains close to a Gibsonian approach to affordance perception, others have departed further from this framework. Julia Lupton (2014) argues that "Gibson's commitment to a model of immediate perception can seem at odds with the humanities' commitment to culture, language, and history" (617). She provides an overview of how affordances have been taken up by researchers in theater and performance studies, many of whom emphasize the guiding role of the agent's intentionality and the perception of affordances, quite literally, as *possibilities* for action. This includes symbolic and creative considerations that are especially difficult to fit into a Gibsonian model. Lupton brings attention to ways affordance theory has been used to understand how theater texts are meaningful in different social and historical periods. We provide an extended example here to illustrate this point, which has important implications for sport contexts.

Evelyn Tribble's (2011) research on distributed cognition in Elizabethan theater draws on affordance theory in her analysis of historical performance and rehearsal practices. She considers the dynamic and woven affordances of multiple artifacts, the architecture of the performance space, and the actions of other people for the ways they scaffold memory and collaborative performance processes when players performed up to six different productions a week. Drawing on the work of Simon Palfrey and Tiffany Stern (2007), Tribble (2011) describes the way that an actor's part was circulated, including only the actor's lines and the preceding cue words rather than the entire text of the play. This affords a particular way of "understanding the unfolding shifts in passion of an individual character. The playbook by contrast affords comparisons between temporal moments in the play and a grasp of the structures of the scene" (68). This historic distribution of parts, reflective of an era long before photocopiers and iPads, contrasts greatly with the detailed knowledge of the shape of a particular scene, or even the details of an exchange between two characters, that actors study in rehearsal and have access to today.

An especially interesting aspect of this is that Shakespeare wrote his plays with these performance processes in mind. Tribble draws attention to a passage from act 3, scene 3 in *The Merchant of Venice* in which the cue words, "have my bond" appear five times in thirteen lines of text spoken by the character Shylock. This would have elicited an increasingly irritated (or perhaps exasperated, comical, or forceful) response from the actor playing Solanio, whose part simply indicates his next line comes immediately after these words. This clever direction from Shakespeare heightens the emotional pitch and the physical action of the performance on stage. Since contemporary actors follow very different rehearsal processes, *what these cue words originally afforded is often lost to the modern eye*.

Tribble's research shows that an understanding of affordances can be used historically, to understand patterns of movement and awareness far removed from our contemporary sensibilities, and reinforces the importance of considering cognitive aspects of affordance perception, especially in the creative, intentional exploitation of affordance perception. This kind of exploitation also plays important roles in sport. One form this can take is deceiving an opponent, for example with a feint or by simulating tiredness.

Reflective understanding of affordance perception also plays a role in the design of equipment and the selection of equipment by individuals. Justin Spinney (2006) argues that technology influences our relationship to the environment, our perception of what it affords, and shapes our bodies in response. Consider the way new biking technologies, such as suspension and lighter, stronger frame materials, reshape what riders can do onboard. This changes how they perceive the taskscape and the skill sets they develop, and has effects on the design and wear and tear of the trails. Paul Barratt (2011) describes the rock climber's shoes as mediating the body-environment-affordances triad. As the climber's grip is enhanced on the rock, new routes become available. At the same time, the amount of skill needed to climb those routes decreases. Climbers choose equipment, such as their shoes, to decrease some risks while retaining the sensations of others (Barratt 2011). These ethnographic observations reveal a central role for affordance awareness in mediating larger interactions among technological changes, changes in sport activities, socially informed values and desires, reflective equipment choices and action planning, and individual abilities.[4] We now turn to an example of individual performance that likewise exhibits considerable richness, including sophisticated forms of reflective affordance awareness.

5 Getting Dirty: A Case Study from Mountain Biking

Most research on affordance perception has focused on relatively simple actions and performance conditions. Since the problem of selecting the right actions at the right times will be greatly affected by the complexity of the task and situation, this may obscure processes that contribute to affordance awareness. It is important therefore to investigate cases where there is high complexity. We now examine a case study from elite mountain bike racing that reveals some of the features of affordance awareness in a demanding real-world sport situation.

The following piece of writing is from Paul van der Ploeg, 2013 UCI World Mountain Bike Cross-Country Eliminator champion and multiple Australian champion (including Olympic distance under-23 cross-country in 2008, 2010, 2011, and cyclo-cross in 2015).[5] In this excerpt he describes his own racing experiences at a particularly muddy cross-country round of the UCI Mountain Bike World Cup in Bromont, Canada. He published this account on his own website shortly after the race.[6] While van de Ploeg's experiences can't be taken as representative of the experiences had by all mountain bikers while racing, they provide a useful sample and raise important issues for further theoretical analysis and empirical investigation.[7] We have included our notes clarifying some insider terminology in square brackets.

> The gun went and people were all over the [start] grid trying to clip in [to their pedals], I fluked a good clip and picked my way through the madness straight into the killer climb. After getting blinded by waves of mud several times I was regretting leaving the Oakleys [sunglasses] back at the start line. The barrow mud [tires] instantly showed me why "MUD" was written on the side walls.[8] As all riders dismounted due to lack of traction I stayed clipped in in a swarm of slipp-running riders and I couldn't help but smile. [Teammate, Nathan] Haas called out "Yeah dogg, smack that hill" because he witnessed the superior traction I was getting. The real test came soon after on the small chutes on the climb and after riders rag dolling it into the bushes [crashing] I was happy to be keeping it rubber side down....
>
> The descent was looser than I could have ever imagined but the "New" Geax Gato was biting though the slop and finding hope where I had none. I was pleased to be keeping on the wheels of the crazy Canadians who live and breathe these conditions....
>
> At the top of the jump line on the 5th lap I pulled the brakes on and it was suddenly evident that my NEW brake pads were down to the metal backing plates! This would have been

> "negative goodness." I hit the steep sections and applied the point and shoot technique, when I found both [brake] levers pulled straight into the bars it was all I could do. I opened my eyes at the bottom still on track, thanked my lucky stars and kept going. (van der Ploeg 2009)

In this description, van der Ploeg demonstrates an acute awareness of many factors present in the performance situation. The muddy conditions have a strong impact, and van der Ploeg mentions his tires several times, reflecting, with surprise, on their superior performance. While there is likely to be an element of sponsor promotion in this, his awareness of the good performance of the tires appears to have a significant influence on his race strategy. In particular, he continues to ride up a climb when many others are dismounting and pushing their bikes, giving him a substantial advantage, and altering his strategic approach to subsequent sections of track as a result. Thus, in this report we see evidence of van der Ploeg's observations on the affordances of equipment (well-used and never used) influencing his in-race strategies and decisions, alongside observations on physical ability, as well as sociocultural comparisons (between himself and his teammates, competitors, and Canadian riders) in order to recalibrate his own performance goals and expectations.

The fine-grained, goal-oriented awareness of the conditions, his equipment, and the other riders that van der Ploeg exhibits is not atypical, given the high performance levels required at an elite level. Relatively small differences can have significant effects, and riders need to understand how each component relates to the whole. Riders heavily customize their bikes and suspension, for instance choosing different tires for different types of dirt and adjusting the air pressures in the tires in relation to specific course designs, their own riding style, and the speed they plan to take through certain obstacles in anticipation of specific race and training runs, and future trail degradation (Flow Mountain Bike 2015; Graves 2013). This level of awareness, preparation, and top-down consideration suggests that riders do not simply rely on unreflective, intuitive responses. Reflective awareness and problem solving is of course important in training, but this preparation and sustained engagement in the sport also contributes to rapid reflective processes during performance. We argue that such preparation builds rich anticipation of race conditions that reduces cognitive load during racing and allows for a more focused ability to respond to additional demands that arise in this context. We now turn to a discussion of some of the cognitive mechanisms that may play a role.

5.1 A Causal Control Model

Above we suggested that the processes involved in affordance awareness will be influenced by task complexity, and in van der Ploeg's description we've now seen some of the kinds of complexity that can arise in an elite sporting context. One effect of complexity will be to make the problem of tracking affordances and selecting between them particularly challenging, because affordances are highly context-sensitive and influenced by a wide range of variable factors. And one consequence of this will be that immediate perceptual information will often be ambiguous. As discussed above, representational processes can reduce ambiguity by integrating multiple sources of information, including information from multiple perceptual sources and from memory. Christensen et al. (2015) propose that a particular kind of representation—a *causal control model*—plays a role in helping the individual track key factors that influence performance. Theoretically we can interpret van der Ploeg's awareness as, in part, updating his causal control model, which represents the capacities of his equipment and himself as they relate to the performance conditions. In the case of the tires, this includes traction, grip, the way they interact with the mud, the slope of the hill, and the power produced through his legs.

Because the causal control model tracks relations among these factors, it plays a key role in the awareness of what actions are possible or, in other words, the affordances that are available at any given point. As van der Ploeg learns about the properties of the tires in these conditions, he can adjust his expectations for what he can do, including the ways he can intervene in specific movement sequences to achieve a given outcome. To extend the arguments made in a previous paper (Bicknell 2010), in which Drew Leder's (1990) concept of incorporation is used to discuss the ways skills become part of a bodily or phenomenological "I can," what we see here is a process of attuning that incorporation—to (and through) a sensing of place, and of equipment.

A further concept that builds on the notion of the causal control model is awareness of the *performance envelope*. This is awareness of the relation between the current state and the limits of performance. These limits can include the outer bounds of what is possible as well as narrower ranges defining success in the context. The actions that can be performed at a given point and the performance envelope are interdependent: some actions are not possible because they will take the performance state outside the limits of the performance envelope, and some actions may be required in order to keep the performance state within the performance envelope. For example, van der Ploeg's awareness of the limits of his traction very likely influenced his awareness of how much power he could put down on different parts of the course, and the distribution of body weight in relation to the gradient of any uphills, while maintaining a forward momentum. Awareness of the limited traction available in the conditions is also likely to have led him to monitor the space between himself and other riders, rather than following them too closely. If another rider came to a fast halt immediately in front of him it could force van der Ploeg off his bike too.

5.2 Keeping It Rubber Side Down: Staying Safe and Adjusting on the Fly

The failure of van der Ploeg's brakes and his response to the problem is a dramatic illustration of the ability, and oftentimes, necessity, to be able to adjust to changing circumstances on the fly. During the race, van der Ploeg found that his levers "pulled straight into the bars," which he interprets as indicating that his brake pads are worn away (they were down to the metal backing plates, meaning the levers pull farther toward the handlebars before the backing plates touch the rotor).[9] In other words, van der Ploeg observed that pulling the levers *no longer* afforded braking. This assessment combines knowledge of the equipment with the sensation felt through the levers, and it serves as a cue to adjust performance.[10] He describes himself as riding down the steep sections by applying "the point and shoot technique." Whether or not he did close his eyes as claimed, his description indicates that he wasn't confident at the time that he would ride the obstacle without crashing. Nevertheless, he succeeded, and we can see here again the dynamic, context-sensitive nature of affordances and the need to rapidly adjust action control, or intervene in well-learned action repertoires, in response. A notable aspect of this is the way that immediate awareness can drive long-range anticipatory adjustments—as soon as van der Ploeg discovers that his brakes don't work, he must change his whole riding approach. The causal control model helps to explain this kind of flexibility by representing these interdependencies and focusing attention on relevant factors. In contrast, it isn't clear how just the right interdependencies could be captured by nonrepresentational mechanisms, especially in complex situations that have substantial novel elements and hence where learned responses will tend to break down. By highlighting relevant factors, the causal control model can drive flexible attention and rapid problem solving during performance, for example when equipment fails.

We aren't suggesting, however, that these representational models are solely responsible for affordance awareness. The kinds of perceptual-motor links described by Fajen may well play an important role, as may the kind of dynamical self-organization of the perceptual-motor system that Rietveld points to. We doubt, however, that these kinds of processes operate without cognitive influence. We argue that representations can track complex relations and thus help resolve the perceptual ambiguities that arise in complex tasks and situations. Research on declarative memory has provided an extensive body of evidence and theory indicating that humans and other animals do form representations that capture the structure of situations, which can be used to guide action in tasks like variable maze problems. It is very likely that athletes similarly draw on declarative memory to represent the structure of the performance situation to form anticipations, such as of what is around the corner or the consequences of a brake failure on performance and strategy. This allows them to exert sophisticated instrumental control, adjusting actions in relation to shifting goals and changing circumstances. In addition, though, the lower-level processes described by cognitive research that we reviewed will also make a contribution. Fatigue and other bodily factors will alter the perception of affordances. Action selection is likely to occur at multiple levels, with the low-level processes described by Cisek being modulated by the higher-level processes we have discussed. On a larger scale, sociocultural and historical processes reshape sport activities, technologies, values, practices, and ideas.

Thus, it may be that all extant approaches capture important aspects of affordance awareness. For this reason, rather than argue for one approach to the exclusion of others, it may be more productive to look for potential complementarities, and to push to develop our theories further—it is virtually inevitable that our current understanding is at the least simplistic. Equally, we should regard all approaches with a degree of healthy skepticism and tackle theory development in a pragmatic and open-minded way.

6 Conclusion

Gibson's concept of affordances has been taken up in a wide range of academic fields in ways that he might not have imagined and, in many cases, would not have agreed with. His work was pioneering in part because he conceptualized the perceiver as an active agent—moving through the environment and interacting with it—rather than as the immobile viewer of a scene. While we've suggested that the anti-representational approach that he pioneered might not yield a complete account of action control, we strongly endorse the idea that we should understand affordance perception in terms of the active agent. A central issue that arises when approaching affordances from this perspective is the high degree of sensitivity of action to a welter of situational factors. We've suggested that cross-fertilization between multiple approaches can help us develop a fuller picture, and we conclude by focusing on a specific aspect of this. There is a danger that laboratory-based research on affordance perception can overlook the complex, dynamic processes of affordance perception in real-world action, such as racing bikes in sloppy mud. Equally, philosophical investigation conducted from the armchair may provide only limited insights into the complex phenomenology and action-control processes of elite athletes whose expertise and experiences are far removed from those of the philosopher. For these reasons, direct empirical investigation of sporting performance in its natural environment is an essential component of an evolving research matrix. This will not only further contribute to a more unified understanding of affordances, but also extend other research into skilled action, embodied cognition, and anticipatory control.

Notes

1. Our thanks to Massimiliano Cappuccio, John Michael, Tom McClelland, and John Sutton for helpful suggestions that have greatly improved the chapter.

2. Or, indeed, the very appearance of the humble platypus.

3. This research is controversial because of methodological challenges inherent in the experiment design. For a review see Philbeck and Witt (2015).

4. For further discussion on equipment design, embodied experiences, and perceptions of risk, expanding on some of the concepts described here, see Bicknell (2016).

5. The UCI or Union Cycliste Internationale is the world governing body for cycling.

6. Minor typos have been edited for clarity. See van der Ploeg (2009) for the original, extended report.

7. Bicknell (2013) describes the value of rider self-reports as a window into the phenomenological experience of racing at this level. Because of the close proximity of the writing to the race, this report provides evidence concerning some elements of the individual rider's awareness and experience at the time of racing. This is a valuable source of information given the difficulty of sampling these thoughts from racers during the events themselves. Of course, this evidence can be influenced by extraneous factors. There is, for example, an assumed obligation to mention sponsor's products in a positive way. Nevertheless, van der Ploeg's discussion of his experiences during the race is detailed and, plausibly, fairly accurate.

8. Van der Ploeg provides more information on the tire, and the fact that he has never used it before, earlier in the report: "Luckily for me I packed the ultimate weapon in the last second rush out the door. It is in the form of un-tested Geax TNT Barrow MUD 1.7 inch (very narrow) tractor tire! This was a tough decision but with the conditions it was worth a try and I will tell you now it saved my whole race." He also describes his own pre-race skepticism, and that of his team coach, about whether it would work on that particular course.

9. As described in a section of his report that we haven't included here, he subsequently confirmed this by inspecting his brakes after the race.

10. See Sutton (2007) and Bicknell (2011) on "performance nudges" that encourage an embodied adjustment to skilled performance.

References

Barratt, Paul. 2011. "Vertical Worlds: Technology, Hybridity and the Climbing Body." *Social and Cultural Geography* 12 (4): 397–412.

Berti, A., and F. Frassinetti. 2000. "When Far Becomes Near: Remapping of Space by Tool Use." *Journal of Cognitive Neuroscience* 12 (3): 415–420.

Bhalla, Mukul, and Dennis R. Proffitt. 1999. "Visual-Motor Recalibration in Geographical Slant Perception." *Journal of Experimental Psychology: Human Perception and Performance* 25 (4): 1076–1096.

Bicknell, Kath. 2010. "Feeling Them Ride: Corporeal Exchange in Cross-Country Mountain Bike Racing." *About Performance* 10:81–91.

Bicknell, Kath. 2011. "Sport, Entertainment and the Live(d) Experience of Cheering." *Popular Entertainment Studies* 2 (1): 96–111.

Bicknell, Kath. 2013. "Everybody's Writing." In *Proceedings of the 5th Australian Cycling Conference*, edited by Peter Lumb, Katie Gillfillan, and Jennifer Bonham, 89–96. Adelaide: The Science Exchange.

Bicknell, Kath. 2016. "Technology, Equipment and the Mountain Biker's Taskscape." In *Women in Action Sport Cultures*, edited by Holly Thorpe and Rebecca Olive, 237–258. Global Culture and Sport Series. London: Palgrave Macmillan.

Brain, W. Russell. 1941. "Visual Orientation with Special Reference to Lesions of the Right Cerebral Hemisphere." *Brain: A Journal of Neurology* 64 (4): 244–272.

Bruineberg, Jelle, and Erik Rietveld. 2014. "Self-Organization, Free Energy Minimization, and Optimal Grip on a Field of Affordances." *Frontiers in Human Neuroscience* 8 (August): 599.

Chapman, Seville. 1968. "Catching a Baseball." *American Journal of Physics* 36 (10): 868–870.

Christensen, Wayne, Kath Bicknell, Doris McIlwain, and John Sutton. 2015. "The Sense of Agency and Its Role in Strategic Control for Expert Mountain Bikers." *Psychology of Consciousness: Theory, Research, and Practice* 2 (3): 340–353.

Cisek, Paul. 2007. "Cortical Mechanisms of Action Selection: The Affordance Competition Hypothesis." *Philosophical Transactions of the Royal Society of London B: Biological Sciences* 362 (1485): 1585–1599.

Cisek, Paul, and John F. Kalaska. 2010. "Neural Mechanisms for Interacting with a World Full of Action Choices." *Annual Review of Neuroscience* 33 (1): 269–298.

Davies, Nicholas B., John R. Krebs, and Stuart A. West. 2012. *An Introduction to Behavioural Ecology*. Hoboken, NJ: John Wiley and Sons.

Dicks, Matt, Keith Davids, and Chris Button. 2010. "Individual Differences in the Visual Control of Intercepting a Penalty Kick in Association Football." *Human Movement Science* 29 (3): 401–411.

di Pellegrino, Giuseppe di, and Elisabetta Làdavas. 2015. "Peripersonal Space in the Brain." *Neuropsychologia* 66 (January): 126–133.

Eichenbaum, H. 2000. "A Cortical-Hippocampal System for Declarative Memory." *Nature Reviews: Neuroscience* 1 (1): 41–50.

Fajen, Brett R. 2005. "Perceiving Possibilities for Action: On the Necessity of Calibration and Perceptual Learning for the Visual Guidance of Action." *Perception* 34 (6): 717–740.

Flow Mountain Bike. 2015. "Bike Check: Chris Panozzo's Trek Remedy 9.8 Enduro Beast." *Flow Mountain Bike*, November 9. http://flowmountainbike.com/features/bike-check-chris-panozzos-trek-remedy-9-8-enduro-beast/.

Gibson, James Jerome. 1979. *The Ecological Approach to Visual Perception*. Boston, MA: Houghton Mifflin.

Graves, Jared. 2013. "Jared Graves—UCI World Championships." YETI. http://www.yeticycles.com/blog/?p_3460.

Ingold, Tim. 2011. *The Perception of the Environment: Essays on Livelihood, Dwelling and Skill*. London: Routledge.

Leder, Drew. 1990. *The Absent Body*. Chicago: University of Chicago Press.

Lee, David N. 1976. "A Theory of Visual Control of Braking Based on Information about Time-to-Collision." *Perception* 5 (4): 437–459.

Lupton, Julia Reinhard. 2014. "The Affordances of Hospitality: Shakespearean Drama between Historicism and Phenomenology." *Poetics Today* 35 (4): 615–633.

Matzel, Louis D., and Stefan Kolata. 2010. "Selective Attention, Working Memory, and Animal Intelligence." *Neuroscience and Biobehavioral Reviews* 34 (1): 23–30.

Michaels, Claire F. 2003. "Affordances: Four Points of Debate." *Ecological Psychology* 15 (2): 135–148.

Milner, A. D., and Melvyn A. Goodale. 1995. *The Visual Brain in Action*. Oxford: Oxford University Press.

Milner, A. D., and Melvyn A. Goodale. 2008. "Two Visual Systems Re-Viewed." *Neuropsychologia* 46 (3): 774–785.

Palfrey, Simon, and Tiffany Stern. 2007. *Shakespeare in Parts*. Oxford: Oxford University Press.

Philbeck, John W., and Jessica K. Witt. 2015. "Action-Specific Influences on Perception and Post-perceptual Processes: Present Controversies and Future Directions." *Psychological Bulletin* 141 (6): 1120–1144.

Pijpers, J. Robert, Raôul R. D. Oudejans, and Frank C. Bakker. 2007. "Changes in the Perception of Action Possibilities while Climbing to Fatigue on a Climbing Wall." *Journal of Sports Sciences* 25 (1): 97–110.

Reid, R. Clay. 2003. "Vision." In *Fundamental Neuroscience*, 2nd ed., edited by Larry R. Squire, Floyd E. Bloom, Susan K. McConnell, James L. Roberts, Nicholas C. Spitzer, and Michael J. Zigmond, 727–754. San Diego, CA: Academic Press.

Rietveld, Erik, and Julian Kiverstein. 2014. "A Rich Landscape of Affordances." *Ecological Psychology* 26 (4): 325–352.

Spinney, Justin. 2006. "A Place of Sense: A Kinaesthetic Ethnography of Cyclists on Mont Ventoux." *Environment and Planning D: Society and Space* 24 (5): 709–732.

Squire, L. R. 1992. "Memory and the Hippocampus: A Synthesis from Findings with Rats, Monkeys, and Humans." *Psychological Review* 99 (2): 195–231.

Sutton, John. 2007. "Batting, Habit and Memory: The Embodied Mind and the Nature of Skill." *Sport in Society* 10 (5): 763–786.

Tribble, E. 2011. *Cognition in the Globe: Attention and Memory in Shakespeare's Theatre*. New York: Springer.

Turvey, Michael T. 1990. "The Challenge of a Physical Account of Action: A Personal View." In *A Natural-Physical Approach to Movement Control*, edited by H. T. A. Whiting, O. G. Meijer, and P. C. W. van Wieringen, 57–93. Amsterdam: Free University Press.

Van der Ploeg, P. 2009. "Bromont World Cup ... Full Details." Paul van der Ploeg: Travelling adventures and racing stories. http://www.paulvanderploeg.com/2009/08/bromont-world-cup full-details.html.

Wagman, Jeffrey B. 2012. "Perception of Maximum Reaching Height Reflects Impending Changes in Reaching Ability and Improvements Transfer to Unpracticed Reaching Tasks." *Experimental Brain Research* 219 (4): 467–476.

Warren, William H. 1988. "Chapter 14: Action Modes and Laws of Control for the Visual Guidance of Action." In *Complex Movement Behaviour: "The" Motor-Action Controversy*, vol. 50, edited by Onno G. Meijer and Klaus Roth, 339–379. Advances in Psychology Series. Amsterdam: Elsevier.

Withagen, Rob, and Anthony Chemero. 2009. "Naturalizing Perception: Developing the Gibsonian Approach to Perception along Evolutionary Lines." *Theory and Psychology* 19 (3): 363–389.

Withagen, Rob, Harjo J. de Poel, Duarte Araújo, and Gert-Jan Pepping. 2012. "Affordances Can Invite Behavior: Reconsidering the Relationship between Affordances and Agency." *New Ideas in Psychology* 30 (2): 250–258.

VII Predictive and Anticipatory Skills: Imagination, Improvisation, and Creativity in Sport

23 Imagery, Expertise, and Action: A Window into Embodiment

Tadhg E. MacIntyre, Christopher R. Madan, Noel E. Brick, Jürgen Beckmann, and Aidan P. Moran

1 Introduction

In 1890 William James discussed the "idea that sensations modify the nervous system, and enable mental reproductions to emerge in the mind" (Park and Kosslyn 1990, 183). Furthermore, he categorized people on the basis of individual differences in their modality-specific imagery ability (e.g., visual and motor types). In 1990, Park and Kosslyn duly described how William James (1890) had been prescient in his synthesis of the key challenges in mental imagery research a century earlier. They asserted that his ideas on "the sensory-perceptual aspects of the mind have largely been neglected" (Park and Kosslyn, 1990, 183). Now, a quarter of a century after Park and Kosslyn's remarks, we have witnessed not only the proliferation of motor imagery research (Gabbard 2013; Glover and Baran 2017; Madan and Singhal 2012a; Moran et al. 2012) but also the emergence of embodied cognition approaches in the past two decades (Glenberg 2015; Loeffler, Raab, and Cañal-Bruland 2016; Wilson and Golonka 2013; Wilson 2002). This latter paradigm shift is at the forefront of cognitive science, as demonstrated by the surge in related research topics (Borghi and Pecher 2011; Lynott, Connell, and Holler 2013) and handbooks (e.g., Calvo and Gomila 2008; Shapiro 2011) and the emergence of a variety of approaches to the embodied cognition approach (Wilson 2002).

In this chapter, we explore the aforementioned paradigm shifts and how they offer an avenue for new research. We first elucidate what precisely "mental imagery," the parent construct of motor imagery, is and explain the research milestones that have elucidated our understanding of this complex topic. The construct of motor imagery has become a thriving research topic thanks to the development of the action simulation model by Marc Jeannerod, which provided a framework in which imagery and movement are viewed as part of an action continuum (Jeannerod 1994, 2006).

Three key pivots occurred over two decades of motor imagery research, relating to conceptual issues, measurement challenges, and the application of the expertise paradigm; each is explained in turn. Subsequently, the potential for grounded cognition accounts to explain the interactions among our cognition, action, and emotional systems is evaluated (Shapiro 2011). The grounded cognition approach to investigating motor imagery arguably provides an opportunity for the interdisciplinary investigation of questions on the nature of representation with implications for researchers and practitioners alike. Finally, new directions for both scientists and practitioners are addressed, with the emphasis on athletic samples, including those suffering from sport injury. First, we consider the construct of mental imagery and its link to expertise and skill acquisition.

William James (1890) wrote how your imagination could allow you *learn to swim* in winter and *learn to skate* in summer. This application of imagery, as we shall see later in this chapter, is known as *mental practice*, and while understanding the utility of imagery as a simulation process was central to scientific interest since James's first musings, mental imagery and its motor equivalent are also of interest for theoretical reasons. For example, research on visual imagery has elucidated our understanding of visual perception (Kosslyn, Thompson, and Ganis 2006). Similarly, findings from motor imagery (the simulation of action) have enhanced our knowledge of action-control mechanisms in both healthy and pathological brains (de Lange, Roelofs, and Toni 2008). Understanding action is important because, historically, it has been a neglected topic in psychological science (Rosenbaum 2005). Among the reasons for its neglect is the "dumb-jock hypothesis," which, according to Rosenbaum, (2005) suggests that "one does not have to be highly intelligent, as measured by IQ tests, to move well" (311). The work of Bartlett (1932) on motor schema provided a welcome exploration from cognitive perspective on action concepts (Moran 2012). However, this was an exception among psychology researchers who had largely been "preoccupied with disembodied perceptions … and indifferently concerned with translating perceptions and higher processes into action" (Adams 1987, 66).

Inspired by the ecological approach of Gibson (1979), the development of direct-perception explanations for action spawned an alternative theoretical account. These approaches were no longer dominated by a concern with the internal representations and computations underlying action prevalent in disembodied perspectives (e.g., Newell and Simon 1972) that had led to the exclusion of embodied cognition approaches previously.

Embodied cognition is the idea that cognitive representations are "grounded in, and simulated through, sensorimotor activity" (Slepian et al. 2011, 26) or that mental processes that evolved to control action can also be used off-line to simulate motor skills and knowledge (Wilson 2002). It has been described as a "multifaceted theoretical proposition that (1) cognitive processes are influenced by the body, (2) cognition exists in the service of action, (3) cognition is situated in the environment, and (4) cognition may occur without internal representation" (Goldinger et al. 2016, 959). To explain, Lorey et al. (2009) proposed that body-related experiences also shape processes such as imagery formerly conceptualized as purely "cognitive" or disembodied. Conflicting evidence has led to researchers varying in the degree to which their explanations are in fact embodied. These range from grounded cognition to enactivism, and conflicting evidence has emerged that has been discussed in preceding chapters. Emerging accounts of grounded cognition outline how sensation, motor activity, and perceptual imagery shape cognitive processes ranging from object representation to emotion recognition (Slepian et al. 2011).

Research on aspects of embodied cognition in sport has been one impetus for the return of action research to the realm of interdisciplinary scientific discovery. Philosophers (Cappuccio 2015) and neuroscientists concerned with action (Beilock 2008), language (Bergen 2012), and concepts (Barsalou 2008) have all looked to sport to explain the implications of embodied cognition approaches (see also Shapiro and Spaulding, this volume).

2 What Is Mental Imagery?

To illuminate how motor imagery offers a window into embodied cognition, it is necessary to revisit how mental imagery, the overarching construct, has been operationalized. Our capacity to reexperience scenarios or events that we've encountered previously is remarkable, perhaps superseded only by our ability to "experience objects or events that do not exist in the world through our imagination" (Pearson and Kosslyn 2013, 5). According to Pearson and Kosslyn, this ability is critical to our capacity to reanalyze our past, plan our future goals and actions, and even simulate events that may never occur.

Mental imagery has been operationalized in a myriad of ways since William James's chapters on imagination were written (1890). The diverse definitions of mental imagery to date reflect both the dominant paradigm of the time and the orientation of the researchers involved (i.e., whether experimental or applied in focus). For example, cognitive scientists have proposed that mental imagery can be defined as the cognitive simulation process by which we can represent perceptual information in our minds in the absence of appropriate sensory input (Munzert, Lorey, and Zentgraf 2009). An array of terms have been employed to explain the application of mental imagery, including *visualization, mental rehearsal, symbolic rehearsal, covert rehearsal, mental practice, visuo-motor behavior rehearsal (VMBR),* and *motor imagery* (see Moran et al. 2012). To explain, one of the earliest studies was conducted by Vandell et al. (1943), in which they explored the efficacy of mental practice in enhancing free-throw performance. Mental practice is "the systematic use of mental imagery to rehearse an action in the minds' eye without engaging the actual physical movements involved" (Moran 2012, 349), and it has been shown to be an effective performance-enhancement strategy, according to meta-analytic reviews with sport samples (Driskell, Copper, and Moran 1994) and randomized controlled trials with surgeons (Arora et al. 2011). Similarly, VMBR was developed by Richard Suinn (1972) and describes a procedure that combines relaxation and mental practice (Suinn 1997). From this we can conclude that mental imagery is a covert process, but it has been used to encompass a range of cognitive and behavioral processes including relaxation. Consequently, the operationalization of the term is challenging for researchers.

Not surprisingly, researchers have noted that "there continues to be no consensus on the definitions of imagery" (Schack et al. 2014, 5). Schack et al. (2014) explained that "imagery refers to a collection of abilities, including, for example, visual imagery, kinesthetic imagery, imagery of movements or combinations of imagery modalities" (5). This multisensory approach is supported by a long line of mental imagery research (Betts 1909; Belardinelli et al. 2004, 2009; Madan and Singhal 2012a; Sheehan et al. 1967). Sport psychologists have focused on the potential multisensory nature of the imagery experience and have defined it as "a symbolic sensory experience that may occur in any sensory mode" (Hardy, Jones, and Gould 1996, 28). This contrasts with the emphasis on imagery as a representation by cognitive scientists. For instance, Wraga and Kosslyn (2002) describe it as "an internal representation that gives rise to the experience of perception in the absence of the appropriate sensory input" (466).

The above debate, whether imagery is conceptualized as a *quasi-perceptual phenomenological experience* or as a *mental representation,* was central to it becoming a legitimate area of study in the zeitgeist (Cornoldi and De Beni 2012). The complex and ephemeral nature of phenomenological accounts of imagery led to imagery being a neglected topic of study during the era of behaviorism. Even within the cognitive revolution, the topic generated a controversy that became known as the imagery debate (see Pylyshyn 2002). While the focus of the neuroscience research conducted by Stephen Kosslyn and other proponents of the analogical account of imagery was on the nature of the representation underlying visual imagery experiences (Kosslyn, Thompson, and Ganis 2006), motor imagery was also central to the illumination of the construct. This latter concern with action and imagery opened a window for the exploration of embodied cognition perspectives. Before we address the embodied nature of these representations, it is worthwhile to ascertain what precisely we mean by the term *motor imagery* and to evaluate whether there is agreement among researchers with regard to operational definitions of the term.

2.1 What Is Motor Imagery?

William James neatly summed up the embodied complexity of motor imagery when he wrote that "every representation of a movement awakens in some degree the actual movement" (1890, 526). Consequently, one can infer that, within the mental imagery construct, "motor imagery" refers to the mental representation of an action without engaging in its actual execution (Madan and Singhal 2012b; Moran et al. 2012). Again, we are confronted with a disembodied account of motor imagery. And the entropy only increases, as motor imagery typically occurs in conjunction with visual imagery, for example, rather than in isolation. On the other hand, visual imagery is commonly reported without other senses (Kosslyn et al. 1990). The interaction between visual and motor imagery only blurs the conceptual clarity further.

2.2 Is Motor Imagery *Limited* by Visual Imagery Perspective?

The dual visual viewpoint that one can adopt during imagery (whether first- or third-person) led to findings in which it was assumed that motor imagery was limited to an egocentric or first-person viewpoint (see Moran et al. 2012). This artifact, in which visual perspective during imagery was conflated with the presence or absence of motor imagery, created further confusion among researchers. Moran et al. (2012) refer to this issue as the "limited perspective problem." Only in recent decades have researchers reconciled this issue, as both neuroscience evidence (Fourkas, Ionta, and Aglioti 2006) and phenomenological studies with elite performers has confirmed the possibility of motor imagery from a third-person perspective or allocentric viewpoint (Callow and Roberts 2010; Moran and MacIntyre 1998).

Thus the definitional dilemma erroneously linked to visual perspective has been averted to some degree (Moran et al. 2012). One definition provides further clarity by specifying that motor imagery is a dynamic mental state during which the representation of a given motor act or movement is rehearsed in working memory without any overt motor output (Guillot and Collet 2010). The term *overt motor output* is used to highlight that it's not the absence of movement per se but the activation at the muscular level that should be absent. For example, gripping a basketball in your hand while standing on the free-throw line will entail a degree of motor activation (e.g., postural activation, isometric force to grip the ball, and so on) even without any *overt movement.* One may expect that this increased level of conceptual clarity provides a solution for researchers and practitioners alike. However, William James wasn't wrong when he suggested that mental imagery of movement *awakens* to some extent the *actual movement*. This *contamination* of a cognitive simulation technique by motor processes, as we discuss later, has been termed *quasi-movements* by Nikulin et al. (2008) and is central to the argument in this paper that motor imagery is a construct highly relevant in advancing our accounts of grounded cognition.

3 Movement in Measurement Research

Since William James's (1890) early treatise, in which he discussed the nature of individual differences in imagery, the topic of mental imagery had been hampered in its quest for legitimacy until an innovation in imagery measurement by Shepard and Metzler (1971). They devised the mental rotation paradigm, which was an implicit objective measure of what had been previously viewed only as a subjective experience impenetrable to rigorous measurement. Briefly, mental rotation involves the comparison of two 3-D block figure objects, which are presented in different orientations. To compare whether the two objects match, it was hypothesized that participants would *mentally rotate* one object to see if matched the criterion object. Response times increased linearly with increased differences in angular disparity. In other words, a second-order isomorphism existed, in that physical properties of objects influenced our operations on them in our mental world. Interestingly, "kinesthetic" sensations appeared to be present during mental rotation for some subjects, according to Jackie Metzler (coauthor with Roger Shepard, 1971). So visual imagery investigations were recognized as potentially involving the *motor* system. Kosslyn and Sussman later argued that "visual mental images are transformed in part via motor processes" (1995, 345). If this were the case, it would have implications for studies that were concerned with the localization of mental rotation processes at a neural level.

One question that emerged was whether the involvement of motor processes in mental rotation was due to a voluntary strategy adopted by participants. A subsequent neural study employed positron emission tomography (PET) while subjects mentally rotated either their hands or the original 3-D block objects (Kosslyn et al. 1998; also see Ganis et al. 2000). The results highlighted that two mechanisms could be applied: "one mechanism that recruits processes that prepare motor movements and another that does not" (Kosslyn et al. 1998, 151; also see Madan and Singhal 2012a). Was this a case of embodied cognition? Again we turn to a mental rotation study comparing animate versus inanimate stimuli for answers. Kosslyn et al. (2001) had subjects engage in a familiarization training condition prior to the mental rotation experiment. Participants viewed a 3-D block object being moved by an electric motor (exogenous force) or, in the alternative condition, were required to twist the object with their right hand to orient it (endogenous force).

The familiarization process influenced the strategy adopted by participants in the study, and only in the latter condition (endogenous force) was the primary motor cortex activated. Recent studies have also examined mental rotation of human figures, with results indicating an effect of embodiment (Madan and Singhal 2012c, 2014, 2015). These finding provided tentative evidence for grounded cognition in action simulation, a conclusion that became stronger as further empirical evidence to demonstrate that motor imagery was grounded in the physical experiences of the imager accumulated. The theoretical backdrop to these findings is now discussed in advance of the evaluation of the recent empirical evidence.

3.1 From Ideomotor Theory to Motor Cognition

William James had expounded on *ideomotor* theory, which he remarked "combined the driving force of a dominant idea with the resulting involuntary motor activity" (1890). This concept resonates clearly with the thrust of the current theoretical accounts from simulation theory. In the past two decades, a new domain of study called "motor cognition" has emerged (Jeannerod 1994, 2006). This field of study explores how the mind plans, simulates, and produces goal-directed movements. Specifically, it is concerned with the "preparation and production of actions as well as the processes involved in recognizing, anticipating, predicting and interpreting the actions of others" (Jackson and Decety 2004, 259).

An important distinction is made between the terms *movement* and *action*. "Action" is posited to have both covert stages (action simulation including motor imagery) and overt stages (movement execution), and movement related to when the activation leads to the displacement of a limb in space (i.e., proximal or distal). Within this approach, motor imagery is predicted to be functionally equivalent to action because it has been shown to share common neurological mechanisms, and information is processed in comparable ways. The discovery of mirror neurons stimulated research on the neural basis of action representations (Rizzolatti, Fogassi, and Gallese 2001).

According to Jeannerod (2006), the action continuum predicts that the difference between the simulation of an action and its executed counterpart is one of degree and not one of kind. Consequently, the continuum posits that at one end of the spectrum is an action representation and at the other end is intentional movement. This conceptualization, although not without criticism (Gallese and Sinigaglia 2011; Glover and Baran 2017) is of particular interest from an embodied cognition perspective, and it has implications for psychological science and applied psychology.

3.2 Is Motor Imagery Uncoupled from Action?

The motor cognition paradigm undoubtedly returns the study of action to psychology (Moran et al. 2012; MacIntyre et al. 2013). In addition, the motor cognition account questions the artificial decoupling of motor imagery from movement by providing an action spectrum encompassing imagery and motor execution. Traditionally, imagery, by definition, occurred in the absence of movement. Empirical evidence and practice-based evidence have questioned this decoupling. For example, at least one contemporary model of imagery in athletes postulates that movement *is* possible during imagined action (Holmes and Collins 2001). We now focus our attention on this issue.

Morris, Spittle, and Watt (2005), in their monograph on the topic of imagery in sport, state that imagery "may be considered as the creation or re-creation of an experience generated from memorial information, involving quasi-sensorial, quasi-perceptual and quasi-affective characteristics, that is under the volitional control of the imager, and which *may* occur in the absence of the real stimulus antecedents normally associated with the actual experience" (19, emphasis added). This definition retains key elements of traditional definitions (e.g., multisensory, conscious experience) but is novel in that it includes the possibility that imagery and action may co-occur.

The traditional definitions of mental imagery presuppose that the simulation occurs in the absence of actual perception or movement execution. However, as we discovered with motor imagery in mental rotation, the complexity of these processes means they are not easily dissociable. In the visual imagery literature, for example, it has been suggested that there is no such thing as immaculate perception (Kosslyn and Sussman 1995). Thus, visual imagery was seen to be central to perception in providing top-down knowledge that influenced our visual recognition abilities. Indeed, early studies by Perky (1910) attempted to answer the question of the role of imagery in perceptual recognition by projecting a faint illustration of objects during imagery of either congruent or incongruent objects. While debate over the methods continues, the principle that imagery can facilitate visual recognition processes remains.

In the motor context, *quasi-movements*—a term used by Nikulin et al. (2008) to describe volitional movements that are suppressed during motor imagery and thus are neither movement execution nor motor imagery per se—have been recorded. The inhibition of such movements is integral to motor imagery processes (Guillot et al. 2012), and these movements are described as part of what has been termed *dynamic imagery* (MacIntyre and Moran 2010). Again, by definition, motor imagery is said to occur in the absence of any overt movement or motor output (Guillot and Collet 2010). However, on the basis that athletes often engage in movements while engaging in imagery, sport psychologists have recommended that performers apply *dynamic imagery* in their imagery practice (Holmes and Collins 2001). Researchers had noted that athletes engaged in either *synchronous movements* (e.g., moving the appropriate limbs to simulate the executed skill) or *asynchronous movements* (e.g., other movements in which, for example, their hand may simulate the carving movement of a surfboard) during imagery (MacIntyre and Moran 2010). Interestingly, a broad definition of mental imagery encompasses coactivation of simulation and motor execution processes to account for dynamic imagery (Morris, Spittle, and Watt 2005).

A number of studies within sport psychology suggest that motor imagery is superior to visual imagery in improving athlete's performance (Driskell, Copper, and Moran 1994). Guillot, Moschberger, and Collet (2013) conducted a study with twelve elite high-jump athletes to test the hypothesis that movement during imagery would enhance the participants' imagery. Their measure was temporal accuracy—the comparison between duration of simulation and motor execution of the run-up jump and landing for dynamic imagery and motionless imagery. They reported a significant difference between imagery and actual times when participants performed motionless imagery. In contrast, they achieved temporal congruence during dynamic imagery. Furthermore, ratings on the quality of their imagery supported previous quasi-experimental findings (Callow, Roberts, and Fawkes 2006) and qualitative reports. For instance, in another study. one elite-level canoe-slalom competitor explained, "It can help … if you move your arms in a similar motion as you're going to move them in the boat, it can help with the timing a little bit more and you can sort of feel how you're anticipating" (MacIntyre and Moran 2007). While one can tentatively conclude that the evidence suggests athletes find this beneficial, it requires further study.

The implications of these findings go beyond the performance-enhancement role, however, and question the traditional definitions of motor imagery as occurring without *any* overt motor output. Jeannerod's (1994, 2006) action-simulation model proposes that imagery processes are involved in motor planning (covert process), and this enables the off-line simulation of action. As noted earlier, motor imagery is part of the action spectrum, with other simulation activities on this spectrum including *shadow shots* (e.g., a low-amplitude post-execution practice swing) and *action-observation*, which have varying degrees of motor activation, potential for motor output, and visual cognition. As we shall see later in this chapter, sport experts have demonstrated specific metacognitive expertise that enables them to control and manage their action-simulation processes. These expertise effects have consequences for our future research directions. First, we should consider the breadth of evidence supporting the grounded cognition approach within motor imagery research.

Ionta et al. (2012) reported that variations in the hand position of participants during mental rotations tasks influenced the latencies for congruent stimuli. They concluded that sensorimotor and postural information coming from the body might influence mental rotation of body parts according to specific, somatotopic rules. These preliminary findings were congruent with the *body-specificity hypothesis*, which claims that body-specific patterns of motor experience shape the way we think (Casasanto 2011, 2014). An interesting study tested this same concept of the *body-specificity hypothesis* using the mental travel paradigm. Body position was controlled across different conditions to be either congruent or incongruent with the action (e.g., standing: congruent with walking; sitting: incongruent with walking), and the duration of the motor imagery was compared across the conditions (Saimpont et al. 2012). Using both elderly and youth samples, the researchers reported that simulation times in the congruent (standing) position were closer to actual walking times, and this effect appeared to be maintained across the lifespan. Furthermore, research by Ionta and colleagues (2013) has provided evidence that motor constraints—for example, anatomically plausible versus illusory posture—affects the mental rotation of body parts. Imagery of heavy objects has been demonstrated to increase the duration of response times relative to motor imagery of lighter objects (Ionta et al. 2012). Furthermore, future findings from this line of inquiry may have ramifications for the recent accounts of embodiment and cognition (Borghi and Cimatti 2010; Gallese and Sinigaglia 2011).

Providing further evidence that cognition is embodied, rather than merely being fully explained by an information-processing approach, is a range of findings that demonstrate an interaction between motor and cognitive processes. For example, Gentilucci and Gangitano (1998) demonstrated this directly, wherein people differentially reached toward blocks that had the words "long" and "short" printed on them. Specifically, peak reaching acceleration, velocity, and deceleration were higher for the "long" block, even though the two blocks were identical in physical dimensions. Similarly, Gentilucci et al. (2000) observed differences in reaching toward blocks that had the words "near" and "far" printed on them, but not in a control condition in which the words on the block were unrelated to motor actions. Glover et al. (2004) demonstrated that these effects of language on motor actions are not constrained to words directly related to motor actions, but that words representing the names of relatively large and small graspable objects (e.g., "apple" and "grape," respectively) can influence peak grip aperture. These differences provide evidence that cognitive processes can influence overt motor execution. Functional properties of objects represented by words and images have been shown to influence later memory (Madan and Singhal 2012c) and have been associated with automatic motor simulations (Madan, Chen, and Singhal 2016).

4 What Can We Learn from Experts?

Individual differences in imagery abilities have been acknowledged by researchers since the time of Galton (1880). Evidence for consistent differences in imagery abilities related to sporting expertise has emerged (Milton et al. 2007). For example, studies with elite performers have indicated that they have more advanced imagery abilities than their non-elite counterparts (MacIntyre et al. 2013; MacIntyre and Moran 2010). This also includes metacognitive knowledge (Dunlosky and Metcalfe 2009) or, more specifically, meta-imagery, which is athletes' knowledge of, and control over, their own mental imagery skills and experiences (Moran 2002). Imagery ability is a moderating variable in the mental practice effect (Driskell, Copper, and Moran 1994). In other words, those with greater proficiency on imagery ability tests gain more from mental practice than their less-proficient counterparts. This may be due to more experienced performers having a more accurate representation of their movement. For example, a novice may not have knowledge about the grip, stance, and target area during mental practice of a free throw and thus may gain little from the rehearsal. Mental travel research, in which the duration of simulated and executed motor skills are compared, also supports expertise effects (Guillot and Collet 2008). Not surprisingly, numerous studies have shown motor imagery ability to be a promising indicator of an athlete's success (Madan and Singhal 2012a).

The aforementioned expertise effects provided an impetus for motor cognition researchers to explore the natural laboratory of sport. This emphasis on investigating the abilities of experts has been termed the *strength-based approach* (MacIntyre et al. 2013). It augments the prototypical *deficit-based approach*, which comprised both patients and healthy subjects and may have overlooked the potential for unique insights from those who are highly skilled on imagery ability measures. Rather than replacing traditional paradigms, this approach simply widens the net based on specific criterion for expertise (MacIntyre et al. 2013). The strength-based approach isn't simply preselecting athlete samples or those who excel on a task. It includes those who demonstrate specialist learning and abilities.

One such example is the patient IW, who suffered from chronic deafferentation and had been a participant in over two decades of research. A recent case study with the patient IW used mental rotation of animate versus inanimate stimuli to investigate if his imagery abilities reflected his impaired motor system (Horst et al. 2012). The authors reported that IW's motor imagery processes were impaired but that visual imagery processes were enhanced compared with controls. This relative expertise is important to recognize, as in this case it helped the patient overcome the fundamental challenge to his motor system by developing his visual imagery ability.

Similarly, much is still to be learned from the comparison of patient and non-patient groups, as recent mental travel research has demonstrated (Fusco et al. 2014, 2016). The implications of research using the strength-based approach are even greater for those engaged in performance domains, for example, participants in elite sport (Beilock 2008; MacIntyre et al. 2013) and professional dance (Bläsing, Puttke, and Schack 2010; Calvo-Merino et al. 2005, 2006: Nordin and Cumming 2005). A potential bidirectional benefit may occur from research insights with these participants, as not only may theories be tested but, moreover, knowledge that may benefit performance also may arise from such research (Cappuccio 2015).

5 Five Questions to Be Answered

5.1 To What Extent Is Our Knowledge Constrained by Neural Operations That Embody Previous Actions and Experiences?

Those with extensive motor skill experience in a particular domain should represent information in that domain quite differently than those without such experiences, even when there is no intention to act. Is motor imagery grounded in our prior experiences? Tentative evidence suggests that this is the case with regard to expert-novice differences (Jansen and Lehmann 2013; Olsson and Nyberg 2012). Expertise effects among mental imagery abilities have been demonstrated among dancers (Bläsing, Puttke, and Schack 2010). Furthermore, Olsson and Nyberg (2012), in their comparative study of a wheelchair athlete and a control sample, used fMRI of motor imagery of stair walking and wheelchair slalom to show that only tasks that we have physical experience of recruit the motor system. More recently, Jansen and Lehmann (2013), in a mental rotation study, reported higher mental rotation accuracy for human figures compared to cubed figures for athletic samples compared to non-athletes. They concluded that their study added to the literature of the coupling of perception and action and deserves further attention in the literature on embodied cognition. They recommended taking consideration of prior expertise in body representation in future investigations of the extent to which cognitive processes are rooted in the body and its interaction with the world.

One question for researchers is whether we need to measure movement abilities to study motor imagery. It may be necessary not only to account for current body posture during a motor imagery protocol but also to evaluate participant abilities for specific movements. For example, if exploring golfers' expertise, it may be useful to measure their putting ability and consistency prior to a study on simulated putting (MacIntyre et al. 2013). This may be of particular interest in illuminating our understanding of the developmental trajectory of cognitive abilities, including motor imagery, that may be influenced by developmental milestones in motor capacity (Gabbard 2013).

5.2 Can Measures of Imagery Ability Be Used to Advance Our Understanding of Embodied Cognition?

As a complementary approach to manipulating motor imagery within a cognitive task, inter-individual ability can be evaluated using questionnaires. The most common questionnaires of motor imagery ability were inspired by the Vividness of Visual Imagery Questionnaire (VVIQ) (Marks 1973), which asked participants to imagine a visual scene and then to judge the vividness of the imagery on a Likert scale. The related motor imagery questionnaires are the Vividness of Movement Imagery Questionnaire (VMIQ) (Isaac, Marks, and Russell 1986; also see Roberts et al. 2008) and the Movement Imagery Questionnaire (MIQ) (Hall and Pongrac 1983; Hall, Pongrac, and Buckholz 1985; also see Gregg, Hall, and Butler 2010). Eton, Gilner, and Munz (1998) found that the VMIQ, but not the VVIQ, differed between athletes and nonathletes. Furthermore, VMIQ scores were significantly correlated with self-assessments of imagery use (e.g., "Do you use mental imagery to enhance sport performance?"). Unfortunately, because these questionnaires are subjective, non-imagery factors may also influence responses. For instance, participants may calibrate their vividness responses to be consistent with their own views of their deliberate use of motor imagery and motor skills.

As an alternative approach, objective measures of motor imagery—in which there is a correct response, rather than a subjective Likert scale—may provide a less biased assessment of the role of motor imagery in sports. One such measure is the Test of Ability in Movement Imagery (TAMI) (Madan and Singhal 2013, 2014). In the TAMI, participants are instructed to imagine a series of five movement instructions that manipulate the head, arm/hand, torso, or leg/foot. After reading the instructions, participants flip to the response page and must select from a set of five body-positioning images, along with the options "none of the above" and "unclear." The TAMI consists of ten questions, preceded by a practice question.

The TAMI was further refined to a weighted-scoring procedure, wherein more difficult questions are weighted more heavily, specifically to improve sensitivity for use with athlete populations (Madan and Singhal 2014). The general procedure of the TAMI was inspired by the Controllability of Motor Imagery Test (CMI) (Nishida et al. 1986). There are a variety of motor imagery tests, and consideration is needed when determining which may be the most appropriate measure for a given research question. For instance, while it is well known that there are sex differences in the mental rotations test (Parsons 1987; Peters et al. 1995; Voyer 2011), sex differences were not found in the TAMI (Madan and Singhal 2015). The literature contains many useful measures of inter-individual ability in motor imagery, including some designed specifically within the domain of sport psychology. Careful consideration is necessary when selecting the appropriate measures (both subjective and objective) for evaluating imagery ability, and future research is necessary to understand how these imagery questionnaires relate to extant approaches for studying embodied cognition.

5.3 Can Motor Imagery and Embodied Cognition Provide a Portal into Our Emotional State?

Previously researchers have utilized embodied cognition perspectives to elucidate our understanding of choking behavior in sport (Beilock 2008; Cappuccio 2015; see also Montero, Toner, and Moran, this volume). Interestingly, recent research has demonstrated that motor retardation, a symptom of depression, is also evident during motor imagery tasks (Chen et al. 2013). To explain, a slowdown in motor execution has been reported in mental rotation studies that compared differences between the response times for two sets of stimuli. Briefly, in a study with patients with unipolar depression, their mental rotation of animate stimuli reflected slower reaction times in comparison with the latencies for another condition that used inanimate stimuli (e.g., block objects). This raises an interesting question for researchers: Does this impairment reflect our negative emotional state through embodied cognition? Evidence for these effects are accumulating (Bennabi et al. 2014), but research is required with those with less-profound emotional distress to explore whether our action system and simulation processes convey mood disturbances across the spectrum (i.e., positive and negative mood). For example, injured athletes compared with those in flow state may differ vastly both in their emotional state and their ability to react to stimuli; the possibility of developing implicit measures of mood state from motor imagery research remains.

5.4 Can Embodied Cognition Perspectives Help Optimize Injury Recovery and Rehabilitation?

Mental imagery more broadly and, indeed, motor imagery have been widely recommended as interventions for injury recovery for athletes (Callow and Roberts 2010; Driediger, Hall, and Callow 2006). The psychological consequences of sport injury are often profound, with psychological distress commonly reported (Brewer 2010). For example, in a qualitative study with injured athletes, Driediger, Hall, and Callow (2006) reported that athletes experienced negative or debilitative images (e.g., imagining failing to return to play). This type of imagery may increase athletes' fear of reinjury and provide a significant obstacle in their return to play by reducing their adherence to rehabilitation protocols. Thus it is paramount that, if an imagery intervention is employed, specific recommendations are followed to enhance the psychological recovery (i.e., reduce fear of reinjury). Limited evidence supports mental imagery being applied as a global recovery strategy, as individual differences in imagery ability, among other factors, should be considered. Imagery rescripting (reediting the imagery to ensure it's facilitative) offers a promising therapeutic strategy that has been previously demonstrated among clinical patients (Holmes et al. 2015). It is necessary to develop specific protocols for performance enhancement to ensure the goals set are achieved. For example, McIsaac and Eich (2004) reported that traumatic images retrieved from a third-person perspective were experienced as less emotional than those retrieved from a first-person perspective. An interesting topic for study would be the evaluation of the relative efficacy of different perspectives (which may involve different levels of embodiment) in rescripting imagery interventions. Moreover, the role of prospective positive images (e.g., return to play) may be more valuable than simply using imagery of skill acquisition (Brewer 1994). For example, Baird, Smallwood, and Schooler (2011) found that positive constructive daydreaming tends to be future-oriented and that those with greater working memory assets are more likely to engage in future-oriented daydreaming. Thus, idle working memory resources are essential to adaptive, prospective daydreaming. Whereas retrospective mind wandering tends to be loosely related to personal goals, Baird, Smallwood, and Schooler (2011) conclude that spontaneous prospective thought is adaptive because it advances personally relevant goals, and embodied cognition may be central to elucidating our understanding of such daydreaming or spontaneous mental imagery (McMillan, Kaufman, and Singer 2013).

The implications for recovery from sport injury may also have consequences for those with impairments to their neural function (e.g., stroke patients). Motor imagery has been employed in stroke rehabilitation with varying degrees of success (Grangeon et al. 2012). A greater understanding of the role of embodiment in cognition undoubtedly has implications for the application of mental imagery as an injury-recovery strategy and rehabilitation strategy.

5.5 Does Our Perception of Our Environment Have Implications for Our Cognition and Emotional State?

Adams and Galinsky (2012) proposed the concept of *enclothed cognition* to illustrate the interaction between what we wear and our cognition. They posited that the term *enclothed cognition* encompassed "the effects of clothing on people's psychological processes" which "depend on both a) the symbolic meaning of the clothes and b) whether people are actually wearing the clothes" (919). The broader environment may indeed have a wider influence on our cognition than has been previously thought. For example, exercise and physical activity in natural spaces—what has been termed *green exercise*—has distinct effects on our attentional capacity and emotions (Barton and Pretty 2010). Emerging evidence suggests that even rambling on a forest trail can enhance working memory capacity (a process called *attention restoration*; e.g., Kaplan 1995) relative to the similar physical activity in an urban setting. The differences between urban and rural settings are potentially substantial in terms of visual stimuli, social factors (i.e., whether solitary or social activity), and environmental factors like air pollution and noise, but other factors may also be at play here. Walking is a complex motor behavior with a special relevance in social interactions (for review, see Pavlova 2012). By observing walking, people can extract a considerable amount of information, including emotional states and intentions of the agent (Dalla Volta et al. 2015). Natural environments provide a rich sensory experience, often without the threat (e.g., crime) or risk (e.g., traffic) obvious in other settings. Walking supports various psychological mechanisms for reconciliation, including creativity, locomotion motivation, and embodied notions of forward progress (Webb, Rossignac-Milon, and Higgins 2017). Another possibility is that the vividness of our memories of these natural experiences (e.g., walk along a beach), mediated by embodied cognition, provides a multisensory episodic procedural memory that gives green exercise its *sticky behavior effect* (i.e., increased adherence and higher propensity for future engagement). Embodied cognition should be considered a worthy framework from which to investigate green exercise and other nature-based solutions for well-being.

6 Conclusion

One commonality between embodied cognition and motor imagery is their long past in philosophical discourse but relatively short empirical history within psychology. Nevertheless, criticism still abounds, and scientific debate is seldom far from both imagery (Madan and Singal 2012a; Pylyshyn 2002) and embodied cognition (Gallese and Sinigaglia 2011; Glenberg 2015; Mahon and Caramazza 2008). Nevertheless, a notable benefit of the shared interest in these topics from psychologists (including practitioners), neuroscientists, and philosophers is the potential synergies that arise from the interdisciplinary discourse. This arguably will develop new avenues of research with the potential to create more comprehensive understanding of the human mind (Denis 2012). It is possible that transdisciplinary approaches will emerge from the fusion of research questions from both paradigms. As Stock and Stock (2004) noted in their historical review of ideomotor theory, we should not forget to learn from its past. It is apparent that William James's research, which expounded on the confluence of action and motor imagery, has finally come of age.

References

Adam, H., and A. D. Galinsky. 2012. "Enclothed Cognition." *Journal of Experimental Social Psychology* 48 (4): 918–925. http://dx.doi.org/10.1016/j.jesp.2012.02.008.

Adams, Jack A. 1987. "Historical Review and Appraisal of Research on the Learning, Retention, and Transfer of Human Motor Skills." *Psychological Bulletin* 101 (1): 41–74. doi:10.1037//0033-2909.101.1.41.

Arora, Sonal, Rajesh Aggarwal, Pramudith Sirimanna, Aidan Moran, Teodor Grantcharov, Roger Kneebone, Nick Sevdalis, and Ara Darzi. 2011. "Mental Practice Enhances Surgical Technical Skills: A Randomized Controlled Study." *Obstetrical and Gynecological Survey* 66 (6): 336–338. doi:10.1097/ogx.0b013e31822c17e1.

Baird, B., J. Smallwood, and J. W. Schooler. 2011. "Back to the Future: Autobiographical Planning and the Functionality of Mind-Wandering." *Conscious and Cognition* 20:1604–1611. doi: 10.1016/j.concog.2011.08.007

Barsalou, Lawrence W. 2008. "Grounded Cognition." *Annual Review of Psychology* 59:617–645.

Bartlett, Frederic. 1932. *Remembering: A Study in Experimental and Social Psychology*. Cambridge: Cambridge University Press.

Barton, Jo, and Jules Pretty. 2010. "What Is the Best Dose of Nature and Green Exercise for Improving Mental Health? A Multi-Study Analysis." *Environmental Science and Technology* 44 (10): 3947–3955.

Beilock, Sian L. 2008. "Beyond the Playing Field: Sport Psychology Meets Embodied Cognition." *International Review of Sport and Exercise Psychology* 1 (1): 19–30. doi:10.1080/17509840701836875.

Belardinelli, Marta Olivetti, Rosalia Di Matteo, Cosimo Del Gratta, Andrea De Nicola, Antonio Ferretti, Armando Tartaro, Lorenzo Bonomo, and Gian Luca Romani. 2004. "Intermodal Sensory Image Generation: An fMRI Analysis." *European Journal of Cognitive Psychology* 16 (5): 729–752. doi:10.1080/09541440340000493.

Belardinelli, M. Olivetti, M. Palmiero, C. Sestieri, D. Nardo, R. Di Matteo, A. Londei, A. D'Ausilio, A. Ferretti, C. Del Gratta, and G. L. Romani. 2009. "An fMRI Investigation on Image Generation in Different Sensory Modalities: The Influence of Vividness." *Acta Psychologica* 132 (2): 190–200. doi:10.1016/j.actpsy.2009.06.009.

Bennabi, Djamila, Julie Monnin, Emmanuel Haffen, Nicolas Carvalho, Pierre Vandel, Thierry Pozzo, and Charalambos Papaxanthis. 2014. "Motor Imagery in Unipolar Major Depression." *Frontiers in Behavioral Neuroscience* 8 (December): 413. doi:10.3389/fnbeh.2014.00413.

Bergen, Benjamin K. 2012. *Louder than Words: The New Science of How the Mind Makes Meaning*. New York: Basic Books.

Betts, George Herbert. 1909. *The Distribution and Functions of Mental Imagery*. New York: Teachers College, Columbia University.

Bläsing, Bettina, Martin Puttke, and Thomas Schack. 2010. *The Neurocognition of Dance: Mind, Movement and Motor Skills*. London: Psychology Press.

Borghi, Anna M., and Felice Cimatti. 2010. "Embodied Cognition and Beyond: Acting and Sensing the Body." *Neuropsychologia* 48 (3): 763–773. doi:10.1016/j.neuropsychologia.2009.10.02.

Borghi, Anna M., and Diane Pecher. 2011. "Introduction to the Special Topic: Embodied and Grounded Cognition." *Frontiers in Psychology* 2 (August): 187. doi:10.3389/fpsyg.2011.00187.

Borghi, Anna M., Claudia Scorolli, Daniele Caligiore, Gianluca Baldassarre, and Luca Tummolini. 2013. "The Embodied Mind Extended: Using Words as Social Tools." *Frontiers in Psychology* 4 (May): 214. doi:10.3389/fpsyg.2013.00214.

Brewer, Britton W. 1994. "Review and Critique of Models of Psychological Adjustment to Athletic Injury." *Journal of Applied Sport Psychology* 6:87–100.

Brewer, Britton W. 2010. "The Role of Psychological Factors in Sport Injury Rehabilitation Outcomes." *International Review of Sport and Exercise Psychology* 3 (1): 40–61. doi:10.1080/17509840903301207.

Bufalari, I., A. Sforza, P. Cesari, S. M. Aglioti, and A. D. Fourkas. 2010. "Motor Imagery beyond the Joint Limits: A Transcranial Magnetic Stimulation Study." *Biological Psychology* 85 (2): 283–290. doi:10.1016/j.biopsycho.2010.07.015.

Callow, Nichola, and Ross Roberts. 2010. "Imagery Research: An Investigation of Three Issues." *Psychology of Sport and Exercise* 11 (4): 325–329. doi:10.1016/j.psychsport.2010.03.002.

Callow, Nichola, Ross Roberts, and Joanna Z. Fawkes. 2006. "Effects of Dynamic and Static Imagery on Vividness of Imagery, Skiing Performance, and Confidence." *Journal of Imagery Research in Sport and Physical Activity* 1 (1). doi:10.2202/1932-0191.1001.

Calvo, Paco, and Toni Gomila. 2008. *Handbook of Cognitive Science: An Embodied Approach*. Amsterdam: Elsevier Science.

Calvo-Merino, B., D. E. Glaser, J. Grèzes, R. E. Passingham, and P. Haggard. 2005. "Action Observation and Acquired Motor Skills: An FMRI Study with Expert Dancers." *Cerebral Cortex* 15 (8): 1243–1249. doi:10.1093/cercor/bhi007.

Calvo-Merino, Beatriz, Julie Grèzes, Daniel E. Glaser, Richard E. Passingham, and Patrick Haggard. 2006. "Seeing or Doing? Influence of Visual and Motor Familiarity in Action Observation." *Current Biology* 16 (22): 2277. doi:10.1016/j.cub.2006.10.065.

Cappuccio, Massimiliano L. 2015. "Introduction: When Embodied Cognition and Sport Psychology Team-Up." *Phenomenology and the Cognitive Sciences* 14 (2): 213–225. doi:10.1007/s11097-015-9415-1.

Casasanto, Daniel. 2011. "Different Bodies, Different Minds." *Current Directions in Psychological Science* 20 (6): 378–383. doi:10.1177/0963721411422058.

Casasanto, Daniel. 2014. "Bodily Relativity." In *Routledge Handbook of Embodied Cognition*, edited by L. Shapiro, 108–117. London: Routledge.

Chen, J., L. Q. Yang, Z. J. Zhang, W. T. Ma, X. Q. Wu, Zhang X. R., D. H. Wei, et al. 2013. "The Association between the Disruption of Motor Imagery and the Number of Depressive Episodes of Major Depression." *Journal of Affective Disorder* 150 (2): 337–343. doi:10.1016/j.jad.2013.04.015.

Cornoldi, C., and R. De Beni. 2012. "Foreword." In *Essays in Honour of Michel Denis: From Mental Imagery to Spatial Cognition and Language*, edited by V. Gyselinck and F. Pazzaglia, ix–x. Sussex: Psychology Press.

Dalla Volta, Riccardo, Fabrizio Fasano, Antonio Cerasa, Graziella Mangone, Aldo Quattrone, and Giovanni Buccino. 2015. "Walking Indoors, Walking Outdoors: An fMRI Study." *Frontiers in Psychology* 6 (October): 1502. doi:10.3389/fpsyg.2015.01502.

De Lange, Floris P., Karin Roelofs, and Ivan Toni. 2008. "Motor Imagery: A Window into the Mechanisms and Alterations of the Motor System." *Cortex* 44 (5): 494–506. doi:10.1016/j.cortex.2007.09.002.

Denis, Michel. 2012. "Decades of Images: Reminiscences of a Shared Scientific Journey." In *Essays in Honour of Michel Denis: From Mental Imagery to Spatial Cognition and Language*, edited by V. Gyselinck and F. Pazzaglia, 203–244. Sussex: Psychology Press.

Driediger, Molly, Craig Hall, and Nichola Callow. 2006. "Imagery Use by Injured Athletes: A Qualitative Analysis." *Journal of Sports Sciences* 24 (3): 261–272. doi:10.1080/02640410500128221.

Driskell, James E., Carolyn Copper, and Aidan Moran. 1994. "Does Mental Practice Enhance Performance?" *Journal of Applied Psychology* 79 (4): 481–492. doi:10.1037//0021-9010.79.4.481.

Dunlosky, J., and J. Metcalfe, eds. 2009. *Metacognition: A Textbook of Cognition, Educational, Life Span, and Applied Psychology*. Thousand Oaks, CA: Sage.

Eton, D. T., F. H. Gilner, and D. C. Munz. 1998. "The Measurement of Imagery Vividness: A Test of the Reliability and Validity of the Vividness of Visual Imagery Questionnaire and the Vividness of Movement Imagery Questionnaire." *Journal of Mental Imagery* 22:125–136.

Fourkas, Alissa D., Silvio Ionta, and Salvatore M. Aglioti. 2006. "Influence of Imagined Posture and Imagery Modality on Corticospinal Excitability." *Behavioural Brain Research* 168 (2): 190–196. doi:10.1016/j.bbr.2005.10.015.

Fusco, Augusto, Maria Chiara Gallotta, Marco Iosa, Giovanni Morone, Luigi Iasevoli, Domenica Trifoglio, Vincenzo Maria Saraceni, Stefano Paolucci, Carlo Baldari, and Laura Guidetti. 2016. "The Dynamic Motor Imagery of Locomotion Is Task-Dependent in Patients with Stroke." *Restorative Neurology and Neuroscience* 34 (2): 247–256. doi:10.3233/rnn-150573.

Fusco, Augusto, Marco Iosa, Maria Chiara Gallotta, Stefano Paolucci, Carlo Baldari, and Laura Guidetti. 2014. "Different Performances in Static and Dynamic Imagery and Real Locomotion:

An Exploratory Trial." *Frontiers in Human Neuroscience* 8 (October): 760. doi:10.3389/fnhum.2014.00760.

Gabbard, Carl. 2013. "The Role of Mental Simulation in Embodied Cognition." *Early Child Development and Care* 183 (5): 643–650. http://dx.doi.org/10.1080/03004430.2012.681649.

Gallese, Vittorio, and Corrado Sinigaglia. 2011. "What Is So Special about Embodied Simulation?" *Trends in Cognitive Sciences* 15 (11): 512–519. doi:10.1016/j.tics.2011.09.003.

Galton, Francis. 1880. "Statistics of Mental Imagery." *Mind* 19:301–318.

Ganis, G., J. P. Keenan, S. M. Kosslyn, and A. Pascual-Leone. 2000. "Transcranial Magnetic Stimulation of Primary Motor Cortex Affects Mental Rotation." *Cerebral Cortex* 10 (2): 175–180. doi:10.1093/cercor/10.2.175.

Gentilucci, M., F. Benuzzi, L. Bertolani, E. Daprati, and M. Gangitano. 2000. "Language and Motor Control." *Experimental Brain Research* 133 (4): 468–490. doi:10.1007/s002210000431.

Gentilucci, Maurizio, and Massimo Gangitano. 1998. "Influence of Automatic Word Reading on Motor Control." *European Journal of Neuroscience* 10 (2): 752–756. doi:10.1046/j.1460-9568.1998.00060.x.

Gibson, James J. 1979. *The Ecological Approach to Visual Perception*. Boston: Houghton Mifflin.

Glenberg, Arthur M. 2015. "Few Believe the World Is Flat: How Embodiment Is Changing the Scientific Understanding of Cognition." *Canadian Journal of Experimental Psychology / Revue Canadienne de Psychologie Experimentale* 69 (2): 165–171. doi:10.1037/cep0000056.

Glover, Scott. 2004. "Separate Visual Representations in the Planning and Control of Action." *Behavioral and Brain Sciences* 27 (1): 3–24; discussion 24–78.

Glover, Scott, and Marek Baran. 2017. "The Motor-Cognitive Model of Motor Imagery: Evidence from Timing Errors in Simulated Reaching and Grasping." *Journal of Experimental Psychology: Human Perception and Performance* 43 (7): 1359–1375. doi:10.1037/xhp0000389.

Goldinger, Stephen D., Megan H. Papesh, Anthony S. Barnhart, Whitney A. Hansen, and Michael C. Hout. 2016. "The Poverty of Embodied Cognition." *Psychonomic Bulletin and Review* 23 (4): 959–978.

Grangeon, M., P. Revol, A. Guillot, G. Rode, and C. Collet. 2012. "Could Motor Imagery Be Effective in Upper Limb Rehabilitation of Individuals with Spinal Cord Injury? A Case Study." *Spinal Cord* 50 (10): 766–771. doi:10.1038/sc.2012.41.

Gregg, M., C. Hall, and A. Butler. 2010. "The MIQ-RS: A Suitable Option for Examining Movement Imagery Ability." *Evidence-Based Complementary and Alternative Medicine(eCAM)* 7 (2): 249–257. http://doi.org/10.1093/ecam/nem170.

Guillot, Aymeric, and Christian Collet. 2008. "Construction of the Motor Imagery Integrative Model in Sport: A Review and Theoretical Investigation of Motor Imagery Use." *International Review of Sport and Exercise Psychology* 1 (1): 31–44. doi:10.1080/17509840701823139.

Guillot, Aymeric, and Christian Collet. 2010. *The Neurophysiological Foundations of Mental and Motor Imagery*. Oxford: Oxford University Press.

Guillot, Aymeric, Franck Di Rienzo, Tadhg Macintyre, Aidan Moran, and Christian Collet. 2012. "Imagining Is Not Doing but Involves Specific Motor Commands: A Review of Experimental Data Related to Motor Inhibition." *Frontiers in Human Neuroscience* 6. doi:10.3389/fnhum.2012.00247.

Guillot, Aymeric, Kevin Moschberger, and Christian Collet. 2013. "Coupling Movement with Imagery as a New Perspective for Motor Imagery Practice." *Behavioral and Brain Functions* 9 (February): 8. doi:10.1186/1744-9081-9-8.

Hall, C. R., J. Pongrac, and E. Buckolz. 1985. "The Measurement of Imagery Ability." *Human Movement Science* 4: 107–118.

Hall, Craig R., and J. Pongrac. 1983. Movement Imagery Questionnaire. In Craig Hall, John Pongrac, and Eric Buckholz, "The Measurement of Imagery Ability." *Human Movement Science* 4 (June 1985): 107–118. doi: 10.1016/0167-9457(85)90006-5.

Hardy, Lew, J. Graham Jones, and Daniel Gould. 1996. *Understanding Psychological Preparation for Sport: Theory and Practice of Elite Performers*. Chichester, UK: J. Wiley.

Holmes, Emily A., Lalitha Iyadurai, Gitta A. Jacob, and Susie Hales. 2015. "Mental Imagery in Psychological Disorders." In *Emerging Trends in the Social and Behavioral Sciences: An Interdisciplinary, Searchable, and Linkable Resource*, edited by Stephen M. Kosslyn, Robert A. Scott, and Marlis C. Buchmann, 1–15. Hoboken, NJ: John Wiley and Sons. doi:10.1002/9781118900772.etrds0216.

Holmes, Paul S., and David J. Collins. 2001. "The PETTLEP Approach to Motor Imagery: A Functional Equivalence Model for Sport Psychologists." *Journal of Applied Sport Psychology* 13:60–83.

Horst, Arjan C. Ter, Jonathan Cole, Rob van Lier, and Bert Steenbergen. 2012. "The Effect of Chronic Deafferentation on Mental Imagery: A Case Study." *PLoS ONE* 7 (8): e42742. doi:10.1371/journal.pone.0042742.

Ionta, Silvio, David Perruchoud, Bogdan Draganski, and Olaf Blanke. 2012. "Body Context and Posture Affect Mental Imagery of Hands." *PLoS ONE* 7 (3): e34382. doi:10.1371/journal.pone.0034382.

Ionta, Silvio, Anna Sforza, Mariko Funato, and Olaf Blanke. 2013. "Anatomically Plausible Illusory Posture Affects Mental Rotation of Body Parts." *Cognitive, Affective and Behavioral Neuroscience* 13 (1): 197–209. doi:10.3758/s13415-012-0120-z.

Isaac, Anne, David F. Marks, and David G. Russell. 1986. "An Instrument for Assessing Imagery of Movement: The Vividness of Movement Imagery Questionnaire (VMIQ)." *Journal of Mental Imagery* 10 (4): 23–30.

Jackson, Philip L., and Jean Decety. 2004. "Motor Cognition: A New Paradigm to Study Self-Other Interactions." *Current Opinion in Neurobiology* 14 (2): 259–263. doi:10.1016/j.conb.2004.01.020.

James, William. 1890. *The Principles of Psychology*. New York: Henry Holt.

Jansen, Petra, and Jennifer Lehmann. 2013. "Mental Rotation Performance in Soccer Players and Gymnasts in an Object-Based Mental Rotation Task." *Advances in Cognitive Psychology* 9 (2): 92–98. http://doi.org/10.2478/v10053-008-0135-8.

Jansen, Petra, Jennifer Lehmann, and Jessica Van Doren. 2012. "Mental Rotation Performance in Male Soccer Players." *PLoS ONE* 7 (10): e48620. https://doi.org/10.1371/journal.pone.0048620.

Jeannerod, Marc. 1994. "The Representing Brain: Neural Correlates of Motor Intention and Imagery." *Behavioral and Brain Sciences* 17 (2): 187–202. doi:10.1017/s0140525x00034026.

Jeannerod, Marc. 2006. *Motor Cognition: What Actions Tell the Self.* Oxford: Oxford University Press.

Kaplan, Stephen. 1995. "The Restorative Benefits of Nature: Toward an Integrative Framework." *Journal of Environmental Psychology* 15 (3): 169–182. doi:10.1016/0272-4944(95)90001-2.

Kosslyn, Stephen M., Gregory J. Digirolamo, William L. Thompson, and Nathaniel M. Alpert. 1998. "Mental Rotation of Objects versus Hands: Neural Mechanisms Revealed by Positron Emission Tomography." *Psychophysiology* 35 (2): 151–161. doi:10.1111/1469-8986.3520151.

Kosslyn, Stephen M., Carol Seger, John R. Pani, and Lynn A. Hillger. 1990. "When Is Imagery Used in Everyday Life? A Diary Study." *Journal of Mental Imagery* 14:131–152.

Kosslyn, Stephen M., and A. L. Sussman. 1995. "Roles of Imagery in Perception: Or, There Is No Such Thing as Immaculate Perception." In *Cognitive Neurosciences,* edited by Michael S. Gazzaniga, 1035–1042. Cambridge, MA: MIT Press.

Kosslyn, Stephen M., William L. Thompson, and Giorgio Ganis. 2006. *The Case for Mental Imagery*. Oxford: Oxford University Press.

Kosslyn, Stephen M., William L. Thompson, M. Wraga, and Nathaniel M. Alpert. 2001. "Imagining Rotation by Endogenous versus Exogenous Forces: Distinct Neural Mechanisms." *NeuroReport* 12 (11): 2519–2525. doi:10.1097/00001756-200108080-00046.

Loeffler, Jonna, Markus Raab, and Rouwen Cañal-Bruland. 2016. "A Lifespan Perspective on Embodied Cognition." *Frontiers in Psychology* 7 (June): 845. doi:10.3389/fpsyg.2016.00845.

Lorey, Britta, Matthias Bischoff, Sebastian Pilgramm, Rudolf Stark, Jörn Munzert, and Karen Zentgraf. 2009. "The Embodied Nature of Motor Imagery: The Influence of Posture and Perspective." *Experimental Brain Research* 194 (2): 233–243. doi:10.1007/s00221-008-1693-1.

Lynott, Dermot, Louise Connell, and Judith Holler. 2013. "The Role of Body and Environment in Cognition." *Frontiers in Psychology* 4 (July): 465. doi:10.3389/fpsyg.2013.00465.

MacIntyre, Tadhg E., Eric R. Igou, Mark J. Campbell, Aidan P. Moran, and James Matthews. 2014. "Metacognition and Action: A New Pathway to Understanding Social and Cognitive Aspects of Expertise in Sport." *Frontiers in Psychology* 5 (October): 1155. doi:10.3389/fpsyg.2014.01155.

MacIntyre, Tadhg, and Aidan Moran. 2007. "A Qualitative Investigation of Imagery Use and Meta-Imagery Processes among Elite Canoe-Slalom Competitors." *Journal of Imagery Research in Sport and Physical Activity*, 2 (1). doi: 10.2202/1932-0191.1009.

MacIntyre, Tadhg, and Aidan Moran. 2010. "Meta-Imagery Processes among Elite Sports Performers." In *The Neurophysiological Foundations of Mental and Motor Imagery*, edited by A. Guillot and C. Collet, 227–244. New York: Oxford University Press.

MacIntyre, Tadhg E., Aidan P. Moran, Christian Collet, and Aymeric Guillot. 2013. "An Emerging Paradigm: A Strength-Based Approach to Exploring Mental Imagery." *Frontiers in Human Neuroscience* 7 (April): 104. doi:10.3389/fnhum.2013.00104.

Madan, Christopher R., and Anthony Singhal. 2012a. "Motor Imagery and Higher-Level Cognition: Four Hurdles before Research Can Sprint Forward." *Cognitive Processing* 13 (3): 211–229. doi:10.1007/s10339-012-0438-z.

Madan, Christopher R., and Anthony Singhal. 2012b. "Using Actions to Enhance Memory: Effects of Enactment, Gestures, and Exercise on Human Memory." *Frontiers in Psychology* 3 (November): 507. doi:10.3389/fpsyg.2012.00507.

Madan, Christopher R., and Anthony Singhal. 2012c. "Encoding the World around Us: Motor-Related Processing Influences Verbal Memory." *Consciousness and Cognition* 21 (3): 1563–1570. doi:10.1016/j.concog.2012.07.006.

Madan, Christopher R., and Anthony Singhal. 2013. "Introducing TAMI: An Objective Test of Ability in Movement Imagery." *Journal of Motor Behavior* 45 (2): 153–166. doi:10.1080/00222895.2013.763764.

Madan, Christopher R., and Anthony Singhal. 2014. "Improving the TAMI for Use with Athletes." *Journal of Sports Sciences* 32 (14): 1351–1356. doi:10.1080/02640414.2014.889847.

Madan, Christopher R., and Anthony Singhal. 2015. "No Sex Differences in the TAMI." Cognitive Processing 16 (2): 203–209. doi:10.1007/s10339-014-0644-y.

Mahon, Bradford Z., and Alfonso Caramazza. 2008. "A Critical Look at the Embodied Cognition Hypothesis and a New Proposal for Grounding Conceptual Content." *Journal of Physiology, Paris* 102 (1–3): 59–70. doi:10.1016/j.jphysparis.2008.03.004.

Marks, David. F. 1973. "Visual Imagery Differences in the Recall of Pictures." *British Journal of Psychology* 64:17–24.

McIsaac, Heather K., and Eric Eich. 2004. "Vantage Point in Traumatic Memory." *Psychological Science* 15 (4): 248–253. doi:10.1111/j.0956-7976.2004.00660.x.

McMillan, Rebecca L., Scott Barry Kaufman, and Jerome L. Singer. 2013. "Ode to Positive Constructive Daydreaming." *Frontiers in Psychology* 4 (September): 626. doi:10.3389/fpsyg.2013.00626.

Milton, John, Ana Solodkin, Petr Hlustík, and Steven L. Small. 2007. "The Mind of Expert Motor Performance Is Cool and Focused." *NeuroImage* 35 (2): 804–813. doi:10.1016/j.neuroimage.2007.01.003.

Moran, Aidan. 2002. "In the Mind's Eye." *Psychologist* 15 (8): 414–415.

Moran, Aidan. 2012. "Thinking in Action: Some Insights from Cognitive Sport Psychology." *Thinking Skills and Creativity* 7 (2): 85–92. doi:10.1016/j.tsc.2012.03.005.

Moran, Aidan, Mark Campbell, Paul Holmes, and Tadhg MacIntyre. 2012. "Mental Imagery, Action Observation and Skill Learning." In *Skill Acquisition in Sport: Research, Theory and Practice*, edited by N. Hodges and M. A. Williams, 94–111. London: Routledge.

Moran, Aidan, Aymeric Guillot, Tadhg MacIntyre, and Christian Collet. 2012. "Re-Imagining Motor Imagery: Building Bridges between Cognitive Neuroscience and Sport Psychology." *British Journal of Psychology* 103 (2): 224–247. doi:10.1111/j.2044-8295.2011.02068.x.

Moran, Aidan, and Tadhg MacIntyre. 1998. "'There's More to an Image than Meets the Eye': A Qualitative Study of Kinaesthetic Imagery among Elite Canoe-Slalomists." *Irish Journal of Psychology* 19 (4): 406–423. doi:10.1080/03033910.1998.10558203.

Morris, Tony, Michael Spittle, and Anthony P. Watt. 2005. *Imagery in Sport*. Champaign, IL: Human Kinetics.

Munzert, Jörn, Britta Lorey, and Karen Zentgraf. 2009. "Cognitive Motor Processes: The Role of Motor Imagery in the Study of Motor Representations." *Brain Research Reviews* 60 (2): 306–326. doi:10.1016/j.brainresrev.2008.12.024.

Newell, Allen, Herbert Alexander Simon. 1972. *Human Problem Solving*. Vol. 104. Englewood Cliffs, NJ: Prentice-Hall.

Nikulin, Vadim V., Friederike U. Hohlefeld, Arthur M. Jacobs, and Gabriel Curio. 2008. "Quasi-Movements: A Novel Motor-Cognitive Phenomenon." *Neuropsychologia* 46 (2): 727–742. doi:10.1016/j.neuropsychologia.2007.10.008.

Nishida, T., A, Katube, K. Inomata, Y. Okazawa, M. Ito, S. Kayama, K. Tsuru- hara, and Y. Yoshizawa. 1986. "A New Test for Controllability of Motor Imagery: The Examination of Its Validity and Reliability." *Japan Journal of Physical Education* 31:13–22.

Nordin, Sanna M., and Jennifer Cumming. 2005. "Professional Dancers Describe Their Imagery: Where, When, What, Why, and How." *Sport Psychologist* 19 (4): 395–416. doi:10.1123/tsp.19.4.395.

Olsson C. J., and Lars Nyberg. 2010. "Motor Imagery: If You Can't Do It, You Won't Think It." *Scandinavian Journal of Medicine and Science in Sports* 20 711–715 10.1111/j.1600-0838.2010.01101.x

Olsson, C. J., and Lars Nyberg. 2011. "Brain Simulation of Action May Be Grounded in Physical Experience." *Neurocase* 17 (6): 501–505. doi:10.1080/13554794.2010.547504.

Park, Sohee, and Stephen M. Kosslyn. 1990. "Imagination." In *Reflections on "The Principles of Psychology": William James after a Century*, edited by G. Johnson and T. B. Henley, 183–196. Hillsdale, NJ: Erlbaum.

Parsons, Larry M. 1987. "Imagined Spatial Transformation of One's Body." *Journal of Experimental Psychology: General* 116:172–191.

Pavlova, Marina A. 2012. "Biological Motion Processing as a Hallmark of Social Cognition." *Cerebral Cortex* 22 (5): 981–995. doi:10.1093/cercor/bhr156.

Pearson, Joel, and Stephen M. Kosslyn. 2013. "Mental Imagery." *Frontiers in Psychology* 4 (April): 198. doi:10.3389/fpsyg.2013.00198.

Perky, Cheves West. 1910. "An Experimental Study of Imagination." *American Journal of Psychology* 21 (3): 422–452. doi:10.2307/1413350.

Peters, M., B. Laeng, K. Latham, M. Jackson, R. Zaiyouna, and C. Richardson. 1995. "A Redrawn Vandenberg and Kuse Mental Rotations Test: Different Versions and Factors That Affect Performance." *Brain Cognition* 28 (1): 39–58.

Pylyshyn, Zenon W. 2002. "Mental Imagery: In Search of a Theory." *Behavioral and Brain Sciences* 25 (2): 157–182; discussion 182–237. doi:10.1017/s0140525x02000043.

Rizzolatti, G., L. Fogassi, and V. Gallese. 2001. "Neurophysiological Mechanisms Underlying the Understanding and Imitation of Action." *Nature Reviews: Neuroscience* 2 (9): 661–670.

Roberts, R., N. Callow, L. Hardy, D. Markland, and J. Bringer. 2008. "Movement Imagery Ability: Development and Assessment of a Revised Version of the Vividness of Movement Imagery Questionnaire." *Journal of Sport and Exercise Psychology* 30:200–221.

Rosenbaum, David A. 2005. "The Cinderella of Psychology: The Neglect of Motor Control in the Science of Mental Life and Behavior." *American Psychologist* 60 (4): 308–317. doi:10.1037/0003-066x.60.4.308.

Saimpont, Arnaud, Francois Malouin, B. Tousignant, and Phillip L. Jackson. 2012. "The Influence of Body Configuration on Motor Imagery of Walking in Younger and Older Adults." *Neuroscience* 222 (October): 49–57. doi:10.1016/j.neuroscience.2012.06.066.

Schack, Thomas, Kai Essig, Cornelia Frank, and Dirk Koester. 2014. "Mental Representation and Motor Imagery Training." *Frontiers in Human Neuroscience* 8:328. doi:10.3389/fnhum.2014.00328.

Shapiro, Lawrence. 2011. *Embodied Cognition*. London: Routledge.

Shapiro, Lawrence, and Shannon Spaulding (this volume). "Embodied Cognition and Sport." In *Handbook of Embodied Cognition and Sport Psychology*, edited by Massimiliano Cappuccio. Cambridge, MA: MIT Press.

Sheehan, Peter Winston 1967. "A Shortened Form of Betts' Questionnaire upon Mental Imagery." *Journal of Clinical Psychology* 23 (3): 386–389.

Shepard, Roger N., and Jackie Metzler. 1971. "Mental Rotation of Three-Dimensional Objects." *Science* 171 (3972): 701–703. doi:10.1126/science.171.3972.701.

Slepian, Michael L., Max Weisbuch, Nicholas O. Rule, and Nalini Ambady. 2011. "Tough and Tender: Embodied Categorization of Gender." *Psychological Science* 22 (1): 26–28.

Stock, Armin, and Claudia Stock. 2004. "A Short History of Ideo-Motor Action." *Psychological Research* 68 (2–3): 176–188. doi:10.1007/s00426-003-0154-5.

Suinn, Richard M. 1972. "Behavior Rehearsal Training for Ski Racers." *Behavior Therapy* 3 (3): 519–520. doi:10.1016/s0005-7894(72)80191-6.

Suinn, Richard M. 1997. "Mental Practice in Sport Psychology: Where Have We Been, Where Do We Go?" *Clinical Psychology: Science and Practice* 4 (3): 189–207. doi:10.1111/j.1468-2850.1997.tb00109.x.

Vandell, Roland A., Robert A. Davis, and Herbert A. Clugston. 1943. "The Function of Mental Practice in the Acquisition of Motor Skills." *Journal of General Psychology* 29 (2): 243–250. doi:10.1080/00221309.1943.10544442.

Voyer, D. 2011. "Time Limits and Gender Differences on Paper-and-Pencil Tests of Mental Rotation: A Meta-Analysis." *Psychonomic Bulletin & Review*, 18:267–277. doi:10.3758/s13423-010-0042-0.

Webb, Christine E., Maya Rossignac-Milon, and E. Tory Higgins. 2017. "Stepping Forward Together: Could Walking Facilitate Interpersonal Conflict Resolution?" *American Psychologist* 72 (4): 374–385.

Wilson, Andrew D., and Sabrina Golonka. 2013. "Embodied Cognition Is Not What You Think It Is." *Frontiers in Psychology* 4 (February): 58. doi:10.3389/fpsyg.2013.00058.

Wilson, Margaret. 2002. "Six Views of Embodied Cognition." *Psychonomic Bulletin and Review* 9 (4): 625–636. doi:10.3758/bf03196322.

Wraga, Maryjane, and Stephen M. Kosslyn. 2002. "Imagery." In *Encyclopedia of Cognitive Science* 2, 466–470. London: Nature Publishing Group.

Wraga, Mary-Jane, and Stephen M. Kosslyn. 2006. "Imagery." In *Encyclopedia of Cognitive Science* 2, edited by Lynn Nadel, 466–470. Hoboken, NJ: John Wiley and Sons.

24 Predictive Processing in the Control of Interceptive Motor Actions

David L. Mann

1 Introduction

In the mid-1980s, the French movement scientist Hubert Ripoll found something quite striking when examining where skilled table tennis players look when hitting a ball. Ripoll and colleagues (Ripoll and Fleurance 1988; Ripoll, Fleurance, and Caseneuve 1987; Ripoll 1989) recruited five of the best table tennis players in France and used what would be now considered to be quite primitive equipment to track where the players were looking when playing against an opponent. It was widely expected that the players would "keep their eyes on the ball" by directing their central vision toward the position of the ball throughout its flight, yet the results revealed that these elite players often directed their gaze *ahead* of the approaching ball. In particular, they followed the initial part of the ball-flight with their central vision, but after a short period of tracking performed a fast eye movement called a *saccade* to move their eyes to where they *expected* the ball would bounce in the future. This showed that the athletes used the motion-trajectory information to predict the imminent position of the ball, and it would later turn out that these predictions are highly accurate and are associated with the level of skill that athletes possess when hitting a fast-moving target such as a baseball or cricket ball.

Although the potential implications of the findings may not have been entirely clear at the time, the outcomes helped contribute to a growing debate about the nature of predictions and predictive processing when intercepting fast-moving targets. The aim of this chapter is to examine the nature of these predictions and to consider whether they may help us better understand the growing interest in predictive processing in perception.

The issue of prediction in visual-motor control is a controversial one. Early work in fast-ball sports in the 1970s and 1980s relied on chronometric analyses of when movements were initiated, in an effort to uncover how skilled athletes such as baseball and cricket batsmen were able to hit a fast approaching ball (Glencross and Cibich 1977;

Howarth et al. 1984). When doing so, humans must account for the inherent visual-motor delay required for a movement to be modified on the basis of visual information (thought to be approximately 150–200 ms; Georgopoulos, Kalaska, and Massey 1981; Saunders and Knill 2003).

Yet, at the time, it was also sometimes assumed that the movements produced by these batters were "preprogrammed" and unlikely to be altered once initiated. So to account for the visual-motor delay *and* the time it would take to execute the movement, it was surmised that a skilled batsman would have to make a very early prediction about where and when an approaching ball would arrive. As a result, the chronometric analyses suggested that athletes, when performing some of the most challenging visual-motor tasks, would need to predict the outcome either very soon after the initiation of ball-flight, or in some cases even before the ball initiated its flight (see Howarth et al. 1984). In essence, it was thought that skilled athletes had a repertoire of actions that they could produce, and knowing the time it would take to execute each action, the key role of the athlete would be to, on the basis of their predictions, know simply what action to execute and when to initiate it.

Crucially, these analyses suggested that skilled athletes should possess a highly refined ability to generate very accurate and early predictions. However, this scenario seemed highly unlikely to some interested in visual-motor control, and it saw the birth of very influential work that sought to dispel the idea that skilled movements were preprogrammed, and therefore that predictions would be necessary when performing those actions.

David Lee, an influential psychologist from the University of Edinburgh in Scotland, presented quite compelling findings to help dispel the idea that movements were preprogrammed. Lee and colleagues (1983) asked participants to jump and punch a ball that fell toward them from above. If the movements were preprogrammed, then it was predicted that the jumps should be highly repeatable and therefore would be initiated at some set time prior to the time at which the performer made contact with the ball. Instead, Lee found considerable variation in the delay from when the jump was initiated to when the ball was hit. Moreover, the participants were found to adapt their movements while in the air by dynamically coordinating the knee and elbow joints during each jump. In essence, the participants were not producing preprogrammed movements, but instead dynamically altering their movements on the basis of continuing visual information available throughout the jump. In addition, the finding that movements could be altered in a relatively on-line fashion helped fuel the idea that the human visual-motor delay may be much shorter than had previously been assumed (closer to 60–150 ms).

Although the results of some aspects of the findings from Lee's studies remain controversial (for a wider discussion, see Wann 1996), they led to wider acceptance that movements were not as preprogrammed as had been initially assumed, and questioned the need for very early predictions when performing these types of interceptive actions. The results also led to a wealth of work that sought to better understand *how* interceptive actions are guided and controlled on the basis of real-time visual information.

Perhaps the most influential of the follow-up studies was that performed, again in table tennis, by Reinoud Bootsma and Piet van Wieringen at Vrije Universiteit in Amsterdam. In their seminal study, Bootsma and van Wieringen (1990) performed a kinematic analysis of the arm movements of skilled table tennis players when hitting an approaching ball. Their findings also revealed that, instead of producing perfectly reproducible movements, each shot differed. In particular, there was considerable variation in both the time and place that the shot was initiated (relative to when and where the ball was hit), and there was a "funneling" effect, wherein the shots looked progressively more similar as the bat approached the moment of bat-ball contact. Bootsma and van Wieringen concluded that the players were able to use the time to contact with the ball in a real-time fashion to dynamically alter the acceleration of the arm movements to ensure accurate bat-ball contact (though see, van Soest and Beek 2010; van Soest et al. 2010; Bootsma et al. 2010). Again these findings helped question the notion of skilled actions being preprogrammed, and placed further doubt on the necessity for predictions of the future location of the moving target well in advance of its arrival (i.e., soon after or even before the ball initiates its flight).

Given the converging evidence that early predictions might not be necessary for accurate visual-motor control in interception, Hubert Ripoll's results on the *gaze behavior* of table tennis players posed an interesting conundrum. Skilled performers appeared to be controlling actions in a relatively on-line fashion, yet were found to be generating predictions of where the ball would be in the future. Before delving any further into what we know about predictive behavior on the basis of studies of gaze, it is worthwhile taking a wider look at some background information on the growing interest in predictive processing in perception, and then a consideration of how studies of visual gaze help us better understand the embodied nature of cognition and motor actions.

2 Predictive Processing in Perception

The discussion centering on the role of prediction in perceptual-motor control is pertinent given the recent interest in the use of predictive models to explain human perception (Hohwy 2013; Clark 2013). The classic view of perception is one of bottom-up processing, in which, in the case of vision, a sensory signal arriving at the eye is constructed from low-level sensory stimulation (at the early visual cortex) and then progressively "put together" at higher-order areas in the brain. This means that changes in the bottom-up visual input generate changes in perception, and that there may be little need for top-down influences to explain what we "see" in our surrounds. Yet there are problems with this bottom-up conceptualization of perception, perhaps most notably that it cannot explain very well situations where the causes of visual input are ambiguous. There are many examples of visual ambiguity, but a good recent example has been the case of "the dress" (Lafer-Sousa, Hermann, and Conway 2015; Gegenfurtner, Bloj, and Toscani 2015; Winkler et al. 2015), in which a washed-out image of a dress went viral online because of the apparent ambiguity of its colors: to some it was seen as being black and blue, and to others as being white and gold. It is challenging when viewing this conundrum from a bottom-up perspective to conceptualize why the same image would be interpreted differently by different people, or even differently at different moments by the same person. Instead, there is a growing view that perception may be better explained by a top-down process whereby the brain is a "hypothesis-testing" organ that seeks to make inferences about our surrounding environment, and that prediction is at the heart of how these hypotheses are tested.

The idea that the brain uses inferences to perceive is useful when seeking to better understand the concept of the hypothesis-testing brain (Hohwy 2013). The brain at any moment has access only to sensory information and must infer from that input what has actually caused that information. This is challenging because there is not a one-to-one relationship between a cause and its sensory consequence: different causes can result in the same sensory input, and different sensory inputs can result from the same cause. A small model airplane located close to the eye could theoretically produce the same retinal image as a real airplane located farther away in the sky. And conversely, the model airplane viewed from the side will result in different retinal input than when it is viewed from behind. Yet our brain is capable of differentiating the different scenarios and correctly attributing what is a model and what is a real plane. The inconsistency in the cause-effect relationship means that, to do so, the brain must make inferences about what is being seen.

An increasingly popular explanation for how perceptual inferences are made is that the brain must rely on prior beliefs and act in a way that is consistent with Bayesian inference. According to the Bayesian approach (Knill and Pouget 2004), the brain would generate hypotheses about what may cause a particular perceptual experience and would weigh the different hypotheses according to how well they can explain the cause. Ultimately, the brain would settle on the hypothesis that best explains the cause. According to Bayes rule, the weighting would be performed by combining the likelihood of the hypothesis, that is, the probability that the cause would actually result in the observed effect, and the prior probability, that is, the probability of the hypothesis actually occurring at all in advance of the effects being observed. Moreover, this process is understood to occur at a *subconscious level* so that the person generating the hypotheses is unaware that this process is taking place. Although the details of this process are not important to the central story here (and so can be read elsewhere; I recommend Hohwy 2013), the key message according to this view is that the brain would make inferences about the surrounding environment by generating hypotheses and weighting them according to how likely they are to explain what is perceived.

The central mechanism for inference is thought to be that the brain generates internal models of the world that are capable of predicting and explaining familiar perceptual input. And crucially, these models are said to be developed and refined on the basis of *prediction error minimization*. According to this framework, a specific model (i.e., hypothesis) is developed to predict what the perceptual information should be, and is then tested when faced with the appropriate scenario. The predicted input is compared with the actual input to determine the error in the model, and on the basis of this prediction error, the parameters of the model (i.e., the priors) are refined, in an effort to improve the model and thereby minimize error in the future. As a result of this process, the bottom-up perceptual information available from the environment is used as feedback as part of a self-supervising system that tests and refines the model to ensure more accurate predictions in the future.

The actions produced as a result of agency provide a very useful way for the brain to further test and refine its internal models. By means of *active inference*, action is used to actively test the predictions made by the brain. Because a person should be able to predict what would be the sensory consequences of a particular movement, action allows the person to actively sample the world so that those predictions can be tested to better understand and refine the model. Ultimately this leads to the proposition that movement can be controlled in an on-line fashion by attunement to prediction error, moving in a way that minimizes prediction error and leads the person toward the goal state. Importantly in the context of perceptually guided motor actions, this suggests that people generate models that predict what they expect to perceive, and actively test these models as a means of improving their predictions in the future.

3 Gaze and the Embodied Nature of Motor Actions

It has been known for some time that gaze behavior changes according to the demands of a task, and this can help us better understand the manner in which both perceptual and motor tasks are performed. In his classic book, translated into English in 1967,

Alfred Yarbus (1967) recorded the eye movements of observers asked to perform different perceptual tasks while viewing the same image. Observers viewed an image of people in a living room, but in one condition were asked to guess the ages of the people in the room, in another condition to memorize the position of the people and objects in the room, and in another to estimate the material circumstances of the people in the room. The findings revealed that the way that the participants searched the image (i.e., the movements of their gaze direction) differed in each condition, showing that gaze is adapted according to the demands of the task. Although this finding might now seem somewhat obvious, it helped to demonstrate that the examination of gaze can provide a potentially powerful means of uncovering how task demands can alter behavior when performing that task.

More recently, the examination of visual gaze has been used to demonstrate the embodied nature of visual-motor control in interception. Matt Dicks and his colleagues (Dicks, Button, and Davids 2010) asked skilled football (soccer) goalkeepers to attempt to "save" penalty kicks performed by an opponent while manipulating two key task constraints: (1) the type of response performed by the goalkeepers (a verbal, joystick, or actual movement response); and (2) the manner in which the opponent was presented to the goalkeeper (an actual opponent in-situ versus a video projection of the same opponent). Dicks, Button, and Davids' findings revealed unique patterns of gaze behavior in each of the conditions. Specifically, the way that gaze was controlled was unique when producing an interceptive movement as opposed, in particular, to a simple verbal prediction of the outcome, with much more time spent viewing the ball and less time on the body of the kicker. Moreover, gaze differed when facing a real opponent instead of a video projection of that opponent, even when responding in the same manner (verbally or by moving a joystick).

Given the findings of Yarbus (1967), the results of Dicks and colleagues show that the way that the goalkeeping task was performed differed according to the constraints of that task. Crucially, it is consistent with the idea that the way that a visual-motor action is performed may be embodied, and that simplified task demands such as requiring a verbal instead of motor response, or observing a video rather than live opponent, may lead to a misunderstanding of how visual-motor tasks are actually performed (see also Mann, Abernethy, and Farrow 2010). As a case in point, previous research performed using video displays of penalty takers had recommended that skilled goalkeepers should spend extended periods of time observing the movements of the kicker's hips and supporting leg prior to the kick (Savelsbergh et al. 2005). Yet Dicks, Button, and Davids' findings show that those recommendations found when observing a video display do not necessarily extend to what is or should be done when facing a live opponent. A true understanding of visual-motor control (and the gaze behavior associated with it) should, wherever possible, be conducted in conditions that accurately represent those experienced in the performance environment (see Pinder et al. 2011).

4 Predictive Gaze during Interception

Given the notion that the examination of visual gaze provides a valuable means of understanding the embodied nature of visual-motor control, it is now worth returning to our consideration of gaze during interception, and what it helps to reveal about the nature of predictions in interception. Almost fifteen years after Ripoll's original findings, Michael Land and Peter McLeod performed a more modern replication of Ripoll's work, albeit in cricket batsmen, but importantly looking at whether gaze behavior differed across batsmen of different levels of proficiency in batting (a professional, intermediate, and novice batsman) when hitting balls projected from a ball machine at a moderate speed. In what has become a classic study published in *Nature Neuroscience*, Land and McLeod (2000) revealed that the gaze behavior of the batsmen differed commensurate with their level of skill, with progressively earlier saccadic eye movements (*predictive saccades*) being made toward the location of ball-bounce as the level of skill of the batsman increased. This suggests that better batsmen have a capacity for superior prediction, and that they act out those predictions in the form of earlier eye movements to the location of ball-bounce. Moreover, Land and McLeod reported that after the bounce, batsmen were unable to track the ball up to the moment of bat-ball contact, with gaze typically falling behind the ball before it reached them, irrespective of their skill level. On the basis of these gaze findings, Land and McLeod (2000) presented a mathematical model that posited skilled batsmen need only ball-flight information available immediately after release, and at the moment of bounce, to make predictions about the likely time and location that the ball would arrive. The claim that skill in prediction played an important role in the level of proficiency of the batsmen helped reignite the debate about whether predictions are necessary during interception, and if so, what purpose they might serve in facilitating accurate interception.

The most popular explanation for the role of the predictive saccades was originally that they must be required because a fast-moving ball might simply move too fast to be accurately pursued by the eyes, and so the saccades would prevent gaze from falling behind the location of the ball (Ripoll and Fleurance 1988; Bahill and LaRitz 1984). In an effort to uncover the threshold speed above which saccades would be required, James Croft and colleagues in New Zealand examined the gaze of junior cricket batsmen who attempted to hit balls projected toward them at a range of different ball speeds (Croft,

Button, and Dicks 2010). To their surprise, though, the changes in ball speed did not alter the gaze behavior of the batsmen in any systematic way. Different batsmen used different patterns of gaze, but those strategies remained largely unchanged in response to the manipulations in ball speed.

I and some colleagues in Australia more recently examined the gaze of two of the world's best-ever cricket batsmen, who hit balls at speeds that were representative of a competition scenario (Mann, Spratford, and Abernethy 2013). We found that the elite batsmen produced not one but *two* predictive saccades in most scenarios. The batsmen almost always produced the saccade to ball-bounce found by Ripoll and others, but they also often, immediately after ball-bounce, produced a second saccade to where they would ultimately make contact with the ball. As a result, those batsmen were sometimes spending more time with their gaze ahead of the ball than they were with their gaze directed toward it. Crucially, we also showed that although the elite batsmen directed their gaze ahead of the ball, the direction of their *head* was almost always accurately directed toward the *real-time* position of the ball. That is to say that, even though their gaze was ahead of the ball, the batsmen coupled the downward rotation of their head to the position of the ball so that the ball remained in a consistent egocentric direction relative to the head. By way of analogy, if the batsmen were to be wearing a "miner's torch" on their forehead while batting, and the torch were to be shone toward the ball at the moment of release, the elite batsmen rotated their head in a fashion that ensured that the light would have remained on the ball throughout its ball-flight. In contrast, two competent but much-less-proficient batsmen were less capable of doing so, with their head direction starting to lag behind the ball soon after the initiation of ball-flight, and with the lag progressively increasing through to the moment of bat-ball contact. This notion of head-ball coupling is important on a number of fronts. In particular, it shows that the predictive saccades were not required to compensate for ball speeds that exceeded what could be tracked by the eyes. Rather, the central vision of the batsmen would have been guided directly toward the ball throughout ball-flight if the batsmen had simply rotated their heads and kept their eyes perfectly still within the head. Yet the batsmen still produced the predictive saccades that moved their gaze ahead of the ball, suggesting that the saccades perform some other role during interception.

Another popular explanation for the role of the saccades has been that saccades may be required to assist in the tracking of the ball after it has bounced. From the viewpoint of an observer, a ball will undergo a very rapid change in its velocity following bounce, and so a saccade may help account for the necessary change in velocity by placing the gaze to "lay in wait" for the ball to track it more accurately after bounce. Mary Hayhoe and colleagues (2012) examined the gaze of skilled squash players during on-court rallies and found behavior that supports this idea. The squash players initiated saccades before the ball hit the wall and before it hit the ground, with results showing that post-bounce tracking in each case was initiated faster when earlier saccades were performed. This provides support for the hypothesis that saccades facilitate post-bounce tracking, though it does not appear to offer a viable explanation for why the elite cricket batsmen in the Mann, Spratford, and Abernethy (2013) study performed a second saccade—immediately after ball-bounce—to the anticipated location of bat-ball contact. Those batsmen did not track the ball after bounce, undermining the idea that the saccade was performed to assist in post-bounce tracking. Moreover, the batsmen did not track the ball immediately after it was hit either, instead, in many cases, holding their gaze at the location of contact well after hitting the ball. Again, the saccade to bat-ball contact did not help facilitate faster post-contact tracking. These observations suggest that there may be some other functional reason for the predictive saccades to be made, though unfortunately at this stage a suitable explanation remains largely unclear.

That predictive saccades occur during interception is particularly surprising given results from lab-based studies which suggest that pursuing a target as closely as possible with the eyes *should* provide the best chance of intercepting it. Brenner and Smeets (2011) manipulated where participants looked while moving a stylus on a touch screen to intercept a small rectangular target that moved in a straight line: in one condition participants pursued the target closely, while in another condition participants looked ahead to where they should make contact with the target. The results revealed that looking ahead to where interception should occur resulted in a *decrease* in the accuracy of interception. Instead, interception was most accurate when the target was followed as closely as possible by the eyes. In support, Spering et al. (2011) found that when accurately tracking a moving target with the eyes, movement information from the extraocular muscles that move the eyes may improve accuracy by providing additional information that helps to anticipate where the target will be in the future. Given that watching the target closely *should* provide the best chance if hitting it, it remains unclear why saccades are performed. What is clear is that those lab-based studies have used objects that move using linear trajectories—not acting under gravity, and not bouncing off a surface. Perhaps the saccades are required to somehow facilitate performance in conditions where the moving object moves in a less-predictable manner and/or undergoes abrupt changes in direction.

While the exact role of the saccades remains unclear, what has become clearer is that those predictions can be remarkably precise—seemingly much more that what might have previously been thought. Gabriel Diaz and colleagues in the United States conducted a study in which they tracked the gaze of *novice* participants asked to hit approaching racquetballs that bounced in front of them in a virtual environment (Diaz et al. 2013). Although a virtual environment may be less representative of a real-life scenario where an actual ball is hit (see Mann and Savelsbergh 2015; Mann, Abernethy, and Farrow 2010; Dicks, Button, and Davids 2010), this approach does offer the opportunity to use more sophisticated eye-tracking equipment that is capable of tracking not one but both eyes, and at a higher temporal precision, when compared to most mobile eye trackers used to track eye movements when hitting a ball. Diaz and colleagues examined the predictive saccades performed immediately before bounce when participants hit virtual balls that approached at one of three velocities. Participants made predictive saccades, but rather than moving gaze toward the exact point at which the ball bounced, the saccades redirected gaze to a location where the ball would be a short time *after* it bounced.

Moreover, Diaz et al. (2013) found something quite extraordinary. Irrespective of the ball speed, the predictive saccades redirected gaze to where the ball would be at a particular yet consistent time (≈170 ms) after ball-bounce. In an elegant experimental manipulation, the elasticity of the ball was altered to change the velocity of the ball *after* it bounced without any change in the pre-bounce velocity. Even more remarkable, the results revealed that the novice racquetball players still, after only a few trials, produced predictive saccades that relocated gaze to where the ball would be ≈170 ms after it bounced. This means that the participants, who were novice in the task, were able to adjust their saccades to account not only for differences in real-time ball velocity but also for a change in post-bounce velocity in a highly accurate way. Diaz and colleagues reasoned that the participants were relying on an internal model of motion trajectory that produced predictions on the basis of both real-time and prior information in the form of information about ball-flight and ball-elasticity, respectively.

The striking findings of Diaz et al. (2013) highlight the manner in which predictions rely on contextual information. Predictive eye movements are not made just on the basis of what is seen in the present, but also on the basis of what has been observed or experienced in the past. Moreover, the predictions also take into account what *might* happen in the future. In support, Vishnu Sarpeshkar and his colleagues (Sarpeshkar, Abernethy, and Mann 2017; Sarpeshkar and Mann 2011) examined the gaze of skilled cricket batsmen who hit balls again projected by a ball machine. Sarpeshkar, Abernethy, and Mann were particularly interested in how the context in which the batting was performed might influence the gaze behavior of the batsmen. In one condition, batsmen hit balls that followed only a straight trajectory, while in a second condition, those straight trajectories were interleaved with trials that swung following a curved flight path. The gaze behavior observed when batsmen faced only straight trials was very similar to that observed in previous studies, in particular with predictive saccades made in advance of the bounce of the ball on the ground. However, the *possibility* of ball-swing in the second condition had a profound effect on what the batsmen did when facing the straight trials. Their gaze behavior was more novice-like and less predictive, with a delay in the timing of the saccades to ball-bounce, an overall decrease in the number of saccades to both bounce and bat-ball contact, poorer head tracking, and a decrease in the proportion of trials in which gaze was aligned with the ball at contact. Ultimately these changes resulted in a significant decrease in batting performance when there was a possibility of ball-swing. These findings show that predictions are altered according to the context in which they are performed. And in this case it appears that the possibility of additional possible outcomes in the form of the presence (or absence) of ball-swing may have moderated the ability to generate accurate predictive saccades.

The accuracy with which eye movements are performed can also be altered by the possibility of reward. Brielmann and Spering (2015) asked participants to track a moving target on a screen with their eyes, with greater accuracy in one condition leading to monetary reward, and in another condition leading to no monetary reward. The results showed that participants tracked the target more accurately when a monetary reward was on offer, with control conditions showing that the finding could not be explained by other factors such as better preparation or motivation. Although not specifically looking at predictive eye movements per se, the findings help to reinforce the pervasive effect that a range of different contextual influences can have on eye movements. These eye movements, and the predictions sometimes associated with them, are not generated just on the basis of real-time information, but the way in which they are performed is influenced by a range of different contextual influences, including what has happened in the past and what might happen in the future.

5 A Dissociation between Gaze and Conscious Awareness

Clearly humans are capable of making very precise predictions when intercepting objects, but it is interesting to ask how *aware* we might be that we are making these types of predictions. Take a moment to think about it. Very few of us would be skilled in a task like racquetball, yet Diaz et al.'s (2013) findings suggest that we should be capable of making remarkably precise predictions about motion trajectories that allow us to know where an approaching racquetball would be at a very specific point in its future flight path. I suspect that very few of us (if any) would know that we are making these types of predictions, let alone know how those predictions are being made. Even on this anecdotal account it appears that at least some of our predictions revealed by eye movements may be performed outside of conscious awareness. And there is a growing body of evidence to support the idea that we have very little voluntary awareness of many of the different eye movements that we perform.

A number of laboratory-based studies have sought to examine the potential dissociation between gaze and perception. In one elegant example, motion perception and eye movements were compared when viewing two orthogonally drifting gratings that were each presented to one of the observer's two eyes (Spering, Pomplun, and Carrasco 2011). When viewing the two gratings simultaneously (e.g., one with leftward drift, and the other with downward drift), participants generally reported seeing motion in the direction that matched the vector average of those two gratings (i.e., in this example, down and to the left). However, the relative strength of the two gratings was manipulated by adapting participants to one of the gratings through an extended period of exposure to that grating, let's say the one with leftward drift, resulting in a reduction in sensitivity to motion in that direction. Participants would therefore perceive motion to be headed toward the direction in which they were not adapted; in this case, resulting in a downward direction. Yet the results of the study revealed that the reflexive eye movements tracked the direction represented by the real vector average (down and to the left) rather than the direction of the perceived motion. That is to say, the participants thought that the grating was moving in one direction (leftward), even though their eye movements told them otherwise. The authors concluded that the dissociation between perception and gaze implies that the signals that guide eye movements do so in the absence of conscious awareness. Moreover, the converging evidence that eye movements often occur in the absence of voluntary awareness is consistent with a model whereby information for eye movements and perception are processed in different areas of the brain, or at least in different populations of neurons within the same area (Spering and Carrasco 2015).

The dissociation between what our eyes do and what we consciously perceive can help explain other interesting social phenomena. For instance, Kuhn and Land (2006) examined the gaze of observers who watched a magician perform the *vanishing ball illusion,* where a person juggling pretends to throw a ball in the air but does not actually release it from their hand. The juggler uses other social cues such as their own gaze direction to give the indication that they had released the ball and that it must have disappeared at the top of its flight. Most observers who watch this trick are indeed fooled by the illusion, and report that they saw the ball vanish at the top of its flight. Yet surprisingly, their gaze was not fooled; although observers would typically follow the ball with their gaze when it *was* thrown in the air by the juggler, Kuhn and Land found that the observers *didn't* move their eyes away from the ball when the ball was not released. Observers *say* that they saw the ball disappear from a particular position in space, yet they weren't even looking there. Their expectations of the ball being released (from previous observations) and the social cues from the gaze of the juggler override what the oculomotor system is telling them, further highlighting the strong dissociation between gaze and what is reported as being seen.

Returning to the consideration of gaze in interception, the studies performed with elite cricket batsmen suggest that the batsmen too possess little awareness of where they are looking when hitting the ball (see also Koedijker and Mann 2015). In fact, our studies originated from a discussion with Justin Langer, who was, at the time, the batting coach of the Australian cricket team, and a former international player. Langer struggled to believe the claim that batsmen do not watch the ball at the moment they hit it, because he felt that he—when batting well against a ball-projection machine—could clearly see markings on the ball at the moment he hit it (balls used in ball-projections machines have small dimples on their surface). After several robust discussions on the topic, we measured Langer's gaze while batting and found that he did indeed have his gaze directed toward the ball at the moment of contact, using the same two-saccade strategy (to bounce and contact) later reported in Mann, Spratford, and Abernethy (2013). Intriguingly, Langer had no conscious awareness that he was performing these saccades. His conscious experience was that he tracked the ball throughout its flight path, though he was less certain of this claim than he was of watching the ball at contact. We too tested another batsman, one of the best batsman to have ever played the game, and just like Langer, he used the two saccades on most trials and clearly had his gaze directed toward the ball at contact. Yet, he was adamant that he *does not* watch the ball at contact, and that he felt it was in fact impossible to do so. Here we see two elite batsmen who used what was essentially the same gaze strategy, yet had very different conscious experiences of where they looked when batting. It seems that elite batsmen such as Justin Langer (and most likely others) have, as a result of their training, developed an ability to generate better predictions than others, yet are not consciously aware that they do so and have almost certainly not used any sort of conscious strategy to improve these predictions during their development.

6 Gaze as a Model of Predictive Processing in Perception?

Predictive saccades performed during interception are skill-related, remarkably accurate, generated using real-time and prior information, and occur subconsciously. When reflecting on the predictive processing framework outlined earlier as a means of understanding human perception (Clark 2013; Hohwy 2013), what we now know of the saccades does raise the question of whether these predictive saccades reflect the brain's process of prediction-error minimization as a means of testing its own model of ball-flight, and even to possibly use the prediction error to control action in an on-line fashion. Although the precise role of the saccades remains unclear, one potential explanation has been that they may provide a useful means of providing feedback about the success of a prediction and the ensuing interception (Mann, Spratford, and Abernethy 2013). The case of the saccades to bat-ball contact provides an intriguing conundrum. Because of the inherent visual-motor delay when performing a visually guided action, visual information at the moment of bat-ball contact will not help improve the quality of the real-time action being performed, unless the saccade to contact better allows peripheral vision to be used to refine the visually guided action as late as is permissible by the visual-motor system. Rather, it could be that the saccade to contact is being used to provide feedback about the predicted and actual time and place of ball arrival to refine the predictions made in the future. This sounds very similar to what would be expected on the basis of prediction error minimization: using active inference through action (eye movements) to test the brain's model of, in this case, predicted ball-flight. That way error in the form of misjudgments about the place and time of arrival of the ball could be used to refine model parameters (priors) to improve predictions in the future.

The pressing challenge is to uncover the functional role of the predictive saccades. If they do play a role in detecting errors and exploiting those errors to modify future predictions, then clever manipulations in the error feedback (for instance, manipulations in ball-flight possible when using virtual reality) may help determine whether subsequent predictions are altered in the presence of the saccades. Recent evidence in the form of recorded brain activity has been presented as support for predictive coding in perception, and this too may help uncover the role of the saccades. It has been shown that areas within the inferior temporal cortex encode information about probabilities and prediction errors (Bell et al. 2016), with neural signals in the visual system actively altering the activity on the basis of the predictions made about the sensory environment. This type of approach may too provide an opportunity to understand whether the saccades are associated with predictive processing and the attenuation of activity in the visual cortex.

If predictive saccades were to provide an observable outcome of the error minimization process, then this would offer a very promising model from which we could test hypotheses about the "hypothesis-testing brain." For instance, the very specific nature of the predictions made in the form of where and when the ball will be in the future offers the opportunity to understand how manipulations to real-time and prior information alter the predictions and therefore the internal model being used to generate those predictions. Specifically, manipulations of the statistics of prior information (e.g., the mean and the variability of the prior information; Burr and Cicchini 2014; Narain et al. 2013) could reveal what information is being used to generate predictions, and what parameters skilled performers refine in order to improve the nature of their predictions (Cicchini et al. 2012). Moreover, this could offer a means of better comprehending and intervening in conditions where motor coordination fails, for instance in developmental coordination disorder in children.

7 Conclusion

Most people expect that skilled athletes would track a moving ball as closely as possible when trying to hit it, but instead it turns out that they perform fast saccadic eye movements that move gaze ahead of the ball. These predictions improve when athletes refine their hitting ability, with skilled batters capable of performing earlier predictions than lesser batters do. Yet even novice performers are still capable of remarkably accurate predictions that must take into account both real-time and prior information about ball-flight characteristics. Moreover, these predictions occur at a subconscious level, with the performer typically unaware that they are making predictions or acting them out in the form of saccadic eye movements. If these saccades are revealed to be a reflection of active hypothesis-testing in the brain, then they hold promise as a means of better understanding how the embodied brain makes its predictions when performing motor actions.

References

Bahill, A. Terry, and Tom LaRitz. 1984. "Why Can't Batters Keep Their Eyes on the Ball?" *American Scientist* 72 (3): 249–253.

Bell, Andrew H., Christopher Summerfield, Elyse L. Morin, Nicholas J. Malecek, and Leslie G. Ungerleider. 2016. "Encoding of Stimulus Probability in Macaque Inferior Temporal Cortex." *Current Biology* 26 (17): 2280–2290.

Bootsma, Reinoud J., Laure Fernandez, Antoine H. P. Morice, and Gilles Montagne. 2010. "Top-Level Players' Visual Control of Interceptive Actions: Bootsma and van Wieringen (1990) 20 Years Later." *Journal of Experimental Psychology: Human Perception and Performance* 36 (4): 1056–1063; discussion 1064–1066.

Bootsma, Reinoud J., and Piet C. Van Wieringen. 1990. "Timing an Attacking Forehand Drive in Table Tennis." *Journal of Experimental Psychology: Human Perception and Performance* 16 (1): 21–29.

Brenner, Eli, and Jeroen B. J. Smeets. 2011. "Continuous Visual Control of Interception." *Human Movement Science* 30 (3): 475–494.

Brielmann, Aenne A., and Miriam Spering. 2015. "Effects of Reward on the Accuracy and Dynamics of Smooth Pursuit Eye Movements." *Journal of Experimental Psychology: Human Perception and Performance* 41 (4): 917–928.

Burr, David, and Guido Marco Cicchini. 2014. "Vision: Efficient Adaptive Coding." *Current Biology* 24 (22): R1096–1098.

Cicchini, Guido Marco, Roberto Arrighi, Luca Cecchetti, Marco Giusti, and David C. Burr. 2012. "Optimal Encoding of Interval Timing in Expert Percussionists." *Journal of Neuroscience* 32 (3): 1056–1060.

Clark, Andy. 2013. "Whatever Next? Predictive Brains, Situated Agents, and the Future of Cognitive Science." *Behavioral and Brain Sciences* 36 (3): 181–204.

Croft, J. L., C. Button, and M. Dicks. 2010. "Visual Strategies of Sub-Elite Cricket Batsmen in Response to Different Ball Velocities." *Human Movement Science* 29 (5): 751–763.

Diaz, Gabriel, Joseph Cooper, Constantin Rothkopf, and Mary Hayhoe. 2013. "Saccades to Future Ball Location Reveal Memory-Based Prediction in a Virtual-Reality Interception Task." *Journal of Vision* 13 (1): 1–14. doi:10.1167/13.1.20.

Dicks, Matt, Chris Button, and Keith Davids. 2010. "Examination of Gaze Behaviors under in Situ and Video Simulation Task Constraints Reveals Differences in Information Pickup for Perception and Action." *Attention, Perception and Psychophysics* 72 (3): 706–720.

Gegenfurtner, Karl R., Marina Bloj, and Matteo Toscani. 2015. "The Many Colours of 'the Dress.'" *Current Biology* 25 (13): R543–544.

Georgopoulos, Apostolos P., John F. Kalaska, and Joe T. Massey. 1981. "Spatial Trajectories and Reaction Times of Aimed Movements: Effects of Practice, Uncertainty, and Change in Target Location." *Journal of Neurophysiology* 46 (4): 725–743.

Glencross, D. J., and B. J. Cibich. 1977. "A Decision Analysis of Games Skills." *Australian Journal of Sports Medicine* 9 (1): 72–75.

Hayhoe, Mary M., Travis McKinney, Kelly Chajka, and Jeff B. Pelz. 2012. "Predictive Eye Movements in Natural Vision." *Experimental Brain Research* 217 (1): 125–136.

Hohwy, Jakob. 2013. *The Predictive Mind.* Oxford: Oxford University Press.

Howarth, C., W. D. Walsh, B. Abernethy, and C. Snyder. 1984. "A Field Examination of Anticipation in Squash: Some Preliminary Data." *Australian Journal of Science and Medicine in Sport* 16 (3): 6–10.

Knill, David C., and Alexandre Pouget. 2004. "The Bayesian Brain: The Role of Uncertainty in Neural Coding and Computation." *Trends in Neurosciences* 27 (12): 712–719.

Koedijker, Johan M., and David L. Mann. 2015. "Consciousness and Choking in Visually-Guided Actions." *Phenomenology and the Cognitive Sciences* 14 (2): 333–348. doi:10.1007/s11097-014-9398-3.

Kuhn, G., and M. F. Land. 2006. "There's More to Magic than Meets the Eye." *Current Biology* 16 (22): R950–R951.

Lafer-Sousa, Rosa, Katherine L. Hermann, and Bevil R. Conway. 2015. "Striking Individual Differences in Color Perception Uncovered by 'the Dress' Photograph." *Current Biology* 25 (13): R545–546.

Land, M. F., and P. McLeod. 2000. "From Eye Movements to Actions: How Batsmen Hit the Ball." *Nature Neuroscience* 3 (12): 1340–1345.

Lee, D. N., D. S. Young, P. E. Reddish, S. Lough, and T. M. Clayton. 1983. "Visual Timing in Hitting an Accelerating Ball." *Quarterly Journal of Experimental Psychology A: Human Experimental Psychology* 35 (Pt 2): 333–346.

Mann, D. L., and G. J. P. Savelsbergh. 2015. "Issues in the Measurement of Anticipation." In *Routledge Handbook of Sport Expertise*, edited by J. Baker and D. Farrow, 166–175. Oxon, UK: Routledge.

Mann, David L., Bruce Abernethy, and Damian Farrow. 2010. "Action Specificity Increases Anticipatory Performance and the Expert Advantage in Natural Interceptive Tasks." *Acta Psychologica* 135 (1): 17–23.

Mann, David L., Wayne Spratford, and Bruce Abernethy. 2013. "The Head Tracks and Gaze Predicts: How the World's Best Batters Hit a Ball." *PLoS ONE* 8 (3): e58289.

Narain, Devika, Robert J. van Beers, Jeroen B. J. Smeets, and Eli Brenner. 2013. "Sensorimotor Priors in Nonstationary Environments." *Journal of Neurophysiology* 109 (5): 1259–1267.

Pinder, Ross A., Keith Davids, Ian Renshaw, and Duarte Araújo. 2011. "Representative Learning Design and Functionality of Research and Practice in Sport." *Journal of Sport and Exercise Psychology* 33 (1): 146–155.

Ripoll, H. 1989. "Uncertainty and Visual Strategies in Table Tennis." *Perceptual and Motor Skills* 68 (2): 507–512.

Ripoll, H., and P. Fleurance. 1988. "What Does Keeping One's Eye on the Ball Mean?" *Ergonomics* 31 (11): 1647–1654.

Ripoll, H., P. Fleurance, and D. Caseneuve. 1987. "Analysis of Visual Patterns of Table Tennis Players." In *Eye Movements: From Physiology to Cognition*, edited by J. K. O'Regan and A. Levy-Schoen, 616–617. Amsterdam: Elsevier Science.

Sarpeshkar, Vishnu, Bruce Abernethy, and David L. Mann. 2017. "Visual Strategies Underpinning the Development of Visual-motor Expertise when Hitting a Ball." *Journal of Experimental Psychology: Human Perception and Performance* 43:1744–1772.

Sarpeshkar, Vishnu, and David L. Mann. 2011. "Biomechanics and Visual-Motor Control: How It Has, Is, and Will Be Used to Reveal the Secrets of Hitting a Cricket Ball." *Sports Biomechanics / International Society of Biomechanics in Sports* 10 (4): 306–323.

Saunders, Jeffrey A., and David C. Knill. 2003. "Humans Use Continuous Visual Feedback from the Hand to Control Fast Reaching Movements." *Experimental Brain Research* 152 (3): 341–352.

Savelsbergh, Geert J. P., John Van der Kamp, A. Mark Williams, and Paul Ward. 2005. "Anticipation and Visual Search Behaviour in Expert Soccer Goalkeepers." *Ergonomics* 48 (11–14): 1686–1697. doi:10.1080/00140130500101346.

Spering, Miriam, and Marisa Carrasco. 2015. "Acting without Seeing: Eye Movements Reveal Visual Processing without Awareness." *Trends in Neurosciences* 38 (4): 247–258.

Spering, Miriam, Marc Pomplun, and Marisa Carrasco. 2011. "Tracking without Perceiving: A Dissociation between Eye Movements and Motion Perception." *Psychological Science* 22 (2): 216–225.

Spering, Miriam, Alexander C. Schütz, Doris I. Braun, and Karl R. Gegenfurtner. 2011. "Keep Your Eyes on the Ball: Smooth Pursuit Eye Movements Enhance Prediction of Visual Motion." *Journal of Neurophysiology* 105 (4): 1756–1767.

van Soest, A. J. (Knoek), and P. J. Beek. 2010. "Similar Findings, Different Interpretations: A Response to the Commentary by Bootsma et al. (2010)." *Journal of Experimental Psychology: Human Perception and Performance* 36 (4):1064–1066.

van Soest, A. J., Ljr Casius, W. De Kok, M. Krijger, M. Meeder, and P. J. Beek. 2010. "Are Fast Interceptive Actions Continuously Guided by Vision? Revisiting Bootsma and van Wieringen (1990)." *Journal of Experimental Psychology: Human Perception and Performance* 36 (4): 1040–1055.

Wann, J. P. 1996. "Anticipating Arrival: Is the Tau Margin a Specious Theory?" *Journal of Experimental Psychology: Human Perception and Performance* 22 (4): 1031–1048.

Winkler, Alissa D., Lothar Spillmann, John S. Werner, and Michael A. Webster. 2015. "Asymmetries in Blue—Yellow Color Perception and in the Color of 'the Dress.'" *Current Biology* 25 (13): R547–548.

Yarbus, Alfred L. 1967. "Eye Movements during Perception of Complex Objects." In *Eye Movements and Vision*, 171–211. New York: Springer.

25 Embodied and Enactive Creativity in Sports

Zuzanna Rucińska and Kenneth Aggerholm

1 Introduction

Creativity on the field is thought to be a useful skill, though one that is hard to achieve. We want to know how performance is not just improved, but actually pushed to a new, higher level (Hristovski et al. 2011). For example, in football, in the situation of attacking or advancing, on-the-spot creative maneuvers that can surprise the defendant can be beneficial to the game. As Memmert, Baker, and Bertsch (2010) claim, "Creativity entails varying, rare and flexible decision-making in complex game situations ... [but] it is not clear how this type of thinking is developed" (3). Similarly, Hristovski et al. (2011) identify a problem, in that, "Creativity in sport performance has seldom been the subject of systematic research. This state of affairs is exemplified by the absence in sport science of established theoretical rationales for studying and explaining creative behavior" (176).

Creativity in sport can manifest in various ways, and calling an act *creative* can refer to substantially different acts, depending on which discipline we study and which theoretical perspective we apply to it. For example, there is not one set of criteria that would sufficiently determine creativity in such various contexts as dancing, boxing, basketball, snowboarding, or golf. Hence, our aim in this chapter is not to create a taxonomy of the great variety of creative ways of performing in practice. It is rather to showcase the ways in which creativity in sport has been conceptualized in the (sport) literature and to propose our own reconceptualization, in line with the embodied and enacted accounts of cognition.

First, in this chapter we aim at shedding light on the understanding of creativity and various approaches of its study and development. Second, we promote a new embodied and enactive creativity account (EECA in short), focusing on the role of the agent in its context and the environmental affordances to better understand creativity. Third, we suggest applications for the EECA in the context of sport. The chapter contributes to the debate on creativity in sports as it applies the principles of enactivism and phenomenology to better understand the potential for creative performance in practice.

2 Creativity in Theory: State of the Art

Here we introduce the topic of creativity by providing a brief discussion of the mainstream creativity concepts and accounts, found in both philosophy and sport psychology. We look at how creativity has been conceptualized and operationalized, setting the stage for a proposal of how to understand creative capacities in the sport context.

2.1 Defining Creativity

What is creativity? Philosophical questions about creativity refer mainly to questions about its nature. One set of important questions that have recently been raised is, What is the bearer of creativity? Is it a person that is creative, is it a process in which one takes part, or is it a product of this process that we refer to as creative? Moreover, is creativity an objective value (realism), or does it depend on social acceptance (constructivism)? Is creativity context-dependent? Finally, is creativity an inherent part of any activity, or is it reserved to exceptional innovations? (Klausen 2010; Amabile 1996; Beghetto and Kaufman 2007). There is no single accepted way of defining creativity. As Klausen (2010) notices, "The standard definition of creativity is problematic and maybe in an even worse state than is generally acknowledged by creativity researchers themselves" (347). Creativity, whatever it may be, is not a concrete and immediately identifiable phenomenon.

Yet, the most commonly found definitions propose to explain creativity as an umbrella term that encompasses key characteristics. These characteristics are novelty, originality (understood as statistical rareness), flexibility, and usefulness. Another aspect of creativity scholars agree on is that being creative is posited as juxtaposed to following a routine. Creativity has also been understood as the production of something that is both novel and appropriate. While many focus on novelty or originality as a key factor to creativity (see Amabile 1996), Klausen (2010) stresses the normative aspect of creative behavior. As he points out,

> Creativity requires novelty; the obvious contrast to creativity is mere repetition and replication. But not every kind of novelty will do; diverging from established practice is not considered creative if it does not lead to a positive result. Hence, creativity is about breaking with norms or practices, doing something unexpected or unpredictable, but still meeting certain—albeit

> more liberal—constraints.... The novelty and usefulness requirements cannot be split; what we are after is a qualified usefulness, probably a novel kind of usefulness. (349–350)

Thus, Klausen proposes that only together do novelty and usefulness form the key conditions for creativity. While a creative act need not necessarily reduce to a successful act ("It should be possible to engage in a genuinely creative process which, for some reason or another, nevertheless fails to produce a result that is accepted as tenable, useful, or satisfying," 349), some form of normativity, or appropriateness to context, of the creative act is important. In line with antirealist positions, Klausen (2010) claims that creativity is highly context-dependent; the product of creativity is to be considered only in the context of an appropriate audience and suitable conditions.[1] This approach to creativity is in line with the affordance-based explanation of creativity that we propose in part 3.

2.2 Operationalizing Creativity

When it comes to operationalizing creativity, psychologists have considered: What is required for creativity? *What are the necessary and/or sufficient conditions under which creativity occurs?*[2] Many propose that some form of representing the situation is required. This suggests that creativity is a process, which is rooted in the head of an individual.

It is typical to think of creativity as requiring "stopping" with the routine and "thinking" about alternatives. When the familiar circumstances and routine actions break down, we turn to the representational models of cognition. The assumption is that in the case of unproblematic circumstances, attention disrupts the fluid pattern of a familiar routine, while in problematic scenarios attention is required to improvise a new problem-solving strategy. The latter expresses expertise and skill just because it efficaciously employs attentive detached self-monitoring for purposes of problem solving and creative improvisation. Expert skills are "characterized by superior capabilities of decision making, problem solving, and creative improvisation in problematic or unfamiliar situations" (Cappuccio et al., this volume, chapter 5). In other words, what is taken for granted is that in problematic (or novel) circumstances, attention (self-monitoring) or problem-solving capacities are posited.

Problem-solving capacities and creative improvisation have been considered as explicitly representational in character. When we are creative or engage in improvisation, representational processes such as full-blown "thinking" is said to be taking place; as Runco and Pina state, creativity "involves thinking that is removed from the reality" (in Taylor 2013, 381). Such contrasts are common in philosophy: for example, "creative imagination" is contrasted with "recreative imagination" as the one that requires explicit representing (Currie and Ravenscroft 2002). Creative imagination is said to be "combining ideas in unexpected and unconventional ways.... We see it when someone puts together ideas in a way that defies expectation or convention: the kind of imaginative 'leap' that leads the creation of something valuable in art, science, or practical life" (9). Similarly, Beaty et al. (2016) claim that "creativity researchers have long speculated that creative thought involves a two-stage process of idea generation and idea evaluation" (90), emphasizing the role of cognitive control together with the role of default neural networks in creative processes. Beaty et al. (2016) ask, "How does the brain produce creative thought?" suggesting that creative thought involves dynamic interactions of large-scale brain systems (87). They have studied the brain patterns to identify "a network of brain regions associated with divergent thinking," divergent thinking understood as thinking that involves "generating several possible solutions to an open-ended problem, such as inventing creative uses for common objects" (88). Such understanding of creativity as stemming from thinking invites consideration of creativity as a representational process.

2.3 Creativity in Sports

In sport psychology, creativity seems to be defined through its measurability. Most commonly, Guilford's (1967) creativity measuring scale is endorsed. The scale involves *originality* (it denotes the unusualness, innovativeness, statistical rareness, or even uniqueness of tactical solutions to a sport game-related task) and *flexibility* (it characterizes the ease with which someone changes between thoughts, generates different hypotheses, or modifies information; Memmert and Roth 2007). Flexibility is measured by counting diversity of tactical solutions over different game situations. At times, *fluency of thinking* is counted; it is defined as the number of adequate solutions to one given situation produced by an individual (in Memmert and Roth 2007, 2). Others propose that novelty (i.e., originality) and functionality (i.e., usefulness, effectiveness, appropriateness, success, or adequacy) are the two key dimensions that co-characterize a creative product or behavior (Hristovski et al. 2011).

One suggestion of how these criteria translate into specific sport contexts can be proposed with an example of a boxer. Consider a boxer practicing his moves before a tournament. *Originality* or novelty of a move would occur in the context where he has a repertoire of practiced moves 1 through 4 (left hook, right jab, left uppercut, right cross), and a new and original "move 5" emerges. *Flexibility* or ease of combining or changing between the moves would occur with the boxer bringing about novel combinations of his moves unexpectedly; instead of going through with the routine 1 through 4, the boxer quickly shifts between the moves, 1, 4, 3, 1, 2, 2, 3, and so on, creating a new unexpected pattern for action yet with the same original movements.

Fluency of thinking or functionality would occur in a case where the boxer chooses, in a specific situation *S*, to target a specific move, "3," because he considers it the best move to make. This consideration is judged, or reasoned, to be the most efficient one for the goal at hand.

These aspects of creativity have contrasting criteria: they allow creativity to be defined both at the behavioral level and at a cognitivist level (Memmert, Baker, and Bertsch 2010). As such, it is open to interpretation which theoretical framework can best describe these aspects of creativity. Again, the representational approaches have always been favored. *Originality*, *flexibility*, and *fluency of thinking* are all, in their descriptions, considered as characteristics of a thought process. Sport psychologists have proposed to classify these aspects of creativity into "divergent" and "convergent" thinking. As Memmert, Baker, and Bertsch (2010) claim,

> Convergent thinking refers to the ability to find the ideal solution to a given problem, whereas divergent thinking is defined at the behavioral level as the unusualness, innovativeness, statistical rareness, or even uniqueness of solutions to a related task. In sports, this latter form of thinking relates to tactical creativity, that is, varying, rare, and flexible decisions in different kinds of situations. Conversely, expert decision-making describes the general ability to find the best tactical solution in any specific situation. (4)

Tactical creativity is one example of a creative behavior in sports. It is an example of divergent thinking that has to do with *originality* and *flexibility*. *Originality* tends to be understood as the ability to "*think* outside the box," and *flexibility* as changing "between thought levels" and "generating different hypotheses" (Memmert and Roth 2007, 2). For example, in the situation of attacking or advancing (as opposed to defending) in a game, when the action is initiated, it would show as the on-the-spot creative maneuver that surprises the defendant. Convergent thinking, or the *fluency of thinking* aspect of creativity, here remains to be best characterized as a type of thought, as it seems to require cognitive processes like evaluation to aim at the "best" possible maneuver. There seem to be correctness conditions to be satisfied; planning to make the best move possible seems to require making some sort of judgment of what is the best move available, and that judgment can be right or wrong. As such, we can call this process representational, as one represents the world and the best outcome of acting in the world in advance of the action. It also follows the classical computational model: "sense→model→plan→act." For example, a footballer is sensing the ball in his presence, modeling the environment in which he acts (considering where is the goal or the next player), planning the appropriate action, and acting accordingly. While the representational process is happening sub-personally, or beyond conscious thought, the creative process may also be considered to take place in the individual, planning segment of the cognitive act.

2.4 Looking for Alternatives

As clarified, the typical way of operationalizing creativity, whether in general or in sport context, is by recourse to mental representations. What is often not clarified is how the term "mental representation" is being used. The traditional and most commonly used notion is that mental representations are semantic content-bearing vehicles.[3] This sense of mental representations is most adequate for explaining thought processes and, in extension, creativity understood as such a thought process.

Yet, this characterization of mental representations does not reflect the commitments of many theorists who speak of creativity. For example, Van Leeuwen (2011) suggests that imagination involves making a *forward model*, "an internal representation of motor commands that anticipates the consequences of those commands on bodily motion" (56) that is supposed to be nonlinguistic. He links his theory to observations from sports, claiming that "a basketball player who imagines her free-throw motion from a first person perspective prior to taking the shot is imaginatively constructing such a forward model" (68). If creativity is parasitic on imagination, and imagination is explained with the use of such forward models, then a case could be made for understanding aspects of creativity in such a manner as well. This way of conceptualizing creativity would be to appeal to most minimal kinds of representations, ones that are not conscious, intentional, or conveyed through propositions. Consider, as an example, explaining flexibility (one feature of creativity) on this model. Tactical creativity that requires maneuvering between a set of skills could be explained through the computational "sense-model-plan-act" mechanism, wherein one's cognitive process would have to only "sense" the environment and then model various movements, plan the action, and move the body to act according to the plan.

In short, there is a difference in kind between language-like representations that form propositional attitudes and non-propositional, action-oriented representations or motor representations. Recourse to the weak notion of representations is often proposed to explain various cognitive acts in sports, such as when the "embodied knowledge representations" are used to explain the role of motor skills in predictive imagining of the expert athlete (Beilock 2008).

Yet, some argue that such "representations" are not in fact representations at all, as they do not traffic any contents (Hutto and Myin 2013, 2017). Moreover, it is unclear whether forward models must be cashed out as mental representations, or whether imaginings that are said to underlie creativity have conditions of satisfaction. For example, it is not clear how percepts are "encoded" by the brain or how "forward models" work; more work has to be done to show what role, if any, they play in creative processes. Re-creating can have novel and creative elements to it, and there is no way of telling whether it "matches" what actually has been seen. Considering that one can imagine anything one wishes, there would be nothing constraining whether the imagining was done correctly or incorrectly; the worry is that without some kind of semantic description, the models allow "anything" to go (Langland-Hassan 2015). Hence, images alone might not be enough; it is what one can do with them that accounts for how one acts creatively.[4]

Importantly for this chapter, what the positions promoting either notion of representation lack is reference to the *embodied, social,* and *interactive* aspects of creativity. The shortcomings of the representational accounts of creativity are their focus on individualism and overintellectualization of creativity. Individualism shows in the focus on one person's expressions of creativity considered as an innate cognitive process, whereas wider context in which the creative act takes place is not considered. The potentially detrimental roles of the body, the environment, and the others in a context promoting creativity are not fully accounted for, which leaves a gap to promote a new proposal of how to operationalize creativity, one that gives constitutive power to the body and the environment in considering cognition. Intellectualization shows in considering the creative process to be a cognitive activity that requires planning of action and modeling of the environment, tools that may not be needed when engaging in creative acts. Another possibility is to consider creativity in terms of responsiveness to affordances. Clarification of this explanatory tool will be made in part 3 below.

3 Introducing the Embodied and Enactive Creativity Account (EECA)

In contrast to the representational accounts of cognition, the embodied and enactive accounts of cognition endorse the key role of interacting with the environment in shaping our cognitive processes. In line with this approach, a creative act can be recharacterized as necessarily an embodied and situated act that involves novelty and flexibility in movement as well as its usefulness and appropriateness in the context of that movement (the normative aspect of creativity). The novel account proposes to think of creativity of a person as an aptitude or responsiveness to the available affordances of the situation, involving the capacity to let new affordances, or possibilities for action, emerge in situations. It proposes a new, interactive model of a "body (including the brain) $\leftrightarrow$ environment $\leftrightarrow$ other" dynamic, while emphasizing that this model is not static or fixed; at times, the body, the environment, or the other in the context can play a bigger role in shaping the creative response.

To properly account for the novel approach to creativity, the embodied and enactive creativity account (EECA), we first clarify key terms in the field of embodied and enactive literature, linking its origin to phenomenological proposals of creativity.

3.1 Embodied and Enactive

Embodied and enactive accounts of cognition denote distinct yet related concepts that contrast traditional frameworks of philosophy of mind and cognitive science. Embodied cognition refers to the idea that cognition is constrained as well as regulated and grounded by our sensorimotor system, by the specific characteristics of our own brain-body system. Enactive cognition emphasizes in turn the active role of the agent and the environment in co-constructing cognition. It recognizes a crucial interdependency between an autonomous agent and the world he or she inhabits. The environment is again a crucial aspect of the cognitive process. Cognitive activity is defined neither by the agents nor their environment, but is actively emergent from their interaction. The outcome of taking an embodied and enactive approach to cognition is that it finds mentality in the interactions between organisms and environments, not in mental representations.[5] These approaches focus on dynamic interactions of the agents with their environments, which shape their cognition (Varela, Thompson, and Rosch 1991; Chemero 2009; De Jaegher and Di Paolo 2007; Hutto and Myin 2013, 2017).

3.2 Phenomenological Roots

The Structure of Behavior by Merleau-Ponty (1963 [1942]) is a good starting point for pinpointing the roots of aspects of the embodied and enactive cognition view. In the passage below, Merleau-Ponty describes the experience of a football player in the field:

> [For] the player in action the football field is not an "object," that is, the ideal term which can give rise to an indefinite multiplicity of perspectival views and remain equivalent under its apparent transformations. It is pervaded with lines of force (the "yard lines," those which demarcate the "penalty area") and sectors (for example, the "openings" between the adversaries) which call for a certain mode of action and which initiate and guide the action as if the player were unaware of it. The field itself is not given to him, but present the immanent term of his practical intentions; the player becomes one with it and feels the direction of the "goal," for example, just as immediately as the vertical and the horizontal planes of his own body.... Each maneuver undertaken by the player modifies the character of the field and establishes in it new lines of force which the action in turn unfolds and is accomplished, again altering the phenomenal field. (168–169)

According to Merleau-Ponty, we have to abandon a description of the playing field as an "object." Instead it should be conceived of as a "phenomenal field," or a situation. Here objects of perception are first and foremost lived as realities rather than known as, for example, conceptual objects. Yet, according to Merleau-Ponty, the situation is not a range of objective stimuli that causes the player to act in specific ways. Performance cannot be reduced to a causal effect of external stimuli. There is a difference between the sensations of the situation and the meaning of the situation, and in *Phenomenology of Perception,* Merleau-Ponty drew on this insight to distinguish between a *spatiality of position* (that of external objects), and a *spatiality of situation* (1962 [1945], 114–115). This latter spatiality is not an objectifiable external space but a bodily space that serves as the background and the horizon for any perception and/or movement to occur.[6]

In this passage, Merleau-Ponty shows that neither a behaviorist nor an intellectualist approach can capture the experience of the player. This holds implications for the way we understand the relation between the player and the field, which can inform our understanding of performance in various sports, and which forces us to reconsider the understanding of creative performance as "divergent thinking" as described in contemporary approaches in sport psychology. Rather, it invites describing creativity as a general aptitude, a kind of responsiveness of the player(s) to alter situations and let new possibilities emerge. Such possibilities of action can be described as *affordances,* which is a central notion in ecological psychology that relates to the embodied and enactive approaches.

With Merleau-Ponty's notion of creativity further developed later, next we briefly clarify the modern descriptions of affordances, including an application of one of the affordance theories to a sport context.

3.3 Affordances

Affordances, in the most general terms, can be understood as possibilities for action that the environment affords to the agent. While there is no consensus as to what affordances are, and many interpretations have been proposed (including Gibson 1979; Turvey 1992; Chemero 2009; Withagen et al. 2012; Rietveld and Kiverstein 2014; see Rucińska 2017 for an overview), we will draw on an understanding of affordances as relational aspects of the environment. Importantly to our story, affordances alone are not enough to account for any action. Affordances of the environment must be complemented by agent's *effectivities* in a specific context in order for the affordances to *solicit* or *invite* any actions to come about.[7]

Affordances and effectivities also do not explain behaviors, including creative behaviors, on their own. Any object can have an almost infinite number of possibilities for action (affordances) and any agent has just as many effectivities. Often it is the relevant context, including other people in this context, who are actively engaging with the agent or only present in the background, which allows for the relevant affordance-effectivity pair to invite actions. The thought experiment below will elucidate this point with an example.

3.4 Thought Experiment: Kobe versus LeBron

Consider a hypothetical case of a basketball player (let us call him Kobe) who has the capacity to slam-dunk the ball during high-profile games. Kobe is very confident and secure with his skill. In normal game context (in the presence of known defenders), the hoop invites slam-dunking (for Kobe, who likes to establish his superiority over these defenders). However, the presence of one particular defender in a game (let us call him LeBron), who, as Kobe previously experienced, is often successful at blocking Kobe's dunks, affects the hoop as uninviting the dunk to Kobe. The mere presence of LeBron could be considered as the relevant change of context that actualizes the new hoop affordance–Kobe effectivity pair: the hoop becomes more inviting from afar, inviting shooting three-pointers. Importantly, it is not necessarily the hoop itself or Kobe's skills that invite slam-dunking; it is the additional presence of LeBron that makes a difference in what action occurs.

Thus, calling on other people in the immediate context of play is just one possible way to explain why certain affordance-effectivity pairs strongly invite and drive our actions. This is not the only way to step away from one practice to another; we respond to affordances all the time, and so we could switch about even without the presence of others, but because of some new occurrence in our contexts. Also, we may change our moods or attitudes about what practice we take ourselves to be in, and that change could bring about different affordances as inviting as well.[8] Yet, the fact that situational factors such as the presence of other people, and not just individual concerns, moods, intentions, or explicit choices can affect the context needs to be stressed; it is the environment that can also play the relevant role.

The context, including other persons, forms the relevant context for new affordances to be discovered. It shapes and structures the responsiveness of the individual, allowing for his or her creative responsiveness to available affordances of the environment. In connection with individual's capacities and history of interactions with the environment, the context accounts for novel affordances to be brought forth in the agent's phenomenal field.

3.5 Accounting for Normativity

As mentioned earlier, creativity in sport context requires accommodating the idea of normativity. Affordances, understood as mere possibilities for action found in the environment, on their own are not normative; they do not specify what the action is good for.[9] One cannot go wrong in acting on affordances; one *just acts* on different affordances. However, affordance-effectivity pairs actualized in a context can be regarded as normative. Actualized affordances solicit, or invite (but do not mechanically cause) particular action to take place. *Solicitations* have been introduced into our theoretical vocabulary as those affordances that invite action. They are relevant to the agent's concerns (Rietveld and Kiverstein 2014, 342) and have a "demand character." When affordances do invite or select particular behaviors, we can think of this selection process as based on the world and partly on the way the organism has developed to respond to certain aspects of it.[10] Introducing solicitations is an important contribution to the field, as it shows that this selection is not just mind-to-world that cries out for mental representations; rather, there is no direction of fit, as the agent's capacities and environment mutually affect each other in dynamical interaction.

Withagen et al. (2012) as well as Rietveld and Kiverstein (2014) suggest that solicitations are normative in the phenomenological sense, because they strongly invite behaviors that lead to what Merleau-Ponty called an "optimal grip." Solicitations point to the relations between aspects of the environment and abilities in a form of life, suggesting that there is an appropriate fit between the agent and the object. Such normativity can take place only in the context of the mutuality of the agent and the environment. There is a better or worse "grip" one can have on events, and novel ways of performing in one's situation can be more or less valuable or appropriate.

3.6 Motor Intentionality and Bodily Meaning

The understanding of having an optimal grip, or grip directed at the best situation, as well as of the "embodied space," as mentioned with reference to Merleau-Ponty, rests on the classic phenomenological understanding of consciousness: it is *of* something, it is directed and, hence, intentional at the outset. Following Husserl, Merleau-Ponty (1962 [1945]) argued that we must acknowledge, prior to the intentionality of representations, an operative intentionality (xx, 486, 498), which is the practical intentionality that he also refers to as motor intentionality (127, 159, 169, 370). It describes how the body as a motor power mediates between the intentional object and the actual movement in a way that makes them inseparable.

This understanding of bodily space and motor intentionality can inform an understanding of performance that rests on pre-reflective, bodily, and motor responsiveness to situations, which are prior to engagement in reflection or representation. In light of this, and in accordance with Hamrick's (1994) analysis of creativity in Merleau-Ponty, an embodied understanding of creative performance in sport can in general terms be described as creation of new *bodily meaning* in one's situation, which can also be described as revealing and/or expressing new motor significance in one's performance.

Such creation of bodily meaning can be explained by following the phenomenological insight that intentional objects can be both actual and possible, which means that agents can be intentionally related to real objects in the situation, as well as to virtual or nonexistent objects (Merleau-Ponty 1962 [1945], 128). Merleau-Ponty's notion of motor intentionality can describe how relating to, or shifting between, these levels of bodily space need not involve mental representation of either the situation or one's own body (body image). Rather, "the body is available not only in real situations into which it is drawn. It can turn aside from the world, apply its activity to stimuli which affect its sensory surfaces, lend itself to experimentation, and generally speaking take its place in the realm of the potential" (125).

This enactment is thus a dimension of the lived body, which Merleau-Ponty also describes as a "virtual body" (291) capable of "abstract movements" (128), such as pointing and expressing oneself in relation to possibilities in one's situation. In sport, such kind of movement is evident, for example, when players perform feints in football (Aggerholm, Jespersen, and Ronglan 2011) or when athletes in general perform "dramatic expressions" (Aggerholm 2015, 120–145).

3.7 Effect: Embodied and Enacted Creativity

What the above-mentioned positions in embodied and enacted cognition and phenomenology suggest is that agent's actions are affected by the mutuality of the environmental affordances and agent's effectivities in the right context. It is the variety in the context that affects various behaviors, including creative behaviors on the field, to occur. Following the embodied and enactive account suggests that creativity could be understood as a result of having new embodied experiences, rather than putting together disembodied ideas. Creativity is not a skill (know-how) or a specific knowledge (knowledge proper), but, as Merleau-Ponty puts it, it has more to do with a general aptitude to the situation, or *creative responsiveness*. This creative responsiveness is a result of interaction with solicitations, which can relate to both actual and possible aspects of one's situation that shape and delineate the potential actions for an agent. Creativity is thus not in the first place solely a cognitive trait of the agent, but a result of the interaction between the agent's effectivities and environmental affordances that make up solicitations for actions.

Similarly, Merleau-Ponty's description of abstract movement refers to that which transcends what is present and expected; it homes in on the potential or virtual. Creativity, in similar respect, is said to go beyond what is immediate, transcending the routine actions into a sphere of novelty. Explaining this is where recourse to mental representations often takes place, but with Merleau-Ponty's account it is possible to understand how dealing with the "abstract" is also an aspect of embodiment, a form of movement, and not a mental representation or another cognitive addition to the actual movement. It is a general human ability to be bodily directed toward a field of possibilities. It can thus describe more expressive forms of creativity, such as originality, expression of new meaning, or pretense and deception as creative acts in relation to others, without recourse to mental representation.

In short, there is much more in sensorimotor skills than we usually imagine, and there is enough space to accommodate the particular kind of intelligence that we usually call creativity.[11] This proposal cannot be translated into a simple explanatory model. There is no direct route to explain how one individual can act in a creative manner and another cannot, or why the same individual can at times act creatively and at another times gets stuck in a rote. However, the advantage of this proposal is that solicitations can account for the normative aspect of creativity in sport. A creative action must be an appropriate action that aims at advancing in the game and is within the bounds of the rules of the game. There is a successful way of acting in a creative way that is determined by the particular situation. The normative aspect of embodied action in sport accounts for the fact that there is improvement or competitive advantage that follows from (or perhaps is even central to) the creative act.

Thus, with the embodied and enactive account of cognition available, there exists a motivation to challenge the standard representational takes on analyzing creativity and suggest another approach as a viable alternative, if not a more promising one, to understanding emergence and development of creativity on the field. This proposal can also suggest ways to develop one's responsiveness that need not require representational capacities. How creative responsiveness can be developed is addressed in part 4.

3.8 Coda: Between Dreyfus and McDowell

One clarification is necessary at this stage. It may seem that the EECA has a natural affinity with Dreyfus's (2002) notion of *absorbed coping*, whereby agents in the midst of the activities in which they have expertise do not need to represent what they are doing (or in any demanding way "think" about their actions). Instead, they are directly immersed in the *flow* of the activity (Csíkszentmihályi 1990), utilizing their embodied *know-hows*. This is a familiar theory applicable to sport professionals, but also applicable in dance, theater, and practical skills in many daily activities (e.g., driving a car).

However, we should not assume that following the embodied and enactive route necessarily leads to fully committing to Dreyfus's position on embodied rationality, seen as a matter of absorbed coping that he deems to be *mindless*; it is not a non-mental practical activity without experiential content, where an absorbed agent "ceases to be a subject" (Dreyfus 2007, 373) or is "in a way like a sleepwalker" (Dreyfus 2013, 38). In response to the Dreyfus-McDowell debate, Zahavi (2013) proposes a middle position, wherein embodied rationality is understood as more than nonconscious automatic responding but less than a conceptual or linguistic activity of deliberation (McDowell 2007); it involves an experiential aspect related to pre-reflective subjectivity (326–331; see also Aggerholm 2015). According to Thompson (2005), pre-reflective subjectivity or bodily self-awareness is implicit and non-intentional; our perceptual experience involves such awareness. It corresponds to one's experience of one's body as perceiving and acting, rather than as perceived. Also, according to Gallagher (2015), embodied rationality can be understood as a form of *thinking-without-thinking-about-it*, a form of intelligent, embodied, and situated reflection that is embedded in a context and may be accomplished with others, yet need not require consulting rules (143). This middle position between mindless and mental accounts of coping is much in line with the embodied and enactive approach we have sought to outline above, and this, we argue, can provide a fruitful account of the enactment of creativity in sport.

4 Implications: EECA in Sports

Here we consider what implications follow from the embodied and enactive creativity account (EECA) in our understanding of tactical creativity and its development in sport contexts. We consider what follows from treating creativity as a form of responsiveness to the environment. We propose that creativity understood as embodied and enactive responsiveness will make a difference with respect to the methodology of training creativity.

4.1 Training Creativity

The considerations about how to frame creativity in sports lead to the question of whether creativity can be developed, trained, or in any way practiced. It may be hard to conceive of creativity as trainable as, on the face value, creativity clashes with routine-based activity; it is common to think of creativity as requiring "stopping" with the routine in order to "come up with" something that the routine does not encompass, whereas training involves repeating a routine in order to gain new bodily habits. Moreover, as we train mainly through drills or routinizing a set of skills, it seems that creativity cannot be something that is trainable. However, this is a misconception that the EECA will tackle.

It must be cautioned that the theory outlined above does not in itself prescribe direct ways of facilitating the development of creative athletes. What EECA highlights is the important role of the interaction of the body, environment, tools, and other people in structuring agent's creativity in a particular context. As performance is context-dependent, no one rule for how to train creativity can be proposed. Prescribing how to become creative is in some sense contradictory; creativity itself cannot be instructed. Nonetheless, EECA can inform some general guidelines on how to facilitate creative responsiveness. A central point is that an embodied and enactive approach to creativity means that the development of creativity is part of practice in the field—and hence not a matter of engaging in mental training detached from the practical engagement or by testing and exploring other kinds of sport. EECA does not refer to any representational capacities, whether linguistic, imagistic, motor, or other. It focuses solely on understanding creativity through recourse to sensorimotor capacities, interactionism, and dynamical systems theory. Under this account, to paraphrase Currie and Ravenscroft (2002), creativity would entail combining bodily *experiences* (not *ideas*) in unexpected and unconventional ways, as that forms creative responsiveness. Putting these experiences together, in turn, would be a result of cultivating knowing how to act in original and flexible ways achieved through acting in the environment. Achieving creativity on the field then requires engaging in bodily acts as opposed to mere mental training. A concrete example of a sportsman engaging in creative responsiveness is proposed in part 4.5 (The Case of a Boxer) below.

Current literature on creativity is divided with respect to the issue of how to train creativity. Most suggestions have been proposed in the literature based on the qualitative analysis of the proposals for *deliberate play* and *deliberate practice*. On the one hand, proposals are made for deliberate play, a form of nonspecific training of creativity; on the other hand, deliberate practice is emphasized, which involves focusing on the developing of the expert skills within one discipline. In what follows, we expand on both types of measures for enhancing creativity, after which we propose our suggestion.

4.2 Developing Creativity via Deliberate Play

According to Memmert and Roth (2007), deliberate play designates a form of nonspecific training that can lead to improved "general creativity." They focus on unstructured play as a source of great variety of experiences across different sports. Indeed, as Ford et al. (2009) claim, "There is some evidence to suggest that play is important in the development of soccer game intelligence, such as anticipation and decision-making, as well as creative tactical responses" (1040). Arguments for deliberate play have informed hypotheses for late specialization, also referred to as *early diversification*. For example, in the sampling years of sport training (age 7–12), children are encouraged to engage in several sports; play-focused training is valued over goal-oriented, hard training in the specific discipline.

As Memmert, Baker, and Bertsch (2010) suggest, "Current theoretical approaches regarding the development of creativity support the view that gathering diversified experience over years (the time spent in unstructured play activities) is an ideal medium for creative thinking" (3). Reasons for engaging in deliberate play are based on an idea of the benefits of "transfer of skills." What enhances tactical creativity is gathering diversified experience by *physical involvement* in a diverse range of sport activities; *versatility in activities* (extending the activities to participating in unstructured games) that allows for transfer of learning; and a wide range of *environmental variability* that may increase capability to deal with situations that occur unexpectedly. For example, Memmert, Baker, and Bertsch (2010) mention the beneficial role of *constantly changing* materials (e.g., hockey stick, tennis racquet), balls (e.g., softballs, handballs, balloons), and parts of the body mainly used (hand, foot, head, or racquet) in every lesson. They thus suggest that coaches could ensure short-term varied experiences as part of the training.

This position is in line with the affordance-based account; there are many environmental affordances that can be explored, which allows for novel affordance-effectivity pairs to come about, allowing for novel ways of acting to develop. Deliberate play reveals new possibilities for action. In deliberate play, where one is participating in various playful, unstructured engagements and is exposed to a myriad of situations, one can train the skill of pushing the boundaries of what is acceptable in a game. Playful variations may be of value: for example, participating in different sports (structured games), in the same sport but being placed on different positions, or participating in various other, unstructured games could allow new sets of skills to be developed, which are likely to be transferable to the another context. But, while we agree with the unquestionable benefits of exploring the various environmental affordances, focusing solely on deliberate play seems to undermine the role of developing good bodily habits necessary for expert skills. Memmert, Baker, and Bertsch (2010) distinguish creativity from expertise to argue that creative players are often at a lower level of expert decision making. However, this need not be necessary; we look at expert practice below.

4.3 Developing Expertise via Deliberate Practice

Deliberate play is often described as a contrast to deliberate practice, which is an approach to talent development that argues for seeing expertise level as a result of practice hours rather than inborn talent (see, e.g., Baker, Côté, and Deakin 2005; Helsen, Starkes, and Hodges 1998; Hodges et al. 2004; Law, Côté, and Ericsson 2007; see also Ericsson 1998, 2014; Ericsson, Krampe, and Tesch-Römer 1993). Arguments for deliberate practice have informed arguments for early specialization, as advocated by Ericsson and colleagues (e.g., Ericsson, Krampe, and Tesch-Römer 1993). Their famous claim is that 10,000 hours of deliberate practice are needed to become an expert. Ericsson has been a key proponent for this view and has, as part of the deliberate-practice paradigm, advanced what Simonton (2000) calls the creative-expertise hypothesis, which states how individual differences in creative achievements can be ascribed to the amount of effort and time a person has devoted to domain mastery (284).

This is relevant for creativity in sport and the role of practicing is also a central aspect of EECA. At the same time, an embodied and enactive account is very different from deliberate practice. First, deliberate practice is governed by empirical cognitive psychology; its result is physical adaptation and acquisition of more refined cognitive and/or physical skills. Specific training is said to be able to lead experts to achieve refined representations, making them capable of performing creatively in sport and other domains (Ericsson 1998).[12] Deliberate practice is also said to develop long-term working memory (Ericsson and Kintsch 1995) and is described as improving perceptual and cognitive skills, such as anticipation or decision making. Second, and related to this, deliberate practice objectifies the process of practicing. While highlighting important aspects of development of athletes—for example, the role of effort and repetition in their development of expertise—it does so in an objectifying and instrumental fashion, when it argues that the motivation for practice is purely extrinsic (such as achieving goal or improving skills) and that the process of practicing is not inherently meaningful (Ericsson, Krampe, and Tesch-Römer 1993, 371–372).

A more qualitative and phenomenologically informed understanding of practicing can help challenge this instrumental understanding of practicing repetitions found in deliberate practice (see Aggerholm 2015, 52–57 and 170–197; Aggerholm 2016). Repetition does not presuppose doing something by rote; on the contrary, repeating toward new variations and improvements are part of engagement in practicing new moves and skills. As Hristovski et al. (2011) claim with respect to the case of a boxer who developed a new movement with respect to the punching bag, "Even a repetition of a movement is actually an exploration of some small set of movement configurations. Because of small differences in initial conditions (i.e., specific task constraints) of the action, each repetition is actually slightly different from others" (187). Such qualitative insights can help describe how repetition and practicing can be central to developing creativity.

4.4 Our Suggestion

There is a clear compatibility between EECA and engagement in deliberate play as a way to develop creativity on the field. EECA proposes that, in line with deliberate-play proposal, creativity could be enhanced through active exploration of the tools (such as various balls and instruments in sport), through which novel affordance-effectivity pairs can be developed. This in some sense requires breaking with a routine (the mechanistic application of previous skills), yet it does not necessarily require application of cognitive capacities such as inference or calculating. What is needed is exposure to novel situations, where new habits can develop.

However, in our view, creative performance should be linked to expertise, in line with deliberate-practice proposal. Creative performance marks a step up in the level of performance, such as in invasion games, when unpredictability is a key element of high-level performance. In this respect, creativity need not only be considered in relation to novelty, but also in relation to *flexibility* found within engaging in one sport and *usefulness* in a particular sport one is an expert in. Therefore, it is not sufficient to describe creativity on the field as developed solely by engaging in different sports or random play.

4.5 The Case of a Boxer

Consider the example of the boxer who runs sequences of movements 1 through 5 during training. Hristovski et al. (2011) showed that *relaxing task constraints* during deliberate practice in one sport can be deemed useful in enhancing the boxer's tactical creativity. In his experiment, boxers were asked to perform sixty punches at a static heavy-bag from ten different scaled distances. Later the heavy-bag was stochastically moved by an assistant to the left and right. Participants used existing classical boxing repertoire, while changing the scaled distance to the target. Hristovski comments:

> Jabs, hooks and uppercuts were afforded at scaled distances from the heavy-bag, which showed that the learned repertoire was adjusted accordingly to the affordance of the heavy-bag.... [What followed was that] 2 out of 4 performers created a novel outward-directed, arched striking movement with their right arms when the heavy-bag was displaced at widths greater than the widths of their right shoulders. These observations signified an emergence of a qualitatively different, i.e. innovative, divergent fist-target angle action configuration, with respect to the central visual line. (193)

This suggests that relaxing task constraints may give rise to a creative cross-fertilization of actions. Such relaxation of task constraints, symptomatic of playful contexts, is a direct effect of the presence of and responsiveness to new affordances in the same environment in which one is masterfully engaging. Hence, both deliberate play and deliberate practice can hold valuable insights regarding development of creativity, and as part of EEAC, these two dimensions of training should be balanced.[13] Such EECA explanation of creative responsiveness dominates over classic representational explanations, as it acknowledges the mutual effects of play and practice in shaping the creative responsiveness.

The EECA, therefore, has the advantage of utilizing the agent-environment dynamic to account for creativity in sport context; the environment is, crucially, both of play and of practice. It proposes that creativity is not an individualistic achievement of a person decontextualized from her environment; the environment plays a constitutive role in creativity, as it allows creative responses to occur. Aside from taking under consideration the capacities of the agent, an important explanatory role is played by the shape of the agent's interaction with the environment. Through deliberate play one gains flexibility, and through deliberate practice one benefits from repetition and can achieve novelty in action. Both deliberate play and deliberate practice are actions in the world, where the novel affordances, or possibilities for action, can show up to the agent.

4.6 Follow-Up: Environments for Creativity

Here we consider further the role of the environment in accounting for developing creativity in practice. Some suggestions for development of creative skills, in line with EECA, propose changes to the environmental context. For example, the players can participate in exchanges, as "individuals are always situated in and acculturated by their socio-cultural environment," whereas different clubs have different "traditions" and "classical techniques" to teach (Hristovski et al. 2011, 181). Also, these techniques draw on the notion of environmental affordances and various social contexts as the potential enabling tools for acquiring creativity. Furthermore, physical engagement with different objects (rackets, balls, etc.) plays a crucial role (as the interaction theory predicts), which could mean that mere mental training to play would not be as beneficial to practicing being creative as actual engagement in the play. As Carr (2015) writes, "Achieving goals through unusual means might very well be a goal-directed task activity that can be practiced and routinized, at least to some degree. The routinized result would be that the performer does 'absorbed coping' in Dreyfus' sense, and demonstrates 'enactive creativity' ala' Rucińska. But only if the conditions of practice are constantly varying, and trying different actions in response to those conditions is encouraged as part of the goal during practice" (232).

The idea is simply that acting in unusual situations allows one to be responding to various affordances, and the response may be creative. Thus, such responding is itself a skill that can benefit from training and practice. As Carr (2015) suggests, it may be important to introduce scrimmages to the training routines, because playing is usually like a full, contextualized performance, rather than like a structured drill, and so engaging in play like scrimmage would allow practicing creative responding in a situation most similar to that on the field.

Furthermore, interacting with what the world affords alone is almost certainly not the whole story. Otherwise everyone who is older, who had more chance at engaging in various situations, should by definition be more creative (which we know need not be the case). One proposal of what could be enhancing the worldly interactions is narrative practices. Narrating (such as engagement in storytelling) plays a key role in shaping what affordances we see (Rucińska 2016; Hutto 2008). Narratives open up new fields of possibilities, also in sport contexts. For example, explaining how to make a hand movement to dunk a basketball with a reference to reaching for cookies from a highly placed cookie jar works as an additional way to develop novel movements. The narrative practices play an active role in imagining new possibilities for action; as narrative practices are part of the social practice, narratives can be considered as further worldly social affordances that open up new possibilities for creative responsiveness.

Gallagher's (2015) notion of embodied thinking can explain why even recourse to narrative practices need not involve purely representational powers. Even when thinking does occur, it in itself need not be seen as a disembodied activity. As Gallagher (2015) helpfully writes, there is a form of embodied thinking in which we engage:

> Reflective thinking, insofar as it is an *embedded* or *situated* reflection … is a *skill* as much as the physical coping involved in skiing is, for example. Indeed, reflective thinking can be a form of embodied coping. Reflection in the downhill skier is not disconnected from the performance or the skier's expertise, but is part of it—a dimension of the flow rather than something different from it … the expert skier should know when to reflect and when not to; and what to reflect about—and that is a skill, and a way of coping with her environment. (140; emphasis original)

Thus, EECA can inform some general guidelines on how to facilitate creative responsiveness. What can be done to enhance possibility of creative response is enhancement of the environmental affordances and development of new agential effectivities, so that creative response can be solicited in the context of sport. The suggestion is that such enhancement of affordance-effectivity pairs points neither at engaging solely in deliberate play, nor at engaging solely in deliberate practice. There are environments for practicing creative responsiveness that can be part of the training of the athlete, which representational models that focus solely on individualistic capacities have not predicted.

5 Conclusion

Clarifying the spectrum of different approaches to studying creativity is important for two reasons. First, it opens up logical space for a new understanding of creativity, making space for the embodied and enactive account of creativity to emerge. Our new approach to creativity proposes an ecological dynamics account of the emergence of creative behaviors. It pertains to the embodied and enactive cognition. It emphasizes that bodily movement and its repetition in training triggers new possibilities for action to be acted on.

With the reconceptualization of creativity, we gain new ideas with respect to how it occurs. What follows about tactical creativity in sport context is that it need not be seen as a form of thinking. The two aspects mentioned under "divergent thinking"—originality and flexibility—need not be considered as thought processes. Another possible way to understand them is as enactive skills. Calling unusualness, innovativeness, or statistical rareness of behavior any form of "thinking" may already lead astray from the possibility that this process does not involve thinking in the traditional sense, but an intelligent embodied response to the environment.

This is not to say that creative thinking never occurs; EECA does not propose that athletes and players cannot stop and reflect from time to time when responding to a situation creatively. Certainly, some of the most creative acts in the history of sport, such as Dick Fosbury's invention of a new style (the Fosbury flop) in high jump, probably involved careful considerations and rational planning. Yet, rational planning can hardly account for the many creative ways of performing in sport; our proposal was that the embodied responsiveness to myriad of affordances accounts for most creative (yet subtle) activities in sport practice.

Thus, while the classic testing methods of creativity in sports are on par with conceptualizing creativity as a form of thinking, some novel approaches to creativity ask for a different characterization of creativity in line with dynamical systems account. Such characterization can be proposed by the theories of embodied and enactive cognition and enriched with an account considering phenomenology of sport. As Hristovski et al. (2011) notice, "Explanations of innovative behavior, based on internalized inferential mechanisms represented in neurobiological nervous systems, have recently been criticized leading to an ecological dynamics account of the emergence of creative behaviors" (Hristovski et al. 2011, 176). The enactive account of creativity proposes one way to support the ecological dynamics account. We propose an understanding of creativity as trainable and potentially shared and interactive.

Moreover, reconceptualization of creativity inspires different methods of operationalizing creativity and working with it in practice, such as training in sports. With respect to testing creativity, EECA shows that developing creative skills cannot be reduced to one fixed model or method. It is important to transcend the empirical studies of creativity focusing merely on divergence (originality and flexibility). If we follow EECA, creativity is always to be studied in a specific context; it may be futile to seek "universal" tests of creativity, as creativity is always situated in a specific context. However, some suggestions can be proposed with respect to how to arrange one's environment to enhance the chances of developing creative responsiveness. Ultimately, engagement in both deliberate play and deliberate practice can be beneficial for development of creativity in sport. How different athletes in different sport domains vary with respect to development of creativity in their fields is only to be assessed on individual bases, in contextualized settings.

Notes

1. "This seems to be what we are after: Creativity appears to be a response-dependent property in much the same way a color is. A creative product is something that would appear creative to an appropriate audience under suitable conditions" (Klausen 2010, 354).

2. Asking for necessary and sufficient conditions is a specific philosophical requirement for a definition. We could define creativity as whatever is "new" or "unexpected," but such characterization would make creativity contingent on another.

3. First, they are theoretical entities, posited for explanatory purposes. Second, they are nothing short of objects with semantic properties. They have contents, which fulfill some condition of satisfaction, whether truth, accuracy, correctness, or the like, as the world is taken (or "claimed") to be in a certain way that it might not be in. In short, mental representations have conditions of satisfaction (Chemero 2009). They are the vehicles of such truth-evaluable contents.

4. See Rucińska (2016) for further argument.

5. As Varela, Thompson, and Rosch (1991) claim, "[Enactivism] questions the centrality of the notion that cognition is fundamentally representation.... The second is that we pick up or recover these properties by internally representing them.... We propose as a name the term *enactive* to emphasize the growing conviction that cognition is not the representation of a pregiven world by a pregiven mind but is rather the enactment of a world and a mind on the basis of a history of the variety of actions that a being in the world performs" (9).

6. The signification of the situation holds an immanent motor value, which is to say that performance is, in a fundamental way, embodied and situated. We have an awareness of the situation and are situated before we explicitly know of it. Thus, according to Merleau-Ponty, performance should not be analyzed as an idea, a choice, or a judgement; rather, it is closely tied to the agent's embodiment.

7. We follow a framework inspired by Turvey (1992) that introduces the conception of affordance-effectivity pairs. For each affordance in the environment, there must be a complementary effectivity of the agent. Effectivities encompass all sorts of moods, capacities, biological setups, cultural history, and individual history (including training) of the agent that shape up the agent's responsiveness to affordances. Importantly for the EECA, none of these factors need to be seen as mental representations.

8. For example, moods or current concerns could be referred to in shaping the playful context. They are also likely to affect which affordances present themselves as inviting. For example, they determine the perception of the amount of effort that would have to be put by the agent to act on the affordance. In a situation of having to go to the top floor of a building, an agent feeling lazy would feel no inclination to climb a steep staircase if the lift was also present. However, if an agent is feeing active and seeks a challenge or an exercise, such steep staircase would solicit climbing.

9. Szokolszky (2006) explains that while Gibsonian affordances are meaningful, they do not tell us how to best act on the objects or the environment, contrasting them to functional properties of the environment. As she proposes, "Traditionally, functional properties are taken to be predetermined properties of objects that define what the object is good for—pillows are for sleeping, and knives are for cutting. Affordances, on the other hand, are defined as action potentials in relation to the particular actor at a more basic level of on-line coordination with the object world" (2006, 68). Hence, although meaningful, affordances are not normative; they are not "good for" anything, or do not lead to a "better action."

10. This fits with Withagen et al.'s (2012) understanding of solicitations as referring to the agent-environment dynamic. They claim, "How are we to understand these invitations? Are invitations environmental properties, mental properties, or do they, like affordances, 'cut across the dichotomy of subjective-objective' (Gibson 1979/1986, 129). We are inclined to a mutualist perspective on invitations—they depend on the relation between the physical properties of the environment and the agent" (255).

11. Thanks to the editor Max Cappuccio for this comment.

12. As Ericsson (1998) claims, "According to the expert-performance framework, training is necessary for students to acquire mental representations that allow them to imagine and create their products and achievements" (94–95).

13. Following Memmert, Baker, and Bertsch (2010), "Collectively, these results indicate the need for a balance between the play necessary for motivation, the development of creative thinking, and the practice necessary for highly specific adaptations to task-relevant demands" (12), except our suggestion is that the development of creative thinking is not a third achievement beyond deliberate play and practice, but a result of engagement in them both. Both types of games are also good from medical perspective, too, as they are helpful in "avoiding one-sidedness or muscular imbalances during a child's development" (Memmert and Roth 2007, 8), and retain motivation of players in pursuing the chosen sport.

References

Aggerholm, Kenneth. 2015. *Talent Development, Existential Philosophy and Sport: On Becoming an Elite Athlete*. London: Routledge.

Aggerholm, Kenneth. 2016. "On Practising in Sport: Towards an Ascetological Understanding of Sport." *Journal of the Philosophy of Sport* 43 (3): 350–364.

Aggerholm, Kenneth, Ejgil Jespersen, and Lars Tore Ronglan. 2011. "Falling for the Feint—An Existential Investigation of a Creative Performance in High-Level Football." *Sport, Ethics and Philosophy* 5 (3): 343–358.

Amabile, Teresa. M. 1996. *Creativity in Context.* Oxford: Westview Press.

Baker, Joseph, Jean Côté, and Janice Deakin. 2005. "Expertise in Ultra-endurance Triathletes Early Sport Involvement, Training Structure, and the Theory of Deliberate Practice." *Journal of Applied Sport Psychology 17* (1): 64–78.

Beaty, Roger E., Mathias Benedek, Paul J. Silvia, and Daniel L. Schacter. 2016. "Creative Cognition and Brain Network Dynamics." *Trends in Cognitive Sciences* 20 (2): 87–95.

Beghetto, Ronald A., and James C. Kaufman. 2007. "The Genesis of Creative Greatness: Mini-c and the Expert Performance Approach." *High Ability Studies* 18 (1): 59–61.

Beilock, Sian L. 2008. "Beyond the Playing Field: Sport Psychology Meets Embodied Cognition." *International Review of Sport and Exercise Psychology* 1 (1): 19–30.

Carr, Thomas H. 2015. "Strengths and Weaknesses of Reflection as a Guide to Action: Pressure Assails Performance in Multiple Ways." *Phenomenology and the Cognitive Sciences* 14 (2): 227–252.

Chemero, Anthony. 2009. *Radical Embodied Cognitive Science*. Cambridge, MA: MIT Press.

Csíkszentmihályi, Mihaly. 1990. *The Psychology of Optimal Experience*. New York: Harper and Row.

Currie, Gregory, and Ian Ravenscroft. 2002. *Recreative Minds: Imagination in Philosophy and Psychology*. Oxford: Clarendon Press.

De Jaegher, Hanne, and Ezequiel Di Paolo. 2007. "Participatory Sense-Making." *Phenomenology and the Cognitive Sciences* 6 (4): 485–507.

Dreyfus, Hubert L. 2002. "Refocusing the Question: Can There Be Skillful Coping without Propositional Representations or Brain Representations?" *Phenomenology and the Cognitive Sciences* 1 (4): 413–425.

Dreyfus, Hubert L. 2007. "Response to McDowell." *Inquiry* 50 (4): 371–377.

Dreyfus, Hubert L. 2013. "The Myth of the Pervasiveness of the Mental." In *Mind, Reason, and Being-in-the-World*, edited by J. K. Schear, 325–352. Oxford: Routledge.

Ericsson, K. Anders. 1998. "The Scientific Study of Expert Levels of Performance: General Implications for Optimal Learning and Creativity." *High Ability Studies* 9 (1): 75–100.

Ericsson, K. Anders. 2014. *The Road to Excellence: The Acquisition of Expert Performance in the Arts and Sciences, Sports, and Games*. London: Psychology Press.

Ericsson, K. Anders, and Walter Kintsch. 1995. "Long-term Working Memory." *Psychological Review* 102 (2): 211.

Ericsson, K. Anders, Ralf T. Krampe, and Clemens Tesch-Römer. 1993. "The Role of Deliberate Practice in the Acquisition of Expert Performance." *Psychological Review* 100 (3): 363–406.

Ford, Paul R., Paul Ward, Nicola J. Hodges, and A. Mark Williams. 2009. "The Role of Deliberate Practice and Play in Career Progression in Sport: The Early Engagement Hypothesis." *High Ability Studies* 20 (1): 65–75.

Gallagher, S. 2015. "The Practice of Thinking." In *Phenomenology of Thinking: Philosophical Investigations into the Character of Cognitive Experiences*, edited by Thiemo Breyer and Christopher Gutland, 134–146. London: Routledge.

Gibson, James Jerome. 1979. *The Ecological Approach to Visual Perception*. Boston: Houghton Mifflin.

Guilford, J. P. 1967. *The Nature of Human Intelligence*. New York: McGraw-Hill. http://psycnet.apa.org/psycinfo/1967-35015-000.

Hamrick, William S. 1994. "Merleau-Ponty's View of Creativity and Its Philosophical Consequences." *International Philosophical Quarterly* 34 (4): 401–412.

Helsen, Werner F., Janet L. Starkes, and Nicola J. Hodges. 1998. "Team Sports and the Theory of Deliberate Practice." *Journal of Sport and Exercise Psychology* 20 (1): 12–34.

Hodges, Nicola J., Tracey Kerr, Janet L. Starkes, Patricia L. Weir, and Angela Nananidou. 2004. "Predicting Performance Times from Deliberate Practice Hours for Triathletes and Swimmers: What, When, and Where Is Practice Important?" *Journal of Experimental Psychology: Applied* 10 (4): 219.

Hristovski, Robert, Keith Davids, Duarte Araujo, and Pedro Passos. 2011. "Constraints-Induced Emergence of Functional Novelty in Complex Neurobiological Systems: A Basis for Creativity in Sport." *Nonlinear Dynamics, Psychology, and Life Sciences* 15 (2): 175–206.

Hutto, Daniel D. 2008. *Folk Psychological Narratives: The Sociocultural Basis of Understanding Reasons*. Cambridge, MA: MIT Press

Hutto, Daniel D., and Erik Myin. 2013. *Radicalizing Enactivism: Basic Minds without Content*. Cambridge, MA: MIT Press.

Hutto, Daniel D., and Erik Myin. 2017. *Evolving Enactivism: Basic Minds Meet Content*. Cambridge, MA: MIT Press.

Klausen, Søren Harnow. 2010. "The Notion of Creativity Revisited: A Philosophical Perspective on Creativity Research." *Creativity Research Journal* 22 (4): 347–360.

Langland-Hassan, Peter. 2015. "Imaginative Attitudes." *Philosophy and Phenomenological Research* 90 (3): 664–686.

Law, Madelyn P., Jean Côté, and K. Anders Ericsson. 2007. "Characteristics of Expert Development in Rhythmic Gymnastics: A Retrospective Study." *International Journal of Sport and Exercise Psychology* 5 (1): 82–103.

McDowell, John. 2007. "Response to Dreyfus." *Inquiry* 50 (4): 366–370.

Memmert, Daniel, Joseph Baker, and Claudia Bertsch. 2010. "Play and Practice in the Development of Sport-specific Creativity in Team Ball Sports." *High Ability Studies* 21 (1): 3–18.

Memmert, Daniel, and Klaus Roth. 2007. "The Effects of Non-Specific and Specific Concepts on Tactical Creativity in Team Ball Sports." *Journal of Sports Sciences* 25 (12): 1423–1432.

Merleau-Ponty, Maurice. [1942] 1963. *The Structure of Behavior*. Translated by A. L. Fisher. Boston: Beacon Press.

Merleau-Ponty, Maurice. [1945] 1962. *Phenomenology of Perception*. Translated by C. Smith. London: Routledge.

Rietveld, E., and J. Kiverstein. 2014. "A Rich Landscape of Affordances." *Ecological Psychology* 26 (4): 325–352.

Rucińska, Zuzanna. 2016. "What Guides Pretence? Towards the Interactive and the Narrative Approaches." *Phenomenology and the Cognitive Sciences* 15 (1): 117–133.

Rucińska, Zuzanna. 2017. "14: The Role of Affordances in Pretend Play." In *Embodiment, Enaction, and Culture: Investigating the Constitution of the Shared World*, edited by Christoph Durt, Thomas Fuchs, and Christian Tewes, 257–277. Cambridge, MA: MIT Press.

Simonton, Dean Keith. 2000. "Creative Development as Acquired Expertise: Theoretical Issues and an Empirical Test." *Developmental Review* 20 (2): 283–318.

Szokolszky, Agnes. 2006. "Object Use in Pretend Play: Symbolic or Functional?" In *Doing Things with Things: The Design and Use of Everyday Objects*, edited by A. Costall & O. Dreier, 67–86. Farnham: Ashgate.

Taylor, Marjorie. 2013. *The Oxford Handbook of the Development of Imagination*. New York: Oxford University Press.

Thompson, Evan. 2005. "Sensorimotor Subjectivity and the Enactive Approach to Experience." *Phenomenology and the Cognitive Sciences* 4 (4): 407–427.

Turvey, Michael T. 1992. "Affordances and Prospective Control: An Outline of the Ontology." *Ecological Psychology* 4 (3): 173–187.

Van Leeuwen, Neil. 2011. "Imagination Is Where the Action Is." *Journal of Philosophy* 108 (2): 55–77.

Varela, Francisco J., Evan Thompson, and Eleanor Rosch. 1991. *The Embodied Mind: Cognitive Science and Human Experience*. Cambridge, MA: MIT Press.

Wallas, Graham. 1926. *The Art of Thought*. New York: Harcourt, Brace.

Withagen, Rob, Harjo J. De Poel, Duarte Araújo, and Gert-Jan Pepping. 2012. "Affordances Can Invite Behaviour: Reconsidering the Relationship between Affordances and Agency." *New Ideas in Psychology* 30: 250–258.

Zahavi, Dan. 2013. "Mindedness, Mindlessness and First-Person Authority." In *Mind, Reason and Being-in-the-World*, edited by Joseph K. Shear, 320. London: Routledge.

26 Prefiguration, Anticipation, and Improvisation: A Neurocognitive and Phenomenological Perspective

Nelson Mauro Maldonato, Alberto Oliverio, and Anna Esposito

1 Introduction

In recent decades, the study of the relation among perception, action, and anticipation has received considerable attention both in sport psychology and in other fields of research related to cognitive science (Cappuccio 2015). A large number of studies inspired by an embodied approach to cognition show that perception and action are closely related and are interdependent, as they recruit largely overlapping neurocognitive structures (Beilock et al. 2004; Berthoz 2000; Garbarini and Adenzato 2004; Holt and Beilock 2006). This happens because the nervous system directly encodes the perceptual properties of the physical world in terms of action possibilities. Familiarity with action possibilities, in turn, binds our perceptual and attentional processes, fine-tuning them to the situational contingencies in order to succeed in the task at hand (Gibson 1979; Gray 2014). This shared cognitive architecture reflects how our sense of familiarity with the world and our confident ability to efficaciously adapt to its changes depend on the consolidation—during recurrent explorative and interactive experiences—of action-perception feedback loops. The most fundamental relationship of humans with their environment is essentially one of sensorimotor interaction and bodily engagement.

This relationship is constitutive of our embodied presence in the world as expert agents situated in an open horizon of action possibilities. That is why becoming familiar with the physical objects in the external world—such as a football—means first of all recognizing them as opportunities to deliver appropriate motor actions, such as catching the ball in the air, kicking it to score a goal, passing it to a teammate, and improvising the whole range of movements and gestures that an experienced football player must be able to perform rapidly, effectively, and without hesitation. It is widely agreed that a good sport performance depends not only on excellent technical execution, defined by the physical components of well-trained motor routines (precision, coordination, velocity, endurance, etc.), but also—and above all—on the perceptive, decision-making, and anticipatory readiness of the subject. This responsive and adaptive capability reflects our promptness to predict, recognize, and understand the transformations occurring in the environment as they are generated by our actions, predicting their impending or potential effects.

The ability to immediately predict and anticipate the effects of a skillful action depends on, and is deeply rooted in, our familiarity with the execution of that kind of action. But how does our brain behave when faced with unforeseen situations, that is, situations that cannot be predicted or decoded by simply relying on familiar motor routines? And how can our brain quickly execute new motor sequences that are appropriate to the immediate contingencies, even if we don't hold any direct familiarity or stored memory related to those contingencies? What problem-solving strategies do we enact, as cognitive agents and decision makers, to promptly respond to these situations?

For a long time, little attention was paid to this problem. Improvisation was for the most part studied under the label of executive functions and considered as a particular aspect of classic motor control theory (Adams 1971; Rosenbaum 1991; Cooper and Shallice 2006). This theory sees the execution and the control of particular sets of movements as instrumental to the implementation of goal-oriented action plans aimed at realizing a particular transformative intention. Motor functions primarily serve the implementation of these intentional action plans and the achievement of their specific motor goals. Secondarily, they contribute to the monitoring (and, if necessary, anticipating and correcting) of the sensorimotor effects generated by one's movements, so as to adapt the course of one's action to contingent changes in the environment. Several mutually coordinated subroutines serve this purpose: for example, the inhibition of a response at an inappropriate moment (or its postponement to a more appropriate moment); the step-by-step segmentation or holistic reconfiguration of articulated movement sequences (motor chains). These sequences can be specifically designed to be flexibly integrated within an overarching goal structure or even a conceptual representation of the task's goal/purpose based on the information (memorized or immediately perceived) associated with the desired result/end state (Diamond 2013).

The associative cortex of the frontal lobe supervises these functions at three different levels of operation: (1) at the dorsomedial level, it supervises the usage of the working memory necessary for the selection and implementation of motor goals through intentional behaviors, (2) at the mesial level, it controls the integration of the emotional and motivational aspects necessary for the continuation of the action, and (3) at the orbital level, it triggers the inhibition of incongruous behaviors and instinctual impulses. These areas coordinate with the frontal lobes, the cerebellum, the basal ganglia, and the spinal cord for the effective execution of the movement and its completion (Cotterill 2001).

In the picture advanced by classic motor control theory, the creation of new sequences of action is only implemented, but *not invented*, by the low-level mechanisms of motor control. According to this picture, such mechanisms hold only an instrumental function, without playing any decisional role: the cognitive space that produces real improvisation is one in which the procedures of error correction are controlled top-down, imposed by a superior order (more general, related to intentions and goals) on an inferior one (more particular, related to the movement execution and secondary adjustments to environmental contingencies). In this picture, individual instances of particular movements are combined according to pre-given action plans, forming nested hierarchies of routines and subroutines instrumentally designed to produce the intended goal-directed action through stratified levels of action control. This hierarchical model renders the motor functions subordinate to higher levels of brain activity and drastically reduces our comprehension of how new sequences of action originate from motoric skill and expertise. In fact, this model doesn't offer appropriate explanatory tools to enable us to understand how the contingent details of bodily movement itself (even when not organized in a clear plan according to a precise goal) are already capable—in themselves and by themselves—of drawing the trajectory of a meaningful project of action, suggesting a possible direction of intentional development through creative improvisation and on-line reconfiguration of one's purposes and goals. To overcome the intrinsic limitations of the traditional approach to motor control theory, Adams (1976) proposed the existence of "traces of perceptual memory," that is, semi-independent motoric representations that, in the absence of central supervision, would initiate the automatic correction of execution errors as soon as they occur during the course of an action. With the definitive proceduralization of the skills due to the acquisition of fully automatized motor routines, this on-line correction process would reduce the dependence of the movements on abstract planning and explicit intention (Namikas 1983). This view reduces the primacy of top-down intentional control, attributing a greater importance, for the correct execution of semi-improvised goal-oriented actions, to the unconscious prediction of the effects of the action based on the consideration of the motoric and implementational details of the action itself.

Against this view, Bernstein (1967) had already shown that the explicit planning of a motor action necessarily presupposes the implicit anticipation of upcoming situations. This anticipatory capability, rooted in the reciprocal coordination of top-down and bottom-up control mechanisms, can be best understood in the light of the long evolutionary background that led to the rise of *Homo sapiens*. This evolutionary path has shaped the anatomical and functional architecture of the human skeletal and muscular systems; it has calibrated the selective properties of the sensory receptors and equipped the brain with enormous decision-making capabilities. Furthermore, it has endowed the human cognitive systems with efficient and versatile predictive models capable of anticipating the events quickly occurring in the body and the world, so as to ensure the most efficacious adaptation of our reflexive responses to rapidly changing and potentially risky situations (Maldonato 2014).

Bernstein was one of the first researchers to attempt to overcome the traditional theory of motor control as a linear sequence of anticipation, preparation, execution, and evaluation phases. His action-perception cycle model consists of three key functions, recurring in a loop: (1) the system determines the mismatch between the anticipated and the executed movement, comparing the latter with the former; (2) when there is no mismatch, the system recognizes that the intended act was completed, triggering the passage to the next phase of the motor sequence, which allows for a quick and smooth transition from one action context to another; (3) when faced with an unexpected situation, the system introduces on-line corrective interventions to quickly restore a typical plan of action, reducing the deviation between ongoing movements and what is sensed as an optimal action sequence.

According to this model, the postural reactions and the anticipatory movements of the body are not reducible to stereotyped action templates, as they are not governed by fixed sets of rules; rather, they emerge as the dynamic balance between excitatory and inhibitory tendencies, depending on a real-time negotiation between the agent's proactive intention and the context in which the action takes place. The decision-execution-completion sequence of the movement, generated by the comparison between a predetermined model of action and its final effects, exploits fluid dynamics of constant control and sensorial stabilization guaranteed by feedback and reflex systems.

Half a century before, Jackson (1884) had hypothesized that the brain knows the body's movements more than the groups of muscles that implement them (Critchley and Critchley 1998); Bernstein (1967), in turn, maintains that the brain plans its actions primarily in terms of motor goals and practical purposes, not single movements or means detached from the overall intention of the action. This intuition has been further developed through the idea of a "dictionary of motor actions" that, according to Rizzolatti, Fogassi, and Gallese (2001) is encoded in the motor cortex: according to this metaphor, the lexicon of the dictionary would be represented by populations of neurons, while the single entries would primarily describe the purposive dimension of the action (the goals of the action, such as grasping, ripping, pulling, etc.), and only secondarily the particular component movements necessary to achieve those goals (which muscle has to contract at a given time, for example).

With his "theory of motor skills," Schmidt (1976) hypothesized the existence of a general system that selects flexible patterns of movement to modulate the action according to the context. Other theories, connected to his own, hypothesize the existence of a "system of unity of action" (Allport 1980), or of "organizational invariants" (Kugler, Kelso, and Turvey 1980), inspired by Gibson's "ecological model" (1979) and by Prigogine's "dissipative structures" (1967). Applied to motor action, this means that the required models of coordination of the neuromuscular events and properties tend to overcome the particular constraints imposed by the specific situations and tasks (Saltzman and Kelso 1987), giving rise each time to general solutions that can be adapted to many specific situational problems.

Such hypotheses, as productive as they are, require the support of empirical evidence. For example, the theory of "organizational invariants" seems to reflect more the principles of classical motor control than those of high-level decision making (Mogenson, Jones, and Yim 1980; Morris et al. 2006). In fact, the latter requires competencies open to the broadest possibilities of interaction with the external environment. Even if every action involves discrete and serial aspects, modulating a familiar action within unknown situations requires complex abilities, that is, the characteristics that best epitomize expertise: adaptability, efficiency, fluidity, flexibility and—in social contexts—expressiveness (Welford 1976; Shaffer 1980; Sparrow 1983). Feedback and forward mechanisms play a generic role in action control, but seem insufficient to explain the unique specificity of the nonlinear dynamics involved in the creation of original behaviors, as these dynamics closely depend on a personal reinterpretation of the experiential path followed by a well-trained expert during the process of acquisition and improvement of his/her skills.

An executive control for higher levels of decision making, as noted by Jeannerod (2001), presupposes distributed cortical-subcortical structures, in which each level influences both the preceding and the subsequent one. This distributed system, based on a circular dynamic that influences the entire sensorimotor processes, must be supported by a shared workspace for decision making and prefiguration capable of generating a consistent representation of future actions on the basis of a comprehensive knowledge of past actions. This representation combines the analysis of the action goal, the selection of the means necessary to achieve it, and the calculation of its consequences for the organism and the external world. Generating this representation, our brain anticipates the effects of our actions and those of others, becoming able to articulate its own goals and plans and understand the actions and emotions of others (Jeannerod 2001).

2 Biological Algorithms for the Invention of New Sequences of Action

In the complex system of executive functions, the basal ganglia play a major role. They control cognitive activities such as spatial memories and the execution of motor actions in specific practical contexts, as well as motivational elements of learning and knowledge consolidation (Coccurello et al. 2000; Cotterill 2001). The cortex and the basal ganglia are closely linked and control, also through the cerebellum, the motivational aspects of movement (the preparation for the action), the contextual aspects that trigger the action (the initialization of the movement), and the status of its execution (Graybiel 1997).

In what way does this complex system contribute to the generation of rapid and unexpected behaviors? Catching a flying rugby ball, hitting a fast-moving baseball with a bat, pronouncing long sentences with great fluidity, or playing a piano require such short execution time that the possibility of correction by means of on-line sensory feedback is virtually excluded most of the time. This kind of ballistic movement may succeed or fail, depending on whether it was appropriately calibrated during action planning, but because of the time constraints it cannot be further corrected once the motor program is launched (Oliverio 2009). Therefore, in what way can the brain trigger such rapid muscle action sequences, to the point of overcoming the temporal limits of the neural circuits? This question concerns both hand and leg movements, as well as the precise articulation of words that are generally produced with very fast rhythms and yet without execution errors that might alter the comprehension of the meaning (Oliverio 2009).

There are analogies between speech production and other domains of motor activity, for example fast sport disciplines and martial arts. Karate is one of the sport disciplines that may help us better understand such dynamics. Here, the cognitive decision about the action to be executed must be almost simultaneous to the exploration of the available possibilities of movement and the comprehension of their implications. Only the simultaneous occurrence of motor intention and execution can allow, on the one hand, the efficacious completion of a ballistic action (a karate fist) and, on the other, the differential analysis between intention, perceived result, and correction of the error, which is at the basis of a sense of agency and intentional control (Kickert, Bertrand, and Praagman 1978).

In the case of an improvised action, the possibility for error is constant in all of the phases of its execution: from the perception of the opponent (e.g., for a feint) to action selection (e.g., the best kind of karate move to counter an attack) and from the planning to the implementation of the movements. During a *kumité*, which sees two athletes take each other on at a distance of about two meters, it is necessary to achieve the maximum stability with the minimum expenditure of energy. The karate expert, then, does not limit herself to reacting to expected events: she operates in the future, by means of anticipatory and compensatory strategies that generate postural responses, thus safeguarding stability and allowing her own muscles to rapidly contract before the voluntary control of movement (Won and Hogan 1995). The efficiency and effectiveness of these mechanisms improves with constant practice and correlates with the quantity of skills and techniques memorized (Schechner 1995), which allow the expert to develop a sort of internal algorithm that permits her to instantly calculate the variables in play and prepare the most appropriate reaction according to her own predictions (Berthoz 2000, 2006).

It must be said, nevertheless, that the fluidity and effectiveness of the performances of experts do not derive only from the greater familiarity with the task, or from having imagined at length oneself in action, but also from the capacity to distance oneself from sentiments, desires, worries, or thoughts that could interfere with the performance. To avoid such an eventuality, the expert naturally tends to recreate a state of flow, which can be characterized as a form of liberation from unnecessary cognitive burdens and negative emotional constraints. In normal conditions, such burdens and constraints may limit the spontaneity of the action, reducing the capacity for instantaneous adaptation and improvisation that are based on preconscious anticipation (Maldonato and Dell'Orco 2012). Sensorial and cognitive interferences risk reactivating conscious control, compromising the fluidity of the movement and bringing the action back under the control of explicit decision making (Jackson and Csíkszentmihályi 1999). It is by filtering out these unnecessary stimuli that concentration and, therefore, the effectiveness of an action, may reach the highest levels. For an actor, a dancer, or a musician—so absorbed by their action as to be entirely identified with their own task—concentration, automatisms, and imagination build on the real-time flow of action itself (i.e., the intrinsic capability of automated goal-oriented actions to anticipate their own bodily outcomes), rather than on a detached representational schema of the movement to be executed (Limb and Braun 2008; Jackson and Csíkszentmihályi 1999).

But what makes the invention of new sequences of action distinctively intelligent and original? Can we consider such invention an expression of human creativity? Classical neurobiological studies examined creativity starting from the different functions of the cerebral hemispheres: traditionally, the logico-symbolic and linguistic functions have always been linked to the left hemisphere of the brain, whereas the holistic-generalist-emotive functions were primarily associated with the right hemisphere

(Oliverio 2012). Although the mechanisms underlying hemispheric lateralization (Geschwind and Galaburda 1985; Gazzaniga 1995) are certainly very complex and still poorly understood, there is little doubt about the primacy of the left hemisphere in symbolic-linguistic activities and in logico-mathematical problem solving (Kolb and Whishaw 1996). This is important for understanding how the key preconditions for creative behavior spontaneously arise: various studies on hemispherical asymmetries, through fMRI, suggest that creativity is correlated, on the one hand, with a standby of the left hemisphere and, on the other, to an intense activity in the right hemisphere—probably subserving the formation of associations and semantic connections, primarily through metaphors and analogies, that would offer new critical perspectives on things (Levy 1979).

The role of the right hemisphere in the discovery of new explanations is demonstrated by its involvement in a series of functions such as perception, imagination, and artistic creation, in both the visual and the musical domains (Zaidel 2014). The sudden insight that preludes the discovery of the solution to a given problem is consistently associated with the activation of the right hemisphere (Oliverio 2008). For example, the moment of the correct response in a test (cognitive or noncognitive) coincides with a rapid activation of the right temporal lobe, in particular of the right anterior superior temporal gyrus, which is preceded by a sudden change in the patterns of activation of the prefrontal cortex, the area primarily involved in higher-level cognitive and executive tasks (Kandel 2012). These different hemispherical properties have led to the hypothesis that the creative, emotional, and intuitive processes enacted by the right hemisphere are distinct from, and in a sense complement, the rational ones, which are epitomized by the logico-symbolic and semantic-cognitive faculties controlled by the left hemisphere.

A central feature of creativity that shows the complementarity of intuitive (insightful) and rational (analytical) ways of thinking captured by the hemispheric lateralization doctrine is the active process of recombination of known contents and stored information that is enacted through the formation of original associations. New creative ideas originate from the discovery and exploration of unexpected relationships among known facts, even when such facts were initially deemed unrelated or mutually contradictory. The possibility to discover these secret or unexpected relationships and their power to generate new possibilities of interpretation and meaning lies not in deductive reasoning, but in mental imagery articulated as a quasi-pictorial process of visualization (Kosslyn 1994). Analogies, in particular, reveal organizational correspondences and iconic similarities among objects, events, and facts. Detecting such correspondences and similarities allows us to solve a puzzle or overcome an apparently nonsensical situation, or find meaning in it. This happens by comparing knowledge of the current situation with information acquired during previous heterogeneous experiences.

The process of abstraction enacted through analogical reasoning discloses original models of reality, or ways of making sense of experience, that cannot be explicitly represented because of their fundamental distance from our senses (Oliverio and Maldonato 2014). Artists would have a natural propensity to tangibly portray the ideas that escape the minds of common people, as artistic thinking allows them to express multimodal concepts that cannot be translated into formal (amodal) linguistic representations. This tendency to generate new meanings from the recombination of familiar sensorial experience and past memories shows how the representational function of the mind is not essentially meant *to mirror* the external world (producing an internal model), but *to invent* it (revealing concrete opportunities for action and new practical approaches to decision making).

Deploying strategies that allow us to see beyond what is known, the mind captures images and metaphors to extract and generalize information. Improvisation is not reducible to the mere work of combinatorial probability or to retrospective fantasy (which may be the sign of regressive tendencies to escape into an inward-looking universe). On the contrary, it is a proactively structured process of imagination that primarily makes use of analogies to design a meaningful project of intervention in the world. Unlike formal logical processes, which contingently imprison and limit the flow of free associations, the exercise of analogical thinking increases the probabilities of generating creative results (Hofstadter 2001).

The associative and prefrontal cortical regions are the ones involved in the production of analogies. The latter is much more extended in humans than in other primates. As is well known, the associative cortex creates synthetic connections among different kinds of sensorial stimuli that relate to, or are generated from, the same experience. For example, the process of recognizing someone is possible if one has memorized their facial features, their voice, the circumstances in which one has met them, the emotional reactions experienced during the encounter, and so on (Schacter 1987). Such diverse experiential elements are subsequently recombined by the associative cortex to ensure the creation of integrated memory contents that include complex bundles of particular sensorial memories (Oliverio 2009). Once the dedicated bundle for a certain known person is available, the associative cortex can retrieve the critical aspects related to that person's face, how he expresses emotions through gesture and behavior, and so on. The retrieval process can begin from any specific cue, such as the tone of the voice.

The prefrontal cortex, on the other hand, functions as an archive of synthetically structured representations from which the particular elements that are useful for responding to specific requests are recovered (Lewis 1979). When analogies come into play, the prefrontal cortex selects the contextual information relevant to the task at hand, or the demands related to the current situation, while the associative cortex connects the characteristics of the current situation to networks of similar or contiguous elements, immediately linking one's subjective experience to semantically interconnected conceptual categories such as "night," "sleep," and "darkness," among others.

That is why patients with lesions to the left angular gyrus, while being capable of understanding the literal meaning of a proposition, most often struggle to grasp the figurative meaning of metaphors (Ramachandran 2003). For example, most of them would interpret "all that glitters is not gold" as "you need to be careful when you buy jewels." In its most elementary form, analogical thinking favors the transition from a known fact to one that is unknown. When grappling with a new problem, our mind automatically looks for situations similar to the new circumstances, proposing adaptable solutions—just like a scientist who, when facing a new problem, resorts to analogies based on previously acquired knowledge (Hofstadter 1996).

Analogical thinking is supported by a modality of reasoning that is different from the formal one: it is not filtered by rigorous deductions meant to evaluate the plausibility or utility of a certain explanatory model; rather, it solicits the formation of open-ended interpretative matrices that apply at the same time to familiar and unknown phenomena, constituting and connecting all of them in a continuum of imaginative variations. This imaginative connection facilitates the articulation of original explanations of the phenomena and effective predictions about the possible outcomes of current actions.

3 From Secondary to Primary Processes

Creative thinking, like analogical thinking, promotes the original recombination of the information available to the system. What are the neural and cognitive correlates of the creative process? In the brain there are two distinct systems, each of which deals with a different type of information: one emotional and the other cognitive. These pathways, reaching the thalamus, trigger two different sequences: an initial emotional sequence, processed in the amygdala, and a subsequent affective sequence, processed in the cingulate cortex and in the ventromedial prefrontal cortex (Oliverio 2008). The cognitive system, on the other hand, involves other limbic structures—chiefly the hippocampus and the temporal, occipital, and parietal cortices (Tanji and Hoshi 2008). There is broad agreement on the fact that this circuit is the seat of the long-term memory.

The full integration of emotional and cognitive information depends on the convergence of these two types of processing, emotional and cognitive, on the dorsolateral prefrontal cortex (Groenewegen et al. 1990). This region not only intervenes in the execution of motor functions but also integrates the information necessary to allow upper functions such as abstract thinking, cognitive flexibility, planning, and awareness. Also, this region is recruited in the formulation of plans and strategies for appropriate conduct and action execution, through the motor cortices (Baddeley 1996).

Finally, cognitive functions such as working memory, temporal integration, and sustained selective attention, which allow for the most complex cognitive functions, depend on this cortical zone. Neural integration in this area is made possible by two different systems involved in the acquisition (learning), memorization, and representation of information: the explicit system and the implicit system (Dienes and Perner 1999). The first is conscious and may be expressed verbally, using linguistic rules and content; the second is unconscious and cannot be expressed verbally, as it is based on practical capabilities and transformative know-how (Schacter 1987).

From a neural point of view, the explicit system is associated with the superior cognitive functions of the frontal and prefrontal lobes and of the medial temporal lobe; the implicit system, on the other hand, is more efficient and is associated with abilities supported mainly by the basal ganglia (Doya 2000). The evolutionary origin of the explicit system is quite recent, as it is distinctive of primates with a highly developed prefrontal cortex. In this information-processing architecture, most sophisticated mental abilities, such as the representation of explicit knowledge, depend on a higher-order structure: the prefrontal cortex.

Obviously, a rigid separation between explicit and implicit knowledge, and the corresponding nervous structures on which these cognitive abilities depend, would be simplistic (Oliverio 2008). Indeed, both systems can be activated in parallel and the striatum (a fundamental structure of the basal ganglia) is also involved in explicit cognitive functions; its activity is usually coordinated with the cognitive functions of the prefrontal cortex and works in harmony with it, also because of the complex connections that link it to the prefrontal cortex. Moreover, the striatum combines the information deriving from the different cortical areas for the convergence of their respective terminal nerve fields (Alexander, DeLong, and Strick 1986).

It has been suggested that stimuli revealed in new or unexpected contexts activate the ventral striatum and that the basal ganglia verify the reliability of the predictions formulated in the prefrontal cortex (Kotz, Schwartze, and Schmidt-Kassow 2009). The expectations can be either cognitive or motor in nature, and it is reasonable to assume that the basal ganglia are heavily involved in the activation of the chemical signals emitted in response to stress, evoked by dissonance or discrepancies between perceptions and expectations (Posner 1989). According to the system's immediate needs, the ventral striatum can intervene also in the adaptation of cognitive strategies to rapidly evolving contexts. It is in this way that the subcortical reinforcement mechanisms, through their interaction with the frontal cortex and the limbic and striatal systems, play a key function in planning, in the selection of the most appropriate actions, and in the relevant decision-making processes (Hikosaka 1994). Furthermore, it is well-known that the frontal cortex is involved in different levels of aware activity or vigilance. For example, sleepiness is associated with a low level of vigilance, while the response to sudden stimuli requires a strong cortical activation, which reaches more intense levels during negative emotions such as anger, fear, and so on. It should be added that easy tasks are compatible with significant emotional levels, while a high level of concentration requires lower levels of cerebral activation. The transition from wakefulness to daydreaming (reverie) and, finally, to full sleep entails a decrease in the level of vigilance (Tononi and Cirelli 2006). Indeed, EEG waves become increasingly slower, while their tension increases (Vaitl et al. 2005). The primary processes of thought, such as free associations or daydreaming—from which original analogies and creative ideas often emerge—take place at an intermediate level of activation, while the secondary processes (in which cognition is abstract, logical, and orientated toward reality) require attention with a higher level of activation (Hobson, Pace-Schott, and Stickgold 2000). It has been suggested that the activation of the prefrontal cortex disregards irrelevant mental associations and instead facilitates purpose-oriented behaviors such as problem solving (Oliverio 2012).

The dimension along which cognition varies consists of the primary process/secondary process continuum: that is, creative individuals tend to have a more pronounced ease of movement between these two dimensions of thinking (Fromm 1978). Creative intuition (Kris 1952) tends to provoke a transition toward a primary state of consciousness facilitating the discovery of new combinations of elements, while creative processing tends to lead one back to the secondary process, in which abstract and logical thinking prevails and which is oriented toward the real world, typical of waking consciousness, implying a greater activation of the prefrontal cortex. It is plausible that creative people have easier access to primary thinking processes (Oliverio 2012; Martindale 1999). The primary processes (such as the associations that characterize the dream state and even altered states of consciousness from which analogy and creative associations can emerge) happen at medium-low levels of activation and occur at an unconscious level.

Ultimately, the production and the selection of creative ideas tend to occur according to this sequence: the implicit striatal system reacts to novelty and generates a range of new responses to deal with new situations (Martindale 1999; Cotterill 2001); but subsequently it is the prefrontal cortex that selects the recently acquired behaviors and governs them. On the basis of a continuous competition-collaboration between subcortical structures that generate novelty and the prefrontal cortex that analyses them, creativity can be identified as a Darwinian process based on the classical procedure of variation-selection. The basal ganglia generate innovation in all of the key situations that are at the root of creativity, such as explorative behaviors, infantile pretend play, and analogical thinking, while the prefrontal cortex is the mechanism that selects and can transform the change into truly creative behaviors.

4 Flow, Spontaneity, and Creativity

Years ago, Csíkszentmihályi (1996) hypothesized the existence of "flow," an underexcited and almost automatic state of mind linked to reduced prefrontal activity, characterized by the absence of tension, that recurs in mental or physical activities with a high level of concentration. This is a sort of direct contact with a primary reality, ordinarily masked by rationality. It is unpredictable, in continuous evolution, and draws on cues, associations of unused ideas, intuitions, and movements, recombining them through different "emotional sets" (Bastick 1982). Such activity (unconscious) would call into question the implicit cognitive systems that depend on the basal ganglia, over which the prefrontal cortex has no influence whatsoever. With their implicit strategies and memories, the basal ganglia continuously give rise to new neural events, while the prefrontal cortex transforms the new events into creative behaviors (Oliverio 2008). In this sense, the rich associative network that allows the striatum to integrate the motivational, cognitive, and emotional information, originating from different cortical areas, and to transmit them to the prefrontal cortex, represents a generative instrument (Oliverio and Maldonato 2014). Its activity can explain both the transformation of the motor and explorative experiences into cognitive schemas and the production of analogies at the basis of creative discoveries (Kandel 2012).

Flow may also be considered as a temporal interval during which a routine ability or a well-trained cognitive function operate without the interference of the explicit system: this way of operating is characterized by a state of lesser activity of the prefrontal lobe, in such a way that the analytical capacities of the explicit system are temporarily "switched off" (Nakamura 1988). However, as we shall see below, the condition of flow requires explicit attention in order to endure and, therefore, an extended status of flow requires the activation of the frontal neural network. Within certain limits, flow is compatible with a decrease in the prefrontal function and a weaker self-awareness. Indeed, flow is often interpreted as a lower level of frontal activity that allows the mind to focus on a target causing the standby of the other executive and cognitive abilities of the prefrontal cortex (Hampshire et al. 2010; Wulf 2013). Now, if the attentional focus on the current activity allows the implicit system to function at the maximum level of efficiency, creativity emerges from the involvement of different cerebral circuits.

As we have already argued, the new event is first generated within the implicit system (ventral striatum) and then analyzed and processed by the prefrontal cortex, which transforms the new local neural events into responses to critical variables and into creative behaviors (Oliverio 2012). As made evident by martial and dynamic arts, the reduction of the time lag between action and reaction corresponds to the reduction of the cognitive processing in the execution of a motor program, to the extent that it becomes simultaneous in exceptional cases. By facilitating the transition from a state of voluntariness to free instinctivity (Rietveld 2008), the centroencephalic structures generate the mental representation of the ego (Maldonato 2017) when the ego is fully absorbed in routine abilities (although they were originally acquired through conscious efforts and exercise). The phenomenology of fluid, flexible, and original sequences of action, brought about by the weakening of awareness (and of attention), is heterarchical and allows for the rapid passage between cortical and subcortical modular structures (Dietrich 2004). It is plausible that innate clusters of action codified in archaic neural matrices are activated by interaction with the environment, giving birth to new flexible and original sequences of action, even if only a limited number of them prevail. According to this hypothesis, more flexible executive functions could create original motor combinations out of indeterminate, unpredictable, and nonlinear results (Li and Yorke 1975), using open dynamics not linked to complete and detailed knowledge of the environmental variables, for flexible and adaptively advantageous decisions.

Consider now the experience of musical improvisation: an elective embodied activity in which the performer gives himself over to the spontaneity of the composition and the creation of melodies in real time. How can a set of dissonances, digressions, and isolated and connected variants flow in a spontaneous harmonious order without a score, without preestablished repertoires, or without the guidance of the conductor's baton? What neural circuits and what cerebral areas give a musical shape to improvised sounds? How can they create such harmony and rhythm, if they can't rely on previous codifications or preexisting narrative/morphological structures? It should be clear by now that improvisation is made possible by a plurality of structures coordinated in real time, whose functional characterization is not reducible to the traditional left/

right hemisphere dichotomy (although this dichotomy can tell us something about the basis of creativity as reuse and imaginative variation). Defining improvisation as a process of spontaneous production, reducible to the selection, execution, and original recombination of known auditory-motor sequences, appears insufficient, because this definition doesn't include the specific temporal structure that characterizes improvisation as a creative event that is tied to the phenomenology of present experience: this temporal structure involves not only a reinterpretation of past knowledge, but also an anticipation of the future (Bengtsson, Csíkszentmihályi, and Ullén 2014).

The scientific literature offers a large number of *brain imaging* studies on musical cognition, particularly on perception and musical development (Zatorre, Chen, and Penhune 2007), but few focus on musical invention. The others are, for the most part, confined to the study of already memorized performances (Bengtsson and Ullén 2006). Only very few studies deepen the nature of musical improvisation as a real-time activity. In a brilliant work, some years ago, Limb and Braun (2008) asked ten pianists to memorize a melody. They then had them lie in the tube of a suitably modified magnetic resonance machine and, once they were connected to a keyboard, managed to have them reproduce the melody they had just learned, make a simple scale, and, finally, improvise. Limb and Braun saw that the improvisation was correlated to the activation of a neural network that included, among other things, structures such as the inferior left frontal gyrus, the anterior cingulated cortex, and the medial prefrontal cortex.

The most interesting result was the widespread "turning off" of the prefrontal areas, which are generally correlated with the conscious control of the activities in progress. These areas often interfere with one's capacity for concentration. This experience of "turning off," which is not yet sensorial or perceptive, is not an experience of emptiness, but corresponds to the activation of mental images that anticipate the ideation of a specific action (Kosslyn, Ganis, and Thompson 2001), which in turn solicits an internal emulation of the planned motor actions, very similar to what takes place in reality. As recently shown by Ridderinkhof and Brass (2015), in a study involving the activity domain of football, the comparison between the effects of the anticipated action and the effects predicted by an internal emulation generates an error signal that guides the on-line correction of the motor performance, even without the execution of real movements.

However, during the average episode of improvisation, the frontal areas involved in the conscious control of action are never entirely "turned off." Some of them are, in fact, very active. Although the brain does not dedicate the same amount of reflective attention to every aspect of its spontaneous activity, at a lower level of unconscious processing it continuously monitors, assesses, and selects all the intervening ideas, evaluating the thoughts that emerge during the creative process as valid opportunities for action (Berkowitz and Ansari 2008). This critical function probably requires the intervention of the frontal lobes (above all prefrontal), which exert control over motor actions. This would explain why some parts of the frontal lobes are not entirely "turned off." This sort of internal generator of thoughts and ideas, memories and images, that crop up spontaneously and often unexpectedly in the consciousness, is related to the so-called *default mode network* (Mason et al. 2007; Beaty 2015). The activation of this network tends to mitigate the "turning off" of conscious control. In particular, partial conscious control is needed when a partial or almost total focus on one's own stream of thoughts becomes necessary, for example because it is requested as part of the task. Such a situation is characterized by an intense concentration on the task in progress and by the elimination of the awareness of the passing of time (Pinho et al. 2014; Beilock and Carr 2004).

Now, performative competence is definitely a necessary condition for efficacious and rich improvisation—without a lot of experience, indeed, there is no possibility of high-level automatisms, hence no opportunity to trigger the involuntary memory and, subsequently, no space for enacting creative play through the imaginative exploration of possible worlds. That is why expert performers show a more marked capacity for deactivating their selective attention, compared with budding musicians and non-musicians. The cerebral area called on for such blended modulation of conscious and unconscious control is the temporoparietal junction, which has the function of screening, filtering out, or inhibiting information, allowing the performers to integrate ordinary (semi-automatic) thought processes within the problem-solving processes required by more challenging tasks, thus maintaining their attention while keeping at bay potentially disturbing external thoughts, ideas, and perceptions (Berkowitz and Ansari 2010).

The suspension of the conscious monitoring of one's movement confers on the hands a relative autonomy, guided by the musical subject matter at hand (Pressing 1984). In improvised music, as with sport and other ordinary actions such as walking or eating, the "subject matter" consists of the timbre and complexity of the gesture, its aesthetic-emotional sensitivity, and its expressive design. It emerges in free contexts that are highly structured, and during independently selected tasks (Welford 1976). Nevertheless, automatic processing produced by constant practice does not reduce, per se, demands on the attention necessary to successfully complete the task: it only reduces the need to pay attention to one's own movements and, in general, to oneself. In other words, in order to produce peak performance or efficacious improvisation, an expert needs (as does the novice) to focus on the task at hand and dedicate his attentional resources to it—especially the resources needed for strategical reflection and prediction of the effects of one's own actions (Wulf 2013; Beilock et al. 2004). However, only the expert needs to turn his attention away from the component movements and the procedural aspects of his own actions, because that kind of reflective self-awareness disrupts the fluidity of the action and interferes with his capability to richly adapt to the contingent circumstances.

5 Beyond Thought: Spontaneity and Improvisation

The variability of action through an open range of imagined possibilities is decisive in improvisation, and is a key component in all performances by experts (Schmidt 1983). The ability to produce free variations is more complex than the simple musical repetition performed by a musician who plays on the basis of her inner ear. The mind of a jazz player absorbed in a process of improvisation is deeply rooted in the perception of the specific possibilities and limitations offered by her own instrument, in ways that the performer of scores never really experiences. In either case, the expressive capacity of a performer is fostered by access to her own "productive" (creative) or "reproductive" (mnestic) *tonal imagery*: a field of consciousness that includes experiences and internal images that can be combined, distorted, associated, while possibly competing with one another (Maldonato 2017).

In the highly original form of life that is jazz, narrating means following the direction of the temporal arrow and being completely absorbed in its rhythm and melody: it is a living experience made out of epiphanies and introversions, of intuitions and revelations, of syncopated rhythms and aesthetic insights, which appear and disappear on the edge of interference between the conscious and the unconscious mind (Berliner 1994; Montuori 2011). The performing urgency of gestures, voices, and sounds highlights the differences between individual performances (D'Errico 2015). In this intense activity of opposition and resolution, the performer's experience becomes an unstable territory that rests on the capacity of the body to remember, decide, anticipate, and invent (Gallagher and Zahavi 2012). The ego reveals itself as an emerging expression of our neural structures. Whether or not conscious awareness could be attributed to improvisation, its role is certainly secondary (Zeman 2001), because the unity of the ego implies a fundamental form of rhythmic coordination even before the establishment, or even the possibility, of conscious self-awareness. The unity of the experiential flux, traversed by the conscious ego, plays a role in musical improvisation insofar as it is the rhythmic expression of the living body engaged in the exploration of its action possibilities (Varela, Thompson, and Rosch 1991). While the content of consciousness is the object of study of phenomenological research, the very possibility of the ego and the causes of its psychological unity are fundamentally rooted in biological processes and depend on the organic functions and the anatomical structure of the body itself.

Improvisation reveals the truly incarnated dimension of the ego because it calls into question the sovereignty of consciousness, a phenomenon that doesn't have a fixed territory, but contingently emerges in a swarm of sensations, thoughts, and memories, in a constant dialogue with new experiences, networks of incipient ideas, and bits of sensorial information received from the periphery of the body (Thomson 2007; Bengtsson and Ullén 2006). While deeply rooted in its incarnated dimension, individual freedom of expression exists as a dialectic between assimilation and rejection. Expression requires that the performer get rid of every obstacle, every resisting element that stands in the way of the creative process. That is because every known structure, convention, or familiar phrase can represent a constraint and a limitation to one's originality. Obviously enough, at the same time, these elements represent the repertoire of an expert and the very material in which her expertise is realized: if they didn't exist, it would be impossible for the performer to construct new associations, intuitions, and give voice to her unknown inner languages and unexplored, deep, and unconscious memories (Nisenson 1995).

These materials can become vehicles of improvisation, rather than obstacles to it, only on the condition that they are subsumed within a subconscious flux of activity, so that they can be accessed and used without explicit processing and without directly referring to them: in order to become effectively usable, these mnestic traces must become elements of a subroutine, an implicit background of the performing process rather than constitutive building blocks of the performance outcome. This is why an expert performer always starts with a known motif and abandons it shortly after. Only by abandoning what is known and leaving it in the background can she express herself spontaneously through the composition. In a continuous search for her own expressive language, the performer must conduct the difficult job of selection and exclusion, a job that is even harder because it cannot be conducted explicitly, while consciously thinking about it. This oscillation between rhythmic regularity and desired originality reveals a dimension of cognition that is beyond explicit thought, to which consciousness can have only indirect, mediated, or delayed access.

What about group improvisation? Here obviously the practical constraints in the use of brain imaging make experimental study even more arduous. With respect to solo improvisation (Limb and Braun 2008), a lesser activation of the default mode network in group situations has recently been reported (Kuhn et al. 2014). There is reason to believe that the necessary harmonization of emerging materials, typical of a group performance, hinders the "turning off" of the prefrontal structures and, on the contrary, raises the level of conscious attention (Benedek et al. 2014). Moreover, the unexpected variations require significant voluntary modulations and a minimum tempo of about 300–500 ms (Welford 1976), during which the musicians react to the changes introduced by the other performers. This is a continuous self/hetero-monitoring, a temporo-spatial parametric supervision of the performance that reintroduces expressive and compositional decision-making control (Parsons et al. 2005). In the overall production, the decision-making procedures recruited by the improvisational process derive from the efficiency of the perceptive transformation and accurate selection of the relevant information.

The efficiency in processing and selecting musical material is filtered and somehow constrained by the limitations of the performer's individual skill. His skill is seriously tested when he has to promptly react to a new set of sensory inputs that emerge, partly unexpected and contingently, from the interaction with the other musicians. We find similar phenomena of selection and coordination in team sports, where the decisions necessary to produce an efficacious performance are far more complex than in individual activities. An intensification of the executive and decision-making control (Vestberg et al. 2012) and, therefore, the activation of prefrontal structures is entailed every time a great ability to direct one's attention is needed: for example, when volleyball players need a refined capacity to read" the "vertical space" of their coordinated actions (Castiello and Umiltà 1988), or when professional football players need to closely monitor every technical-tactical sequence of their teammates, anticipating their consequences and rapidly adapting to them (though the discourse may be broadened to all other group sports).

Improvisational skills of a higher order require an increasingly more efficient use of the available information, which can occur only with the reduction of the redundant data and the accurate recognition of the relevant ones. In music, the continuous shifts in the focus of attention mark the difference between a scripted performance and one that is improvised. During improvisation, this dynamic evolves toward minimum levels of attention (Liu et al. 2012). At the point of deepest absorption, the musician has ceased to reflect—but that doesn't mean that she has stopped thinking or imagining. Indeed, the automatism is what liberates her expressive capabilities from the obstacles created by her own ego. Involuntary memory, intensified by emotional and cognitive processes, allows the performer to recognize the trajectory of every emerging harmonic and rhythmic variation and instantly evaluate their potential relevance as a possible future development of the melody (McPherson and Limb 2013). Each arrangement is subject to continuous atemporal influences. Also, for this reason improvisation is not to be conceived as occurring in an objective time (to be assessed through chronological measurement), but as a time of corporeal action and absorbed intervention, that is, adaptive conduct dictated by the rhythm of first-person experience, memory, and emotion (Maldonato 2017). The dynamic constitution of this subjective temporal dimension is supported by a stream of poly-rhythms and dissonances, pauses, or syncopated, continuous changes in pitch and scale. The evolutions of this stream are in many ways unexpected and unpredictable exactly because they don't and can't conform to an objectively given temporal structure; rather, they contribute to create their own time (Berliner 1994; Montuori 2011; Berkowitz and Ansari 2008).

In this respect, sport activities involving an advanced tactical dimension are like musical improvisation: intuition, invention, and creativity function as vanguards of the deepest levels of the mind, which enable one to grasp what usually remains invisible to ordinary perception. To explore these deepest levels of mental activity, a new embodied approach to perception—a neurophenomenology capable of recognizing and systematically studying its corporeal roots—is needed (Merleau-Ponty 1945): only with such an integrated approach will we become capable of understanding how great sport champions see the world, and why they can see things that others do not, or imagine quick moves and extraordinary feats of ability that other players can't even conceive of.

6 Conclusion

We have argued, hopefully persuasively, that the creative performance of a sport champion tends to be more effective when it is less aware of its own components and underlying processes (Rietveld 2008). In situations of peak performance and flow, decisions are often semi-unconscious. Of course, in sport, as in other domains of human activity, a well-developed capacity for original invention and creation is one of the accomplishments that most distinctively reveals that the ultimate mastery of skill and the most confident expertise have been eventually acquired. But the explanation of the functioning of a creative mind in action cannot be reduced to rational analysis and planning: for an expert performer who relies on his or her well-trained skills, reflective awareness is never a constitutive component of effective improvisation.

References

Adams, Jack A. 1971. "A Closed Loop Theory of Motor Learning." *Journal of Motor Behavior* 3 (2): 111–150.

Adams, Jack A. 1976. *Learning and Memory: An Introduction.* Homewood, IL: Dorsey.

Alexander, Garrett E., Mahlon R. DeLong, and Peter L. Strick. 1986. "Parallel Organization of Functionally Segregated Circuits Linking Basal Ganglia and Cortex." *Annual Review of Neuroscience* 9 (1): 357–381.

Allport, D. Alan. 1980. "Attention and Performance." *Cognitive Psychology: New Directions* 1:12–153.

Baddeley, Alan. 1996. "Exploring the Central Executive." *Quarterly Journal of Experimental Psychology A* 49 (5): 5–28.

Bastick, Tony. 1982. *Intuition: How We Think and Act.* Chichester, UK: Wiley.

Beaty, Roger E. 2015. "The Neuroscience of Musical Improvisation." *Neuroscience and Biobehavioral Reviews* 51 (April): 108–117.

Beilock, Sian L., Bennett I. Bertenthal, Annette M. McCoy, and Thomas H. Carr. 2004. "Haste Does Not Always Make Waste: Expertise, Direction of Attention, and Speed versus Accuracy in Performing Sensorimotor Skills." *Psychonomic Bulletin and Review* 11 (2): 373–379.

Beilock, Sian L., and Thomas H. Carr. 2004. "From Novice to Expert Performance: Attention, Memory, and the Control of Complex Sensorimotor Skills." In *Skill Acquisition in Sport: Research, Theory and Practice*, edited by A. Mark Williams and Nicola J. Hodges, 309–328. London: Routledge.

Benedek, Mathias, Emanuel Jauk, Markus Sommer, Martin Arendasy, and Aljoscha C. Neubauer. 2014. "Intelligence, Creativity, and Cognitive Control: The Common and Differential Involvement of Executive Functions in Intelligence and Creativity." *Intelligence* 46 (September): 73–83.

Bengtsson, Sara L., Mihaly Csíkszentmihályi, and Fredrik Ullén. 2014. "Cortical Regions Involved in the Generation of Musical Structures during Improvisation in Pianists." In *The Systems Model of Creativity*, by Mihaly Csíkszentmihályi, 257–278. Amsterdam: Springer.

Bengtsson, Sara L., and Fredrik Ullén. 2006. "Dissociation between Melodic and Rhythmic Processing during Piano Performance from Musical Scores." *NeuroImage* 30 (1): 272–284.

Berkowitz, Aaron L., and Daniel Ansari. 2008. "Generation of Novel Motor Sequences: The Neural Correlates of Musical Improvisation." *NeuroImage* 41 (2): 535–543.

Berkowitz, Aaron L., and Daniel Ansari. 2010. "Expertise-Related Deactivation of the Right Temporoparietal Junction during Musical Improvisation." *NeuroImage* 49 (1): 712–719.

Berliner, D. C. 1994. "Expertise: The Wonder of Exemplary Performances." In *Creating Powerful Thinking in Teachers and Students: Diverse Perspectives*, edited by J. Mangieri and C. Block, 161–186. Fort Worth, TX: Harcourt Brace College.

Berliner, Paul F. 2009. *Thinking in Jazz: The Infinite Art of Improvisation.* Chicago: University of Chicago Press.

Bernstein, Nikolai. 1967. *The Coordination and Regulation of Movements.* Oxford: Pergamon Press.

Berthoz, Alain. 2000. *The Brain's Sense of Movement.* Cambridge, MA: Harvard University Press.

Berthoz, Alain. 2006. *Emotion and Reason: The Cognitive Science of Decision Making*. Oxford: Oxford University Press.

Cappuccio, Massimiliano L. 2015. "Introduction: When Embodied Cognition and Sport Psychology Team-Up." *Phenomenology and the Cognitive Sciences* 14 (2): 213–225.

Castiello, Umberto, and Carlo Umiltà. 1988. "Temporal Dimensions of Mental Effort in Different Sports." *International Journal of Sport Psychology* 19:199–210.

Coccurello, Roberto, W. Adriani, A. Oliverio, and A. Mele. 2000. "Effect of Intra-Accumbens Dopamine Receptor Agents on Reactivity to Spatial and Non-spatial Changes in Mice." *Psychopharmacology* 152 (2): 189–199.

Cooper, Richard P., and Tim Shallice. 2006. "Hierarchical Schemas and Goals in the Control of Sequential Behavior." *Psychological Review* 113 (4): 887–916; discussion 917–931.

Cotterill, Rodney M. J. 2001. "Cooperation of the Basal Ganglia, Cerebellum, Sensory Cerebrum and Hippocampus: Possible Implications for Cognition, Consciousness, Intelligence and Creativity." *Progress in Neurobiology* 64 (1): 1–33.

Critchley, Macdonald, and Eileen A. Critchley. 1998. *John Hughlings Jackson: Father of English Neurology*. Oxford: Oxford University Press.

Csíkszentmihályi, Mihaly. 1996. *Creativity: Flow and the Psychology of Discovery and Invention*. New York: HarperCollins.

D'Errico, Francesco. 2015. *Fuor di metafora. Sette osservazioni sull'improvvisazione musicale. Postfazione di M. Maldonato*. Napoli: Editoriale Scientifica.

Diamond, Adele. 2013. "Executive Functions." *Annual Review of Psychology* 64 (1): 135–168.

Dienes, Zoltan, and Josef Perner. 1999. "A Theory of Implicit and Explicit Knowledge." *Behavioral and Brain Sciences* 22 (5): 735–755; discussion 755–808.

Dietrich, Arne. 2004. "Neurocognitive Mechanisms Underlying the Experience of Flow." *Consciousness and Cognition* 13 (4): 746–761.

Doya, Kenji. 2000. "Complementary Roles of Basal Ganglia and Cerebellum in Learning and Motor Control." *Current Opinion in Neurobiology* 10 (6): 732–739.

Fromm, Erik. 1978. "Primary and Secondary Process in Walking and in Altered States of Consciousness." *Altered States of Consciousness* 4:115.

Gallagher, Shaun, and Dan Zahavi. 2012. *The Phenomenological Mind*. Oxford: Routledge.

Garbarini, Francesca, and Mauro Adenzato. 2004. "At the Root of Embodied Cognition: Cognitive Science Meets Neurophysiology." *Brain and Cognition* 56 (1): 100–106.

Gazzaniga, Michael S. 1995. "Principles of Human Brain Organization Derived from Split-Brain Studies." *Neuron* 14 (2): 217–228.

Geschwind, Nicholas, and Albert M. Galaburda. 1985. "Cerebral Lateralization: Biological Mechanisms, Associations, and Pathology: A Hypothesis and a Program for Research." *Archives of Neurology* 42 (7): 428–459.

Gibson, James Jerome. 1979. *The Ecological Approach to Visual Perception.* Boston: Houghton Mifflin.

Gray, Rob. 2014. "Embodied Perception in Sport." *International Review of Sport and Exercise Psychology* 7 (1): 72–86.

Graybiel, Ann M. 1997. "The Basal Ganglia and Cognitive Pattern Generators." *Schizophrenia Bulletin* 23 (3): 459–469.

Groenewegen, Henk J., H. W. Berendse, J. G. Wolters, and A. H. Lohman. 1991. "The Anatomical Relationship of the Prefrontal Cortex with the Striatopallidal System, the Thalamus and the Amygdala: Evidence for a Parallel Organization." *Progress in Brain Research* 85:95–118; discussion 116–118.

Hampshire, Adam, Samuel R. Chamberlain, Martin M. Monti, John Duncan, and Adrian M. Owen. 2010. "The Role of the Right Inferior Frontal Gyrus: Inhibition and Attentional Control." *NeuroImage* 50 (3): 1313–1319.

Hikosaka, Okihide. 1994. "Role of Basal Ganglia in Control of Innate Movements, Learned Behavior and Cognition—A Hypothesis." In *The Basal Ganglia IV: New Ideas and Data on Structure and Function,* edited by Gérard Percheron, James S. McKenzie, and Jean Feger, 589–596. Advances in Behavioral Biology 41. New York: Plenum Press.

Hobson, J. A., Edward F. Pace-Schott, and Robert Stickgold. 2000. "Dreaming and the Brain: Toward a Cognitive Neuroscience of Conscious States." *Behavioral and Brain Sciences* 23 (6): 793–842; discussion 904–1121.

Hofstadter, Douglas R. 1996. *Concetti fluidi e analogie creative.* Milano: Adelphi.

Hofstadter, Douglas R. 2001. "Analogy as the Core of Cognition." In *The Analogical Mind: Perspectives from Cognitive Science,* edited by Dedre Gentner, Keith James Holyoak, and Boicho Kokinov, 499–538. Cambridge, MA: MIT Press/Bradford.

Holt, Lauren E., and Sian L. Beilock. 2006. "Expertise and Its Embodiment: Examining the Impact of Sensorimotor Skill Expertise on the Representation of Action-Related Text." *Psychonomic Bulletin and Review* 13 (4): 694–701.

Jackson, J. Hughlings. 1884. "The Croonian Lectures on Evolution and Dissolution of the Nervous System." *British Medical Journal* 1 (1214): 660–663.

Jackson, Susan A., and Mihály Csíkszentmihályi. 1999. *Flow in Sports: The Keys to Optimal Experiences and Performances.* Champaign, IL: Human Kinetics.

Jeannerod, Marc. 2001. "Neural Simulation of Action: A Unifying Mechanism for Motor Cognition." *NeuroImage* 14 (1 Pt 2): S103–S109.

Jeannerod, Marc. 2006. *Motor Cognition: What Actions Tell the Self.* Oxford: Oxford University Press.

Kandel, Eric R. 2012. *The Age of Insight: The Quest to Understand the Unconscious in Art, Mind, and Brain, from Vienna 1900 to the Present.* New York: Random House.

Kickert, Walter J. M., Jan-Willem M. Bertrand, and Jaap Praagman. 1978. "Some Comments on Cybernetics and Control." *IEEE Transactions on Systems, Man, and Cybernetics* 8 (11): 805–809.

Kolb, Bryan, and Ian Q. Whishaw. 1996. *Fundamentals of Human Neuropsychology.* New York: Freeman.

Kosslyn, Stephen M., Giorgio Ganis, and William L. Thompson. 2001. "Neural Foundations of Imagery." *Nature Reviews Neuroscience* 2 (9): 635–642.

Kosslyn, Stephen Michael. 1994. *Image and Brain: The Resolution of the Imagery Debate.* Cambridge, MA: Bradford.

Kotz, Sonia A., Michael Schwartze, and Maren Schmidt-Kassow. 2009. "Non-Motor Basal Ganglia Functions: A Review and Proposal for a Model of Sensory Predictability in Auditory Language Perception." *Cortex: A Journal Devoted to the Study of the Nervous System and Behavior* 45 (8): 982–990.

Kris, Ernst. 1952. *Psychoanalytic Explorations in Art.* New York: International Universities Press.

Kugler, Peter N., J. A. Scott Kelso, and M. T. Turvey. 1980. "On the Concept of Coordinative Structures as Dissipative Structures I: Theoretical Lines of Convergence." In *Tutorials in Motor Behavior,* edited by George Stelmach J. Requin, 3–47. Advances in Psychology 3. Amsterdam: Elsevier.

Kuhn, Simone, Simone M. Ritter, Barbara C. N. Müller, Rick B. van Baaren, Marcel Brass, and Ap Dijksterhuis. 2014. "The Importance of the Default Mode Network in Creativity: A Structural MRI Study." *Journal of Creative Behavior* 48 (2): 152–163.

Levy, Jerre. 1979. "Psychobiological Implication of Bilateral Asymmetry." In *Hemisphere Function in the Human Brain,* edited by Stuart Dimond and John G. Beaumont, 121–183. London: Elek Science.

Lewis, Donald J. 1979. "Psychobiology of Active and Inactive Memory." *Psychological Bulletin* 86 (5): 1054–1083.

Li, Tien-Yien, and James A. Yorke. 1975. "Period Three Implies Chaos." *American Mathematical Monthly* 82 (10): 985–992.

Limb, Charles J., and Allen R. Braun. 2008. "Neural Substrates of Spontaneous Musical Performance: An fMRI Study of Jazz Improvisation." *PLoS ONE* 3 (2): e1679.

Liu, Siyuan, Ho Ming Chow, Yisheng Xu, Michael G. Erkkinen, Katherine E. Swett, Michael W. Eagle, Daniel A. Rizik-Baer, and Allen R. Braun. 2012. "Neural Correlates of Lyrical Improvisation: An fMRI Study of Freestyle Rap." *Scientific Reports* 2 (November): 834.

Maldonato, Mauro. 2014. *The Predictive Brain: Consciousness, Decision and Embodied Action.* Chicago: Sussex Academic Press. https://www.tandfonline.com/doi/full/10.1080/02604027.2017

.1345247?af=R.Maldonato, Mauro. 2017. "Improvisation: The Astonishing Bridge to Our Inner Music." *World Futures:* 1–17.

Maldonato, Mauro, and Silvia Dell'Orco. 2012. "The Predictive Brain." *World Futures* 68 (6): 381–389.

Martindale, Colin. 1999. *Handbook of Creativity*. Cambridge: Cambridge University Press.

Mason, Malia F., Michael I. Norton, John D. Van Horn, Daniel M. Wegner, Scott T. Grafton, and C. Neil Macrae. 2007. "Wandering Minds: The Default Network and Stimulus-Independent Thought." *Science* 315 (5810): 393–395.

McPherson, Malinda, and Charles J. Limb. 2013. "Difficulties in the Neuroscience of Creativity: Jazz Improvisation and the Scientific Method." *Annals of the New York Academy of Sciences* 1303 (1): 80–83.

Merleau-Ponty, Maurice. 1945. *Phénoménologie de la perception*. Paris: Gallimard.

Mogenson, Gordon J., Douglas L. Jones, and Chi Yiu Yim. 1980. "From Motivation to Action: Functional Interface between the Limbic System and the Motor System." *Progress in Neurobiology* 14 (2/3): 69–97.

Montuori, Alfonso. 2011. "The Complexity of Improvisation and the Improvisation of Complexity: Social Science, Art and Creativity." *Human Relations: Studies towards the Integration of the Social Sciences* 56 (2): 237–255.

Morris, Genela, Alon Nevet, David Arkadir, Eilon Vaadia, and Hagai Bergman. 2006. "Midbrain Dopamine Neurons Encode Decisions for Future Action." *Nature Neuroscience* 9 (8): 1057–1063.

Nakamura, Jeanne. 1988. "Optimal Experience and the Uses of Talent." In *Optimal Experience: Psychological Studies of Flow in Consciousness*, edited by Mihály Csíkszentmihályi and Isabella Selega Csíkszentmihályi, 319–326. Cambridge: Cambridge University Press.

Namikas, Gediminas. 1983. "Vertical Process and Motor Performance." In *Memory and Control of Action*, edited by Richard A. McGill, 95–117. Advances in Psychology 12. Amsterdam: Elsevier.

Nisenson, Eric. 1995. *Ascension: John Coltrane and His Quest*. New York: St. Martin's Press.

Oliverio, Alberto. 2008. "Brain and Creativity." *Progress of Theoretical Physics: Supplement* 173:66–78.

Oliverio, Alberto. 2009. *La vita nascosta del cervello*. Firenze: Giunti.

Oliverio, Alberto. 2012. *Cervello*. Torino: Bollati Boringhieri.

Oliverio, Alberto, and Mauro Maldonato. 2014. "The Creative Brain." *2014 5th IEEE Conference on Cognitive Infocommunications (CogInfoCom)* 5 (7): 527–532.

Parsons, Lawrence M., Justine Sergent, Donald A. Hodges, and Peter T. Fox. 2005. "The Brain Basis of Piano Performance." *Neuropsychologia* 43 (2): 199–215.

Pinho, Ana Luísa, Örjan de Manzano, Peter Fransson, Helene Eriksson, and Fredrik Ullén. 2014. "Connecting to Create: Expertise in Musical Improvisation Is Associated with Increased Functional Connectivity between Premotor and Prefrontal Areas." *Journal of Neuroscience* 34 (18): 6156–6163.

Posner, Michael I. 1989. *Foundations of Cognitive Science*. Cambridge, MA: MIT Press.

Pressing, Jeff. 1984. "Cognitive Processes in Improvisation." *Advances in Psychology* 19:345–363.

Prigogine, Ilya 1967. *Introduction to Thermodynamics of Irreversible Processes*. 3rd ed. New York: Interscience.

Ramachandran, Vilayanur S. 2003. *The Emerging Mind*. London: Profile Books.

Ridderinkhof, K. Richard, and Marcel Brass. 2015. "How Kinesthetic Motor Imagery Works: A Predictive-Processing Theory of Visualization in Sports and Motor Expertise." *Journal of Physiology, Paris* 109 (1–3): 53–63.

Rietveld, Erik. 2008. "Situated Normativity: The Normative Aspect of Embodied Cognition in Unreflective Action." *Mind* 117 (468): 973–1001.

Rizzolatti, Giacomo, Leonardo Fogassi, and Vittorio Gallese. 2001. "Neurophysiological Mechanisms Underlying the Understanding and Imitation of Action." *Nature Reviews: Neuroscience* 2 (9): 661–670.

Rosenbaum, David A. 1991. *Human Motor Control*. San Diego, CA: Academic Press.

Saltzman, Elliot, and J. A. Kelso. 1987. "Skilled Actions: A Task-Dynamic Approach." *Psychological Review* 94 (1): 84–106.

Schacter, Daniel L. 1987. "Implicit Memory: History and Current Status." *Journal of Experimental Psychology: Learning, Memory, and Cognition* 13 (3): 501–518.

Schechner, Richard. 1995. *The Future of Ritual*. London: Routledge.

Schmidt, Richard A. 1976. "Control Processes in Motor Skills." *Exercise and Sport Sciences Reviews* 4 (1): 229–261.

Schmidt, Richard A. 1983. "On the Underlying Structure of Well-Learned Motor Responses: A Discussion of Namikas and Schneider and Fisk." In *Memory and Control of Action*, edited by Richard A. McGill, 145–165. Advances in Psychology 12. Amsterdam: Elsevier.

Shaffer, L. Henry. 1980. "26 Analysing Piano Performance: A Study of Concert Pianists." In *Tutorials in Motor Behavior*, edited by George Stelmach J. Requin, 443–455. Advances in Psychology 1. Amsterdam: Elsevier.

Sparrow, William A. 1983. "The Efficiency of Skilled Performance." *Journal of Motor Behavior* 15 (3): 237–261.

Tanji, Jun, and Eiji Hoshi. 2008. "Role of the Lateral Prefrontal Cortex in Executive Behavioral Control." *Physiological Reviews* 88 (1): 37–57.

Thomson, Scott. 2007. "The Pedagogical Imperative of Musical Improvisation." *Critical Studies in Improvisation / Études Critiques En Improvisation* 3 (2).

Tononi, Giulio, and Chiara Cirelli. 2006. "Sleep Function and Synaptic Homeostasis." *Sleep Medicine Reviews* 10 (1): 49–62.

Vaitl, Dietel, N. Birbaumer, J. Gruzelier, G. A. Jamieson, B. Kotchoubey, A. Kübler, D. Lehmann, et al. 2005. "Psychobiology of Altered States of Consciousness." *Psychological Bulletin* 131 (1): 98–127.

Varela, Francisco J., Evan Thompson, and Eleanor Rosch. 1991. *The Embodied Mind: Cognitive Science and Human Experience*. Cambridge, MA: MIT Press.

Vestberg Torbjörn, Roland Gustafson, Liselotte Maurex, Martin Ingvar, and Predrag Petrovic. 2012. "Executive Functions Predict the Success of Top-Soccer Players." *PLoS ONE* 7 (4): e34731.

Welford, Alan T. 1976. *Skilled Performance: Perceptual and Motor Skills*. Glenview, IL: Scott Foresman.

Won, Justin, and Neville Hogan. 1995. "Stability Properties of Human Reaching Movements." *Experimental Brain Research* 107 (1): 125–136.

Wulf, Gabriele. 2013. "Attentional Focus and Motor Learning: A Review of 15 Years." *International Review of Sport and Exercise Psychology* 6:77–104.

Zaidel, Dahlia W. 2014. "Creativity, Brain, and Art: Biological and Neurological Considerations." *Frontiers in Human Neuroscience* 8 (June): 389.

Zatorre, Robert, Joyce L. Chen, and Virginia B. Penhune. 2007. "When the Brain Plays Music: Auditory-Motor Interactions in Music Perception and Production." *Nature Reviews Neuroscience* 8 (7): 547–558.

Zeman, Adam. 2001. "The Paradox of Consciousness." *The Lancet* 357 (9249): 77.

Biographical Notes on Contributors

Ana Maria Abreu was trained in applied psychology and did her postgraduate studies in neuropsychology in Paris VI and King's College London. In the course of three postdoctoral positions, she investigated the neural correlates of expertise in sports (La Sapienza, Rome), the impact of action observation in action execution (FMH-UL, Lisbon), and perceptual deficits in developmental disorders (ICS-UCP, Lisbon). Currently she teaches and researches at Universidade Europeia–Laureate International Universities, Lisbon. Her main areas of interest are motor expertise and action observation; low-level perceptual deficits in ASD; and the influence of technology in modern-day life. She has published in several international journals, is an editorial member and ad hoc reviewer of numerous sporting, psychological, and neuroscientific journals, and has been invited as keynote and chair of several conferences.

Kenneth Aggerholm is associate professor at the Department of Physical Education at the Norwegian School of Sport Sciences. He is a former professional football player and before his academic endeavors he worked with street football for homeless and excluded people in Copenhagen. He has special expertise in the philosophy of sport, and his research interests are focused mainly on existential and phenomenological approaches to performance, learning, and development in the areas of sport, physical education, and adapted physical activity. He has published articles and reviews in *Sports, Ethics, and Philosophy*; *Journal of the Philosophy of Sport*; *Qualitative Research in Sport*; *Exercise and Health*, and others; written chapters on coaching, ethics and youth sport, and existential philosophy for handbooks and anthologies; and is the author of the 2015 book, *Talent Development, Existential Philosophy and Sport: On Becoming an Elite Athlete*, published in the Routledge Ethics and Sport Series.

Salvatore Maria Aglioti was trained as a behavioral neurologist and is now professor of social and organizational neuroscience at Sapienza University of Rome. He is the head of the laboratories of cognitive and social neuroscience at Sapienza and at Fondazione

Santa Lucia, IRCCS, Rome (http://agliotilab.org). He is the director of the doctoral school of psychology and coordinates the International PhD Program in Psychology and Social Neuroscience. His research interests revolve around a variety of social neuroscience topics, ranging from action perception and understanding in sport and music to empathy for pain and existential neuroscience. Moreover, he launched a program on the neural underpinnings of social group coding driven by race as well as by political and religious affiliation. He has published more than two hundred scientific publications, as well as several chapters and books.

Duarte Araújo is head of the Laboratory of Expertise in Sport of the Faculty of Human Kinetics at University of Lisbon, Portugal. He is president of the Portuguese Society of Sport Psychology and a member of National Council of Sports of Portugal. His research on sport expertise and decision making, and affordances for physical activity, has been funded by the Fundação para a Ciência e Tecnologia. He has published more than a hundred papers in scientific journals, supervises doctoral students from a variety of countries, and has been invited worldwide to talk about expert performance. Araújo collaborates regularly with Portuguese sport federations, associations, and clubs. He is a marathon runner.

Jürgen Beckmann is a professor with the Department of Sport and Health Sciences at Technical University of Munich. He graduated with a degree in social sciences from Bochum University in 1981, majoring in psychology. He earned a PhD in 1984 and acquired his postdoctoral teaching qualification in psychology at the University of Mannheim in 1988. Prior to being appointed as Chair of Sport Psychology at TUM in 2006, he held a professorship position in sport psychology at the University of Potsdam (1997). Beckmann conducts research in the field of sport psychology, focusing primarily on motivation and volition, and performance achievement under stress. His research concerns the neurophysiological processes that underlie motivation, learning, and control of movement in stress situations, with applications for high-performance sport and preventive health.

Kath Bicknell's work draws on ethnographic methods to investigate cognition and skilled action in live performance and day-to-day life. She's infectiously interested in what this teaches us about the world we live in and the bodies we have. With a research and teaching background in performance studies, her academic work draws on her experiences as a mountain bike racer and aerialist as a way into interdisciplinary debates on thinking, doing, people, and places. She has worked part time in the Department of Cognitive Science at Macquarie University since 2014 and for ten years as a freelance media professional cementing an international reputation for her multiplatform work on cycling.

Geoffrey P. Bingham is a professor in psychological and brain sciences and cognitive science at Indiana University in Bloomington, Indiana, where he has been the director of the Perception/Action Lab (http://www.indiana.edu/~palab/) since 1989. His research focuses on discovering the information that is used in human perception to guide actions and perceive both events and the 3-D structure of the surroundings. The research has been funded by NSF, NIH, General Motors, Smith and Wesson, the Swedish Defense College, and the Royal Society, among other sources. He has published over 150 papers on topics including visual event perception, visually guided reaches-to-grasp, long-distance throwing, affordances, nonlinear dynamical models of rhythmic coordination, 3-D shape perception, and visual control of locomotory approach behaviors.

Jens E. Birch is associate professor at the Oslo and Akershus University College of Applied Sciences. He has a master's degree in philosophy from the University of Oslo, specializing in philosophy of mind and Nietzsche, and a PhD from the Norwegian School of Sport Science on the relationship between neuroscience, consciousness, and movement in sports. His research focuses on what and how neuroscientific theories can contribute to philosophical problems of consciousness and skill and pedagogical questions concerning learning, memory, and attention.

Gunnar Breivik is professor emeritus in the Department of Cultural and Social Studies at Norwegian School of Sport Sciences in Oslo. He has a long career in teaching philosophy of sport, including theory of science. His research interests encompass empirical studies of risk sport, elite sport, and physical activity in the general population. His philosophical studies combine phenomenology with analytical and neuroscientific approaches and focus on skill, knowledge, and expertise.

Noel E. Brick is lecturer in sport and exercise psychology at Ulster University. He previously worked as a lecturer in sport and exercise science at the Northern Regional College. He completed an undergraduate degree in sport and exercise science at the University of Limerick in 1997 and an MSc in sport and exercise at Ulster University in 2003. In 2016 he completed a PhD at the University of Limerick. Noel's research interests include the effects of attentional focus, cognitive strategies, and metacognitive processes on the regulation of endurance performance. This work also extends to the role of cognitive strategies and metacognition on longer-term exercise activity adherence. Brick is also a long-distance runner and has completed more than twenty marathons and ultramarathons, including the Marathon des Sables in 2012 and the Irish 24-hour Championships in 2013.

Massimiliano L. Cappuccio (PhD, State University of Pavia) is a research associate at the University of New South Wales, where he is also deputy lead (Knowledge Exchange) of the Values in Defense & Security Technology (VDST) group. He has a secondary affiliation with United Arab Emirates University, where he is associate professor of cognitive science and director of the Cognitive Science Laboratory. His work as a cognitive philosopher and a philosophical psychologist addresses both theoretical and applied issues in embodied cognition and social cognition combining analytic, phenomenological, and empirical perspectives. His publications have covered topics like motor intentionality and phenomenology of skill and expertise; unreflective action and choking effect; joint attention and deictic gestures; empathy and mirror neurons; social robotics and technology ethics; artificial intelligence theory; and implicit knowledge and the frame problem. He is one of the organizers of the annual Joint UAE Symposium on Social Robotics, hosted by United Arab Emirates University and New York University Abu Dhabi, and the International Conference in Sport Psychology and Embodied Cognition, sponsored by the Abu Dhabi Sports Council.

Thomas H. Carr is emeritus professor of cognition and cognitive neuroscience at Michigan State University. He has served as visiting scientist at IBM Thomas J. Watson Research Center and the CNRS Laboratory of Cognitive Neuroscience in Marseille; as Mayborn Professor of Cognitive Studies at Vanderbilt University; as editor of *Journal of Experimental Psychology: Human Perception and Performance*; and as associate editor of *Cognitive Psychology and Frontiers of Psychology: Cognition*. A fellow of AAAS, Association for Psychological Science, Society of Experimental Psychologists, and Midwestern Psychological Association, his research has used mental chronometry, neuroimaging, phenomenological report self-report, and naturalistic observation to investigate how basic cognitive processes are brought to bear on task performance, development of skill, academic learning, and performance under demanding conditions such as pressure to do well.

Alberto Cei, psychologist and psychotherapist, teaches coaching at the University of Tor Vergata, Motor Science Department, Rome, and sport psychology at the School of Sport of the Italian Olympic Committee and San Raffaele University, Rome. Cei attended the last six Olympic Games, working with winners of twelve Olympic medals. He has also worked as a consultant of the Malta Olympic Committee and of Indian athletes in shooting sports. He has written fourteen books in sport psychology and performance development, and is the editorial manager of the *International Journal of Sport Psychology* (www.ceiconsulting.it and blog www.albertocei.com).

Anthony Chemero is professor of philosophy and psychology at the University of Cincinnati. His research is both philosophical and empirical; typically, it tries to be both at the same time. His research is focused on questions related to nonlinear dynamical modeling, ecological psychology, complex systems, phenomenology, and artificial life. He is the author of *Radical Embodied Cognitive Science* (MIT Press, 2009) and, with Stephan Käufer, *Phenomenology* (Polity Press, 2015).

Wayne Christensen is a research fellow at the University of Warwick. His research interests include the evolution of cognition, cognitive control, skill, and social cognition. His two most active current projects are on skilled action and the sense of commitment.

Lincoln J. Colling is a research associate in the Department of Psychology at the University of Cambridge and a postdoctoral affiliate at Darwin College, Cambridge. He received his PhD from Macquarie University, Sydney, and has previously worked at the Donders Institute for Brain, Cognition and Behaviour at Radboud University, Nijmegen. He works at the intersection of experimental psychology, philosophy, neuroscience, and statistics in an attempt to understand not only what the mind is but also how best to study it.

Cassie Comley is ABD in the Sociology Department at the University of Oregon. Her areas of research interests are intersectionality, critical surf studies, sociology of sport, and Chicana/o studies. She is currently residing in Southern California collecting data for her dissertation about Mexican American surfer's experiences with sport, in an attempt to understand whether and how they experience identity-based exclusionary practices and racial microaggressions. She is also interested in exploring whether and how Mexican Americans use sport to contest identity-based ideologies and stereotypes, create a sense of community and identity, and construct empowering/transgressive spaces and identities. Her previous work has focused on women surfer's experiences with marginalization and exclusion in leisurely spaces in Southern California.

Keith Davids is professor of motor learning at the Centre for Sports Engineering Research, Sheffield Hallam University. He has held professorial positions in the United Kingdom, New Zealand, Australia, and Finland (Finnish Distinguished Professor 2012–2016). His research program investigates how skill, expertise, and talent emerge in athletes and sport teams, considered as complex adaptive systems. He also seeks to understand how coaches, trainers, teachers, and sport scientists can use this theoretical information to design practice programs that continually enhance the process of athlete development. His research and collaborations have been conducted with the New Zealand South Island Academy, the Queensland Academy of Sport, the Australian Institute of Sport, Diving Australia, Cricket Australia, the Finnish Olympic Research Committee, Sheffield United F. C. Academy, and the English Institute of Sport.

Matt Dicks is a senior lecturer in the Department of Sport and Exercise Science and member of the Centre for Situated Action and Communication at the University of Portsmouth. His research interests focus on the study of perception and action processes that underpin the acquisition and control of skilled human movement. He has published over thirty journal articles in exercise and sports science and experimental psychology disciplines. He has edited one book, written six book chapters, delivered more than twenty-five keynote and invited lectures in nine countries. He has held research assistant positions at the University of Chichester and Auckland University of Technology, a research associate post at Queensland University of Technology, a postdoctoral research position at the VU University Amsterdam and has been a visiting professor at University of Caen and University of Rouen.

Caren Diehl received her PhD in 2010 from the University of Wolverhampton. She has worked in high-performance sport for ten years. During that time she has worked with a variety of sports such as diving (Olympic silver and bronze medalists), ten-pin bowling (various international medalists), sailing (Olympic athletes), soccer, running, surfing, weight lifting, wheelchair basketball, and many others. Dr. Diehl has worked in Ghana, the United Kingdom, the United States, and the United Arab Emirates and is currently a senior sport psychologist at the National Institute of Sports in Malaysia. Her research interests are emotional intelligence, embodied cognition, mindfulness, and cultural sport psychology.

Karl Erickson is assistant professor in the Department of Kinesiology at Michigan State University. He has published many articles in journals such as *Psychology of Sport and Exercise, International Journal of Sports Science and Coaching,* and *PLoS ONE,* as well as chapters in various anthologies. His research focuses on athlete development and coaching in youth sport and understanding youth sport as a context for personal development. He is interested in the integration of performance, health, and psychosocial outcomes and how interpersonal processes associated with participation in sport influence these developmental outcomes. His work examines the influence of coach-athlete interactions, the learning and development of sport coaches, and the influence of different contexts in which youth sport takes place.

Anna Esposito is currently professor in the Department of Psychology at Università della Campania "Luigi Vanvitelli" and director of the Laboratory of Behavioural

Cognitive Systems. She is a research affiliate of IIASS (Vietri, IT) and NuMe Lab (Università di Udine, IT). Her research interests are focused on cognitive features to decode/encode meaningful interactional exchanges, emotional conduct, and actions/reactions. She has published more than 180 papers in international journals, books, and conference proceedings, including peer reviews and editing/coediting twenty-six international books.

Pedro Tiago Esteves trained in sport science and pursued his postgraduate studies in the same area (FMH-UL, Lisbon). His main research interests focus on the identification of the informational constraints that support sporting behavior; the development of approaches that might potentiate training, and, subsequently, the development of approaches that might potentiate competence and sporting success. Currently he teaches in the domain of training in sports at the Instituto Politécnico da Guarda, Portugal. He has published several scientific papers and book chapters in the field of sport coaching and performance. Esteves has been invited to act as a referee for reputable journals on sports psychology, human behavior, and sport science. He is also intensively involved in knowledge transfer through consultancy within the industry, including national teams and governing bodies.

Mirko Farina is a British Academy postdoctoral fellow in the Department of Philosophy at King's College London. He is also visiting scholar at the National Research University Higher School of Economics in Moscow and at the Institute of Philosophy at Saint Petersburg State University. He holds a PhD in cognitive science from Macquarie University, an MPhil in philosophy of mind from the University of Edinburgh, and an MRes in logic and philosophy of science from the University of Milan. His academic interests fall at the confluence of non-Cartesian cognitive science, philosophy of mind, philosophy of science, cultural psychology, developmental neuroscience, and evolutionary biology.

Giolo Fele is professor of culture and communication studies and teaches graduate courses in qualitative methods for social research at the University of Trento, Italy. His research interests include communication in emergency situations, sport and social actions, and professional tasting.

Among his recent publications are "Olfactory Objects: Describing, Recognizing and Assessing the Features of an Olfactory Object during Professional Tasting Sessions" (in *Objects, Bodies, and Work Practice*, Multilingual Matters, 2017); "Performing Taste and Educating the Client: The Sommelier's Ceremony" (with Pier Paolo Giglioli, in *Affecting Tastes*, Routledge, 2017); "Language in a Cultural Sociological Perspective" (in *Handbuch Kultursoziologie*, Springer, 2016); "Normatividad en deporte: una reespecificación etnometodológica" (with R. Sanchez, in *Empiria: Revista de metodología de ciencias sociales*, Special issue on Sociology of Sport, 2015).

Denis Francesconi received his MEd from the University of Verona and his PhD in cognitive science and education from the University of Trento. He is adjunct professor at University of Verona, where he teaches group dynamics. Since 2014 he has also been visiting professor at Humboldt University Berlin, where he teaches theories of education. He also works as an educational specialists and consultant. He has been visiting scholar at the Harvard Graduate School of Education, the University of Central Florida, and the Institute of Education at University College London. His scientific interests are embodied cognition, body-mind practices, and well-being education.

Shaun Gallagher is the Lillian and Morrie Moss Professor of Excellence in Philosophy at the University of Memphis. His areas of research include phenomenology and the cognitive sciences, especially topics related to embodiment, self, agency, and intersubjectivity. Dr. Gallagher has a secondary research appointment at the University of Wollongong, Australia. He is honorary professor at the University of Tromsø, Norway. He has held visiting positions at the Cognition and Brain Sciences Unit, Cambridge University; the Center for Subjectivity Research, University of Copenhagen; the Centre de Recherche en Epistémologie Appliquée (CREA), Paris; the Ecole Normale Supériure, Lyon; the Humboldt University in Berlin; and, most recently, at Keble College, University of Oxford. Professor Gallagher holds the Humboldt Foundation's Anneliese Maier Research Award (Anneliese Maier-Forschungspreis) (2012–2018). Gallagher is a founding editor and a coeditor-in-chief of the journal *Phenomenology and the Cognitive Sciences*. His publications include *How the Body Shapes the Mind* (Oxford, 2005); *The Phenomenological Mind* (with Dan Zahavi, Routledge 2008; 2nd ed. 2012); *Phenomenology* (Palgrave Macmillan, 2011); and *Enactivist Interventions: Rethinking the Mind* (Oxford, 2017).

Gowrishankar Ganesh received his bachelor of engineering (first-class, Hons.) from the Delhi College of Engineering and his master of engineering from the National University of Singapore. He received his PhD from Imperial College London in 2010, while working as an intern researcher at the Advanced Telecommunication Research (ATR), Kyoto. Following his PhD, he worked at the National Institute of Information and Communications Technology (NICT-Japan) as a specialist researcher before joining as a senior (CR1) researcher at the Centre National de la Recherché Scientifique (CNRS). He is a visiting researcher at AIST in Tsukuba, ATR, in Kyoto, and LIRMM in Montpellier, France. His research interests include human sensorimotor control and learning, robot control, cognitive neuroscience, and robot-human interactions.

Rob Gray is an associate professor of Human Systems Engineering at Arizona State University. He completed his BA in psychology at Queen's University and his MS and PhD in experimental psychology at York University. Gray's research focuses on perceptual-motor control with a particular emphasis on the demanding actions involved in driving, aviation, and sports. His goal is to conduct basic research that can be applied toward the improvement of training, simulation, accident prevention, and human-machine interface development within these contexts. In 2007 he was awarded the Distinguished Scientific Award for Early Career Contribution to Psychology from the American Psychological Association and the Earl Alluisi Award for Early Career Achievement in the Field of Applied Experimental and Engineering Psychology. He also produces and hosts the *Perception and Action Podcast*.

Denise M. Hill is a senior lecturer in sport and exercise psychology at Swansea University. Her research specialty is the examination of catastrophic performance failure under pressure, particularly within the sporting domain. Through the adoption of a phenomenological approach, Hill has published widely on elite athletes' experience of choking under pressure and the associated social, situational, and interpersonal triggers. In addition, she is BPS Chartered Psychologist and a BASES Accredited Sport and Exercise Scientist, and thereby uses her understanding of the choking process to support athletes across sports and perform optimally under pressure.

Daniel D. Hutto is professor of philosophical psychology at the University of Wollongong and member of the Australian Research Council College of Experts. He is coauthor of the award-winning *Radicalizing Enactivism* (MIT Press, 2013) and its sequel, *Evolving Enactivism* (MIT Press, 2017). His other recent books include *Folk Psychological Narratives* (MIT Press, 2008) and *Wittgenstein and the End of Philosophy* (Palgrave, 2006). He is editor of *Narrative and Understanding Persons* (Cambridge University Press, 2007) and *Narrative and Folk Psychology* (Imprint Academic, 2009). A special yearbook, *Radical Enactivism*, focusing on his philosophy of intentionality, phenomenology, and narrative, was published in 2006. He is regularly invited to speak not only at philosophy conferences but also at expert meetings of anthropologists, clinical psychiatrists/therapists, educationalists, narratologists, neuroscientists, and psychologists.

Tsuyoshi Ikegami received a BE in aerospace engineering from Osaka Prefecture University in 2003. He received a MEd and a PhD in physical and health education from the University of Tokyo in 2005 and 2012, respectively. From 2010 to 2013, he was a researcher in Computational Neuroscience Laboratories, Advanced Telecommunication Research (ATR), Japan. From 2013, he has been working as a researcher at Center for Information and Neural Networks (CiNet), the National Institute of Information and Communications Technology (NICT), Japan. His research interests include human sensorimotor control and learning and action understanding.

Jesús Ilundáin-Agurruza is professor and chair of the Philosophy Department at Linfield College, Oregon, where he received the 2011–2012 Samuel H. Graf Faculty Achievement Award and was 2008–2009 Allen & Pat Kelley Faculty Scholar. In 2013–2015 he served as president of the International Association for the Philosophy of Sport (IAPS). He has published *Holism and the Cultivation of Excellence in Sports and Performance: Skillful Striving* (Routledge, 2016), and articles in the *Journal of the Philosophy of Sport, Phenomenology and the Cognitive Sciences, Sports, Ethics, and Philosophy*, and other journals, and book chapters on sports, martial arts, and comparative philosophy. He has coedited a book on philosophy and cycling. An avid cyclist, swimmer, and budding free-diver, he also enjoys sparring with his Regenyei steel longsword.

Geir Jordet is currently professor at the Norwegian School of Sport Sciences, where he conducts research on psychology and elite sport performance, specializing in performing under extreme pressure, visual perception/decision making in complex team sports, and talent development/effective learning. Jordet's work is published in leading sport science, sport psychology, and psychology journals, as well as in major media outlets such as the *New York Times*, *Wall Street Journal*, *The Guardian*, BBC, and *Spiegel*. He is also director of psychology at the Norwegian Centre of Football (Soccer) Excellence, and is a sport psychology consultant specializing in elite and professional soccer, advising national organizations and professional clubs all over Europe.

Adam Kiefer received a BS in exercise and sport science from the University of Wisconsin–La Crosse, an MS in movement science from Barry University, and a PhD in experimental psychology from the University of Cincinnati. He is currently an assistant professor of pediatrics in the Division of Sports Medicine at Cincinnati Children's Hospital and the University of Cincinnati College of Medicine. He is also affiliated with the Center for Cognition, Action and Perception at the University of Cincinnati.

Michael D. Kirchhoff is senior lecturer in philosophy at the University of Wollongong. He works on the free energy principle in neuroscience and cognitive science, the extended mind hypothesis, nonmechanistic explanation, consciousness, life-mind continuity, and related topics. He is the editor of a special issue of *Synthese*, "Predictive Brains and Embodied, Enactive Cognition," to appear in 2017. He is currently writing a book on extended consciousness from the perspective of predictive processing, a treatment of the organization of life in terms of the notions of active inference and Markov blanket, which he will investigate further through the use of computational models and simulations. He has published papers in esteemed philosophy journals such as *Philosophical Studies*, the *Australasian Journal of Philosophy*, and *Philosophy and Phenomenological Research*. He has also published papers in science journals such as *Entropy* and *Frontiers in Human Neuroscience*.

Kevin Krein is a professor of philosophy and director of outdoor studies at the University of Alaska Southeast. He has published several articles and book chapters addressing issues in the philosophy of alternative and nature sports, mind, and the martial arts. Krein is currently working on *The Philosophy of Nature Sports,* a monograph for Routledge's Ethics and Sport Series. His outdoor interests are centered around alpine skiing and ski mountaineering. Krein has two decades of experience guiding skiing and mountaineering in Alaska and around the world. His accomplishments include several first descents and a ski descent of Denali.

Kenneth Liberman is professor emeritus of sociology at the University of Oregon and most recently visiting professor at the Università della Calabria. His current ethnomethodological research includes the local orderliness of turn-taking in surfing, objectivity in coffee tasting, and Tibetan practices of dialectical thinking. He lived two years with Australian Aboriginal people (*Understanding Interaction in Central Australia: An Ethnomethodology of Australian Aboriginal People*, Routledge, 1985, 2017) and four years in Tibetan Buddhist monasteries (*Dialectical Practice in Tibetan Philosophical Culture: An Ethnomethodological Inquiry Into Formal Reasoning*, Rowman and Littlefield, 2004). His book *More Studies in Ethnomethodology* (State University of New York Press, 2013) won a Distinguished Book Award from the American Sociological Association.

Tadhg E. MacIntyre is a lecturer with the Health Research Institute at the University of Limerick and course director for the Masters in Sport, Exercise and Performance Psychology. In addition to his undergraduate psychology degree from University College Dublin, he was awarded a first class honours MSc and subsequently a PhD in 2007. He is also an associate fellow of the British Psychological Society and has conducted funded research for the World Anti-Doping Agency, the British Association of Sports and Exercise Sciences, the British Psychological Society, and Erasmus + European Union funding on topics from metacognition to the benefits of nature-based solutions for well-being. In the past five years, he has published in journals including *Medicine and Science in Sports and Exercise, Exercise and Sport Science Reviews*, and *International Review of Sport and Exercise Psychology*, and, since its inception in 2008, has been an associate editor of *International Review of Sport and Exercise Psychology* (the leading journal in the field by impact factor). He was also the guest editor of the special issue, "Mental Health

Challenges in Elite Sport," for *Frontiers in Psychology: Sport Psychology and Movement Science*, and has recently been appointed to their editorial board.

Christopher R. Madan is an assistant professor at the School of Psychology at the University of Nottingham. He graduated from the University of Alberta, Edmonton, with a BSc specialization in psychology, with distinction (2009) and subsequently completed a PhD in psychology (2014). He has also been a postdoctoral research fellow with Dr. Elizabeth Kensinger at Boston College and a visiting scientist in the Department of Systems Neuroscience at the University Medical Center Hamburg-Eppendorf in Hamburg, Germany. He has been funded by fellowships from the Canadian Institutes of Health Research and Natural Sciences and Engineering Research Council of Canada, among other agencies. His primary research interests are in the study of memory and brain morphology. He is particularly interested in what makes some experiences more memorable than others and how this can manifest in decision making. He answers these questions using a combination of cognitive psychology, neuroimaging, and computational modeling approaches.

Nelson Mauro Maldonato is psychiatrist and professor at Università di Napoli Federico II. His academic formation includes studies at the La Sapienza University (Rome) and Federico II (Naples). He has been visiting professor at Duke University, Universidade de São Paulo (USP), and Pontifícia Universidade Católica (PUC) of São Paulo. His research interests focus on consciousness, decision making, executive functions, and personality. He is an author and curator of volumes and scientific articles published in numerous languages. He is also the scientific director of the International Research Week.

David L. Mann is an assistant professor in the Department of Human Movement Sciences at Vrije Universiteit in Amsterdam. He is a clinical optometrist and performs research in visual-motor skill acquisition and expertise. He is the director of the International Paralympic Committee Research and Development Centre for the Classification of Athletes with Vision Impairment, responsible for improving the way that athletes with vision impairment are classified for Paralympic competition. He previously worked in positions at the University of New South Wales (Sydney, Australia), the Australian Institute of Sport, and the University of Hong Kong.

Rich S. W. Masters received his DPhil from the University of York, in England, and is presently professor of human movement psychology at the University of Waikato in New Zealand. Previously, he held positions at the University of Hong Kong and the University of Birmingham. Masters uses experimental psychology to explore how humans learn and then perform skills. His work in the field of implicit motor learning has been the subject of interest in a range of movement-related domains, including surgery, rehabilitation, sport sciences, speech and hearing sciences, movement disorders, and aging.

Patrick McGivern is a senior lecturer in philosophy at the University of Wollongong, Australia. His research focuses primarily on problems of explanation and modeling in science, in particular where emergent phenomena are involved on different spatial and temporal scales. He is interested in developing philosophically rigorous accounts of emergence that are well-suited to applications in science, and in understanding how such accounts might vary across different areas of science. His work has appeared in journals such as *American Philosophical Quarterly*, the *Journal of Medicine and Philosophy*, *Philosophy of Science*, and *Synthese*.

Doris McIlwain was associate professor in the Department of Psychology at Macquarie University in Sydney. As a personality psychologist, she studied emotion and resilience, movement and memory, and charismatic forms of power in narcissistic leaders. Her book *Impatient for Paradise* offered a new account of who is drawn to new religious movements. Her research on skills was informed by long-term practice in yoga and ceramics, and by her small private practice as a psychologist. Doris McIlwain died in April 2015.

Michele Merritt teaches philosophy at Arkansas State University, where she has been an assistant professor for five years. Her research focuses on cognitive science, gender, and nonhuman animal minds. She is currently writing a book, with the University of Georgia Press, on the human-canine interactions and their implications for the proper study of cognition. Merritt is also a marathon swimmer who has completed a 12.5-mile race around Key West and a 6.5-mile race around Fort Desoto, Florida, among many other long-distance swims. Merritt lives with her partner, son, two dogs, and two cats in Jonesboro, Arkansas.

Christopher Mesagno is a senior lecturer in the faculty of Health at Federation University Australia. Christopher has published numerous articles and book chapters on sport anxiety and choking under pressure and presented at international conferences, including an invited keynote to the German Association for Sport Psychology Conference. Mesagno received the 2007 Association for Applied Sport Psychology Dissertation Award. He is on the editorial board for the *Journal of Sport Psychology in Action* and *Case Studies in Sport and Exercise Psychology* and reviews articles for more than twenty journals. He consults with athletes from more than fifteen sports including, among others, ten-pin bowling, golf, gymnastics, kendo, and orienteering. Follow Christopher on Twitter or download his research from Researchgate.

Vegard Fusche Moe is an associate professor in the faculty of Education, Culture, and Sport at the Western Norway University of Applied Sciences. He works in the intersection between sport philosophy and science to understand various aspects of skilled motor behavior. His research includes projects on movement and intentionality, cognition, and embodied learning in the contexts of sport and education.

Barbara Gail Montero is associate professor of philosophy at the City University of New York and is the author of *Thought in Action: Expertise and the Conscious Mind* (Oxford University Press 2016). Before her career as a philosophy professor, she was a professional ballet dancer.

Aidan P. Moran is full professor of cognitive psychology and director of the Psychology Research Laboratory in University College Dublin, as well as a Fulbright scholar and fellow of the Association for Psychological Science. His research investigates mental/motor imagery, attention (eye-tracking), and the cognitive processes underlying expertise in skilled performance. He has published extensively on these topics in influential international journals in psychology, neuroscience, medicine, and sport science. He has also written sixteen books, the most recent of which (coauthored with John Toner) is *A Critical Introduction to Sport Psychology*, 3rd ed., Routledge, 2017). A former psychologist to the Irish Olympic squad, he has advised many of Ireland's leading professional athletes and teams, such as the Irish rugby team.

David Moreau is a cognitive neuroscientist at the University of Auckland, New Zealand. His research focuses on the dynamics and plasticity of cognitive function, using a range of techniques such as structural and functional neuroimaging, cognitive testing, mathematical modeling, physiological measurements, and genetic testing. This line of work has led to the design and implementation of training interventions to improve cognitive abilities in clinical and nonclinical populations. In particular, Moreau's work suggests that the combination of physical and cognitive demands allows maximizing improvements in a wide range of populations, at both the cognitive and physiological levels, while preserving the ecological components of naturalistic activities.

Hiroki Nakamoto received his bachelor and master of education from the Tokyo Gakugei University. He received his PhD from National Institute of Fitness and Sports in Kanoya (NIFS) in 2008. Following his PhD, he is working at the NIFS as an associate professor. He is a visiting researcher at Vrije University Amsterdam in Netherlands. His research interests include motor learning and control, perception in sports, and sport expertise.

Alberto Oliverio is emeritus professor of psychobiology at the University of Rome, where he works on the neural correlates of learning and memory and teaches psychobiology to postgraduate students of neurobiology. He spent long periods in research institutes such as the Karolinska in Stockholm, the Brain Research Institute in Los Angeles, and the Center for the Neurobiology of Learning and Memory at the University of California, Irvine. His present interests are on the brain and creativity.

David Papineau received a BSc in mathematics and statistics from the University of Natal, followed by a BA in philosophy at Cambridge, and then a PhD there on conceptual change and scientific rationality. After academic posts at the University of Reading (1973–1977), Macquarie University (1977–1979), Birkbeck College (1979–1980), and Cambridge University (1980–1990), he joined King's College London, and since 2015 has also spent the second half of each academic year at the Graduate Center of the City University of New York. He served as president of the British Society for Philosophy of Science for 1993–1995, president of the Mind Association for 2009–1010, and president of the Aristotelian Society for 2013–2014. He has written widely on epistemology, metaphysics, and the philosophy of science and mind. His books include *For Science in the Social Sciences* (1979), *Theory and Meaning* (1990), *Reality and Representation* (1987), *Philosophical Naturalism* (1992), *Thinking about Consciousness* (2002), *Philosophical Devices* (2012), and *Knowing the Score* (2017).

Gert-Jan Pepping is deputy head of the School of Exercise Science, Australian Catholic University, Brisbane. He has over twenty years of international experience in academia as well as doing research in sports medicine and working with sports teams in the United Kingdom, the Netherlands, and Australia. Pepping's academic interests and expertise are in ecological psychology and the perception-action processes for decision making in sport and exercise. His work is published in high-ranking academic journals as well as national and international media outlets.

Miriam Reiner is the founder and head of the Virtual Reality and Neurocognition lab in the Technion–Israel Institute of Technology. She is an associate professor in the faculty of Education in Science and Technology. Her areas of research include integration of virtual and augmented reality with brain measures while participants perform a task in virtual reality, in an attempt to model factors in motor-cognitive optimal performance. She especially studied topics related to motor memory consolidation, learning, neural processes in learning and memory, effects of embodiment, and mental imagery. She also looks at how emerging technologies of virtual/augmented reality combined with brain stimulations and neurofeedback can be applied to identify and enhance underpinning mechanisms for enhanced performance. Miriam Reiner has acted as visiting professor at Stanford University, Nanyang Technological University in Singapore, UBC, UCL, and UNC, and has received several awards on her work. She has acted as a guest editor for a number of special issues on topics such as enhanced human performance and neurofeedback, and edited two books on similar topics.

Ian Renshaw is a senior lecturer at Queensland University of Technology, Brisbane. Ian's teaching and research interests are centered on applications of ecological dynamics to sport settings. Recent research has focused on developing the links between sport psychology and skill acquisition; implementing constraints-led approaches in PE and sport coaching; emotions and learning in sport; talent development; visual regulation of run-ups, and decision making in football referees. Renshaw has worked with numerous sports providing coach education and skill acquisition advice and is currently working as a consultant with the Canadian women's soccer team. Renshaw recently was coauthor of *Non-linear Pedagogy in Skill Acquisition* and is currently leading the development of a series of books that aim to bridge the gap between academics and practitioners in the area of constraint-led coaching.

Michael A. Riley received a BA in psychology from the University of Louisiana-Monroe and a PhD in experimental psychology from the University of Connecticut. He is professor of psychology and director of the Center for Cognition, Action, and Perception at the University of Cincinnati.

Zuzanna Rucińska is a postdoctoral fellow at the Institute of Philosophy and Sociology of the Polish Academy of Sciences, Poland, and a lecturer of philosophy of mind at Leiden University, the Netherlands. She was formerly an early stage researcher of the Marie Curie Initial Training Network, TESIS, in the United Kingdom, working on the embodied and enactive account of pretending. Her research interests include pretend and imaginative play, forms of creativity, embodied and enacted cognition, dynamical systems theory, sensorimotor theory, and theory of affordances. She has currently published on the topic of affordances for pretense in the anthology *Embodiment, Enaction and Culture: Investigating the Constitution of the Shared World* (2017).

Raúl Sánchez-García is lecturer of sociology of sport at the School of Sports Science, Universidad Europea in Madrid, and president of the Sociology of Sport working group within the Spanish Federation of Sociology (FES). His main areas of research are sport and social theory (Elias, Bourdieu, Garfinkel), martial arts/combat sports and violence, and ethnomethodological studies of sport. Selected publications include "Manipulating Task Constraints of Situated Normativity to Study Decision Making in Krav Maga" (with Villarroya and Elrío, in *International Journal of Sport Psychology,* 2016); "Normatividad en deporte: una reespecificación etnometodológica" (in *Empiria*, 2015); "Choking RECtified: Enactive Expertise beyond Dreyfus" (with Daniel Hutto, in *Phenomenology and the Cognitive Sciences*, 2015).

Lawrence Shapiro received his PhD from the University of Pennsylvania and is a professor of philosophy at the University of Wisconsin–Madison. He specializes in topics in philosophy of mind and philosophy of psychology. Among his books are *The Mind Incarnate* (MIT Press, 2004), *Embodied Cognition* (Routledge, 2011), and, with Professor Thomas Polger, *The Multiple Realization Book* (Oxford, 2016).

Paula Silva received a BS in physical therapy and MS in rehabilitation science from the Federal University of Minas Gerais, Brazil, and a PhD in experimental psychology from the University of Connecticut. She is currently an assistant professor of psychology and faculty of the Center for Cognition, Action and Perception at the University of Cincinnati.

Shannon Spaulding is an assistant professor of philosophy at Oklahoma State University. Her general philosophical interests are in the philosophy of mind, philosophical psychology, and the philosophy of science. The principal goal of her research is to construct a philosophically and empirically plausible account of social cognition. She also has research interests in imagination, pretense, and action theory.

John Sutton is professor of cognitive science at Macquarie University in Sydney. He studies memory and skill, and has published on sport, music, and dance. He is coeditor of the collections *Embodied Cognition and Shakespeare's Theatre: The Early Modern Body-Mind* and *Collaborative Remembering: Theories, Research, and Applications*. He has led a research partnership since 2012 with the Australian Cricketers' Association and Cricket Australia on emotional skills and the mental game in professional cricket. He has plied his tedious medium-paced bowling and fragile batting skills in many cricketing countries over the years.

Phillip D. Tomporowski is an experimental psychologist involved in the study of learning and the effects of exercise on mental functions and skill acquisition. Currently a professor in the Department of Kinesiology at the University of Georgia, he leads a 21st Century Community Learning Center project titled Physical Activity and Learning. Dr. Tomporowski has conducted large-scale randomized controlled trials that have assessed the effects of exercise on mental functioning in individuals with developmental disabilities, older adults, and children. He is also an avid martial arts practitioner and teacher.

John Toner is a lecturer in sports coaching and performance science at the University of Hull. His research interests include expertise in sport performance and pedagogy in sport coaching. His recent research has been published in *Phenomenology and the Cognitive Sciences*, *Psychology of Sport and Exercise*, and *Review of General Psychology*.

Andrew D. Wilson is a reader in psychology at Leeds Beckett University, where he heads the Cognition in Action Lab (https://cognitioninaction.wordpress.com/). His work has two main strands. Empirically, he works on the mechanisms underpinning the perceptual control of action and uses tasks such as coordinated rhythmic movement and long distance throwing to explore these mechanisms. Theoretically he is developing and expanding the ecological approach to perception and action into a more comprehensive theoretical framework for embodied cognition research. He can be found on Twitter @PsychScientists.

Audrey Yap is an associate professor in the Philosophy Department at the University of Victoria in Canada. Her primary research interests are in feminist epistemology as well as the philosophy of mathematics. She has also trained and competed in a variety of martial arts and combat sports since the age of seven. Now serving as a martial arts coach and instructor, she is very interested in looking at the ways in which gender and other social factors affect athletes' development and progress in these sports.

Qin Zhu is an associate professor in the Division of Kinesiology and Health at the University of Wyoming. His research interest is broadly defined in human movement science, and he has been specifically trained in domains of motor learning and control, biomechanics, and experimental psychology to study human sensorimotor control and motor skill acquisition. Using the perception-action approach, his research examines how perception and action intertwine in producing skilled and functional movements. The topics of his research include the perception of affordances, perception of action, overarm throwing, bimanual coordination, visual-motor control, and rehabilitation of motor skills.

Index